P9-ELT-290

Calorie, Fat & Carbohydrate Counter

Extra Diet Guides & Counters

Weight Control Tips

✅ Eat Sensibly

- Avoid fad diets. Eat 3 sensible meals daily with adequate fruit and vegetables.
- Limit portion size. Limit fats and high-fat foods, sugar, soda and alcohol. *(Sample Diet Plan ~ Page 11)*

✅ Exercise Daily

- Get active and exercise every day!
- Include muscle-strengthening exercises. You'll lose more fat and keep it off. You'll also feel and look better, and you can eat a little more! *(Exercise Guide ~ Page 12)*

✅ Reshape Eating Behaviors

- Be aware of eating habits and behaviors that lead to overeating.
- Also focus on social and emotional situations that lead you to snack compulsively. *(Extra notes ~ Page 14)*

✅ Keep a Food & Exercise Diary

- A diary helps you see exactly what you eat and drink, and how much you exercise.
- An excellent motivator and proven weight loss aid. Keeps you honest!

✅ Arrange Moral Support

Gain the support of family and friends. Get extra professional help if required, from your doctor, dietitian, psychologist, exercise trainer, or slimming group. Beware of family saboteurs who discourage you from adopting a healthier lifestyle!

DOCTOR CHECK-UP

Ask your doctor to check your blood pressure, blood sugar and blood cholesterol levels.

HEALTHY WEIGHTS
~ MEN & WOMEN ~
(Over 18 Years)

Based on weights with least risk of disease or death from heart disease, diabetes, stroke and cancer.

Based on Body Mass Index of 20-35

BMI calculated as: $\dfrac{\text{Weight (kg)}}{\text{Height (m)}^2}$

Height (No Shoes) Ft Ins		Healthy Weight Range (Pounds)
4'7"	~	86-108
4'8"	~	88-110
4'9"	~	92-114
4'10"	~	97-121
4'11"	~	99-123
5'0"	~	101-127
5'1"	~	105-132
5'2"	~	110-136
5'3"	~	112-140
5'4"	~	114-145
5'5"	~	119-149
5'6"	~	123-156
5'7"	~	127-158
5'8"	~	129-162
5'9"	~	134-167
5'10"	~	138-173
5'11"	~	143-178
6'0"	~	145-182
6'1"	~	149-187
6'2"	~	156-193
6'3"	~	158-198
6'4"	~	162-202
6'5"	~	170-211
6'6"	~	172-215
6'7"	~	175-220

Body Fat Distribution & Health

Moderate amounts of body fat do not compromise health. However, excess fat above the hips carries a far greater health risk than fat on or below the hips - better to be a 'pear-shape' than an 'apple-shape'.

Abdominal obesity greatly increases the risk of developing diabetes, heart disease, high blood fats, hypertension, stroke, sleep apnea, arthritis and some cancers. So-called **'cellulite'** carries no extra health risk.

Waist Circumference directly reflects the increased health risk of abdominal obesity. Waist size associated with a high health risk:
Men ~ Over 40 inches **Women** ~ Over 35 inches

Body Mass Index (BMI)

BMI is a general (but not specific) indicator of body fatness. Although BMI alone is not diagnostic, the higher the BMI, the greater the health risk of developing diabetes, high blood pressure and heart disease. BMI does not apply to heavily muscled persons. BMI is used in a different way for children.

Abdominal obesity greatly increases the risk of ill-health and earlier death.

Check Your BMI: Find your height (no shoes) - look across the row to the weight nearest your own. Then track down to BMI.

Ht	WEIGHT (LBS) ~ ADULTS													
5'1"	100	106	111	116	122	127	132	137	143	148	153	158	185	211
5'2"	104	109	115	120	126	131	136	142	147	153	158	164	191	218
5'3"	107	113	118	124	130	135	141	146	152	158	163	169	197	225
5'4"	110	116	122	128	134	140	145	151	157	163	169	174	204	232
5'5"	114	120	126	132	138	144	150	156	162	168	174	180	210	240
5'6"	118	124	130	136	142	148	155	161	167	173	179	186	216	247
5'7"	121	127	134	140	146	153	159	166	172	178	185	191	223	255
5'8"	125	131	138	144	151	158	164	171	177	184	190	197	230	262
5'9"	128	135	142	149	155	162	169	176	182	189	196	206	236	270
5'10"	132	139	146	153	160	167	174	181	188	195	202	207	243	278
5'11"	136	143	150	157	165	172	179	186	193	200	208	215	250	286
6'0"	140	147	154	162	169	177	184	191	199	206	213	221	258	294
6'1"	144	151	159	166	174	182	189	197	204	212	219	227	265	302
6'2"	148	155	163	171	179	186	194	202	210	218	225	233	272	311
6'3"	152	160	168	176	184	192	200	208	216	224	232	240	279	319
6'4"	156	164	172	180	189	197	205	213	221	230	238	246	287	328
BMI	19	20	21	22	23	24	25	26	27	28	29	30	35	40

BMI Classification:

BMI Below 19
Underweight

BMI 19-24.9
Healthy Weight
(Low Health Risk)

BMI 25-29.9
Overweight
(Moderate Health Risk)

BMI 30-40
Obese (High Health Risk)

BMI Over 40
Morbid Obesity
(Very High Risk)

Interactive BMI Calculator
www.calorieking.com

Calories & Weight Loss

Calories in Food

Calories in food are derived from protein, fat and carbohydrate. Alcohol also provides calories. Vitamins, minerals and water provide no calories.

Calorie Values Per Gram	
Fat/Oil	~ 9 Calories
Carbohydrate	~ 4 Calories
Protein	~ 4 Calories
Alcohol	~ 7 Calories

Note that fats have over double the calories of protein and carbohydrate. The higher the fat content of food, the higher the calories.

Sample Calculation

**QUARTER POUNDER®
WITH CHEESE
has 530 calories
derived from:**

30g Fat (x 9 cals/gram)	= 270
38g Carbohyd.(x 4 cals/gram)	= 152
27g Protein (x 4 cals/gram)	= 108
Total Calories	**= 530**

Calorie Levels for Weight Loss

Start with a calorie-controlled diet that allows a moderate weight loss of $1/2$ - 1 pound per week. Weight loss is usually much greater in the first few weeks due to extra fluid losses.

Note: It is better to increase exercise rather than lessen food calories too drastically.

Suggested Calories for Weight Loss		
Women:	Non-active	1000 - 1200
	Active	1200 - 1500
Men:	Non-active	1200 - 1500
	Active	1500 - 1800
Teenagers:		1200 - 1800

The MyPyramid symbol represents the recommended proportion of foods from each food group and focuses on the importance of making smart food choices in every food group, every day. Daily physical activity is also important. *(More info: www.MyPyramid.gov)*

Examples of Single Serving Sizes

Grains (Eat 6 servings per day):
- 1 slice bread (1 oz)
- $1/2$ bun, small bagel or English muffin
- 4 small crackers or 1 tortilla
- 1 oz ready-to-eat cereal
- $1/2$ cup cooked cereal, rice or pasta

Vegetable (Eat 3-5 servings per day):
- 1 cup raw leafy vegetables
- $1 1/2$ cups raw chopped vegetables
- $1/2$ cup cooked vegetables
- $1/2$ - $3/4$ cup vegetable juice

Fruits (Eat 3-5 servings per day):
- 1 medium apple, orange, banana
- $1/2$ cup canned fruit
- $1/4$ cup dried fruit
- $3/4$ cup fruit juice
- $1/4$ medium avocado

Milk (2-3 servings per day):
- 1 cup (8 fl.oz) milk, soy drink, yogurt
- $1 1/2$ oz cheese or $1/2$ cup cottage cheese

Meat & Beans (Eat 2-3 servings per day):
- 2-3 oz (cooked) lean meat/poultry/fish
- 2 eggs **or** 7 oz tofu **or** $1/4$ cup nuts
- 1 cup (cooked) dried beans **or** chickpeas
- 4 Tbsp peanut butter

Portion Size Counts!

Food portion size is critical to controlling calorie intake for weight control.

Super-sized food servings have become more common when eating out and in the home. This can mean a day's worth of calories being consumed in one meal; or a snack being equivalent to a full meal.

It is easy to underestimate portion size of foods and drinks, and unwittingly consume excess calories – even if the fat content is low or even zero!

To more accurately estimate portion size of different foods, weigh and measure your food with food scales, measuring spoons and cups. Better control of calories will result.

For a visual idea of portion sizes, visit www.CalorieKing.com. See examples (fries and cola) on this page.

Allow for Extra Calories in Packaged Food

The actual weight of packaged foods is usually 5-10% more than the label net weight (the minimum legal weight) - and in some cases up to 50% more. However, manufacturers calculate the calories based on the net weight. For actual calories, weigh the product and calculate the extra calories. **For extra details see www.CalorieKing.com**

Basic 'Tools of the Trade'

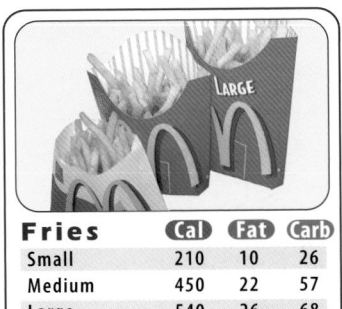

Fries	Cal	Fat	Carb
Small	210	10	26
Medium	450	22	57
Large	540	26	68

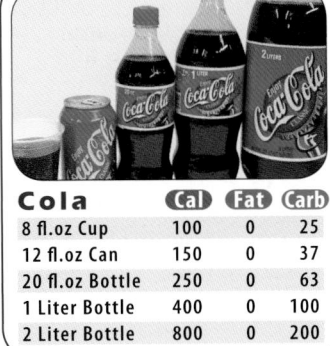

Cola	Cal	Fat	Carb
8 fl.oz Cup	100	0	25
12 fl.oz Can	150	0	37
20 fl.oz Bottle	250	0	63
1 Liter Bottle	400	0	100
2 Liter Bottle	800	0	200

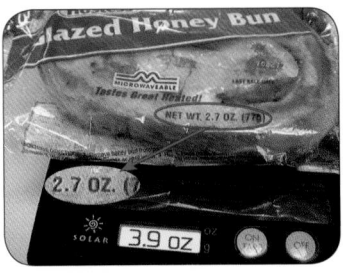

Recommended Fat Intake

Americans consume too much fat with many getting over 40% of total calories from fat – either as fat or oil, or as fat in foods and drinks. A range of 20-30% is healthier.

Fat Intake - Healthy Ranges

Children	~	30-60g
Teenagers (Active)	~	40-80g
Women	~	30-60g
Men: Active	~	40-80g
Heavy Activity/Athlete	~	80-120g

MAXIMUM DESIRABLE FAT INTAKE (Daily)

Calories	Fat	% Fat Cals
1200 cals	30g fat	23%
1500 cals	40g fat	24%
1800 cals	50g fat	25%
2000 cals	60g fat	27%
2200 cals	70g fat	28%
2500 cals	80g fat	29%
3000 cals	100g fat	30%
4000 cals	135g fat	30%

Percentage Fat Calories Formula:

$$\frac{\text{Grams of Fat Per Serving} \times (900)}{\text{Total Calories Per Serving}}$$

Fat Percent Content

(Grams of fat per 100 grams of food)

Don't be fooled by promotion of foods claiming to have a low percentage of fat. **It's serving size and total grams of fat that count.**

For example, whole milk with 3.5% fat sounds low (3.5g fat/100ml) but an 8 fl.oz cup contains 8g fat; and 2 cups contain 16g fat.

Ice cream with 10% fat seems high, yet a regular scoop (3 fl.oz) has only 5g fat.

(Low-fat ice cream has less than 2g fat/serve.)

3 Cookies: **140 calories**

6 oz Muffin: **450 calories**

Reduced fat & fat-free foods are not necessarily low calorie. Portion size is still important.

It is a mistake to think that eating low-fat or fat-free foods allows you to eat double the quantity. You can end up with even more calories than when you eat smaller amounts of regular fat products.

Also fat-free but high in calories are soda drinks, fruit juices, beer, alcoholic spirits, sugar and sugar candy. Bread, rice and pasta also have negligible fat.

Total Calories Count!

Ultimately, **it is food portion size and total calories that count** whether from fat, carbohydrate or protein. Remember, cows get fat on grass!

FOOD LABEL MEANINGS

FDA Nutrition Claim Definitions

(All are on a Per Serving Basis)

Low Calorie: 40 Calories or less

Light or Lite: One third fewer calories or, 50% or less fat than regular product

Fat-Free: Less than half a gram of fat

Low-Fat: 3 grams or less of fat

Reduced Fat: 25% less fat than regular product

Fewer or Less Calories: At least 25% fewer calories than regular product

Hints to Reduce Fat

Meats, Poultry, Fish

- Choose **lean cuts** of meat with little marbling. **Trim all visible fat** from meat and remove the skin from poultry. Removal of fat after cooking, is okay (to prevent dryness). Choose 'extra lean' ground beef.
- **Avoid high-fat meat products** such as salami, bacon, sausage and franks.
- **Broil or bake. Avoid frying in oil.** Allow casseroles to cool and skim off surface fat.
- **Avoid fried fish**, frozen fish in batter and canned fish in oil.

Fats & Oils

- **Use minimal amounts** of all types of fat and oil. All are high in calories.
- **Choose** 'light' and 'reduced fat' spreads but still use sparingly.
- Use minimal amounts of oil when stir-frying. Use no-stick sprays like Pam.

Salad Dressings & Sauces

- **Avoid regular mayonnaise and oil dressings.** Choose 'light', 'reduced fat' or 'fat-free' brands.
- **Choose** low-fat or fat-free sauces (mainly tomato-based). Avoid 'pesto', 'alfredo', 'cheese' and 'creamy' sauces.

Milk, Cheese

- **Choose** low-fat or nonfat milks and yogurts. **Avoid** full-cream milk, cream, Half & Half.
- **Cheese:** Choose fat-free, low-fat and fat-reduced (e.g. cottage, part-skim ricotta). Cheese substitutes can still be high in fat.

Snacks, Cookies, Candy

- **Avoid** high-fat snacks such as potato chips, corn/tortilla chips, cheesy balls, buttered popcorn, chocolate and carob bars.

Desserts/Sweets

- **Avoid high-fat desserts**, such as fruit pies, pastries, cheesecake, cheese board.
- **Choose** fresh fruits, fresh fruit salad, canned fruit in water pack, low-fat ice cream. Use low-fat yogurt in place of cream.

Fast-Foods & Take-Out

Check the Fast-Foods Section of this book for actual fat and calorie counts.

- **Avoid deep-fried chicken**, french fries; onion rings
- **Pizzas:** Avoid sausage/pepperoni. Choose vegetarian topping and modest quantity of cheese. Eat a moderate serving. Eat extra salad and fresh fruit.
- **Hamburgers:** Choose medium size, lower fat burgers. Avoid bacon. Have a side salad (with fat-free dressing).
- **Delis:** Choose sandwiches/bread rolls, pitas with low-fat fillings and plain salad. Limit meat/cheese to small portions.
- **Coffees:** Avoid large sizes of latte and frappuccino. Request nonfat milk and no whipped cream. Avoid cookies.

Extra Information: www.CalorieKing.com

FRYING ADDS FAT!

The greater the surface area of potato exposed to fat or oil, the higher the fat content.

Whole Potato (3 oz)
0g Fat, 65 Cals

Roast Potato (3 oz)
5g Fat, 155 Cals

Fries (Large cut, 3 oz)
12g Fat, 220 Cals

Fries (Small, 3 oz)
15g Fat, 265 Cals

Potato Chips (3 oz)
30g Fat, 450 Cals

Carbohydrates ~ Friend or Foe?

Naturally Friendly Carbs

- **Carbohydrate foods in their more natural forms** (not overly processed) are essential to good health. They are the main source of fuel for the body, and also provide important vitamins, minerals, antioxidants and fiber – all of which help protect against heart disease, diabetes, hypertension, constipation-related ailments and many other diseases.

- Carbohydrates even stimulate production of serotonin, the 'feel good' brain chemical that helps control appetite and overeating. Too little serotonin can lead to mood swings and depression.

Carbohydrates are found in different forms in food as:

- Sugars in fruit, sugar cane, milk
- Starches in whole grains, legumes, nuts, seeds and vegetables
- Dietary fiber – (See Fiber Guide ~ Page 276)
  Glycemic Index & Diabetes ~ Page 20

Low carb diets only work if total calories are reduced.

FAT MATTERS CARBS COUNT BUT CALORIES ARE KING!

Low Carbohydrate Diets

- Popular low carbohydrate diets are extreme in their recommendations to initially cut carb intake to as little as 20 grams per day – the amount in 1 thick slice of bread, or 1 medium apple, or 1 small potato.
  This greatly increases the risk of nutritional deficiencies and compromises health, particularly if fat intake is excessive through fatty meats, high-fat dairy products, and fried foods.

- While overweight Americans do need to reduce carbohydrate intake, it should be done **sensibly as part of reducing portion size and total calories.**

- Simply eating 'low carb' food products without regard to portion size, calories or fats, will do little to promote weight loss or good health.

- **Low carb diets (and indeed any diet) only work if total calories are reduced.**

- Refined sugars should be one of the first targets in moderating carb intake.
  Extra Info ~ www.CalorieKing.com

RECOMMENDED CARBOHYDRATE INTAKE

Calories (Daily)	Carbohydrate (Grams)	Percent Carbohydrate Calories
1200 cals	120g	40%
1500 cals	170g	45%
1800 cals	210g	47%
2000 cals	250g	50%
2500 cals	345g	55%
3000 cals	450g	60%

How Much Do We Need?

- As shown in the chart, well-balanced diets above 2000 calories contain 50-60% of total calories from carbohydrate.
- At lower calorie levels used for weight control (1200-1500 calories), carbohydrates account for as little as 40% of total calories. This is because protein calories have nutritional priority.

Low carbohydrate products may still be high in calories and fat.

- Many overweight, inactive people consume over 500 calories of refined sugars per day either self-added or as part of food products. This is equivalent to over 30 level teaspoons - a significant amount in weight control terms. Halving this amount would be reasonable and worthwhile.

  Note: Naturally occurring sugars in fruits, vegetables and milk are fine when consumed in normal recommended amounts. These foods are also rich in other nutrients.

  Refined sugar is referred to as having 'empty calories' because it supplies calories but negligible nutrients and no fiber.

- **Most sugar in our diet is 'hidden'** in processed foods such as soft drinks, fruit drinks, candy, cookies, cake, jam, sauces, ice cream, desserts, canned foods, and breakfast cereals.

  Certainly enjoy moderate quantities of these foods, but for serious weight control, look for 'low calorie', 'diet' or 'sugar-free'.

  However, be careful not to substitute sugar-rich foods with high-fat foods which might boost calories even more!

- Be aware that sugar comes in different forms such as sucrose, glucose, fructose, malt, high-fructose corn syrup, molasses, honey and maple syrup. Check the label.

- **Sugar alcohols such as sorbitol,** mannitol and maltitol are carb-based and have ½ - ¾ the calories of regular sugar. While not counted as sugar on food labels, they do add to the carb count. Excess amounts can cause bloating, gas and diarrhea.

- **Sugar-free sweeteners** such as *Equal, DiabetiSweet, NutraSweet, Splenda, Sweet'n Low* and *Stevia* make it easy to reduce sugar in drinks and recipes. Use only in moderation.

  Note: Most recipes can be adapted to contain less sugar with little effect on taste or quality.

Extra Info ~ www.CalorieKing.com

Sugar-free snacks and foods may be higher in fat and calories than the regular product.

Example ~ Creme Wafers (3):
Regular ~ 115 cals, 6g fat
Sugar-Free ~ 160 cals, 10g fat

SUGAR CONTENT OF SOME COMMON FOODS

	Teaspoons of Sugar
Coca Cola or *Pepsi,* 12 fl.oz	10
20 fl.oz size	17
Iced Tea, sweetened, 12 fl.oz	8
Chocolate Milk, 12 fl.oz	6
Honey Smacks Cereal, 1 oz	4
Popcorn, caramel, 1 cup	3.5
Chocolate Bar, 1.5 oz	6
M&M's 1.7 oz pkg	7
Muffin, large, 4 oz	6
Choc Chip Cookie, 1 oz	2
Donut, iced	6
Apple Pie, 1 piece	7
Jell-O, ½ cup	4.5
Jam, 1 Tbsp, 20g	2.5
Syrup, maple, 1 Tbsp	3

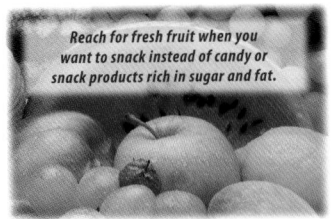

Reach for fresh fruit when you want to snack instead of candy or snack products rich in sugar and fat.

Tips For Overweight Kids & Parents!

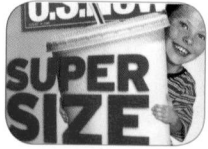

The XL Generation

Some 15% of American kids and adolescents are overweight; and childhood obesity has doubled over the last 20 years. Diabetes, high blood pressure and high cholesterol are major problem areas for overweight children and adolescents, as are depression, low self-esteem, sleep apnea and bone joint problems.

To address this problem, cooperation is required between kids, parents, schools and government. Weight control is a family and community affair.

Some simple tips to get started:

» Watch Soda Intake!

Limit soda and sugary drinks to one serving on the weekends. Soda should not be an everyday beverage. Try water instead. When at fast-food restaurants or using a soda fountain, choose small servings with ice or choose diet soda instead. Schools should provide water and restrict access to soda. Parents need to supervise kids at the soda fountain!

» Cut back on Fast-Foods and Eating Out

Many more calories are consumed when you eat out. Healthy meals prepared at home are best for the whole family.

» Say "No" to Super-Sizing!

Portion sizes are on the increase, and for just a few cents, meals can be upsized - with loads more calories. Choose sensible portion sizes when dining out and at home. Use smaller plates and choose smaller packages.

» Limit Between-Meal Snacking

Watch out for high-fat and high-calorie snacks – they can have more calories than a meal. Keep your eye on portion sizes and limit foods like chips and candy to parties and special occasions. Choose fresh fruit and vegetables instead.

» Get Moving ~ Watch Less TV!

Kids need at least 60 minutes of physical activity every day. Limit time spent in sedentary activities (such as playing computer games or watching TV to just one hour per day.) Also limit the accompanying snacks! Include exercise in family activities.

Note: When kids watch TV in a motionless trance, they burn even less calories than if simply sitting, reading or talking.

For extra information and tips see www.CalorieKing.com

Sample Diet Plan - 1300 Calories

For Overweight Persons. Please Check With Your Doctor.
(Menu contains approximately 30-35 Grams Fat)

 Breakfast (approx. 250 cal)

	1 Small Fruit or ¹/₂ oz Dried Fruit
Plus	Cereal: 1¹/₂ oz Dry (high fiber)
	or 1 cup cooked Oatmeal
Plus	Milk (from daily allowance)

Daily Milk Allowance (160 calories)
2 cups Skim Milk or 1¹/₂ cups Low-fat (1%) Milk
or equivalent Soy Drink, Yogurt, Cheese, Tofu

Fat Allowance (140 calories; 15g Fat)
4 tsp Fat or 6-8 tsp Diet Margarine or 3 tsp Oil
or 1¹/₂ Tbsp Mayonnaise or ¹/₂ medium Avocado
or 1¹/₂ Tbsp Peanut Butter or 30g Nuts/Seeds

 Breakfast ~ Choice 2

	1 Small Fruit
Plus	1 Egg (no added fat)
	or ³/₄ oz Cheese
	or 2 oz Cottage Cheese
	or 1 oz Lean Bacon
Plus	1 Toast or ¹/₂ Muffin (English)

 Lunch (approx. 440 calories)

	2 slices Bread (2 oz) or 1 medium Roll or Bagel
	or 4 Crispbreads/Crackers or 6" Pita
Plus	2 oz lean Meat, Chicken or Turkey
	or 3¹/₂ oz Tuna (in water) or 2¹/₂ oz Salmon
	or 1 oz Cheese or ¹/₂ cup (4 oz) Cottage Cheese
	or ¹/₂ cup (4 oz) Ricotta Cheese (low-fat)
	or ¹/₂ cup (4 oz) Fruit Yogurt (low-fat)
	or ¹/₂ cup (4 oz) Bean Salad
Plus	Large Salad (Oil-free dressing)
Plus	1 small Fruit or ¹/₂ oz Dried Fruit

 Dinner (approx. 360 calories)

	Soup (fat-free)
Plus	3 oz lean Meat (cooked weight)
	or 4 oz Chicken Breast (no skin)
	or 3 oz Chicken Thigh/Leg (no skin)
	or 5 oz Fish (grilled, no fat)
	or ³/₄ cup (6 oz) Beans (Soy, Kidney, Pinto etc)/Lentils
	or Low-fat Entree (e.g. Lean Cuisine) or Recipe Dish
Plus	1 small Potato or ¹/₂ cup Rice/Pasta or 1 slice Bread
Plus	2-3 servings Vegetables/Salad
Plus	1 small Fruit + Diet Gelatin Dessert

 Between Meals Water, Coffee, Tea, Diet drinks,

Fruit from main meals; Raw vegetable pieces, Milk from Allowance

Note: Take a multivitamin/mineral supplement daily while dieting.

Exercise & Weight Control

- **People who exercise regularly lose more weight** and keep it off longer than non-exercisers.

- Exercise also improves general health and well-being. **Mood, confidence and self-esteem are** enhanced by a sense of control and accomplishment.

- **Exercise increases the metabolic rate** of the body even for hours after exercise – a good way to 'wake up' a sluggish metabolism and burn extra fat.

  Exercise compensates for any decrease in metabolic rate with increasing age and also in some heavy smokers who stop smoking.

- **Strength training** further builds muscle and aids body reshaping. You can also eat more food!

Note: It is muscle which burns calories. Each extra pound of muscle burns an extra 100 calories daily – even while you sleep! Weight from exercised muscles is okay. It is surplus fat that is potentially harmful.

- **Avoid injury** by beginning with walking, low impact aerobics, or weight-supported exercise (e.g. swimming, cycling). Avoid competitive sports.

- **How Much?** Start with 10 - 20 minutes/day and progress to 30-45 minutes/day – even if broken into 5-10 minute lots. It all adds up! **Aim to achieve 250-500 calories of exercise daily.**

  Also walk up stairs instead of using elevators. Take a brisk walk at lunch. Use an exercise bike, treadmill or stair machine while watching TV.

- **How Often?** While aerobic fitness requires only 3 - 4 sessions weekly, **weight control is a daily event which requires daily exercise.**

TV CAN BE FATTENING!

Many adults and children watch over 20 hours of television per week (plus computer hours). At the same time, high-calorie snacks and drinks are consumed – potent contributors to obesity.

Are you a TV couch potato? Limit your TV hours and plan healthy physical activities. At least use an exercise bike or treadmill while watching TV!

Be Active Every Day!

Brisk walking each day is a safe and effective way to keep trim and fit. Try it - you'll like it!

Strength-training with light weights helps to retain or rebuild muscle tissue. It enhances weight control.

Middle-age spread has little to do with getting older. Too little exercise is the main culprit.

Daily exercise and sensible eating can minimize middle-age spread.

Calories Used in Exercise

LIGHT
4 Calories/Minute

Walking, slow
Cycling, light
Gardening light
Golf, social
Tennis, doubles
Housework, cleaning
Calisthenics, Yoga
Bowling
Ping-pong, social
Ice Skating
Aquarobics, light
Skate Boarding
Line/Square Dancing

MODERATE
7 Calories/Minute

Walking, brisk
Cycling, moderate
Swimming, crawl
Weight-training, light
Tennis, moderate
Racquetball, beginners
Aerobics, light
Football, Grid Iron
Basketball, Baseball
Walking Downstairs
Snow Skiing (downhill)
Shovelling snow
Dancing (ballroom)

HEAVY
10 Calories/Minute

Walking (power), Jogging
Cycling (vigorous), Spinning
Swimming, strenuous
Weight-training, heavy
Wrestling/Judo, advanced
Racquetball, advanced
Tae Bo, Kick Boxing
Football, training
Basketball (Pro)
Climbing Stairs
Skipping Rope
Skiing (cross country)
Aquarobics, advanced
Dancing (strenuous), Zumba

Note: Only those sports or activities that are sustained over a period of time (e.g running) qualify
for heavy exercise. Stop-start sports such as tennis are considered 'moderate'.

10,000 STEPS PER DAY

PEDOMETERS

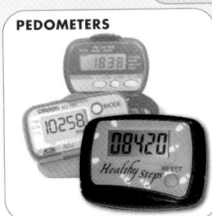

A pedometer can motivate you to be
more active every day.

Different models count steps, miles and
even calories used. It clips to your belt or
waist band and registers each step.

Aim for 8,000 - 10,000 steps per day, instead
of an average of only 3,000 - 4,000 steps.

Ordering Details ~ Page 303

 ## WALKING PROGRAM

Weeks		Distance To Walk	Time Taken	Calories Used (140lb Person)
Weeks 1-2	►	1 mile	20 mins	140 calories
Weeks 3-5	►	1.5 miles	28 mins	200 calories
Weeks 6-8	►	2 miles	35 mins	250 calories
Weeks 9-10	►	2.5 miles	45 mins	310 calories
Weeks 11+	►	3.5 miles	60 mins	420 calories

Reshaping Eating Behaviors

- Eating is a behavior that is largely controlled by people with whom we live or socialize, places in which we carry out our lives, and our emotions. Become aware of those situations that commonly lead to extra food being eaten.

- We may also be unaware of 'bad' eating habits that can lead to excess calorie intake; e.g. eating quickly, large mouthfuls, eating when tense or bored, finishing a large serving of food when not hungry.

Tips to help uncover and correct those 'bad' eating habits:

- **Don't eat while engaged in other activities;** for example, watching TV, reading. Eat only at the table, not at the fridge or while standing.

- **Don't eat quickly.** Chewing slowly allows time to register a feeling of fullness. Don't use fingers, only utensils. Cut food into smaller pieces. Don't load your fork until the previous mouthful is finished.

Practice saying 'NO' politely but assertively.

- **Don't purchase problem high calorie foods.** Shop from a set list to prevent impulse buying. Avoid shopping with children.

- **Buy snack foods** in the smallest package. The larger the serving size or package, the more you are likely to eat or drink.

- **Plan meals in advance.** Stick to a set menu.

- **Plan a strategy to avoid uncontrolled eating** and drinking at social events, or when your emotions urge you to binge.

  Rehearse repeatedly in your mind exactly what you will do in such situations. Remind yourself several times each day that you are in charge of your actions and that you can be strong-willed. Seek counseling or coaching on various strategies.

- **Promise yourself** that when you feel the urge to snack, you will engage in some activity that will distract you away from food (e.g. go for a walk, brush your teeth, phone a friend.)

  If you eat out of boredom, find some new hobby or interest that gets you out of the house. Even enroll in an adult education class.

Do you use food as an emotional crutch? If so, professional counseling may be helpful.

The Value of a Food Diary

The food diary is the most powerful proven aid for dieters. Persons who keep a food and exercise diary not only lose more weight they also keep it off. Here are some of the reasons:

- Recording your eating and exercise habits jolts you into realizing just what you do eat and drink each day; and also whether you exercise sufficiently.

- **Helps you identify problem foods** and drinks with excessive calories and fat.

- **Helps identify moods,** situations and events that lead to excessive eating of unwanted calories. You can then plan to overcome or avoid them.

- **Prevents 'calorie amnesia',** the forgetfulness that leads to rebound weight gain after successful weight loss. Recording puts you back on the right track.

- **Helps you develop greater self-discipline.** You will think twice about overindulging if you have to record it - especially if someone checks your diary regularly. It certainly keeps you honest!

- **Motivates you** to carefully plan your meals and to exercise each day.

- **Serves as a check system** for your doctor, dietitian or counselor to assess your progress and make recommendations.

Write It Down!

"Keeping a diary gives me feedback on exactly what I eat and drink each day.

It helps prevent 'calorie amnesia' and reminds me to exercise each day.

It's a must for successful weight control!"

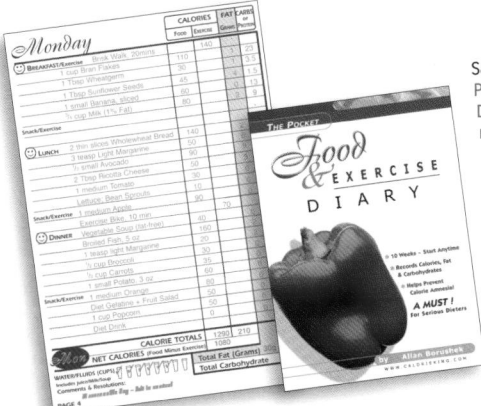

Sample Page from The Pocket Food & Exercise Diary, a 10-week diary to record food and exercise.

At day's end, exercise calories are deducted from food calories.

Includes Weekly Summary Page & Progress Checklist.

EXTRA DETAILS
~ SEE PAGE 302

Diabetes Guide

What is Diabetes?

Diabetes is a disorder in which the body cannot make proper use of carbohydrates (sugar and starches).

- After digestion, sugar and starches are changed into **glucose** – the simplest form of sugar vital for body energy and growth.
- **Insulin** is the hormone which acts like a key that opens the door to body cells and allows glucose to enter.
- **Without sufficient insulin**, unused glucose builds up in the blood and passes into the urine. This produces symptoms of frequent urination, continual thirst and tiredness.
- **Untreated diabetes** increases the risk of damage to nerves and blood vessels. This, in turn, increases the risk of heart disease, stroke, blindness, kidney damage, foot ulcers and gangrene (with amputation), impotence and other complications.

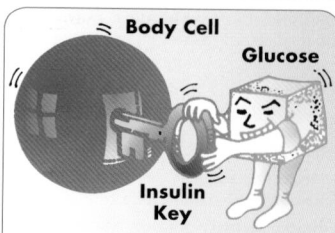

Insulin acts like a key.
It opens the door to body cells and allows glucose to enter.

People with Type-1 diabetes and some with Type-2 have too few or no keys and require insulin injections.

Others (most Type -2) have ample keys but 'misshapen' key holes (insulin resistant) – particularly if obese and inactive.

TYPE-1 DIABETES

Insulin-Dependent Diabetes

- Occurs in 10% of diabetes cases
- Usually in children and young adults
- Pancreas gland produces little or no insulin. Daily insulin injections are necessary, plus:
- Regular meals with even carbohydrate distribution to match insulin dosage. Regular exercise and weight control are also important.

⚠ WARNING SIGNALS

- Frequent urination
- Continual thirst
- Rapid weight loss
- Unusual hunger
- Extreme weakness/fatigue
- Nausea, vomiting, irritability

TYPE-2 DIABETES

Non-Insulin Dependent

- Occurs in 90% of diabetes cases
- Occurs mainly in adults - particularly in overweight and inactive persons
- Insulin is produced but body cells resist its action and glucose cannot enter cells.
- Usually treated with diet and exercise. Sometimes requires medication (tablets or insulin injections).

⚠ WARNING SIGNALS

- Any Type-1 symptom
- Blurred vision
- Excessive itching
- Skin infections with slow healing
- Tingling/numbness in feet

 GESTATIONAL DIABETES • Occurs during pregnancy • Usually disappears on the baby's birth • Over 50% of these mothers develop diabetes within the next 20 years. • Requires weight control, a healthy lifestyle and regular medical checks.

Prediabetes - An Early Warning!

- Prediabetes means you don't have diabetes now but are likely to develop it in the future - if serious preventive action is not taken now! Your risk for heart disease and stroke is also increased by 50%.

- You are prediabetic if your blood sugar level is between 100 and 125 mg/dL (after an overnight fast).

  These levels are higher than normal but not high enough to be diabetes.

- Risk factors for prediabetes include being overweight or obese, a family history of diabetes, high blood lipids, hypertension, and a history of gestational diabetes (during pregnancy).

- Most people with prediabetes can prevent full-blown diabetes (usually Type 2) by adopting a healthier lifestyle. This includes **losing weight if overweight, and exercising for 30 minutes at least 5 days a week.**

- Your doctor and dietitian can plan a preventive lifestyle program for you.

Importance of Weight Control

- **Type-2 diabetes** occurs 2-3 times more often in overweight persons – particularly if inactive.

- Such persons do not usually lack insulin. Rather, their insulin is less effective. As obesity develops, muscle and other body cells may resist insulin in varying degrees. The resultant build-up of blood glucose may lead to diabetic symptoms.

- **Weight loss alone** often corrects this condition in Type-2 diabetes. If overweight, try a moderate diet of 1200-1500 calories **plus daily exercise.**

  Within several weeks, body cells can lose their resistance and become sensitive once again to the effects of insulin. Insulin and blood glucose levels may normalize, and symptoms may disappear.

  Further, the need for oral antidiabetic drugs might be prevented or much lessened in dosage. **So, give diet and exercise a fair chance** – and maintain them to keep symptoms under control.

NEW BLOOD SUGAR CLASSIFICATION FOR DIABETES

(American Diabetes Association, 2003)

NORMAL:
Below 100 mg/dL

PREDIABETES:
100-125 mg/dL

DIABETES:
Over 125 mg/dL

Everyone 45 and over should have a blood glucose test every 3 years.

Get Moving! Everyday, do at least 30 minutes of moderate intensity exercise. It's the key to improving insulin sensitivity.

Add strength-training 3-4 times a week to double the benefits.

Managing Diabetes

Don't battle diabetes alone. Establish a partnership with your doctor, dietitian, certified diabetes educator and pharmacist. **Extra Support:** • *American Diabetes Association* • *American Diabetes Educators Association* • *National Diabetes Education Program*

Hints to keep blood glucose within safe limits:

- **Control your diet.** Know what and when you will eat. Seek referral to a dietitian for expert advice.
- **Exercise regularly.** It assists weight control and can improve sensitivity of body cells to insulin. Plan exercise into your daily routine.
- **Monitor your blood glucose** at home and work – ideally with a portable blood glucose meter. It will help you become familiar with your blood glucose patterns, and the effects of diet, exercise and medication. Insulin pumps can also help control blood glucose levels around the clock.
- **Don't skip prescribed insulin or oral medication.** If on insulin, know what action to take if hypoglycemia (low blood glucose) occurs. Also educate your family and friends.

Medtronic

Accu-Chek (Roche)

Deltec Cozmore   Animas

Blood glucose meters and insulin pumps can greatly improve control of diabetes and lifestyle choices.

Be Heart Smart ~ Know Your ABC's

If you have diabetes, you are at high risk for heart attack and stroke. Heart disease is more likely to strike you – and at an early age – than someone without diabetes.

But you can fight back. Be smart about your heart. **Take control of the ABC's of diabetes** and live a long and healthy live. Talk to your health care provider about your ABC targets.

Be Smart About Your **Heart**
Control the ABCs of **Diabetes**
➤ A1C
➤ Blood Pressure
➤ Cholesterol

National Diabetes Education Program

A is for A1C

The A1C (A-one-C) test – short for hemoglobin A1C – measures your average blood glucose (sugar) over the last 3 months. **Suggested target: below 7**

B is for Blood Pressure

High blood pressure makes your heart work too hard. **Suggested target: below 120/80**

C is for Cholesterol

Bad cholesterol, or LDL, can build up and clog your arteries. **Suggested target: below 100**

A1C VALUES	AVERAGE DAILY BLOOD GLUCOSE
6% ►	**6.5 mmol/L** Excellent Control
8% ►	**10 mmol/L** Needs Treatment Change
10% ►	**13 mmol/L** Poor Control
13% ►	**18 mmol/L** Seriously Out of Control

Guidelines for choosing a healthy diet apply equally to people with or without diabetes. Eating a wide variety of foods that are mainly low in fat and refined sugars, and high in fiber, is recommended.

However, actual food quantities, as well as when you eat, will also influence control of blood glucose. Your dietitian will individualize a diet plan to suit your food preferences, lifestyle and medical status. Here are a few hints:

- **Maintain a healthy weight.** If overweight, even a modest weight loss plus daily exercise can help to normalize blood glucose in Type-2 diabetes.

- **Don't skip meals.** If you take insulin or an oral hypoglycemic agent, regular meals are important.

- **If on insulin,** eat meals at the same time each day. Eat a similar amount of food at each meal. Even distribution of carbohydrate over the day will make best use of the available insulin and prevent wide variations in blood glucose levels.

  Note: Take your rapid-acting insulin no more than 15 minutes before eating. Regular and combination insulins are best taken with about 30 minutes between insulin injection and breakfast.

- **Choose wholegrain breads, cereals and pasta.** Eat fresh fruits, vegetables and legumes. These foods contain more fiber and slow the release of glucose into your blood after a meal.

- **Limit foods high in saturated fat and cholesterol.** Enjoy fish, soy foods, and other foods rich in omega-3 fats. **Extra Notes** ~ *See Fats & Cholesterol Guide, Page 271*

- **Avoid sugars and foods high in added sugar** particularly if overweight. Small amounts of sugar as part of a meal may occasionally be okay. Check with your dietitian. Use *Equal*, *Splenda* and *NutraSweet* – sweetened foods and drinks. **Extra Notes** ~ *See Page 9*

- **Foods (and supplements) rich in antioxidant vitamins C, E and beta-carotene,** as well as omega-3 fats, magnesium, zinc and chromium may help prevent long-term complications of diabetes (such as damage to small blood vessels and nerves). Be sure to check with your doctor.

Eat a well-balanced diet, high in fiber-containing foods and low in saturated fat.

Modest weight loss and daily exercise can greatly improve control of Type-2 diabetes.

***Excess Alcohol** contributes to obesity, diabetes, and high blood pressure.*

The risk of hypoglycemia (low blood sugar) and drug interactions with alcohol is also increased.

19

Diabetes ~ Carbs & Glycemic Index

Carbohydrate Type Affects Blood Glucose

The various forms of carbohydrate affect blood glucose levels in different ways. It is difficult to predict the effect of particular foods, sugars or meals, simply by their carbohydrate content.

Thus the same amount of carbohydrate from different foods may affect blood sugar levels very differently. Many factors affect the rate of digestion and absorption – particularly the type of sugar, starch and fiber; the degree of processing and cooking (which increases digestion rate); and the amount of protein and fat (which slows stomach emptying and digestion).

Glycemic Index (GI)

The GI is a method of ranking carbohydrate foods on a scale (0-100) according to how they affect blood glucose levels. (See next column). The higher the GI value, the greater the food's ability to rapidly raise blood glucose levels and the more insulin needed by the body (not desirable).

Eating low GI foods leads to better control of blood glucose and insulin levels (which in turn lowers the risk of damage to blood vessels and nerves). The slower digestion of low GI foods also helps to delay hunger pangs, and benefit weight control.

Of course, choosing low GI foods is not a licence to eat unlimited amounts – **calorie restriction and portion control for weight control is of prime importance.**

Extra Notes: * GI is not meant to be used in isolation without regard to portion size, and other dietary recommendations for healthy eating. Foods are not good or bad on the basis of their GI.

* The GI concept is yet to be adopted by the American Diabetes Assoc. and American Dietetic Assoc. There are other important aspects to consider for wise use of GI, including GL (Glycemic Load).

Extra Information ~ www.calorieking.com

LOWER GLYCEMIC FOODS

Slower Acting Carbohydrates
These foods are more slowly digested and absorbed. They help maintain more even blood glucose levels, as long as excessive amounts are not eaten. Use these foods regularly but still limit portion size for weight control.
Examples:
- Dried beans, peas, lentils
- Nuts and seeds
- Wholegrain breads and pita
- Bran cereals, oats
- Barley, buckwheat, bulgur
- Spaghetti, pasta, Basmati Rice
- Fresh fruit: apples, avocados, bananas (firm), cherries, grapefruit, grapes, olives, oranges, peaches, pears, plums. Fresh juices.
- Vegetables: sweet potatoes, yam
- Milk, yoghurt, soy drinks
- Sugar alcohols (Sorbitol, Maltitol)

HIGHER GLYCEMIC FOODS

Quicker Acting Carbohydrates
These foods more rapidly raise blood glucose levels. Eat only in moderation.
- White bread, rice cakes, bagels, croissants, doughnuts
- Low fiber cereals: Cornflakes, *Rice Krispies, Froot Loops*
- White potatoes, white rice, corn
- Watermelon, ripe bananas, cantaloupe, pineapple
- Soda, sugar-sweetened sports/energy drinks
- Sugar, Sugar Candy
- Ice Cream (low-fat), Frozen Yogurt

EXTRA INFORMATION
- Book: The New Glucose Revolution by Jennie Brand-Miller
- www.glycemicindex.com
- www.CalorieKing.com

Scales do not distinguish between fat, muscle and fluids.

>> Body Fluid Changes

Body weight fluctuates from day to day. This is mainly due to changes in body fluids which make up around 70% of total body weight. It can be affected by changes in hormone levels, dietary factors such as salt and carbohydrate, and even exercise.

Weight change over several weeks is more likely to reflect changes in levels of fat and muscle rather than fluid. Unfortunately, the scales do not distinguish between weight changes due to water, fat or muscle. This is why **we shouldn't allow every fluctuation in weight to rule our lives.**

To limit fluid retention, avoid salty foods and go easy on the salt shaker. Eating sufficient fruit and vegetables supplies extra potassium which counteracts sodium and encourages fluid loss. However, **do not limit water intake.** Be sure to drink at least 6-8 glasses of water or other fluids per day.

When dining out, be aware that the extra pound or two that might show on the scales the next morning is not the result of a small dietary indiscretion. It is more likely due to fluid retention resulting from more highly seasoned and salty food.

Monthly hormonal changes in women can also account for a build-up of fluids of several pounds prior to menstruation.

>> Menopausal Weight Gains

Most women gain an average of 4-5 pounds in the years leading up to menopause – usually in their middle to late 40's. This can occur even when exercise and eating habits have not changed significantly.

With hormonal changes occurring at that time, body fat also tends to be redistributed from thighs, buttocks and hips to the breast and stomach areas (a greater health risk).

Be sure to eat wisely and continue daily physical activity including strength-training to maintain or build muscles – and to boost metabolism and self-esteem.

>> Underactive Thyroid

Thyroid hormone is made by the thyroid gland in the neck. When insufficient thyroid hormone is made, metabolism and body processes slow down and weight gain can occur.

Symptoms of hypothyroidism can be subtle and easil y overlooked as signs of normal aging. **Early symptoms** may include fatigue, muscle weakness, sluggishness, a swollen tongue that you keep biting, and a puffy face.

As metabolism continues to slow, further **signs can include** chronically cold hands and feet, slow reflexes, constipation, dry skin and coarse hair, brittle nails, heavy menstrual periods, slower pulse, and a husky voice.

Depression-like symptoms may also develop such as forgetfulness, loss of interest, mood swings and irritability.

Weight gains of as much as 10-20 pounds (mainly fluid) can occur, as well as a raised **blood cholesterol level.**

The condition is more common in women, especially following pregnancy, around menopause, or after age 60.

A simple blood test through your doctor can detect hypothyroidism. It is easily treated in most cases with thyroid hormone pills.

Adults 35 and older should have a TSH (thyroid stimulating hormone) test every 5 years. Testing when pregnant is also wise.

Calcium & Osteoporosis Guide

Calcium's Role in the Body

Calcium plays a vital role in nerve and muscle function, clotting of blood, enzyme regulation, insulin secretion and overall bone strength. Bones and teeth store 99% of the body's calcium.

The calcium level in blood is kept at a steady level by the continual exchange of calcium between blood and bone. When insufficient calcium is obtained from food the body draws calcium out of the bones.

This bone loss over a period of years may lead to **osteoporosis** – thinning of the bones (porous bones).

The bones become weak, brittle and easy to fracture, particularly the bones of the wrist, hips and spine. Loss of height and curvature of the spine may also result, as may periodontal disease - the deterioration of the jaw bones that support the teeth.

As osteoporosis progresses after menopause, vertebrae may collapse causing the spine to curve and shoulders to hunch.

Osteoporosis – Common in Women

While osteoporosis also occurs in men, women are particularly vulnerable (1 in 4 by age 60). They have about 30% less bone than men, and a greater bone loss at menopause when estrogen levels drop. Slender framed women are at greater risk. (A woman in her eighties can have lost up to two thirds of her skeleton.)

Insufficient dietary calcium during pregnancy and breastfeeding will see bone reserves drawn upon, increasing the risk of osteoporosis.

Causes of Osteoporosis

The major factors associated with the bone loss of osteoporosis appear to be:
- Hormone changes of menopause
- Insufficient dietary calcium. (Absorption decreases with age)
- Insufficient exercise (weight bearing – such as walking, cycling, weight training)
- Family history of osteoporosis

Other contributing factors may include:
*Excess amounts of alcohol, protein and phosphorus (from excess meats and soft drinks) *smoking *insufficient vitamin D (sunshine, fish, dairy) *insufficient vitamin K, potassium and magnesium (from fruits, vegetables, whole grains, nuts)

RECOMMENDED DAILY INTAKE OF CALCIUM

		Calcium
Infants:		
	0-6 mths ~	210mg
	7-12 mths ~	270mg
Children:	1-3 yrs ~	500mg
	4-8 yrs ~	800mg
	9-12 yrs ~	1300mg
Teenagers:		
	13-18 yrs ~	1300mg
Adults:	19-50 yrs ~	1000mg
	51+ yrs ~	1200mg
Women:		
Pre-menopausal	~	1000mg
Menopausal(beginning)	~	1200mg
Post-menopausal	~	1500mg
Pregnancy/Breastfeeding:		
	Up to 18 yrs ~	1300mg
	19+ yrs ~	1000mg

Calcium & Osteoporosis Guide

Early Prevention Important

Gradual loss of bone begins in the thirties after maximum bone mass is reached. The stronger the bones at that time, the less trouble is likely to occur later. The earlier that prevention or treatment begins the greater the benefit. **The key to prevention is to build strong, dense bones early in life. By age 16,** some 80% of peak bone mass is already reached.

▲ *Osteoporotic Fragile Bone*   ▲ *Healthy Dense Bone*

Young women may lessen the risk by:
*eating high-calcium foods as well as adequate fruits, vegetables, whole grains and nuts
*not engaging in excessive dieting that results in menstrual period cessation (less estrogen)
*taking regular exercise and not smoking

Good Dietary Sources of Calcium
(Eat 3 servings a day of calcium-rich foods)

- Milk, Yogurt, Cheese
- Flavored Milk Drinks, Ice Cream, Custard
- Soy Drinks (calcium-enriched)
- Orange Juice (calcium-fortified)
- Tofu (with calcium coagulant), Miso, Tempeh
- Canned Salmon or Sardines (with edible bones)
- Breakfast Cereals (calcium-enriched): *Total, Wheaties*
- Broccoli, Dried Beans, Baked Beans
- Almonds, Brazil nuts, Hazelnuts, Seeds

For Calcium Counts of common foods, check the CalorieKing.com food database.

> **Calculating Calcium From Food Labels**
> The calcium content of packaged foods and drinks is shown in the Nutrition Facts label as a percentage of the DRI (dietary reference intake) of 1000 mg calcium. To convert this percentage into milligrams of calcium, simply multiply the percent figure by 10 (or add a zero). Examples: 5% = 50 mg calcium; 35% = 350 mg calcium.

Calcium Supplements

Prescribed high doses of calcium (1500-2000mg/day) may benefit persons with osteoporosis - as well as vitamin D, vitamin K, magnesium and zinc. Check with your doctor.

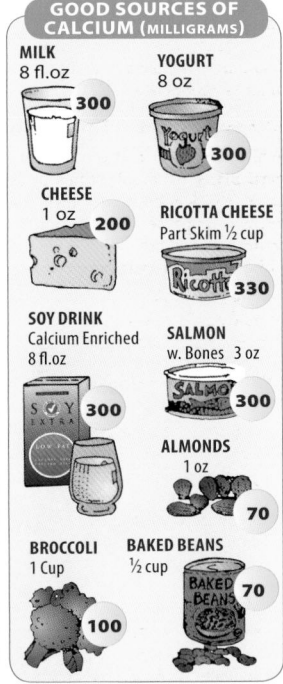

GOOD SOURCES OF CALCIUM (MILLIGRAMS)

MILK 8 fl.oz — 300
YOGURT 8 oz — 300
CHEESE 1 oz — 200
RICOTTA CHEESE Part Skim ½ cup — 330
SOY DRINK Calcium Enriched 8 fl.oz — 300
SALMON w. Bones 3 oz — 300
ALMONDS 1 oz — 70
BROCCOLI 1 Cup — 100
BAKED BEANS ½ cup — 70

Notes, Abbreviations, Measures

» Calorie and fat values have been rounded off. **Calories** ~ to the nearest 5 or 10 calories. **Fat** ~ to nearest half gram. **Note:** Trace amounts of fat (less than 0.3 grams) have been treated as zero.

» **Carbohydrate figures** in this book are for total carbohydrate, and not **Net Carbs** (which deducts fiber, polydextrose and sugar alcohols from total carbs).

» Because manufacturer's figures on labels are rounded off, figures in this book may differ slightly from the label. Serving sizes may also vary.

» Food product formulations change occasionally, and hence the need to regularly update this type of publication. Many products also come and go. Check the food label for any changes.

» **Seek Professional Advice:** This book is intended for educational purposes only. It is not a substitute for professional advice.

» **Feedback Welcome:** Please contact the author directly with your queries, and suggestions for foods to be included in future editions.
Write to: Allan Borushek (Dietitian)
1001 West 17th Street, Suite M, Costa Mesa CA 92627. Email: allan@calorieking.com

» **Food Product Updates:** Check the author's website.

www.CalorieKing.com

C ~ Calories
F ~ Fat (grams)
Cb ~ Carbohydrate (grams)

Abbreviations

tsp	= teaspoon
Tbsp or T	= Tablespoon
oz	= ounce(s)
c	= cup
fl.oz	= fluid ounce(s)
g	= gram(s)
avg	= average
pkg	= package

Volume Measures

(All measures are level)

3 tsp	=	1 Tbsp
2 Tbsp	=	1 fl.oz
½ cup	=	4 fl.oz
1 cup	=	8 fl.oz
2 cups	=	1 Pint
2 Pints	=	1 Quart

Note: 8 oz weight is not the same as 8 fl oz volume (space occupied). Dense foods weigh more per set volume. Examples:
1 cup popcorn weighs ½ oz
1 cup milk weighs 8½ oz
1 cup pudding weighs 10 oz

Metric Conversion

½ oz	=	14 grams
1 oz	=	28.4 grams
2 oz	=	57 grams
3½ oz	=	100 grams
1 fl.oz	=	30 mls
1 cup (8 fl.oz)	=	240 mls
33 fl.oz	=	1 liter (volume)

SOURCES OF INFORMATION

- U.S. Dept. of Agriculture
- Food Manufacturers
- Food Industry Boards & Councils
- Independent laboratory analysis
- Scientific publications
- Overseas food composition tables
- Author extrapolations

Quick Guide | C | F | Cb

Cow Milk ~ Average All Brands

Whole (3.5% fat):

	C	F	Cb
2 Tbsp, 1 fl.oz	20	1	1.5
1 Glass, 6 fl.oz	110	6	8.5
1 Cup, 8 fl.oz	150	8	12
1 Pint, 16 fl.oz	300	16	23
1 Quart, 946 ml	600	32	46

Reduced-Fat (2% fat):

	C	F	Cb
2 Tbsp, 1 fl.oz	15	0.5	1.5
1 Glass, 6 fl.oz	90	4	8.5
1 Cup, 8 fl.oz	130	5	13
1 Pint, 16 fl.oz	260	10	26
1 Quart, 946 ml	520	20	52

Light/Low-Fat (1% fat):

	C	F	Cb
2 Tbsp, 1 fl.oz	12	0.3	1.5
1 Glass, 6 fl.oz	75	2	8.5
1 Cup, 8 fl.oz	120	2.5	14
1 Pint, 16 fl.oz	240	5	28
1 Quart, 946 ml	480	10	56

Light/Low-Fat (½ % fat):

	C	F	Cb
2 Tbsp, 1 fl.oz	12	0.1	1.6

Fat Free/Skim:

	C	F	Cb
2 Tbsp, 1 fl.oz	10	0	1.5
1 Cup, 8 fl.oz	90	0.5	13
1 Pint, 16 fl.oz	180	1	26
w. Replace (Oatrim Fiber): 1 cup	85	0	12

Protein-Fortified:

	C	F	Cb
2% fat, 1 cup	140	5	14
1% fat, 1 cup	120	3	14
Skim, 1 cup	100	0.5	14

Acidophilus: Average All Brands

	C	F	Cb
Reduced Fat (2%), 1 cup	130	5	13
Low-Fat (1%), 1 cup	100	2	13

Buttermilk: Average All Brands

	C	F	Cb
Reduced-Fat (2%), 1 cup	120	5	10
Low-Fat (1%): 1 cup	100	2.5	12

Lactose-Reduced:

	C	F	Cb
Reduced-Fat: Lactaid, 1 cup	130	5	12
Dairy Ease 100, 1 cup	130	5	12
Low-Fat: Lactaid, 1 cup	110	2.5	13
Fat-Free: Lactaid/Lucerne, 1 cup	80	0	13
Lactaid with Soy Protein	110	0	13

Lower Carb Dairy Drinks: Per 8 fl.oz Cup

	C	F	Cb
Carb Countdown (Hood): Regular	130	8	3
2% Reduced-Fat, 1 cup	100	4.5	3
Fat-Free, 1 cup	70	0	3
LeCarb: 2% Low-Fat Dairy, 1 cup	105	4.5	4
Homogenized Dairy	140	9	4

Soy/Non-Dairy Drinks ~ See Page 27

Goat/Sheep Milk, Kefir

Goat's Milk (Meyenberg):

	C	F	Cb
Whole, 1 cup, 8 fl.oz	140	7	11
Light/Low-Fat (1%), 8 fl.oz	90	2.5	9
Evaporated, reconst., 8 fl.oz	145	8	11
Kefir: Steve's Kefir Peach, 1 cup	220	9	25
Nancy's, fruit flavors, avg, 1 cup	200	8	25
Sheep's Milk: Whole, 1 cup	265	17	13

Canned & Dried Milk

	C	F	Cb
Condensed: Reg. 2 Tbsp, 1 fl.oz	130	3	22
Low-Fat (Eagle), 2 Tbsp	120	1.5	23
Fat-Free (Eagle), 2 Tbsp	110	0	24
Evaporated: Whole, 2 Tbsp	40	3	3
Whole, ½ cup	170	10	13
Low-Fat (Carnation), 2 Tbsp, 1 oz	25	0.5	3
½ cup, 4 fl.oz	115	2.5	14
Fat-Free, 2 Tbsp, 1 oz	25	0	4
Dried: Whole, ¼ cup, 1 oz	150	8	11
Skim/Non-Fat, ⅓ cup	80	0	12
Made-up, 1 cup, 8 fl.oz	80	0	12
Buttermilk sweetcream, 1 oz	110	2	13
Non-Fat, 1 Tbsp	25	0	3
Malted (Carnation), dry, 1 Tbsp	30	0.5	6

Whey Drink

	C	F	Cb
Acid: Dry, 1 Tbsp, 3g	10	0	2
Fluid, 1 cup, 8 fl.oz	60	0	13
Sweet: Dry, 1 Tbsp, 8g	25	0	6
Fluid, 1 cup, 8 fl.oz	65	1	13
Nutri Mil: Orig./Low-Fat 8 fl.oz	80	3	11
Chocolate, 8 fl.oz	110	3	19
Fat-Free (Calcium Enriched)	60	0	11

Flavored Milk Drinks

Quick Guide

Chocolate Milk   C   F   Cb
Average All Brands: Per Cup (8 fl.oz)

	C	F	Cb
Whole Milk (3.3%): 1 cup	225	9	26
1 Pint	450	18	52
Reduced-Fat (2%), 1 cup	190	5	26
Low-Fat (1%), 1 cup	160	3	26

Brands ~ Flavored Milk

Ready-To-Drink: Per 8 fl.oz Cup Unless Indicated

	C	F	Cb
Albertson's, low-fat, 1 cup	170	2.5	30
Bodywise, non-fat, 1 cup	180	0	35
Borden Dutch Choc., 1 cup	220	8	28
Bosco, 1 cup	230	8	23
Brown Cow Farm, 1 cup	250	8	39
Carb Countdown (2%), Choc	100	4.5	3
Deans'Chug': Regular	220	9	26
Low-Fat, 1 cup	160	2.5	27
Dominick's Low-Fat, 1 cup	170	2.5	28
Golden Guernsey, 1 cup	130	2.5	15
Grocers Pride Choc D'Lite, 1 cup	120	3	22
Hershey's: Fat-Free Chocolate	165	0	30
Reduced-Fat Chocolate/Strawb.	200	5	31
White Chocolate	130	5	12
MilkShake, avg, 8 oz	285	8	44
Hood: Low-fat (1%), Chocolate	150	2	27
Carb Countdown 2% Reduced-Fat	100	4.5	3
Horizon Organic	160	5	27
Knudsen	200	3	32
Kroger (3.25% milk)	220	9	28
Lactaid (1%)	160	3	26
Land O'Lakes, low-fat (0.5%)	150	1.5	25
Meadow Gold (3.5%)	230	8	31
Nesquik: 16 fl.oz bottle	460	16	64
Banana, 16 fl.oz	385	10	40
Choc., Fat Free, 16 fl.oz bottle	320	0	64
Double Choc., 16 fl.oz bottle	395	10	60
Very Vanilla, 16 fl.oz	370	10	60
Oak Farms, 1 cup	210	8	26
Parmalat (2%)	180	5	28
Ralph's	240	3	34
Sobe Love Bus Chocolate, 8 fl.oz	140	1	28
Viva, Low-Fat	130	2.5	24
Yoo Hoo Choc Drink, 8 fl.oz	130	1	29

Bottled Coffee

See Coffee Section: *Page 164*

Shakes & Smoothies

Smoothies   C   F   Cb
Made Up Ready-To-Drink
(8 fl. oz Milk/Soy + Fruit): *Per 12 fl.oz*

	C	F	Cb
Average all types w. Whole Milk	300	8	50
+ Ice Cream, 1 scoop	400	13	62
with Non-Fat Milk	240	0	50

Freshens; Jamba Juice; TCBY:
   See Fast-Foods Section

Shakes

	C	F	Cb
Regular: Chocolate, 10 fl.oz	360	11	58
Vanilla/Strawberry, 10 fl.oz	320	9	53
Carb Options, 11.3 fl.oz can	185	9	6

Burger King's; McDonald's: See Fast-Foods

Cocoa-Chocolate Mixes

Add extra cals/fat/carbohydrate for milk

	C	F	Cb
Alba '66 Milk Choc, 1 pkg	60	0	14
Carnation Breakfast Drinks: See Page 158			
Ghirardelli: *Per 2 Heaping Teaspoons*			
Choc. Mocha/Hazelnut/Dble Choc	80	1.5	21
Pralines & Creme, 2 Tbsp	90	0	23
Godiva: Chocolixir, no whipped cream			
Dark Choc Decadence, 12 oz	590	23	99
Milk Chocolate Latte, 12 oz	630	23	97
White Choc Raspberry, 12 oz	470	19	73
Hershey's, 1 Tbsp	20	0.5	3
Horlicks, Malt Extract, 1 oz	20	0	3
Land O' Lakes: *Per 1¼ oz Pkg*			
Choc.Mint/Raspb./Supreme	160	5	25
Nescafe Frothe, 3 T., makes 8 fl.oz	15	0.5	2.5
Nestle: French Vanilla, 1 envelope	120	3	22
Hot Cocoa, 2 Tbsp	85	2.5	15
Fat-Free Hot Cocoa, 2Tbsp	25	0	4
w. Marshmallows, 1 envelope	35	0	8
Nesquik Powder *(Nestle): Per 2 Tbsp*			
Choc.; Dble Choc; Strawberry	90	0.5	19
Chocolate, No Added Sugar	40	1	7
Ovaltine Cocoa Mixes, 4 tsp	80	0	20
Swiss Miss: Cocoa Mixes			
Milk Chocolate, 1 oz pkt	110	1.5	22
w. Marshmallows, 1.2 oz pkg	140	3	22
Choc. Sensation, 1.25 oz pkg	150	4	27
Lite, 1 pkg	70	0	18
Diet Cocoa Mix, 1 pkg	25	0	4
Hot Cocoa Sugar Free, 1 pkg	60	0	10
Fat-Free, 0.53 oz	50	0	9
Vending Machine, 1.34 oz pkg	145	2	24
Weight Watchers: Hot Cocoa Mix	70	0	10

Soy ~ Ready-To-Drink

Per 1 Cup Serving (8 fl.oz)

	C	F	Cb
Cereal Match, 1 cup	100	3	17
Eden Blend, 1 cup	125	3	18
Edensoy: Extra Original	130	4	13
Unsweetened	120	6	5
Extra, Vanilla	150	3	23
Carob	170	4	27
Chocolate	175	4	28
Light: Original	100	2	14
Vanilla	120	2	20
8th Continent: Original, Low-Fat	80	3	8
Original, Light	50	1.5	2
Chocolate: Low-Fat	140	3	23
Light	90	1.5	13
Vanilla: Low-Fat	90	3	11
Light	60	1	5
Hain Soy Supreme: Original	80	3	9
Vanilla, 1 cup	100	3	12
Hansen's Soy Smoothies: *See Page 153, 159*			
Harmony Farms: Regular	80	1.5	10
Enriched; Vanilla	80	1.5	10
Health Source: All flavors	150	1.5	23
Health Source Plus	160	1	17
Soy Protein Shake	100	1	4
It's Soy Delicious: Vanilla	110	1	22
Awesome; Chocolate	120	2	22
Lifeway: Slim 6, 8 fl.oz	110	2	3
Soy Treat, 8 fl.oz	160	4	23
Naked Juice: *See Page 155*			
Odwalla Future Shake: Chocolate	160	3	27
Vanilla al'monde	190	6	24
Pacific: Select Plain, Low -Fat	70	2.5	9
Select Vanilla, Low-Fat	80	2.5	11
Organic, Original Unsweetened	90	4.5	4
Ultra (Extra Protein/Calcium): Plain	120	4	12
Vanilla	130	4	14
PowerDream: Mango Passion	320	5	65
Java Jolt, Chai, Vanilla Blast	250	5	42
X-treme Chocolate	260	5	48
Silk *(White Wave):* Plain, regular	95	4	8
Plain, unsweetened	90	4	5
Chai, 1 cup	140	4	19
Chocolate, 1 cup	140	3.5	23
Coffee Soylatte, 1 cup	150	3.5	25
Enhanced, 1 cup	110	5	8
Mocha, 1 cup	140	3.5	22
Spice Soylatte, 11 oz bottle	190	5	27
Vanilla	100	3.5	10
Silk Creamer, 1 Tbsp	15	1	1
Slim-Fast: w. Soy Protein,			
Orange Pinepple Shake, 1 can	220	1	46

	C	F	Cb
SoyDream: Orig./Enriched 8 fl.oz	130	4	17
Carob/Chocolate Enriched	210	3.5	37
Vanilla; Vanilla Enriched	150	3	23
Soy Coffee, 5.5 fl.oz prepared	5	0	0
Soy Fusion: Berry, 1 cup	120	1.5	24
So Nice: Low Carb, 8 fl.oz	65	3	3
Natural, 8 fl.oz	70	3.5	2
Original	80	3	7
Chocolate, 1 cup	145	3	24
Vanilla	100	3	11
SunSoy: Chocolate, 1 cup	150	3.5	26
Creamy Original, 1 cup	100	4	8
Vanilla, 1 cup	100	3.5	12
Vitasoy: Refrigerated, Creamy Orig.	100	4	9
Rich Chocolate	160	4	24
Smooth Vanilla	110	4	11
Long Life: Creamy Original	110	4	11
Classic Original	120	4.5	11
Green Tea Soy Drink	120	4	13
Rich Chocolate	160	4	24
Unsweetened Original	80	4	5
Vanilla Delight	120	4	13
Light: Original	60	2	7
Chocolate	110	2	17
Vanilla Soy Drink	70	2	10
WestSoy: *Plus,* Plain, 8 fl.oz	130	3	13
Plus, Vanilla	130	3	19
100% Organic: Original (2% fat)	130	3.5	18
Unsweetened, Plain	90	4.5	5
Unsweetened, Vanilla	100	4.5	5
Nonfat: Plain, 8 fl.oz	70	0	14
Vanilla	80	0	14
Lite: Plain, 1 cup, 8 fl.oz	90	1.5	15
Chocolate	140	1.5	25
Vanilla	110	1.5	19
Low-fat: Plain	90	1.5	19
Chocolate	140	3	24
Strawberry	160	3	25
Vanilla	120	1.5	21
Soy Slender, avg., all flavors	70	3	5
Chai, Original, 8 fl.oz	130	3	25
Smoothies, all flavors, 8 fl.oz	140	1.5	28
Soy Shakes, Choc; Vanilla	170	3.5	30
Vigor Aid: Vanilla	230	5	37
Chocolate	260	5	42
Juice Bar, average all flavors	120	1.5	24
Vitamite 100: 1 cup, 8 fl.oz	110	5	12
Wild Oats: Original, 1 cup, 8 fl.oz	100	3.5	12
Wildwood: Organic Chocolate	135	3.5	14
Original; Vanilla, 8 fl.oz	105	3	14
Smoothies, 10 fl.oz bottle	130	3.5	18
Zen Soy: Plain, 8 fl.oz	95	3.5	14
Chocolate	170	4	27
Cappuccino	150	3	22
Vanilla	115	3.5	14

Soy Powder Mix

	C	F	Cb
1 oz (¼ cup) mix makes 1 Cup (8 fl.oz)			
Soy Protein Isolate, 1 oz dry	95	1	0
Better Than Milk: Original, 1 oz	100	2.5	16
Light, 1 oz	80	0.5	13
Joy Soy: Extra (Carob/Van.), 2 T.	80	3	11
Revival Soy Shakes: *Per Packet*			
Plain; Chocolate Daydream	110	1.5	2
Flavors, average: with Fructose	225	2	33
Unsweetened or Splenda	130	2	4
Soyagen: Reg./No Sugar, 1 oz dry	130	6	12
Carob, 1 oz dry	130	6	13
Soy Quik *(Ener-g)*, 1 oz dry	100	4.5	8

Rice & Cereal Drinks

	C	F	Cb
Almond Breeze: Original, 8 fl.oz	60	2.5	8
Chocolate, 8 fl.oz	110	3	22
Vanilla, 8 fl.oz	90	2.5	16
Amazake, Almond Light, 8 fl.oz	110	2	20
Horchata: Don José, 8 fl.oz	140	4	25
Kerns, Aguas Frescas, 8 fl.oz	140	3	26
Eden Blend, Rice & Soy, 1 cup	120	3	18
Hain Rice Supreme: Low-Fat Orig.	100	3	16
Low-Fat Cinnamon, 8 fl.oz	130	3	22
Pacific: Multigrain, 8 fl.oz	160	2	30
Organic Oat: Original, 1 cup	130	2.5	24
Vanilla, 1 cup, 8 fl.oz	130	2.5	24
Almond: Original, 1 cup	80	2.5	11
Vanilla, 1 cup, 8 fl.oz	100	2.5	15
Hazelnut: Original, 1 cup	110	3.5	18
Pacific Rice: Low-Fat,			
Plain/Vanilla, 1 cup	130	2	27
Rice Dream: Carob, 1 cup	150	2.5	32
Chocolate; Enriched, 1 cup	170	3	36
Vanilla/Vanilla Enriched, 1 cup	130	2	28
Original/Original Enriched, 1 cup	120	2	25
Westbrae Rice, Plain/Van., 8 fl.oz	110	2.5	20
Wild Oats: Vanilla, 1 cup, 8 fl.oz	120	2	26
Original, 1 cup, 8 fl.oz	100	2	20

Rice/Nut Drink Mixes

	C	F	Cb
Better Than Milk: Light, 19g	70	0.5	14
Original, 23g	100	2.5	14
Nut Quik, 2 Tbsp powder, 18g	110	9	3
Rice Moo, 2 Tbsp powder, 19g	72	0	17
Solait, 3 Tbsp powder, 22g	80	1.5	13
Sun's Up, 2 scoops, 40g powder	160	2	36

Quick Guide

	C	F	Cb
Yogurt			
Average All Brands: Per 8 oz Cup			
Plain Yogurt: Whole, 8 oz	180	7	11
Low-Fat	140	4	16
Non-Fat	110	0	18
Fruit Flavored: Whole, 8 oz	250	6	38
Low-Fat	230	3	32
Non-Fat, regular	150	0	32
Non-Fat, no sugar added	120	0	32
Goat's Milk Yogurt ~ *Same as Regular Yogurt*			

Yogurt ~ Brands

	C	F	Cb
Alex Rod: Fat-Free, all flav., 8 oz	70	0	12
Albertson's (Low-Fat):			
Swiss, avg. all flavors, 8 oz	280	2.5	54
Fruit on the Bottom (low-fat):			
Average all flavors, 8 oz	260	2.5	49
Alta Dena: *Per Cup (8 oz)*			
Low Fat: Average all flavors	220	2	41
Non-Fat: Fruit Flavors, average	190	0	38
Plain	110	0	16
Vanilla	160	0	30
America's Choice: Swiss Style	210	2.5	41
Non-Fat, all flavors, 8 oz	100	0	15
Berkeley Farms: Non-Fat, avg.	100	0	16
Low-Fat: Boysenberry/Cherry	230	2.5	46
Raspberry	220	2.5	43
Strawberry, Lemon, Vanilla	270	2.5	52
Blue Bunny: Lite85, 6 oz	80	0	14
Low-Fat, average all flavors, 6 oz	85	3	5
Swirl'n Magic, Strawb. & Cherry, 4 oz	75	1	12
Yo-Pals, Strawb. & Banana, 4 oz	125	3	19
Breyers: Fruit On The Bottom, 8 oz	240	2	46
Non-Fat varieties, avg., 8 oz	115	0	21
Low-Fat varieties, 4 oz	115	1.5	22
Creme Savers, 4 oz	115	1.5	22
Smooth & Creamy, avg., 8 oz	240	2	48
Brown Cow: *Per 8 oz*			
Cream Top: Plain	170	10	12
Chocolate	250	8	39
Creamy Coffee, Vanilla	210	9	25
Fruit Flavors, average	230	8	35
Low-Fat: Plain	130	3	18
Flavors, average	220	3	41
Non-Fat: Plain	115	0	17
Fruit Flavors, average	190	0	39
Cabot: Plain, 8 oz	140	4	16
Flavors, 8 oz	220	3	42
Cascade Fresh: Low-Fat, 6 oz	140	2	23
Fat-Free, all flavors, 6 oz ctn	110	0	20
Whole Milk, 8 oz	170	8	12

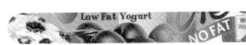

Yogurt ~ Brands (Cont)

	C	F	Cb
Carb Countdown (Hood)			
Average all flavors, 6 oz	80	1.5	4
Colombo			
Light, all flavors, 8 oz	110	0	20
Classic, avg. all types, 8 oz	220	3	41
Fat-Free, Plain, 8 oz	110	0	16
Continental: Vanilla, 8 oz ctn	190	0	38
Fruit on the Bottom, 8 oz	190	0	38
Crowley: Low-Fat Blueberry, 8 oz	240	2.5	48
Dannon: Plain (Natural), 8 oz	170	8	14
Danimals: Super Creamy, 4 oz	120	1	18
Squeezable, 2 oz	140	5	20
Drinkable, 3.3 fl.oz	120	0	22
Fruit Blends: Blueberry, 6 oz	170	1.5	33
Creamy, avg., 6 oz	170	2	32
Strawberry Blueberry, 4 oz	110	1	21
Fruit on the Bottom, 6 oz ctn	160	1.5	29
Frusion Smoothie, 10 fl oz bottle	280	3.5	53
la creme: Avg. all flavors, 4 oz	150	5	21
Mousse, all flavors 2.6 oz	120	5	15
Light 'n Fit (0% Fat): Avg., 6 oz	95	0	16
Carb Control, 4 oz	60	3	3
Creamy, avg. all flavors, 6 oz	100	0	17
Smoothie, 7 fl.oz bottle	80	0	15
w. Fiber, 4 oz	70	0	13
Natural, avg. all flavors, 6 oz	160	2.5	22
Sprinkl'ins, all flavors, 4.1 oz ctn	120	1.5	22
Whipped, avg. all flavors, 4.6 oz	160	3	28
Dominick's: Low-Fat, 8 oz	230	2	40
Fruit on the Bottom, avg, 8 oz	230	2	40
Fat-Free 80 Calories, 8 oz	80	0	13
Plain: Low-Fat, 8 oz	130	2.5	15
Non-Fat, 8 oz	120	0	17
Friendship: Regular type, 6 oz	190	5	31
Grocer's Pride: Low-Fat, 4.4 oz	140	1.5	28
Hood: Fat Free, Plain, 8 oz	130	0	18
Flavors, average, 8 oz	190	0	40
Horizon Organic			
Whole Milk, Plain Vanilla, 8 oz	220	6	32
Low-Fat: Blended, 6 oz cup	165	2	30
Tubes (1)	65	1	12
Fat-Free, all varieties, 6 oz	132	0	26
32 oz Carton, Plain, 8 oz	110	0	15
Yo Yo's, 4 oz	105	1	20
Jerseymaid (Vons)			
Fruit on the Bottom, 8 oz	240	2.5	46
Prestirred (low-fat), average	240	2.5	46
Plain, low-fat, 8 oz	140	3.5	18

	C	F	Cb
Jell-O: Spaceship, 4 oz	110	1	22
Hellios: Kefir Organic, 1 cup	120	5	13
Jewel: Low-Fat, average, 8 oz	250	2.5	48
Kemps: 100 Calories Nonfat, 5 oz	100	0	22
Classic Low-Fat, 6 oz	160	1.5	30
Free Non-Fat, 6 oz	90	0	22
Knudsen: 70 Calories, 6 oz	70	0	11
Free, average, 6 oz	170	0	33
Kroger: Per 8 oz Ctn			
Lite (Non-Fat) avg. all flavors	100	0	16
Low-fat: Plain, 8 oz	120	0	17
Flavors, average, 8 oz	250	2.5	47
Fruit on the Bottom, 8 oz	225	3	41
Lactaid: Low-Fat Vanilla, 8 oz	240	2.5	45
La Yogurt: **Light,** avg., 6 oz	90	0	17
Custard Classics, avg., 6 oz	170	2	32
French Style, avg., 6 oz	160	2	32
Fruit on the Bottom, avg., 8 oz	235	2.5	45
Latin Style, avg., 6 oz	180	2	33
LeCarb: YoCarb Plain, 4 oz	55	2.5	3
YoCarb Flavors, 4 oz	45	1	4
Light n' Lively			
Free 50 Calories, 4 oz	50	0	8
Free 70 Calories, 4 oz	70	0	11
Free (Regular): Vanilla, 6 oz	160	0	32
Fruit Flavors, average, 6 oz	180	0	36
Kidpack/Multipack, avg 4.4 oz	140	1	28
Lucerne			
Low-Fat: Plain, 8 oz	150	3.5	18
Fruit flavors, average, 8 oz	240	2.5	47
Vanilla	230	2.5	43
Fat-Free: Plain, 8 oz	130	0	19
Light Fat-Free, fruit, 8 oz	120	0	22
YoCups, avg all flavors, 4 oz	130	1	27
Yo On The Go, 2.25 oz tube	80	2	13
Meadow Gold: Plain, 8 oz	160	5	16
Flavors, average, 8 oz	250	4	42
Mountain High			
Original Style, plain, 8 oz	190	8	18
European Delight, all flavors, 4 oz	115	2	20
Naturally Nutritious, all flavors, 4 oz	95	0.5	18
Low-Fat: Plain, 8 oz	150	2	22
Classic, 8 oz	150	1	29
Fat-Free: Plain, 8 oz	120	0	19
Natural, 8 oz	165	0	24
Mystic Lake Dairy (Goat Milk Yogurt)			
Plain, 1 cup, 8 oz	120	6	9

Yogurt (Cont)

Brands (Cont)   C   F   Cb

	C	F	Cb
Nancy's: *Per 8 oz Serving*			
Whole Milk: Honey, plain, 8 fl.oz	180	8	17
w. Fruit Cup, avg, 9.5 oz	230	8	29
Low Fat: Plain/Lemon/Vanilla, avg	140	3	16
Other flavors, average	180	3	28
Nonfat: Plain, 8 oz	120	0	17
Maple, Vanilla (8 oz ctn)	160	0	27
w. Fruit Cup, avg, 9.5 oz	165	0	29
Vanilla (32 oz ctn), swtn'd, 8 oz	220	0	40
Soy Cultured: (6 oz ctn): Plain	145	3	25
Berry flavors, average	150	3.5	24
Vanilla	120	3	19
Kiwi-Lime; Mango, average	170	3	33
Old Home: 100 Cal., Non-Fat, 6 oz	100	0	20
Velvet Delight, average, 6 oz	240	7	39
Pavel's: Original Russian, 8 oz	140	8	10
Low-Fat Vanilla, 8 oz	120	4	12
Non-Fat Russian, 8 oz	110	0	15
Mountain Dairy, 6 oz	150	1.5	27
Publix: Fat-Free, Plain, 8 oz	140	0	23
Swiss Style (low-fat), 8 oz	240	2.5	41
Redwood Hill Farm (Goat Milk Yogurt)			
Vanilla; Fruit flavors, avg., 8 oz	180	5	28
Plain, 8 oz	125	6	10
Silk (Soy): Plain, 1 cup, 8 oz	135	3	22
Vanilla, 6 oz ctn	170	3	30
Other flavors, average, 6 oz	170	2	31
Sky Hill Napa Valley, Plain, 8 oz	130	8	8
Snackwell's, Non-Fat, 6 oz	160	0	36
Stater Bros: Non-Fat, avg, 8 oz	130	0	16
Stonyfield Farm (Organic)			
All Natural Fat-Free: Plain, 6 oz	90	0	14
Chocolate Underground, 6 oz	185	0	39
Other varieties, 6 oz	130	0	26
Low-Fat: Caramel	190	1.5	38
Plain	95	1.5	13
Other varieties, average	140	1.5	25
Whole Milk Yogurt: Vanilla Truffle	235	5	41
French Vanilla; Mocca-ccino, 6 oz	185	6	27
Other varieties, avg.	170	6	24
Moo-La-La, flavors, avg., 4 oz	160	5	25
Moove Over Carbs, 4 oz	70	3	14
O'Soy: Choc.; Vanilla, avg., 6 oz	160	2	27
Fruit on Bottom, average, 6 oz	180	2	33
Smoothies: Peach, 10 oz	265	3	49
Other varieties, 10 oz	250	3	46
Squeezers, all flavors, 57g	60	1	11
Yo Self, Low-Fat, average, 4 oz	110	1	21
Stop & Shop, Blended Lite, 8 oz	120	0	20

	C	F	Cb
"TCBY" Fat-Free (Fantasies):			
Banana Creme Pie, 6 oz	110	0	18
White Chocolate, 6 oz	90	0	12
Trader Joe's: Low-Fat, 8 oz	230	2.5	44
Non-Fat: Regular, 8 oz	190	0	40
French Village, Vanilla, 8 oz	170	0	32
Organic Vanilla, 8 oz	160	0	27
Organic Low-Fat, average, 6 oz	150	2.5	24
Cultured Soy, all varieties, 6 oz	140	2.5	28
Wallaby (Organic), avg., 6 oz	150	2.5	24
Wildwood: Soyogurt Plain, 6 oz	105	5	6
Other varieties, avg., 6 oz	130	3.5	20
WholeSoy: Plain, 6 oz ctn	140	2.5	24
Other flavors, avg, 6 oz	150	2.5	27
YoFarm, all flavors, avg, 8 oz	220	6	37
YoCrunch: *Low-fat w. Toppings, 6.5 oz Cup*			
Oreo Cookies	190	4	35
Peach/Strawb./Rasp. w. Granola	220	2	46
Average other varieties	240	6	41
Yoplait: Fruit Flavors, 6 oz	165	1.5	33
Coconut Cream Pie, 6 oz	185	3	34
Lemon Burst, 6 oz	180	1.5	36
Pina Colada, 6 oz	170	2	33
Light (Fat-Free): Fruit, 6 oz	95	0	19
Indulgent Desserts, 6 oz	105	0	20
Custard Style, all flavors, 6 oz	190	3.5	32
Go-Gurt, 2.25 oz tube	80	2	13
Grande: Avg. all flavors, 8 oz	250	2.5	48
99% Fat-Free Plain, 8 oz	135	0	19
Healthy Heart, 8 oz	250	1.5	35
Trix, avg., all flavors, 4 oz	120	1.5	23
Ultra Creme, 6 oz	85	2.5	8
Whips!: 4 oz ctn	145	2.5	25
Chocolate Mousse, 4 oz ctn	160	4	26
Yumsters, 4 oz	120	2	21

Yogurt Drinks & Probiotics

	C	F	Cb
Actimel *(Dannon)* Probiotic, 3.3 fl.oz	95	2	16
Alta Dena, Drinkables, 1 cup	220	4	46
Breyers, Creme Savers, 10 fl.oz	185	3	32
Carb Countdown, 10 fl.oz	100	3	4
Carbolite, 8 fl.oz	85	2	8
Creme Savers *(Breyers),* 10 oz	190	3	32
Dannon: Danimals, 3.4 fl.oz bottle	90	1.5	16
DanActive, 3.4 fl.oz	95	1.5	18
Glen Oaks, all flavors, avg, 1 cup	250	4	46
Nouriche: Regular, 11 fl.oz	280	0	60
Light, 11 fl.oz	170	0	33
Stonyfield Farm, 10 fl.oz	250	3	48
WholeSoy, 12 fl.oz bottle	210	3	35
Yo Soy, 8 fl.oz	80	4	4
Yonique: Pina Colada, 6 fl.oz	190	4	30
Peach; Banana; Guava, 6 fl.oz	170	2	30
Yoplait Go Gurt, 4.2 fl.oz	120	0	23

Quick Guide   C F Cb

Ice Cream

Vanilla: *Average All Brands*
Other flavors ~ See Brand Listings.
Regular Ice Cream (10% fat):
(Examples: Borden/Hood)

	C	F	Cb
3 fl.oz scoop	100	5	12
½ cup, 4 fl.oz	130	7	16
1 Pint, 16 fl.oz	520	28	62
½ Gallon (4 Pints)	2100	112	248

Rich (16% fat):

3 fl.oz scoop	130	8	12
½ cup, 4 fl.oz	170	10	17
1 Pint	690	40	68

Super-Rich (20% fat): *(Haagen-Dazs/Ben & Jerry's)*

3 fl.oz scoop	200	14	16
½ cup, 4 fl.oz	270	18	21
1 Pint	1100	72	84

Reduced-Fat/Light (6% fat):
(Breyer's Light/Hood Light)

3 fl.oz scoop	100	3	14
½ cup, 4 fl.oz	140	4	18
1 Pint	560	16	72

Low-Fat (less than 4% fat):
(Healthy Choice/Weight Watchers/Snackwell's)

3 fl.oz scoop	90	2	17
½ cup, 4 fl.oz	120	2.5	22
1 Pint	480	10	88

Fat-Free: *(Baskin-Robbins FF/Borden FF/Breyers FF/Dreyers FF/Hood FF)*

3 fl.oz scoop	75	0	17
½ cup, 4 fl.oz	100	0	22
1 Pint	400	0	88

Soft Serve: Regular, ½ cup

Regular, ½ cup	140	5	20
1 cup	280	10	40
Non-Fat, ½ cup	90	0	23
1 cup	180	0	46

Quick Guide

Frozen Yogurt   C F Cb

Average All Brands

	C	F	Cb
Hard: Low-Fat, ½ cup	140	3	26
Non-Fat, ½ cup	110	0	29
Soft: Low-Fat, ½ cup	120	2.5	28
Non-Fat, ½ cup	100	0	30

Brands: *See Ice Cream & Ices Section*

Quick Guide   C F Cb

Gelato/Ices/Frozen Custard

Gelato: *Per ½ Cup*

	C	F	Cb
Milk base: Vanilla	200	15	18
Choc. Hazelnut	370	29	26
Water base: ½ cup	100	0	25

Frozen Custard: *Per ½ Cup*

Chocolate	140	6	18
Orange Sherbet	105	2	21
Vanilla	130	6	16

Ice (Milk base): Average all flavors

Hard (4% fat), ½ cup	100	3	15
Soft Serve (3% fat), ½ cup	110	2	19
Shaved Ice: Average, 12 fl. oz	160	0	40
Sherbet: Average, ½ cup	120	2	28
Sorbet: Fruit (no fat), ½ cup	120	0	30
Fruit Ice Pops	80	0	20

Tofu Frozen Desserts: *See Page 35*

Sundaes   C F Cb

Denny's: Sundaes,

	C	F	Cb
Single Scoop, no topping	195	14	14
Double Scoop, no topping	385	27	29
Banana Split	930	43	121
Toppings: Blueberry, 2 oz	105	0	26
Chocolate, 2 oz	340	25	27
Fudge, 2 oz	215	10	30
Strawberry, 2 oz	115	1	26

McDonald's: Sundaes,

Hot Fudge Sundae, 6.3 oz	350	12	52
Strawberry Sundae	290	7	50
Toppings: Nut/Sundae, ¼ oz	50	3.5	2

Ice Cream Bars & Pops

See Pages 36-38

Ice Cream, Cones & Cups

Average All Brands   C F Cb

	C	F	Cb
Wafer Cone/Cup, average	20	0	4
Sugar Cone, average	40	0	9
Waffle Cone:			
Small	60	0	11
Large	100	1	22
Brands:			
Oreo Chocolate Cone	50	1	10
Comet Sugar Cone	50	0	11
Keebler Sugar Cone	45	0	11

Ice Cream & Frozen Yogurt (Cont)

Brands

	C	F	Cb
Aspen: Ice Cream, ½ cup	170	0	4
Wow Cow Frozen Yogurt, ½ cup	40	0	8
Atkins: *Per ½ Cup*			
Endulge, average all flavors	130	11	6
Baskin-Robbins: *See Fast-Foods Section*			
Ben & Jerry's: *Per ½ Cup*			
Body & Soul: Cherry Garcia	170	9	22
Chocolate Chip Cookie Dough	190	9	26
Chocolate Fudge Brownie	180	7	25
Half Baked	190	8	29
Singles: *Per Container*			
Cherry Garcia	220	13	22
Chocolate Fudge Brownie	230	11	28
Cookie Dough	240	13	26
Vanilla	200	13	17
Original: Brownie Batter	310	18	32
Butter Pecan	285	21	20
Cherry Garcia	250	14	26
Chocolate	260	16	25
Chocolate Chip Cookie Dough	280	15	32
Chocolate Fudge Brownie	265	13	32
Chubby Hubby	330	20	21
Chunky Monkey	300	18	30
Coffee	240	15	21
Coffee Heath Bar Crunch	290	18	29
Everything But The...	310	19	30
Fudge Central	300	18	31
Half Baked	280	14	34
Karamel Sutra	285	15	33
Mint Chocolate Cookie	260	16	26
New York Super Fudge Chunk	310	20	30
Oatmeal Cookie Chunk	270	15	31
Peanut Butter Cup	360	26	27
Phish Food	280	13	37
Pistachio Pistachio	260	17	21
Primary Berry Graham	270	15	29
Strawberry	230	13	26
Uncanny Cashew	290	19	27
Vanilla	240	16	21
Vanilla Heath Bar Crunch	305	19	29
Vanilla Swiss Almond	290	18	29
Frozen Yogurt: *Per ½ Cup*			
Phish Food	220	4.5	41
Low-Fat: Black Raspberry	140	1.5	28
Cherry Garcia	170	3	32
Chocolate Fudge Brownie	190	2.5	35
Half Baked	190	3	35
Vanilla	130	1.5	25
Sorbet: Average all flavors	110	0	27
Bars/Pops: *See Page 36*			

Blue Bunny	C	F	Cb
Fat-Free, No Added Sugar: *Per ½ Cup*			
Brownie Sundae; Burgundy Cherry	90	0	23
Caramel Toffee Crunch	90	0	24
Average other flavors	80	0	18
Reduced-Fat, No Added Sugar: *Per ½ Cup*			
Banana Split; Butter Pecan, avg.	125	5	20
Rocky Road; Tin Roof, avg.	130	6	20
Turtle Sundae	140	7	20
Other flavors, avg.	120	5	16
Hi Lite: Butter Pecan	120	4.5	17
Caramel Pecan; Fudge Nut	130	4	21
Cookies & Cream; Vanilla	130	3.5	21
Other varieties, avg.	110	2.5	17
Carb Freedom: Vanilla Bean	100	7	10
Mint Chip; Butter Pecan	110	8	11
Choc. Almond Fudge	120	8	13
Double Strawberry	100	6	13
Frozen Yogurt, ½ cup	100	0	21
Bars/Pops: *See Page 36*			
Bon Bon's *(Nestle):* Milk Choc. (8)	330	23	27
Dark Chocolate, (8)	310	21	26
Bresler's: *Per ½ Cup*			
All Flavors Ice Cream: average	230	12	23
Royal Cremes, average	260	16	21
Royal Lites, average	220	0	49
Breyers: *Per ½ Cup*			
HeartSmart: Cookies & Cream	110	1.5	24
Choc. Fudge Brownie	90	1.5	20
Cookies & Cream	110	1.5	24
Vanilla/Chocolate & Strawberry	90	1.5	19
CarbSmart: Chocolate Almond	130	10	10
Strawberry; Vanilla	130	9	10
Other varieties, avg.	155	12	10
98% Fat-Free, average	90	1.5	21
All Natural: Banana Fudge Chunk	160	8	21
Butter Almond/Pecan	160	10	14
Caramel Praline Crunch	170	9	22
Chocolate Chip Cookie Dough	170	9	20
French Vanilla; Coffee; Cherry	145	8	15
Fruit Sherbet, average	130	1.5	26
Mocha Almond Fudge	170	9	18
Lactose Free; Peach; Strawb.	125	7	14
Peanut Butter & Fudge	170	10	17
Rocky Road	170	8	20
Vanilla & Choc. & Strawberry	140	7	16
Vanilla Fudge Brownie; Almond	160	9	19
Other varieties, avg.	155	8	16
Take Two: Vanilla & Chocolate	140	8	16
Vanilla & Orange Sherbet	130	4.5	21
Light: French Vanilla	120	4	18
French Chocolate	140	5	20
Natural Vanilla	110	3	17
Other varieties, avg.	140	5	20

Brands (Cont)

	C	F	Cb
Breyers (Cont): Per ½ Cup			
No Sugar Added: Butter Pecan	120	7	15
Other varieties, avg.	100	4	14
Premium Edition: Turtle Sundae	190	11	20
Caramel Toffee Crunch; Reese's	180	9	22
Deep Chocolate Fudge	205	12	21
CarbSmart Frozen Yogurt, ½ Cup	90	4.5	15
Brigham's: Per ½ Cup			
Ice Cream: Big Dig	215	12	24
Chocolate/Chip; Vanilla	205	13	19
Chocolate Chip Cookie Dough	225	13	24
Mississippi Mud; Mocha Almond	220	14	20
Raspberry Lime Rickey Sherbert	130	2	27
Bruster's: Ice Cream, ½ cup	160	8	20
Frozen Yogurt, ½ cup	110	3	17
Fat-Free Ice Cream, ½ cup	110	0	23
Reduced-Carb Ice Cream, ½ cup	135	7.5	27
Carb Promise (Kemps): Per ½ Cup			
Butter Pecan	130	11	10
Chocolate Peanut Butter Cup	160	12	12
Cow Tracks	130	8	18
Toffee Fudge Chunk	120	9	12
Vanilla	110	8	10
Vanilla Fudge Nut Sundae	140	11	14
CarbSmart: See Breyers			
Carvel Ice Cream: See Fast-Foods Section			
Coldstone Creamery: See Fast-Foods Section			
Colombo: Per ½ Cup			
Frozen, Soft Serve: Non-Fat var.	100	0	22
Slender Sensations varieties	60	0	11
Low-Fat: Old Worlde; Cookies	120	2.5	20
Sorbet: Vanilla	140	0	29
Other flavors	95	0	24
Costco: Frozen Yogurt, ½ cup	95	0	20
CremaLita (Soft Serve)			
Calories will vary with density (air in product) and serving size.			
Best to weigh product and calculate on 25 cals per 1 oz weight.			
Vanilla: Small (4 fl.oz cup),			
If 2½ oz weight	60	0	14
If 4 oz weight*	100	0.5	23
If 6 oz weight*	150	1	35
(*) Most common weights			
Medium (8 fl.oz cup), 11 oz wt	275	1.5	63
Chocolate: Small, 6 oz weight	160	1	36
Dairy Queen/Brazier: See Fast-Foods Section			

	C	F	Cb
Dannon Frozen Yogurt: Per ½ Cup (4 fl.oz)			
Light Soft, all flavors, average	90	1	21
Light 'N Crunchy, all flavors, avg.	110	1	23
Pure Indulgence, all flavors, avg.	150	3	25
Dolewhip (Soft Serve): Per ½ Cup (4 fl.oz)			
Chocolate; Vanilla	100	3	18
Fruit flavors, average	80	0.5	16
Dove: Per ½ Cup			
Beyond Vanilla	260	16	25
Cappuccino Chocolate Thrill	300	19	28
Caramel Pecan Perfection	310	18	32
Chocolate & Brownie Affair	310	20	30
Give in to Mint	310	19	30
Irresistibly Raspberry	240	13	30
Toffee Caramel Moment	320	20	32
Unconditional Chocolate	300	18	31
Vanilla with a Chocolate Soul	300	19	29
Miniatures: Flavor Collection, 5 pces	300	20	30
Milk Chocolate, 5 piece	300	20	30
Original Dove Choc., 5 pieces	300	20	32
Dreyers: Per ½ Cup			
Fat-Free Ice Cream, avg. all flav.	100	0	20
Carb Benefit, average	160	10	13
Grand: Almond Praline	170	8	21
Chocolate; Coffee, avg.	150	8	18
Fudge Tracks; Peanut Butter Cup	185	11	18
Grovestand Peach	120	5	17
Neapolitan	135	7	16
Nestle Drumstick Sundae Cone	180	10	19
Real Strawberry	125	6	16
Toasted Almond	155	9	15
Vanilla; Americans Vanilla, avg.	155	10	14
Vanilla Bean/Chocolate, avg.	140	8	15
Other flavors, avg.	165	9	18
Light: Vanilla	105	3.5	15
Other regular varieties, average	115	4	17
No Sugar Added, average	100	3	13
Fat-Free, average	95	0	20
No Sugar Added: Regular, avg.	100	3	17
Fat-Free, average	95	0	20
Homemade: Chocolate	155	7	19
Grovestand Peach	120	5	17
Mint Choc. Chunk; Van. Custard	160	8	18
Old Fashioned Butter Pecan	155	9	15
Strawberries and Cream	130	6	17
Vanilla	135	7	15
Frozen Yogurt, average	90	0	20
Sherbet, avg. all flavors	130	2	30

33

Ice Cream & Frozen Yogurt (Cont)

Brands (Cont)

	C	F	Cb
Edys: *Per ½ Cup*			
Grand: Choc. Fudge Mousse	160	8	20
Vanilla/Choc.; Espresso	150	8	17
Choc. Fudge Sundae; Dble Fudge	170	9	19
Ice Cream Sandwich	150	7	19
Grand Light: Vanilla	100	3.5	15
Butter Pecan; Choc. Almond	120	5	16
Chocolate	110	3.5	15
Choc. Fudge Chunk	120	4.5	18
Cookie Dough; P'nut Butter Cups	130	5	18
Cookies 'n Cream; Rocky Road	120	5	18
French Silk	130	4.5	19
Fat-Free: Average all flavors	115	0	25
Carb Benefit: Vanilla Bean	140	9	13
Other varieties, average	160	11	13
No Sugar Added: Regular, avg.	100	3	17
Fat-Free, average	95	0	20
Eskimo Pie: *Per ½ Cup*			
Reduced-Fat: Butter Pecan	140	7	16
Choc. Marshmallow	130	4	23
Neopolitan; Vanilla	110	4	18
Other flavors, avg.	120	4	19
Bars: *See Page 37*			
Friendly's			
Ice Cream: Chocolate Almd Chip	170	10	18
Forbidden Chocolate	150	9	14
Fudge Nut Brownie	200	11	23
Vanilla Choc. Strawb.; Vanilla	150	8	16
Vienna Mocha Chunk	180	11	19
Frozen Yogurt: *Per ½ Cup*			
Regular flavors, average	150	4	24
Low-Fat flavors, average	120	3	20
Sundaes: *Per 3 Scoops*			
Apple Pie	700	30	98
Candy Shop Satisfaction Snickers	810	35	100
Dble Deluxe Caramel Fudge Blast	700	30	98
Cyclones: *Per 12 fl.oz*			
Fudge Brownie	790	25	127
Reese's Peanut Cup	880	43	100
Frostline (Soft Serve): Chocolate	90	2	20
Vanilla, ½ cup	90	3	18
Frusen Gladje: *Per ½ Cup*			
Butter Pecan	280	21	16
Chocolate	240	17	17
Strawberry	230	15	20
Swiss Choc. Candy Almond	270	19	18
Vanilla	230	17	16
Vanilla Swiss Almond	270	19	18
Other flavors, average	275	18	22

	C	F	Cb
Gelatida: *Per ½ Cup*			
Almond Biscotti	150	3	26
Amaretto Chocolate	150	4.5	23
Average other flavors	130	2	22
Godiva: *Per ½ Cup*			
Belgian Dark Chocolate	280	17	26
Choc Hazelnut Truffle	350	23	31
Choc Raspberry Truffle; Vanilla	290	16	33
Chocolate Cheesecake	310	17	36
Chocolate w. Chocolate Hearts	330	20	32
Classic Milk Chocolate	290	18	28
Pecan Caramel Truffle	320	19	32
White Choc. Raspberry	260	12	32
Good Humor: *Per ½ Cup*			
Light: Choc. Chip, Toffee Bar Crunch	130	4	20
Cookies n' Crm; Praline Alm. Crnch	130	3	21
Other varieties, avg.	110	3	19
Haagen-Dazs			
Ice Cream, Sorbet, Frozen Yogurt: *See Fast-Foods Section*			
Bars: *See Page 37*			
Healthy Choice: *Per ½ Cup*			
Brownie Bliss	125	2	25
Cookies 'N Cream	130	2	24
Double Karma; Happy Together	140	2	29
Jumpin' Java	130	2	25
Peanut Butter Cup	110	2	19
Praline & Caramel; Rocky Road	130	2	25
Vanilla; Mint Choc Chip	100	2	18
Other flavors, average	120	2	18
Low-Fat, No Sugar Added: Vanilla	90	2	18
Coffee Almond Fudge	110	2	20
Chocolate Fudge Brownie	115	2	20
Mint Chocolate Chip	100	2	18
Hood: *Per ½ Cup*			
Regular Ice Cream: Avg. all flavors	150	8	17
Light Ice Cream: Creamy Vanilla	110	3.5	18
Raspb. Swirl; Heavenly Hash, avg	130	3.5	22
Other flavors, average	140	5	22
No Sugar Added, Low-Fat Ice Cream:			
Vanilla Dream; Classic Trio	100	1.5	19
Choc Frenzy	120	2.5	19
Chocolate Chip	155	2.5	30
Fat-Free Ice Cream: Avg. all flavors	100	0	23
Frozen Yogurt: Avg. all flavors	150	8	17
Non-Fat: Strawb., Old Fashion. Van.	110	0	24
Other flavors, average	120	0	27
Bars: *See Page 37*			
I Can't Believe It's Yogurt: *See Fast-Foods Section*			

Brands (Cont)

	C	F	Cb
Jerseymaid (Vons): *Per ½ Cup*			
After Dinner Mint; Cookies & Crm	170	9	19
Choc Chip; Mint Choc Chip	160	9	17
Heavenly Hash; Nut Chunky Choc.	170	8	22
Mocha Almd Fudge; Rocky Road	160	7	20
Neopolitan; Vanilla	140	7	16
Strawberry	140	6	18
Kilwin's: *Per ½ Cup*			
Butter Pecan	190	13	16
Butter Pecan Yogurt	130	6	17
Chocolate	170	10	17
Average other flavors	190	10	20
Fat-Free Ice Cream, avg. all flavors	100	0	23
Topping: Caramel	160	4.5	31
Fudge	110	6	28
LeCarba: *Per ½ Cup*			
Chocolate Almond	120	9	6
Lemon	90	6	6
Other flavors	100	7	6
Luigi's Real Italian Ice: *Per Cup (6 fl.oz)*			
Chocolate	160	0	40
Other flavors	125	0	31
Swirl, all flavors	155	0	39
Rice Dream *(Non-Dairy):* *Per ½ Cup*			
Vanilla Carob/Choc/Cappuccino	150	6	23
Other varieties	170	8	26
Sealtest: *Per ½ Cup*			
Butter Pecan	160	9	16
Choc. Chip Cookie Dough	160	8	20
Fudge Royal; Heavenly Hash	150	7	20
Vanilla/Choc. Strawberry	140	7	16
Snackwell's: *Per ½ Cup*			
Brownie; Rocky Road; Praline	140	2	28
Vanilla	100	2	18
Soy Delicious (Organic): *Per ½ Cup*			
Novelties: Twisted Van. Orange	120	2	24
Mocha Fudge	150	3.5	27
Other flavors, avg	145	5	23
Fruit Pints: Almond Pecan	160	6	24
Choc Almond/P'Nut Butter	155	5	25
Other flavors, average	130	3	25
Purely Decadent: Zig Zag; Banana	255	13	32
Other flavors, average	215	9	32
Sweet Nothings, avg.	115	0	29
Soy Dream (Non-Dairy): *Per ½ Cup*			
Butter Pecan	160	10	17
Chocolate Fudge Brownie	150	8	20
Mint Chocolate Chip	150	9	19
Average other flavors	140	6	20

	C	F	Cb
Starbucks: *Per ½ Cup*			
Caramel Cappuccino	240	12	30
Classic Coffee; Italian Roast	230	12	29
Coffee Almond Fudge; Java Chip	250	13	26
Mud Pie	240	11	32
White Chocolate Latte	280	15	31
Low-Fat: Mocha Mambo; Latte	170	3	30
Bars*: See Page 38*			
Stonyfield Farm (Organic): *Per ½ Cup*			
Premium: Chocolate	270	18	22
Gotta Have Vanilla	250	18	20
Other flavors, average	260	16	26
Frozen Yogurt:			
Non-Fat: Vanilla Fudge Swirl	110	0	23
Other varieties	90	0	19
Low-Fat: Creme Caramel	120	1.5	23
Cookies 'n Dream; Mint Choc	130	3	22
Sweet Nothings *(Non-Dairy/Fat-Free)*			
Average all flavors, ½ cup, 3 oz	120	0	28
TCBY: *Per ½ Cup*			
Sorbet, ½ cup	95	0	24
Frozen Yogurt: Non-Fat, all flavors	110	0	23
96% Fat-Free, all flavors	140	3	23
No Sugar Added, all flavors	90	0	20
Hand-Dipped Icecrm: Butter Pecan	260	20	17
Chewy Chocolate Fudge	270	16	27
Chocolate Chocolate; Pralines	215	13	21
Choc. Chunk Cookie Dough	210	14	18
Lemon Meringue Pie	235	12	29
Oatmeal Raisin	220	12	16
Vanilla Bean	195	13	17
Very Berry Strawberry	185	11	19
White Macadamia; Mint Choc.	250	16	23
Tasti D-Lite (Soft Serve)			
Calories will vary with density (air in product) and serving size. Best to weigh product and calculate on 25 cals per 1 oz weight.			
Vanilla: Small (4 fl.oz cup), 6 oz wt	180	4	35
Medium (8 fl.oz cup), 11 oz wt	330	7	64
Tofutti Non-Dairy Dessert: *Per ½ Cup*			
Low-Fat Supreme: Average	110	2	25
Too Toos: Vanilla S'wich	215	10	28
Van. Choc. Swirl/Chip S'wich	230	11	30
Premium: Vanilla	190	11	20
Better Pecan; Alm. Bark	220	13	22
Choc. Cookie Crunch	210	11	26
Chocolate Supreme	180	11	17
Van. Fudge; Wildberry	190	9	24
Cutie Pies: Average, 67g bar	250	19	18
Teddy Fudge, 52g bar	70	1	19

Ice Cream Bars & Pops

Brands (Cont)	C	F	Cb
Turkey Hill: Per ½ Cup			
Black Cherry	140	7	18
Butter Pecan	170	11	16
Choco. Mint Chip, Cookies 'n Crm	160	10	17
Rocky Road	170	8	23
Other flavors, average	140	8	16
Lite: Choco Mint Chip	140	5	19
Cookies 'n Cream	130	5	21
Vanilla & Choc., Van. Bean	110	3	18
WholeSoy Glace: Per ½ Cup (70g)			
Mocha Fudge	130	4	21
Swiss Chocolate	180	9	21
Strawberry	150	6	20
Vanilla Bean	190	9	25

Bars & Pops	C	F	Cb
Per Bar/Serving			
Baby Ruth (Nestlé)	180	12	15
Barg's Root Beer & Ice Cream Float,			
4 oz cup	120	3	22
Baskin Robbins: Tiny Toons	140	17	20
Cappuccino Blast, average	120	4	20
Sundae Bar, Pralines 'n Cream	280	17	28
Ben & Jerry's: 'Wich Cookie S'wich	350	18	45
Peace Pops: Cherry Garcia (1)	280	18	29
Cookie Dough (1)	380	22	41
One Sweet Whirled (1)	270	16	28
Vanilla (1)	300	20	24
Vanilla w. Heath Toffee (1)	320	21	30
Novelties: 'Wich Ice Cream			
Cookie Sandwich	350	18	45
Big Bear: See Klondike			
Big Ed's Super Saucer, 10 fl.oz	420	28	32
Blue Bunny: Ice Pops, avg.	40	0	10
Bomb Pops, avg.	45	0	10
Chocolate Cup, 1.7 oz	100	5	12
Fudge Bar, 2.7 oz	110	1.5	21
Health Smart, 2.2 oz	70	0	17
Sweet Freedom S'wich, avg.	160	2	32
Vanilla Nutty Cone, 3 oz	245	10	34
Carb Freedom: Vanilla Bar	140	12	11
Almond Bar	160	13	11
Fudge Bar	90	4	11
Bon Bons (Nestlé): Milk Choc., (8)	330	22	29
Dark Chocolate, 8 pces	310	22	29
Borden: Sundae Cone	210	10	27
Twin Pops	60	0	14
Bounty, all varieties	70	5	7

Bars & Pops (Cont)	C	F	Cb
Per Bar/Serving			
Breyers: Hershey's Almond	270	19	21
All Natural Light: Fudge	90	2.5	14
Other varieties, average	170	9	21
CarbSmart: Almond	180	15	9
Creamsicle Pops	20	1	5
Fudge Bar	100	7	9
Ice Cream Bar	170	15	9
Ice Cream Sandwiches (1)	80	4	10
Fruit Juice Bar	110	0	28
Fruit Swirls, all flavor	50	0	13
Fruit Bar, No Sugar Added	25	0	5
HeartSmart: Fudge	100	1.5	21
Orange & Raspberry Cream	110	1	24
Ice Cream Cups: Chocolate	165	9	19
Vanilla	150	8	16
Premium Bars, average	110	5	14
Sugar Smart Bars, avg.	150	9	18
Tropical Fruit Bar	80	0	20
Butterfinger Bar, 2.5 oz	190	13	16
CarbSmart: See Klondike			
Carnation: Sandwich, all types	240	10	34
Sundae Cups, average	210	10	28
Chipwich Jr: Choc. Chip S'wich	240	10	35
Chiquita: Swirls, all flavors	80	3	12
Cool Creations: Mini Sandwich	110	5	16
Cookies & Cream Sandwich	240	11	34
Pops, all types, 2 oz	60	0	14
Mickey Mouse / 2.5 oz Bar	120	8	10
Creamsicle: Sugar-free pops	25	0	15
Orange, 2.8 fl.oz	110	3	20
Crunch: Caramel	210	14	19
Chocolate & Vanilla	230	16	18
Vanilla Flavored	220	15	18
Reduced-Fat	150	8	17
Crystal Light: Cool 'n Creamy	50	2	7
Dole: Fruit 'N Juice Bars, 2.5 fl.oz	70	0	18
Fruit Juice Variety Pack, all flavors (1)	45	0	11
No Sugar Added varieties	30	0	7
Dove: Caramel Toffee Crunch	270	16	29
Milk Chocolate w. Almonds	340	23	28
Original Dove; Milk Chocolate	320	21	32
Triple Chocolate	340	22	35
Dreyers/Edys			
Dibs: With Chocolaty Coating (26 Pieces)			
Chocolate; Mint; Vanilla	420	32	28
Van. w. Nestle Crunch/Drumstick	380	28	29
Non-Dairy, Fruit Bars, avg.	80	0	20

Bars & Pops (Cont)

Per Bar/Serving	C	F	Cb
Drumstick (*Nestlé*): Chocolate	360	23	33
Original Vanilla	340	21	33
Vanilla Caramel/Fudge	360	21	37
Eskimo Pie			
No Sugar Added: Strawb. Bar	110	6	15
Cookies & Cream Cone, 75g	140	4.5	28
Cookies & Cream Bar, 52g	120	7	17
Vanilla Dark Choc Bar, 49g	120	8	13
Vanilla Crisp Rice Bar, 47g	120	8	13
Bars: Milk/Dark Choc, 50g	160	11	15
Fudge Bar, 55g	60	1	11
Peppermint Pattie, 78g	240	16	21
Thin Mint Bar, 78g	240	17	20
King Size Bar, avg., 75g	220	14	21
Slender Pie Clamshell, avg.	120	1.5	28
Vanilla Sandwich, 65g	160	4	27
Flintstones: Push Up Sherbet	100	2	20
Push Up Pebbles, 2.75 oz	120	6	15
Cool Cream, 2.75 oz	90	2	18
Frosty Dreams (*Nestlé*)	100	2	19
Frosty Pops (*Nestlé*)	40	0	11
FrozFruit: Peach Boost Bar	70	0	17
Banana; Strawb. Crm Bar, avg.	155	8	21
Fruit Bars: Mango	105	0	26
Other varieties, avg.	80	0	20
Fruit A Freeze: Coconut	130	5	20
Lime	65	0	16
Banana; Strawberry	90	1.5	19
Dark Choc-Dipped Strawberry	90	5	14
Fudge Bar (*Nestlé*)	110	1	23
Fudgesicle: Fudge Bar (1)	45	0.5	9
Fat-Free (1)	60	0	13
Fudgetastics Sticks Sundae	220	15	37
Godiva Pecan Caramel Bar	380	23	39
Good Humor: Bubble Play	105	0	26
Candy Center Crunch	315	23	24
Chocolate Eclair	225	11	30
Great White	70	0	18
Hyper Stripe	80	0	19
Number 1	200	11	21
Premium Vanilla	260	17	23
Reese's Peanut Butter Cup	315	21	27
Strawb. Shortcake; Tstd Almd	230	10	35
Cones: Giant King	395	21	44
King	255	13	30
Premium Sundae	265	15	29
Strawberry Shortcake	235	10	34
Sundae Twist	165	2.5	33
Sandwiches: Premium Vanilla	190	7	29
Giant Mississippi Mud	300	14	37
Giant Neapolitan/Vanilla	260	10	37
Premium Cookie	295	13	41

Per Bar/Serving	C	F	Cb
Haagen-Dazs: Brownie Bar	360	24	30
Chocolate & Dark Chocolate	300	21	24
Coffee & Almond Crunch	310	22	23
Dulce de Leche	300	19	28
Raspberry Sorbet & Vanilla Yogurt	90	0	20
Strawberry Sorbet & Banana Yogurt	90	0	20
Vanilla & Almonds	320	12	22
Vanilla & Dark Chocolate	300	21	23
Vanilla & Milk Chocolate	290	21	22
Health Smart (*Blue Bunny*), avg.	80	0	18
Healthy Choice: Fudge Bar	75	1	13
Caramel Swirl Sandwich	145	3	27
Fudge Swirl Sandwich	145	3	27
Strawberry & Cream	80	1.5	13
Vanilla Sandwich	130	3	24
Hood: Chocolate Eclair, 1 bar	150	10	14
Fudge Bar: Chocolate	95	0.5	21
No Added Sugar	60	1.5	9
Dipped Delights	130	8	14
Java Smoothie	95	2.5	17
Hoodsie/Mint Sandwich	105	4	15
Light Sandwich	160	3.5	29
Hoodsie Cup Van./Choc.	100	5	12
Orange Cream Bar	90	1.5	18
Rockets, each	120	5	18
Vanilla Bar	160	12	11
Ice Cream Sandwich (*Nestlé*)	200	8	28
Klondike: Choco Taco, 4 fl.oz	300	16	35
Dark Chocolate Crunch, 2.5 fl.oz	140	6	14
Heath, 5 fl.oz	295	20	26
Ice Cream Cup, 6 fl.oz	280	17	26
Krunch, 5 fl.oz	280	19	25
Mini's Vanilla Ice Cream, 3 fl.oz	170	11	15
Movie Bites, 3 fl.oz	320	22	26
No Sugar Added Red. Fat, 4 fl.oz	180	9	21
Oreo, 3 fl.oz	160	10	17
Original, 5 fl.oz	280	19	24
Planters Caramel & Peanut	310	20	28
Reese's Peanut Butter, 2.9 fl.oz	220	15	20
Slim-a-Bear, 5 fl.oz	270	15	31
CarbSmart: Fudge Bar	105	7	9
Ice Cream Bar	180	15	9
Sandwich	115	4.5	14
Ice Cream Cone	210	16	14
Cones: Big Bear Sundae Cone	315	17	36
Big Bear Vanilla Sundae Cone	300	17	34
Oreo Cone	250	12	32
w. Oreo Cookies	230	9	34
Sandwich: Big Bear	190	7	28
Giant Cookie w. Hershey's	470	20	66
w. Oreo Cookies	230	9	34

Ice Cream Bars & Pops (Cont)

Bars & Pops (Cont)   C   F   Cb

Per Bar/Serving

	C	F	Cb
Kool-Aid Pops	40	0	10
Krispy Frostick	150	10	13
Juice Flavored Sticks	50	0	13
M&Ms Cookie Ice Cream S'wich	220	11	29
Mars Almond Bar	210	14	20
Matterhorn Cone, 10 fl.oz	510	38	19
Milky Way: Choc, Reduced-Fat	140	7	19
Caramel Swirl, 1 bar	180	10	21
Snack Bar, Vanilla/Chocolate	70	4	9
Minute Maid Fruit Juice Pops	60	0	15
Nestlé: Push Up Pop, average	90	1.5	19
Crunch: Vanilla, 3 oz bar	220	15	18
Multipack, 2.5 oz bar	150	8	17
Drumstick: S'Mores, 4.3 fl.oz	310	18	34
Strawberry Cheesecake	260	12	35
Vanilla, 4.6 fl.oz	340	21	33
Fruit 'N Juice Lemonade	70	0	17
Nesquik Pops	115	6	13
Toll House Sandwich: Choc Chip	520	23	72
Choc Choc Chip	550	29	67
Oreo: Big Stuf, 1 sandwich	240	10	33
Cookies n' Cream, 1 bar, 59g	180	12	18
Pathmark Vanilla w. choc. coat.	150	10	14
Polar Bar: Vanilla w. choc. coat.	240	18	15
Choc. Chip Cookie Dough	450	28	48
Pops (water/juice), average	60	0	14
Popsicles: Big Stick Ice Pops	70	0	17
Creamsicle Pop	70	2	13
Crispy Cones, 2.5 fl.oz	150	7	20
Fudgesicle Fudge Pop	90	1.5	16
Firecracker Super Hero; Fruit Shot	40	0	10
Minis Ice Cream Pop	190	13	18
Rainbow Floats, 1.75 fl.oz	60	1.5	11
Sponge Bob Squarepants Pop Up	90	1.5	17
Scribblers Ice Cream: 2 pces	130	7	15
Juice Pops, 2 pces	60	0	16
Ice Pops: 1 pce	45	0	11
Sugar-Free, 1 pce, 1.9 oz	15	0	3
Reese's: Peanut Butter Ice Cream	160	11	22
Rice Dream: Pies, all flavors	320	18	40
Bars: Strawberry	250	13	31
Chocolate, Vanilla	270	15	32
Choc/Vanilla Nutty	270	18	23

Per Bar/Serving

	C	F	Cb
Safeway Select Coffee Almd Bar	270	17	26
Skinny Cow			
Fat-Free Chocolate Fudge	100	0	22
Low-Fat Cookies n' Cream	120	1.5	23
Sandwiches:			
Caramel; Choc. Peanut Butter	140	2.5	27
Other flavors, average	130	2	23
Sundae Cups: Vanilla Strawberry	120	0	28
Chocolate; Vanilla Choc.	130	0.5	29
Slim-Fast: Fudge Bar	110	1.5	22
Ice Cream Sandwich: Vanilla	130	1	27
Chocolate	130	1.5	27
Snackwell: Ice Cream Sandwich	90	1.5	18
Yogurt Bars, 1 bar, 80g	120	2	22
Snickers: Ice Cream Bar	180	11	18
Pralines n' Creme	220	13	22
Ice Cream Bar (The Big One)	250	15	25
Snack, 4 bars	390	25	38
Soy Delicious: Li'l Buddies S'wich	165	4.5	28
Soy Dream (Non-Dairy):			
Dreamwich Vanilla	130	6	15
Heavenly Pies: Mocha; Vanilla	290	14	40
Lil' Dreamers: Choc; Vanilla	60	3	7
Rocket Bars: Choc; Vanilla	220	12	29
Starbuck's Frappuccino Bars, avg.	130	2	25
Starburst Juice Bars	20	0	5
Super Sundae Bar, 86g	310	20	26
3 Musketeers: 2 fl.oz bars	170	10	21
Snack Bars, regular	60	4	16
Tandem (Nestlé) Sandwich	380	21	39
Twin Pop (Nestlé)	60	0	14
Twix Bar	180	10	19
Vitari Soft Serve, 4 fl.oz, average	80	0	20
Weight Watchers			
Chocolate Mousse (1)	60	0.5	14
Fudge Sundae Cups, average	160	1	38
Fudge Sundae Cones, average	140	4	30
English Toffee Crunch	110	6	13
Giant Cookies 'n Cream	140	5	25
Giant Fudge Bar	110	1	25
Sandwich: Chocolate Round	140	2	33
Vanilla	120	2	28
Vanilla Round	140	2	32
Welch's: Fruit Juice Bars, 92g	80	0	19
Tropical Coolers, 92 bar	45	0	11
No Sugar Added, 1 bar	25	0	6
Fruit Smoothie, 1 ctn	240	0	59

Cream & Creamers

Quick Guide

Cream
Average All Brands

	C	F	Cb
Half & Half Cream: 1 Tbsp, 0.5 oz	20	2	0.5
2 Tbsp, 1 oz	40	4	1
Light, coffee/table (20% fat): 1 T.	30	3	0.5
2 Tbsp, 1 oz	60	6	1
Medium (25% fat), 2 Tbsp, 1 oz	40	4	0.5
Sour Cream:			
Regular, 1 Tbsp, 0.5 oz	30	3	0.5
1 cup, 8 oz	490	48	8
Low-fat/Light, 1 Tbsp, 0.5 oz	20	2	1.5
2 Tbsp, 1 oz	40	2.5	2
Half & Half, 1 Tbsp, 0.5 oz	20	2.5	0.5
Fat-Free, 2 Tbsp, 1 oz	20	0	3
Fat Free: *(HeluvaGood),* 2 Tbsp	20	0	6
(Kroger), 2 Tbsp, 1 oz	25	0	5
(Naturally Yours; Oak Farm), 2 T.	20	0	3
(Knudsen), 2 Tbsp, 1 oz	35	0	6
Sour Cream Substitute:			
(Albertson's/IMO), 2 T., 1 oz	60	5	2
(Tofutti) Sour Supreme, 1 oz	50	5	1
Whipping Cream:			
Heavy (37% fat):			
1 Tbsp fluid/2 Tbsp whipped	50	5	1
¼ cup whipped	100	11	2
½ cup fluid/1 cup whipped	400	44	8
Light (30% fat):			
1 Tbsp fluid/2 Tbsp whipped	45	4.5	0.5
½ cup fluid/1 cup whipped	350	37	4

Coconut Cream/Milk

	C	F	Cb
Coconut Cream (Canned):			
Plain/unsweetened, 2 Tbsp, 1 oz	70	6	4
½ cup, 4 oz	280	24	16
Sweetened: Coco Lopez, 1 oz	120	5	20
½ cup, 4 oz	480	20	80
Coconut Milk (Canned):			
Natural Value: Reg., ¼ c., 2 fl.oz	90	9	1
Lite, ¼ cup, 2 fl oz	55	5	1
Thai Kitchen: Reg., ¼ c., 2 fl.oz	125	7	3
Lite, ¼ cup, 2 fl oz	50	3	2
Premium, 2 fl.oz	125	12	3
Coconut Water (Center), 1 cup	45	0.5	9

Whipped Toppings
Average All Brands

	C	F	Cb
Cream (Pressurized): 2 Tbsp	20	2	1
¼ cup	45	4	2
½ cup	90	8	4
Cream Toppings: *(Jewel)* Lite, 2 T.	20	1	2
Cool Whip: Extra Creamy, 2 T.	25	1.5	2
Lite, 2 Tbsp, 9g	20	1	2
Free, 2 Tbsp, 9g	15	0	3
Non-Dairy, 2 Tbsp	22	2	2
Kraft: Whipped, 2 Tbsp	20	2	1
Real Cream, 2 Tbsp	20	2	1
Reddi-Wip: Original, 2 T., 8g	15	1	0.5
Chocolate, 2 Tbsp, 8g	15	1	1
Extra Creamy, 2 Tbsp, 8g	15	1.5	0.5
Fat-Free, 2 Tbsp, 8g	5	0	1

Non-Dairy Coffee Creamers

Powder:

	C	F	Cb
Coffee-Mate/Cremora/N-Rich			
Regular, 1 tsp	20	2	1
1 heaping tsp	25	2	2
Fat-Free, 1 tsp	10	0	2
Lite, 1 tsp	10	0.5	2
Flavors: 1⅓ Tbsp	60	3	9
Fat-Free: Average, 1⅓ Tbsp	50	0	11
Liquid/Refrigerated: *Per Tablespoon*			
Coffee-Mate Non-Dairy Creamer			
Plain: Regular/Plain, 1 Tbsp	20	1	2
Fat-Free, 1 Tbsp	10	0	2
Lite, 1 Tbsp	10	0.5	2
Flavors: All flavors, 1 Tbsp	40	2	5
Fat-Free, all flavors, 1 Tbsp	25	0	5
Crème de la Soy *(Westsoy):*			
Original, 1 Tbsp	20	1.5	2
Amaretto; French Vanilla, 1 T.	25	1	2
Hood (Non-Dairy), 1 Tbsp	25	1.5	2
International Delight: 1 Tbsp	35	1.5	6
Fat-Free flavors, 1 Tbsp	30	0	7
Mocha Mix: Original, 1 Tbsp	20	1.5	2
Fat-Free, 1 Tbsp	10	0	1
Lite, 1 Tbsp	10	0.5	1
Morningstar, 1 Tbsp	40	1.5	7
Rich's Coffee Rich: Regular, 1 T.	25	1	2
Light	15	0.5	0.5
Rich's Farm Rich: Regular, 1 Tbsp	20	1	2
Light/Fat-Free	10	0	0.5
Silk *(White Wave)* Creamer, 1 Tbsp	15	1	1
French Vanilla, 1 Tbsp	20	1	3

Fats, Spreads & Oils

Quick Guide **C** **F** **Cb**

Butter & Margarine
Average All Brands

	C	F	Cb
Regular: 1 tsp (5g)	35	4	0
1 Pat (5g)	35	4	0
1 Tbsp, approx. ½ oz	100	11	0
2 Tbsp, 1 oz	205	23	0
1 Stick, ½ cup, 4 oz	810	92	0
1 Pound, 2 cups, 16 oz	3240	368	0
Light (Regular) 40% Fat:			
1 tsp, 5g	17	2	0
1 Tbsp, ½ oz	50	6	0
2 Tbsp, 1 oz	100	11	0
Whipped Butter (Regular):			
1 tsp (4 g)	27	3	0
1 Tbsp (10g)	70	7.5	0
1 Stick, ½ cup, 2 ⅔ oz	570	60	0
Whipped Light Butter 40% Fat:			
1 tsp, 5g	10	1	0
1 Tbsp, 9g	35	3.5	0
2 Tbsp, 18g	70	7	0
Unsalted: Same as Regular			

Clarified Butter

	C	F	Cb
100% Fat: 1 Tbsp, ½ oz	130	15	0
2 Tbsp, 1 oz	260	30	0

Flavored Butter/Spread

Average All Brands

	C	F	Cb
Honey Butter (60% Fat):			
1 Tbsp, ½ oz	90	7	4
Downey's, 1 Tbsp, ½ oz	60	1	11
Garlic Butter (80% Fat):			
1 Tbsp, ½ oz	100	11	0
Macadamia Butter *(Atkins)*, 1 T.	125	12	2.5
Sweet Cream Butter:			
Regular, 1 Tbsp	100	11	0
Stick (70% Fat), 1 Tbsp	90	10	0
Tub (60% Fat), 1 Tbsp	80	9	0

Other Spreads & Fats

	C	F	Cb
Copha, Dripping, Lard, Suet, Shortening:			
1 Tbsp, ½ oz	120	13	0
Chicken, Duck, Goose Fat:			
1 Tbsp, ½ oz	115	13	0

Light & Reduced Fat Spreads

Per 1 Tbsp, ½ oz (Unless Stated) **C** **F** **Cb**

	C	F	Cb
Benecol: Spread, 1 Tbsp, 14g	80	9	0
Light, Spread, 1 Tbsp, 14g	45	5	0
Blue Bonnet, Homestyle (48% Veg Oil)	60	7	0
Breakstone's, Whipped Butter	60	7	0
Brummel & Brown, Spread	45	5	0
Chiffon, Whipped, 1 Tbsp	70	7	0
Country Crock *(Shedd's):* Regular	60	7	0
Light; Calcium & Vitamins	50	5	0
Country's Delight (70% Veg.)	90	10	0
Country Morning, Light	50	6	0
Downey's, Honey Butter	60	1	0
Dutch Farms, 52% Veg. Spread	70	7	0
Fleischmann's: Soft Spread	80	9	0
Original Stick	100	11	0
Light Spread	40	4.5	0
'I Can't Believe It's Not Butter': Reg.	90	10	0
Light; Sweet Cream	50	6	0
Imperial, Diet, 1 Tbsp	50	6	0
Jewel: Soft Spread	60	7	0
Unbelievably Butter	90	9	0
Kraft, 'Touch of Butter' (bowl)	50	6	0
Land O'Lakes: Fresh Buttery Taste	80	8	0
Honey Butter	90	7	4
Light Butter Whipped	35	3.5	0
Light Butter	50	6	0
Mazola, Diet	50	6	0
Mother's, Mrs Filbert's, 1 Tbsp	70	8	0
Miracle: Soft	60	7	0
Stick	70	7	0
Nucoa, HeartBeat Margarine	25	3	0
Olivio, Vegetable Spread, 1 Tbsp	80	8	0
Parkay: Squeeze, 1 Tbsp	80	9	0
Stick, ⅓ Less Fat	70	7	0
Tub, 1 Tbsp	60	7	0
Tub, Light/Soft Diet	50	6	0
Whipped	70	7	0
Promise: Regular	90	10	0
Extra Light	50	6	0
Buttery Light	45	5	0
Ultra, w. Canola Oil	35	4	0
Smart Balance: Regular, 1 Tbsp	80	9	0
Light, 1 Tbsp	45	5	0
Smart Beat, Fat-Free	10	0	3
Take Control: Regular Spread	80	8	0
Light Spread	45	5	0
Weight Watcher's, Light	45	4	2

## Butter Substitutes	C	F	Cb
Bake It Perfect (Fat-Free Spread), 1 T.	5	0	0
Best O'Butter, ½ tsp	4	0	0
Butter Buds, 1 serving, ½ tsp	4	0	0
Butterlike Saute Butter, 1 Tbsp	35	2	0
Butter Sprinkles (Watkins), 1 tsp	5	0	0
Earth Balance, Non GMO,1 tsp	35	3.5	0
Molly McButter, ½ tsp	5	0	0
Mrs Bateman's Baking Butter, 1 T.	35	1	0
Natural Touch Soy, 1 Tbsp	85	5.5	5

Spreads Comparison

	C	F	Cb
Mayonnaise: Regular, 1 Tbsp	100	11	0
Light, average, 1 Tbsp	50	5	1
Fat-Free, 1 T.	10	0	3
Miracle Whip (Kraft):			
Regular, 1 Tbsp	70	7	2
Light, 1 Tbsp	40	3	3
Free, 1 Tbsp	15	0	3
SmartBeat Dressing: 1 Tbsp	10	0	3

Extra Listings for Mayonnaise & Dressings
~ See Page 89 ~

	C	F	Cb
Avocado, mashed, 1 Tbsp	25	2.5	2
Peanut Butter, 1 Tbsp	100	8	3.5
Nutella, 1 Tbsp	100	5.5	12

New Diet Aid - The Refrigerator Air Bag!

POOF!

## Animal Fats/Lards	C	F	Cb
Average All Types			
Beef Tallow/Drippings, Lard (Pork),			
Chicken, Duck, Goose, Turkey.			
1 Tbsp (13g)	115	13	0
2¼ Tbsp, 1 oz	255	28	0
1 cup, 7¼ oz	1850	205	0
1 pound, 8 oz	2040	227	0
Ghee/Butter Oil: 1 Tbsp, 13g	110	13	0
2¼ Tbsp, 1 oz	250	28	0

Vegetable Shortening

	C	F	Cb
Average All Types (example, Crisco)			
1 Tbsp, 0.44 oz	113	13	0
2¼ Tbsp, 1 oz	250	28	0
1 cup, 7¼ oz	1810	205	0

Vegetable Oils

Includes almond, avocado, canola, corn, coconut, flaxseed, grapeseed, linseed, mustard, olive, palm, peanut, rice-bran, safflower, sesame, sunflower, soybean, wheatgerm. Note: Oil is 100% fat.

	C	F	Cb
1 tsp, 5g	45	5	0
1 Tbsp, ½ oz	120	14	0
2 Tbsp, 1 oz	250	28	0
1 cup, 7¾ oz	1930	205	0

Fish Oils

	C	F	Cb
Average All Types (Includes cod liver, herring, salmon, sardine):			
1 Tbsp, ½ oz	125	14	0

Cooking Sprays/Squeezes

	C	F	Cb
Cooking Sprays (Pam, Mazola, I Can't Believe It's Not Butter, Weight Watchers, Wesson):			
Per serving	2	0	0
1-3 second spray	6	1	0
I Can't Believe It's Not Butter	0	0	0
Parkay Buttery Spray	0	0	0
Squeeze (Parkay), 1 Tbsp, 0.5 oz	70	8	0

Olestra (Olean)

	C	F	Cb
Olestra (Olean)	0	0	0

Olean is Proctor & Gamble's brand name for olestra – a no-calorie cooking oil that gives snacks (like potato chips, tortilla chips and crackers) taste and texture without adding fat or calories.

Cheese

Quick Guide C F Cb

Firm/Hard Cheeses
(American, Cheddar, Colby, Coon, Swiss)

Regular Cheese:

	C	F	Cb
1 oz slice/piece	110	9	0.5
8 oz package	880	72	4
16 oz (1lb) package	1760	144	8
Cubes: 1" cube, ¾ oz	55	5	0.5
1¼" cube, 1 oz slice	110	9	0.5
Diced: 1 cup, 4½ oz	500	40	2
Grated: 1 Tbsp, ¼ oz	27	2	0
Shredded:			
¼ cup, 1 oz	110	9	0.5
1 cup, 4 oz	440	36	4
Sliced: 1 thin (3½" sq.), ¾ oz	85	7	0.5
Rectangular (7"x 4"x ⅛"), 1½ oz	165	14	1
Round (3¼" diam. x ⅛"), ¾ oz	85	7	0.5
Semi-circular, 1¼ oz			
(5½" long, 3½" radius, ⅛" thick) 140	140	11	0.5
Light: Average All Brands, 1 oz	80	5	0.5
Fat-Free: Average All Brands, 1 oz	50	0	2
Low-Fat: Average All Brands, 1 oz	50	1.5	1

Cheese C F Cb

Per 1 oz Unless Indicated

American:

	C	F	Cb
Regular, 1 slice, 1 oz	110	9	1
Kraft, 0.7 oz slice	80	7	0
Shredded, 1 Tbsp, ¼ oz	20	1.5	0
Light: *Borden*, 1 oz	70	4	0.5
Land O'Lakes, 1 oz	70	5	0.5
Smart Beat, 0.6 oz slice	35	2	0
Kraft, (2% Milk), 0.7 oz slice	50	2.5	2
Fat-Free: *Kraft*, 0.75 oz slice	30	0	2
Alpine Lace, 1 oz	45	0	2
HealthyChoice, Singles, 0.7 pce	75	6	0
Weight Watchers, ¾ oz	30	0	3
Babybel (Laughing Cow), 1 oz	90	7	0
Swiss Light Creamy, 21g pce	70	2	10
Bonbel (Laughing Cow), 1 pce	75	6	0
Swiss Light Creamy, 21g pce	70	2	10
Brick, 1 oz	100	8	0
Brie, 1 oz	95	8	1
Camembert, 1 oz	90	7	1
Caraway, 1 oz	105	8	1

Cheddar: (Also see 'Quick Guide') C F Cb

	C	F	Cb
Regular, 1 oz	110	9	0.5
Reduced-Fat/Light, 1 oz	80	5	0.5
Cabot Vermont, 50% Light	70	4.5	1
Weight Watchers, 1 oz	80	5	1
Fat-Free: *Alpine Lace*, 1 oz	45	0	2
Weight Watchers, 1 sl., ¾ oz	30	0	1
Cheese Balls (Kaukauna), 1 oz	100	7	0.5
Cheese Nut, average, 1 oz	100	7	2
Cheese Logs, average, 1 oz	100	7	0.5
Cheshire, 1 oz	110	9	1.5
Colby: Regular, 1 oz	110	9	0.5
Reduced-Fat *(Alpine Lace)*, 1 oz	80	5	1
Colby-Jack, 1 oz	110	9	0.5
Cottage Cheese: *Average All Brands*			
Creamed (4% milk fat): 2 Tbsp, 1 oz	30	1	1
½ cup, 4 oz	120	5	4
w. fruit, ½ cup, 4 oz	130	4	15
Reduced-Fat (2%), 2 T., 1 oz	25	0.5	1
½ cup, 4 oz	100	2	4
Low-Fat (1%), 2 Tbsp, 1 oz	20	.5	1
½ cup, 4 oz	80	1	3
Fat-Free/Non-Fat, 2 Tbsp, 1 oz	20	0	1
½ cup, 4 oz	80	0	3
Borden Dry Curd (0.5%), ½ c., 4 oz	80	0	0
Friendship: Low-Fat P'apple, 4 oz	120	1	17
Non-Fat Plus Peach, ½ c., 4 oz	110	0	15
Pot Style, ½ cup, 4 oz	90	3	3
w. Pineapple, 4 oz	140	4	16
Hood Fruit Stirs, avg, 110g ctn	200	2.5	24
Knudsen: 1.5% Fruit, 4 oz	110	2	12
Free: Non-Fat, ½ cup, 4.3 oz	80	0	7
Low-Fat, 4 oz	85	2	4
Cottage Doubles, avg, 5.5 oz ctn	150	2.5	18
4% Milk-Fat, ½ cup, 4.3 oz	120	5	5
Light N' Lively: Garden Salad, 4 oz	90	2	5
Peach and Pineapple,			
½ cup, 4 oz	120	1	14
Cream Cheese: *See Page 45*			
Dorman's Castello, 1 oz	135	12	1
Edam, Regular, 1 oz	100	8	0
Farmer (Friendship), 2 Tbsp, 1 oz	50	3	0
Feta: Regular, Frigo, 1 oz	100	8	1
Crumbled, ½ cup, 2½ oz	190	15	2.5
Reduced-Fat *(Alpine Lace)*	60	4	1
Fontina (Sargento/Classica), 1 oz	110	9	0.5
Gjetost (Goat's Milk, fresh), 1 oz	85	7	0.5
Sargento, 1 oz	130	8	12
Goat's Milk: Soft: *Chevre*, 1 oz	70	6	0.5
Chavril, 3 Tbsp, 1 oz	60	4.5	0.5

	C	F	Cb
Goat's Milk Cheese (Cont)			
Semi-Soft: 1 oz	100	8.5	1
Hard: *Sargento*, 1 oz	130	10	0.5
Gorgonzola, 1 oz	110	9	0.5
Galbani Dolcelatte, 1 oz	95	8	1
Gouda, 1 oz	100	8	0.5
Gruyere, 1 oz	115	9	0
Havarti, 1 oz	120	11	0
Italian *(Classica Italiano)*, 1 oz	110	10	1
Jarlsberg, 1 oz	100	7	1
Jarlsberg Lite shredded, 1 oz	70	4	1
Kefir, 2 Tbsp, 1 oz	60	4	1
Labneh *(Lebanese cream chse)*, 1.8 oz	70	4	4
Limburger, 1 oz	90	8	0
Mascarpone, 1 oz	130	13	1
Mexican *(Sargento Recipe Blend)*,			
Shredded, ¼ cup, 1 oz	110	9	0.5
Monterey, 1 oz	105	8.5	0
Monterey Jack: Regular, 1 oz	110	9	0
Light Naturals *(Kraft)*, 1 oz	80	5	0
Alpine Lace, Monti-Jack Lo, 1 oz	80	5	0
Weight Watchers, 1 oz	90	6	1
Mozzarella:			
Regular: *Kraft/Dorman's,* 1 oz	90	7	0.5
Land O'Lakes/Polly-O, 1 oz	80	6	0.5
Shredded, ¼ cup, 1 oz	80	6	0.5
Light: *Polly-O Lite,* 1 oz	60	2.5	0.5
Kraft Light Naturals, 1 oz	80	5	0.5
Sorrento Lite, 1 oz	60	3	0.5
Part Skim *(Alpine Lace)*, 1 oz	70	5	0.5
Polly-O, 1 oz	90	6	0.5
Fat-Free: *Healthy Choice,* ¼ c.,1oz	45	0	1
Polly-O, 1 oz	35	0	1
Kraft, shredded, ¼ cup, 1 oz	50	0	2
Muenster: Regular, 1 oz	110	9	0
Reduced-Fat *(Dorman's)*, 1 oz	80	5	0
Myzithra, 1 oz	115	9	1
Neufchatel: *Dominick's,* 1 oz	70	6	2
Philadelphia, 1 oz	70	6	0.5
Flavored: Fruit/Herbs	80	7	1
Chocolate *(Hickory Farms)*, 1 oz	110	8	1
Parmesan: Fresh/Block, 1 oz	110	7	1
Shredded/Grated, 1 Tbsp	22	1.5	0
Grated (Packaged): 1 Tbsp	26	2	0
1 oz quantity	130	9	1
½ cup, 1¾ oz	230	16	2
w. Romano *(Frigo)*, grated, 1 oz	130	9	1
Kraft Reduced-Fat, 1 Tbsp	20	1	2

Note: Packaged grated and shredded Parmesan have more calories (per unit weight) than block Parmesan Parmesan due to lower moisture content.

	C	F	Cb
Pizza Cheese, shredded:			
Regular *(Frigo)* ¼ cup, 1 oz	90	7	1
Low-Fat *(Frigo)*, 1 oz	65	3	1
Port Du Salut, 1 oz	100	8	0.5
Port Wine *(Hickory Farms)*, 1 oz	100	7	2.5
Pot *(Sargento)*, 1 oz	25	0	1
Provolone: Regular, 1 oz	100	8	1
Reduced-Fat, Alpine Lace, 1 oz	70	5	1
Pub *(Hickory Farms)*, 1 oz	95	7	1
Quark: 40% fat, 1 oz	47	3	1
20% fat, 1 oz	32	1.5	1
Skim/Non-Fat, 1 oz	22	0	1.5
Queso: Anego/Asadero/Blanco	105	9	1
Queso Chichuahua/De Papa	110	9	2
Ricotta Cheese:			
Whole Milk, 2 Tbsp, 1 oz	50	3.5	1
½ cup, 4½ oz	225	16	4.5
Part Skim, 2 Tbsp, 1 oz	40	2.5	1
½ cup, 4½ oz	180	12	4.5
Light/Low-Fat, 2 Tbsp, 1 oz	25	1	1
½ cup, 4½ oz	100	2.5	5
Fat-Free, ½ cup, 4½ oz	100	0	4
Knudsen 'On The Go': Low-Fat, 4 oz	90	2	4
Free (Non-Fat), 4 oz container	80	0	6
Baked Ricotta, 2 oz portion	130	9	3
Romano: Block/Loaf, 1 oz	110	8	1
Grated (Pkg), 1 oz	120	9	1
1 Tbsp	26	2	0.5
Roquefort, 1 oz	105	9	1
Slim Jack *(Dorman's)*, 1 oz	90	7	1
Sheep's Milk *(Hollow Rd Farm)*	45	3	1
Smoked: *Sargents,* Smokestick	100	7	1
Hickory Farm, Smoky Lyte, 1 oz	80	6	1
Stilton, 1 oz	118	10	1
String *(Frigo/Kraft/Sargento)*, 1 oz	80	5	1
Light String-Ums, 1 stick	60	2.5	0.5
String Lite *(Frigo)*, 1 oz	60	2	1
Mootown Light *(Sargento)*, 1 stick	50	2.5	0.5
Swiss: Regular, 1 oz	110	9	1
Reduced-Fat: Alpine Lace, 1 oz	90	6	1
Dorman's/Kraft Light Naturals	90	5	1
Weight Watchers, ¾ oz slice	30	0	2
Taco Cheese, shredded, ¼ cup	110	9	1
Tilsit *(Sargents)*, 1 oz	100	7	0.5
Tybo *(Dorman's/Sargents)*, 1 oz	100	7	0.5
Vermont *(Churny)*, 1 oz	100	9	1
Wensleydale, 1 oz	108	9	0
Whey Cheese, 1 oz	125	8	9

Cheese (Cont)

Cheese Products

	C	F	Cb
Cheese Food:			
Average all flavors: ¾ oz slice	70	5	1.5
1 oz slice	90	6	2
Alouette: Fr. Onion/Garl.,2 T., 0.8oz	70	7	1
Light Garlic, 2 Tbsp, 0.8 oz	50	4	1
Cracker Barrel, Cheddar, 1.1 oz	100	8	4
Delico: Alouette Cajun, 2 T., 0.8 oz	70	7	1
Garden Vegetable, 2 T., 0.8 oz	60	6	1
Handi-Snacks			
Cheez'n Breadsticks, 1 pkg	130	7	11
Cheez'n Pretzels, 1 oz pkg	110	6	11
Cheez'n Crackers, 1.1 oz pkg	130	8	10
Mozzarella Stringchse Stick, each	80	6	0.5
Healthy Choice, Amer. Singles, 1 sl.	30	0	2
Heluva Good Cheese:			
American, 1 slice	45	5	2
Cheddar w. H/radish, 2 Tbsp, 1oz	90	7	3
Jalapeno, avg., all brands, 1 oz	90	7	2
Kraft: American grated, 1T., 0.2 oz	25	2	1
Singles, 1 slice, ¾ oz	70	6	1
Free Singles, 1 slice, 0.7 oz	40	3	3
Pimento Spread, 2 Tbsp, 1.1 oz	80	6	3
Velveeta (Process Cheese Spread)			
Regular, ⅜" slice, 1 oz	100	6	3
Light, ⅜" slice, 1 oz	60	3	3
Rip-Ums, 1 strip, 0.75 oz	80	7	0.5
String-Ums (Lite), 1 stick	60	2.5	0.5
Lifeway Farmers Cheese, 2 oz	75	5	2.5
Precious String Chse Stuffsters, 1 oz	70	4.5	1
Roka Blue, 2 Tbsp, 1.1 oz	80	7	2
Rondele: Soft Spread., 2 T., 1 oz	100	9	1
Light, 2 Tbsp, 0.9 oz	60	4	2
SmartBalance Crmy Cheddar, 1 sl.	40	2	2
Spreadery: Vermont, 2 Tbsp, 1 oz	80	5	3
Neufchatel, all flavors, 2 T, 1 oz	80	7	1
Velveeta: Cheese, 1 slice, 1 oz	100	6	3
Light, 1 oz	60	3	3
Shredded, ¼ cup, 1.3 oz	130	9	3
WisPride: Hickory Smoked Cup;			
Port Wine Ball/Cup, 2 T., 1.1 oz	100	7	4
Light, 2 Tbsp., 1.1 oz	80	3	5

Cheese Whiz (Sauce)

	C	F	Cb
Regular, 2 Tbsp, 33g	90	7	2
Light, 2 Tbsp, 33g	80	3	6
Squeezable, 2 Tbsp, 33g	80	6	2

Cheese Substitutes

	C	F	Cb
Per 1 oz Unless Indicated			
Almond Rella (Nu Soya):			
Cheddar; Garlic & Herb, 1 oz	70	3.5	3
Borden, Taco-Mate, 1 oz	100	7	2
Delicia American Colby	80	6	1
Dorman's Lo Chol	100	7	1
Formagg: Cheddar, 1 slice, 0.7 oz	60	4	0.5
American Wh./Yellow, 1 sl. 0.7oz	60	4	0.5
Mozzarella (Old World), 1 oz	60	3	1
Parmesan Grated, 1 Tbsp, ¼ oz	20	1.5	1.5
Provolone (Vintage), 1 oz	60	3	1
Swiss White, 1 slice, 0.7 oz	60	4	0.5
Frigo Cheddar; Mozzarella, 1 oz	90	7	1
Georgio's: Imitation Cheddar;			
Mozzarella, shredded, ¼ c, 1 oz	90	7	1
Golden Image: American, 0.7 oz			
Mild Cheddar, 1 slice, 0.7 oz	70	5	1
Harvest Moon: *Per ¼ Cup, 1.3 oz*			
Shredded: American; Cheddar	120	9	3
Mozzarella	110	9	3
Nu Tofu: Mozzarella, 1 oz	70	4	2
Fat-Free: Mozz./Ched./Jack, 1 oz	40	0	2
Sargento Classic Supreme:			
Cheddar, shredded, 1 oz	90	6	2
Mozzarella, shrd, ¼ cup	80	6	0.5
Smart Beat, Fat-Free, 0.6 oz sl.	35	0	3
Soya Kaas: Regular, 1 oz	70	5	1
Fat-Free, all varieties, 1 oz	40	2	1
Soyco: Almond/Oat/Rice Slices,			
1 slice, 0.7 oz	40	2	1
Veggy Singles, 1 slice, 0.7 oz	40	2	1
Grated Parmesan, 2 tsp, 5g	15	0.5	0
Tofum Rella, avg. all varieties, 1 oz	80	5	3
Tofutti Better Than Cream Cheese	80	8	1
Weight Watchers: Fat-Free Slices,			
All varieties, ¾ oz slice	30	0	3
Grated Italian Topping, 1 Tbsp	20	0	2
White Wave: Soy A Melt,			
Cheddar/Mozz./Mont. Jack, 1 oz	80	5	1
Fat-Free, 1 oz	40	0	3
Singles: Amer./Mozzarella, ¾ oz	60	4	1
Yves, Good Slice, ¾ oz slice, avg.	35	2	1

PHILADELPHIA

Cream Cheese · C · F · Cb

	C	F	Cb
Regular/Soft: 2 Tbsp, 1 oz	100	10	1
3 oz pkg	300	30	2
w. Chives/Herbs/Pimento, 1 oz	90	9	0.5
w. Fruit/Strawb./P'apple, 1 oz	90	8	5
Lox, 1 oz	90	9	0.5
Philadelphia (Kraft): Per 2 Tbsp			
Original, 1 oz	100	10	1
1/3 Less Fat, 1 oz	70	6	1
Light: Plain, 1 oz	60	4.5	2
Strawberry, 0.7 oz	70	7	1
Fat-Free, 1 oz	25	0	2
Flavored: Blueberry/Raspberry, 1 oz	95	8	5
Strawberry, 1 oz	90	8	4
Garden Vegetable, 1 oz	95	9	2
Snacks: Bars, avg, all types (1)	180	11	20
Snack Bites (1) 1 oz	130	7	15
Bagel & Crm Chse To Go, 3.2 oz	240	9	36
Swirls, 2 Tbsp, 1 oz	90	8	4
Whipped: Regular, 2 Tbsp, 0.7 oz	60	6	1
Mixed Berry, 2 Tbsp, 0.7 oz	70	6	3
Alpine Lace, Fat-Free, 2 T., 1 oz	30	0	1
Weight Watchers, 1 oz	40	2.5	1

Dips/Spreads ~ Per 2 Tbsp (1 oz) · C · F · Cb

	C	F	Cb
Avocado/Guacamole	50	4	4
Baba Ghannoush (Eggplant/Sesame)	70	6	2
French Onion Dip, avg. all brands	60	6	3
Guacamole, 2 Tbsp, 1 oz	50	4	4
Hummus: 2 Tbsp, 1 oz	50	1	5
1/2 cup, 4.5 oz	220	4.5	23
Tzatziki (Cucumber/Yogurt Dip)	40	3	1
Best Foods			
Dippin' Sauce: Totally BBQ, 2 T.	110	12	1
Honey Mustard Madness, 2 Tbsp	60	2	10
Rockin' Ranch, 2 Tbsp	90	6	8
Birdseye No-Fat Veggie Dip, 1.1 oz	25	0	5
Breakstone's Sour Cream, all flav.	50	4	4
Chalco: Quéso Quesadilla; Cotija	120	10	0
Fresco, 1 oz	70	8	0
Cheese Fondue, 1/2 cup, 4 oz	210	14	4
Chi-Chi's: Con Quéso, 2 Tbsp	90	7	4
Hot/Medium/Mild/Acante, 2 T.	10	0	2
Cool Cuts: Carrot & Ranch	60	4	5
Celery & Peanut Butter	170	14	9
Frito Lay: Chili Cheese; Jalapeno	50	3	3
French Onion	60	5	3
Bean/Jalapeno Bean	40	1	6
Guiltless Gourmet: Nacho Dip	25	0	5
Other varieties	30	0	5
Heluva Good Cheese: Chse 'N Salsa	80	3	3
Clam/French Onion	50	5	2
Bacon/Homestyle/Ranch	60	5	2
Light Fr. Onion/Jalapeno Cheddar	40	2	3
Hy-Top Pimiento, 1 oz	90	8	3

Dips/Spreads (Cont) · C · F · Cb

Per 2 Tbsp (1 oz)

	C	F	Cb
Kaukauna Nacho Cheese	90	7	4
Knudsen Nacho Cheese	60	4	3
Sour Cream Bacon & Onion	60	5	2
Sour Cream French Onion	50	4	2
Kroger The Big Dipper; all flavors	60	5	2
Kraft: Average all flavors, 2 Tbsp	60	5	4
Philly flavors:			
Bacon & Cheddar	60	5	3
Average other flavors	55	4.5	3
Fat-Free: Strawberry	25	0	2
Garden Veges	30	0	2
Lay's Low-Fat Sr. Cream, Onion	40	1	5
Louise's: (Fat-Free) Honey Mustard	40	0	0
Sour Cream & Onion/White Chse	25	0	0
Luisa's Fiesta Dip, 2 Tbsp	35	2	3
Marie's: Reg, all types	90	9	2
Lite, 2 Tbsp	60	4	4
Nalley's all flavors, average	120	12	3
Naturally Fresh, all flavors, 1 oz	80	0	19
Old Dutch Cheddar, Nacho	35	3	3
Old El Paso: Black Bean	25	0	5
Cheese'n Salsa: Mild; Medium	40	3	3
Low-Fat, medium	30	1.5	3
Chunky Salsa varieties	15	0	3
Jalapeno Dip	30	1	4
Olys Bagel Spread: Berry	100	8	3
Honey Cinnamon; Raisin	100	8	6
Garden Veg; Garlic & Herb	90	9	1
Prices Orig. Pimiento Cheese Spr.	80	7	2
Rite Cream Cheese & Lox Spread	90	8	1
Ruffles French Onion; Ranch	70	6	4
Sealtest French Onion	50	4	2
Snyder's Mustard Pretzel	90	4	13
Stop & Shop: Veggie Dip, 2 Tbsp	110	10	3
Sour Crm French Onion, 2 T.	60	5	2
Supremo Chihuahua: Quéso Bianco	100	8	0
Quéso Fresco; Rancherito	80	6	0
TGI Fridays: Spinach,Chse,Artichoke	45	3.5	2
Black Bean & Cheese Dip	50	2.5	5
T. Marzetti: Blue Cheese	200	21	1
Light Ranch Veggie	70	6	3
Other flavors, average	130	13	2
Toby's Tofu Spread, avg., 2 T	40	2.5	2
Tostitos Dip: Con Quéso	40	2	5
Medium/Mild/Hot	15	0	3
Wise: Jalapeno Bean	25	0	5
Taco	12	0	3
Salsa: See Page 85			

Egg & Egg Dishes

Chicken Eggs

Fresh Eggs

Raw (weight with shell):	C	F	Cb
Small, 40g	65	4	0
Medium, 44g	70	4	0
Large, 50g	75	4.5	0
Extra Large, 56g	80	5	0
Jumbo, 63g	90	5.5	0
Egg Yolk, 1 extra large	63	5	0
Egg White, 1 extra large	16	0	0

Dried Egg Powder

	C	F	Cb
Whole Egg, ¼ cup, 1 oz	170	12	0
1 Tbsp	30	2	0
Egg White, ¼ cup, 1 oz	105	0	0
Egg Yolk, ¼ cup, 1 oz	195	18	0

Egg Substitutes

¼ Cup (Equivalent to 1 Egg) ~ Zero Cholesterol.

	C	F	Cb
Better 'n Eggs (Papetti), ¼ cup, 2 oz	30	0	0
EggBeaters (Fleischmann's) Frozen/Liquid Regular/Flavors, ¼ cup (61g)	30	0	1
Egg Watchers (Tofutti), 2 oz	30	0	1
Eggstra, ½ envelope	50	2	0
Ener-G, Egg Replacer, 1½ tsp, 4 g	15	0	4
Healthy Choice, ¼ cup, 2 oz	25	0	0
Egg Substitute (Jewel), ¼ cup	30	0	1
Scramblers (Morn Star), ¼ cup	35	0	0
Second Nature: Regular, ¼ cup	60	2	3
Fat-Free, ¼ cup, 60ml	30	0	1
Simply Eggs, ¼ cup	35	1	1

Other Eggs

	C	F	Cb
Duck, 1 large, 2½ oz	130	9.5	0
Goose, 1 large, 5 oz	280	19	0
Quail, 3 eggs, 1 oz	42	3	0
Turkey, 1 large, 3 oz	135	9.5	0
Turtle, 1 egg, 1¾ oz	75	5	0

Omega-3 Fat Enriched

	C	F	Cb
Eggs Land's Best, 1 large	70	4.5	0
Eggs Plus (Pilgrim's Pride), 1 large	70	4.5	0

Note: Cholesterol content same as regular eggs, but Omega-3 fats inhibit blood cholesterol increase.
Also see Cholesterol: *Page 271*

Cooked Eggs

	C	F	Cb
Boiled Egg: Same as raw egg			
Fried Egg:			
With fat: 1 large egg	100	8	0.5
2 small eggs	175	13	1
No fat/nonstick pan, 1 large	80	5.5	0
Deviled Egg, 2 halves	145	13	0.5
Eggs Benedict (2) on toast or English muffin	860	56	25
Eggs Florentine (2) on toast or English muffin	890	59	25
Pickled Egg, 1 large	80	5.5	0
Poached Egg, 1 large	65	4	0
Scotch Egg, 1 egg	300	21	16
Scrambled Eggs: 1 large egg:			
w. 1 Tbsp milk + 1 tsp fat	120	9	1
w. 1 Tbsp skim milk/no fat	85	5.5	1
2 large eggs:			
w. 2 Tbsp milk + 2 tsp fat	260	20	2
w. 2 Tbsp skim milk/no fat	180	11	2

Omelets

	C	F	Cb
1 Egg: Plain (w. 1 tsp fat)	125	10	0.5
with ½ oz cheese	175	15	0.5
w. ½ oz cheese + ½ oz ham	200	16	0.5
2 Eggs: Plain (w. 2 tsp fat)	250	20	1
with 1 oz cheese	360	29	2
w. 1 oz cheese+1 oz ham	410	32	2
3 Eggs: Plain (w. 1 Tbsp fat)	360	29	1.5
w. 2 oz cheese	580	47	2.5
w. 2 oz cheese+2 oz ham	680	53	2.5
Extras: Tomato/Onion/Veges	20	0	4.5
Egg Substitute (EggBeaters):			
2 eggs (½ cup) + 1 tsp fat	100	4	2
3 eggs (¾ cup) + 2 tsp fat	160	8	3
Extras: 1 oz cheese	110	9	1
1 oz ham	50	3	1
Tom./Onion/Veges	20	0	4.5

Egg Nog

~ Per ½ Cup (4 fl.oz)

	C	F	Cb
Regular: Borden	160	9	16
Crowley	190	9	23
Hood (Golden)	180	8	22
Light/Low-fat: Borden	120	2	23
Horizon; Hood	140	3	23
Fat-Free: Hood	100	0	21

Breakfast Sides

	C	F	Cb
Toast: Plain, 1 thick slice	85	1	13
with 2 tsp butter/marg.	155	9	13
with 3 tsp/1 Tbsp fat	190	13	13
English Muffin: Plain, 2 oz	130	1	26
with 3 tsp fat	230	12	26
Bacon, 2 strips	70	5	0
Ham, Lean, 2 oz	100	3	0
Hash Browns: ½ cup	125	6.5	14
1 cup serving	250	13	28
Sausages, 2 links (1 oz ea.)	180	16	1.5

Frozen Egg Breakfasts

Aunt Jemima Great Starts: *Per Package*

	C	F	Cb
Breakfast Wraps w. Bacon	240	9	29
French Toast & Sausage Bkfst	330	19	26
Pancakes & Sausage Breakfast	470	25	50
Sausage, Egg & Chse Biscuit	340	21	27
Sausage, Egg & Chse Croissant	350	23	22
Scrambled Eggs & Saus. Bkfst	370	27	18
Jimmy Dean			
Bacon, Egg, Cheese Muffin (1)	230	9	27
Croissant: Egg & Cheese (1)	310	20	23
Egg, Sausage, Cheese (1)	450	33	24
Egg, Sausage, Cheese Biscuit (1)	430	30	28
Omelet: 3 Cheese (1)	290	23	5
Ham & Cheese (1)	280	17	5
Pillsbury: Toaster Scrambles,			
Cheese, Egg & Bacon	180	12	14
Cheese, Egg & Sausage	180	12	14
Red Baron			
Mini Scrambles: Ham, 4 pieces	390	17	45
Bacon, 4 pieces	420	20	45
Swanson Great Starts			
Breakfast Wrap w. Bacon (1)	270	11	30
Hungryman Hearty Breakfast	450	27	35
Weight Watchers: Omelet	220	5	30
Frozen Pancake/Waffles: *See Page 122*			

Frozen Egg Rolls

Chun King/La Choy: *Average All Brands*

	C	F	Cb
Chicken Egg Rolls: Mini, 6 rolls	210	9	25
Restaurant Style, 1 roll, 3 oz	210	9	25
Pork & Shrimp Egg Rolls:			
Mini, 6 rolls, 3 oz	210	9	27
Shrimp Egg Rolls: Mini, 6 rolls	190	6	28
Restaurant Style, 1 roll, 3 oz	180	7	25
Lotus: Pork, 3 oz	180	7	18
Vegetable, 3 oz	70	1.5	13
Kahiki: Pork, 3 oz	190	6	25
Chicken, 3 oz	120	2	16
Vegetable, 3 oz	120	5	23

Fast Food/Restaurants

	C	F	Cb
Au Bon Pain: Egg on a Bagel	400	4	63
w. Bacon & Cheese	560	18	63
Bob Evans: Eggs Benedict	420	20	35
Cheese Omlettes	470	40	3
Bojangles: Egg Biscuit	400	30	26
Bacon, Egg & Cheese Biscuit	550	42	27
Bruegger's Bagels: Breakfast Sandwiches			
Egg & Cheese	480	15	66
Egg & Cheese & Sausage	695	33	66
Burger King			
Egg & Cheese Croissan'wich	300	17	26
Sausage, Egg & Chse Croissan'wich	500	36	26
Western Omelet Sandwich	330	17	28
Carl's Jr			
Scrambled Eggs & Bacon	745	42	69
Chick-Fil-A			
Chicken, Egg & Cheese Bagel	460	18	47
Denny's: Two Egg B'Fast	680	55	20
Country Scramble, no syrup/marg.	1040	62	79
All American Slam, no toast	815	65	3
Eat 'N Park: Cheese Omelet	390	30	2.5
Hardee's: Bacon Platter	980	56	90
Country Ham Platter	970	53	90
IHOP: T-Bone Steak & Eggs	1310	86	63
Country Fried Steak/Eggs	1530	105	73
McDonald's: Egg McMuffin	290	11	30
Bacon, Egg & Cheese Biscuit	440	24	36
Scrambled Eggs (2)	180	11	5
Whataburger			
Breakfast Platter w. Bacon (2 sl.)	685	42	52

Meat & Beef

Note: Cooking reduces weight of meat by 20-45% due to water and fat losses. Average weight loss is 30%. Actual loss depends on cooking method and cooking time. Examples:
4 oz raw wt. = approx. 3 oz cooked wt.
4 oz cooked wt. = approx. 5½ oz raw wt.

What 3 oz Cooked Meat Looks Like
- Half the size of this book (4¼" x 3" x ⅜" thick)
- Rectangular piece (4" x 2½" x ½" thick)
- Deck of cards (3½" x 2½" x ⅝" thick)

Quick Guide

Steak
Sirloin (Choice Grade)
External fat trimmed to ¼"
Broiled, Edible Portion (no bone)

	C	F	Cb
Small Serving, 3 oz (cooked)			
(3 oz cooked, from 4-4½ oz raw)			
Lean + fat (¼"), 3 oz	225	13	0
Lean + marbling, 3 oz	195	10	0
Lean only, 3 oz	160	6	0
(No external fat or marbling)			
Medium/Regular Serving, 5 oz (cooked wt)			
(from approx. 7 oz raw)			
Lean + fat (¼"), 5 oz	350	21	0
Lean + marbling, 5 oz	325	17	0
Lean only, 5 oz	265	10	0
Large Serving, 8 oz (cooked wt)			
(from 11-12 oz raw)			
Lean + fat, 8 oz	600	36	0
Lean + marbling, 8 oz	520	27	0
Lean only, 8 oz	425	15	0
Extra Large Serving, 12 oz (cooked wt)			
(from approx. 16-17 oz raw)			
Lean + fat (¼"), 12 oz	900	52	0
Lean + marbling, 12 oz	740	40	0
Lean only, 12 oz	640	23	0
Pan Fried			
Sirloin (choice), medium serving:			
Lean + fat (¼"), 5 oz	460	32	0
Lean only, 5 oz	340	16	0

Other Steaks

	C	F	Cb
Filet Mignon (Tenderloin):			
1 Medium steak, 6 oz raw wt.			
Broiled, with ¼" fat trim			
Lean + fat (¼"), 4 oz	380	28	0
Lean only, 3½ oz	230	12	0
New York/Club Steak:			
Top Loin/Short Loin			
1 steak, regular (9¼ oz raw, ¼" fat)			
Broiled: Lean + fat (¼"), 6¼ oz	580	43	0
Lean + marbling, 5½ oz	400	25	0
Lean only, 5¼ oz	360	20	0
Porterhouse Steak:			
1 Medium, (6 oz raw wt. no bone), broiled			
Lean + fat (¼"), 4¼ oz	410	33	0
Lean only, 3½ oz	210	11	0
1 Large (12 oz raw wt. no bone), broiled			
Lean + fat (¼") 8½ oz cooked	820	66	0
Lean only, 7 oz cooked	420	22	0
With Bone: See T-Bone Steak			
T-Bone Steak (Broiled/Grilled): wts. include bone			
Medium, 8 oz raw wt. (with bone)			
Lean + fat (¼")	410	32	0
Lean only, 4 oz raw	230	12	0
Large, (12 oz raw wt.) ¼" fat	620	48	0
Supersize, (20 oz raw wt.) ¼" fat	1025	88	0
Also See Fast-Foods & Restaurants Section ~			
LoneStar Steakhouse, Outback Steakhouse, WesterN SizzliN			

Beef - Average All Cuts

Average All Retail Cuts
Edible weight (no bone)

Raw	C	F	Cb
(1 lb raw yields approx. 11-12 oz cooked)			
Lean + fat (¼" trim), 1 oz	70	6	0
½ Pound, 8 oz	560	44	0
Lean only, 1 oz	40	2	0
½ Pound, 8 oz	320	17	0
Fat only, 1 oz	190	20	0
Cooked (No Added Fat)			
Lean + fat (¼"), 1 oz	86	6	0
Small serving, 3 oz	260	18	0
Lean + marbling, (no ext. fat), 1 oz	78	5	0
Small serving, 3 oz	235	15	0
Lean only, 1 oz	60	3	0
Small serving, 3 oz	180	9	0
Fat only, 1 oz	255	28	0

Beef - Individual Cuts

Average All Grades Edible Weight (no bone)	C	F	Cb
Brisket, whole, braised:			
Lean + fat ¼", 3 oz	330	27	0
Lean + marbling, 3 oz	280	21	0
Lean only, 3 oz	250	17	0
Chuck, blade, braised:			
Lean + fat (¼"), 3 oz	295	22	0
Lean + marbling, 3 oz	290	21	0
Lean only, 3 oz	245	21	0
Flank: Raw, 4 oz	175	8	0
Braised, 3 oz	225	14	0
Broiled, 3 oz	155	6	0
Ribs, whole (ribs 6-12): Roasted			
(1 lb raw yields 10¼ oz roasted)			
Lean + fat (¼")			
(3.6 oz w. bone, 3 oz no bone)	305	25	0
Lean only, 3 oz (no bone)	280	22	0
Round, bottom, braised:			
Lean + fat (¼"), 3 oz	190	7.5	0
Lean only, 3 oz	185	6.5	0
Round, eye/tip, roasted:			
Lean + fat (¼"), 3 oz	205	11	0
Lean, 3 oz	145	4	0
Round, top: Per 3 oz (cooked wt)			
Braised, Lean + fat	210	10	0
Lean only	175	5	0
Broiled, Lean + fat	180	8	0
Lean only	155	5	0
Pan-fried, Lean + fat	235	13	0
Lean only	190	7	0

Ground Beef

Ground Beef, Raw: Per 4 oz	C	F	Cb
73% lean (27% fat)	380	34	0
80% lean (20% fat)	290	22	0
85% lean (15% fat)	240	17	0
90% lean (10% fat)	200	11	0
93% lean (7% fat)	170	8	0
96% lean (4% fat)	150	4.5	0
Baked/Broiled: Reg., 3 oz	230	16	0
Lean (80%), 3 oz	230	15	0
Extra lean (90%), 3 oz	185	10	0
Pan-fried: Regular, 3 oz	230	15	0
Lean, 3 oz	230	15	0
Extra lean, 3 oz	195	10	0
Ground Beef Patties: Average (23% Fat)			
Frozen, raw, 4 oz	320	26	0
Broiled, 3 oz	240	17	0

Quick Guide

Roast Beef	C	F	Cb
Round (Eye/Tip, average) Average All Cuts			
Small Serving, 3 oz			
(2 thin slices/1 thick slice)			
Lean + fat (¼"), 3 oz	200	11	0
Lean only, 3 oz	150	5	0
Medium Serving, 5 oz (3-4 thin slices)			
Lean + fat, 5 oz	330	19	0
Lean only, 5 oz	245	9	0
Large Serving, 8 oz (3 thick slices)			
Lean + fat, 8 oz	525	30	0
Lean only, 8 oz	390	14	0

Roast Dinner Extras

	C	F	Cb
Gravy: Thin, 2 Tbsp	20	0.5	3.5
Thick, 2 Tbsp	50	2	0.5
1 Ladle/4 Tbsp	100	4	1
Veges: Beans, green, ½ cup	20	0	5
Cauliflower w. cheese sce, 4 oz	135	9	15
Corn, kernels, ¼ cup	35	0	9
Carrots, ¼ cup	20	0	3
Peas, ¼ cup	35	0	6
Pumpkin baked: w. fat, 4 oz	90	7	5
No added fat, 2 pces, 4 oz	25	0	5
Potato: Roasted w. fat, 1 small	155	8	30
Baked in Jacket, 1 large	280	0	63
with 1 Tbsp whipped butter	350	6	63
with Sour Cream, 2 Tbsp	270	5	64
Sweet Potato/Yam, 1 medium	105	1	24
Beef Kabobs: Beef & Veggies, 2 oz	160	10	4
If very lean meat	100	4	4

"347 ~ 348 ~ 349..."

Meat ◆ Lamb, Veal, Pork

Lamb

C **F** **Cb**

Choice Grade
Leg (Whole), roasted:

	C	F	Cb
Lean + fat, 3 oz	250	18	0
Lean only, 3 oz	155	6	0

Leg (Sirloin Half), roasted:

	C	F	Cb
Lean + fat, 3 oz	250	18	0
Lean only, 3 oz	175	8	0

Leg (Shank Half), roasted:

	C	F	Cb
Lean + fat, 3 oz	190	11	0
Lean only, 3 oz	155	6	0

Loin Chop, broiled:
1 chop (raw wt., 4¼ oz):

	C	F	Cb
	250	17	0
Lean + fat (2¼ oz edible)	180	12	0
Lean only (1.6 oz edible)	85	3.5	0

Rib Chop, broiled/roasted:
1 chop (raw wt., 3½ oz)

	C	F	Cb
Lean + fat (2½ oz edible)	255	21	0
Lean only (1¾ oz edible)	105	6	0

Shoulder (Arm/Blade):

	C	F	Cb
Braised: Lean + fat, 3 oz	290	21	0
Lean only, 3 oz	240	12	0
Broiled: Lean + fat, 3 oz	240	16	0
Lean only, 3 oz	170	8	0
Roasted: Similar to Broiled			

Cubed Lamb (Leg/Shoulder):
For stew or kabob

	C	F	Cb
Raw, lean only, 8 oz	305	12	0
Braised, lean only, 3 oz	190	8	0
Broiled, lean only, 3 oz	160	6	0

New Zealand Lamb (Imported):
Similar calories and fat to domestic.

Veal

Edible Weights

C **F** **Cb**

Leg (Top Round):

	C	F	Cb
Braised: Lean + fat, 3 oz	180	6	0
Lean only, 3 oz	170	5	0
Pan-fried, breaded:			
Lean + fat, 3 oz	195	8	9
Lean only, 3 oz	175	6	9
Pan-fried, not breaded:			
Lean + fat, 3 oz	180	7	0
Lean only, 3 oz	155	4	0
Roasted: Lean + fat, 3 oz	135	4	0
Lean only, 3 oz	130	3	0

Veal (Cont)

C **F** **Cb**

Loin Chop: 1 chop, 7 oz raw wt.

	C	F	Cb
Braised: Lean + fat, 3 oz	240	14	0
Lean only, 3 oz	190	8	0
Roasted: Lean + fat, 3 oz	185	10	0
Lean only, 3 oz	150	6	0

Rib, roasted: Lean + fat, 3 oz

	C	F	Cb
Lean + fat, 3 oz	195	12	0
Lean only, 3 oz	150	7	0

Shoulder, Arm/Blade, roasted:

	C	F	Cb
Lean + fat, 3 oz	155	7	0
Lean only, 3 oz	145	6	0

Sirloin, roasted:

	C	F	Cb
Lean + fat, 3 oz	170	9	0
Lean only, 3 oz	145	6	0

Cubed for Stew, braised:

	C	F	Cb
Leg/Shoulder, lean only, 3 oz	160	4	0

(1 lb raw yields approx. 9¼ oz cooked)

Pork

Figures based on NLMB data (1990)
Fresh Pork (Cooked Wt., no bone)
(4 oz raw wt. = approx. 3 oz cooked wt.)
Blade Steak, broiled:

	C	F	Cb
Lean + fat, 3 oz	220	15	0
Lean only, 3 oz	190	11	0

Country Style Ribs, broiled:

	C	F	Cb
Lean + fat, 3 oz	280	22	0
Lean only, 3 oz	210	13	0

Spareribs, braised: lean & fat, 6 oz

	C	F	Cb
(from 1 lb raw wt)	675	51	0

Leg (Ham), roasted:

	C	F	Cb
Lean + fat, 3 oz	230	15	0
Lean only, 3 oz	180	8	0

(Ham, cured ~ See Cold Meats)
Loin Chops, broiled: Average
(From 1 chop: 5 oz raw wt. w. bone
or 4 oz raw wt., no bone)

	C	F	Cb
Lean + fat, 3 oz	200	11	0
Lean only, 3 oz	165	7	0

Rib Chops, broiled:

	C	F	Cb
Lean + fat, 3 oz	220	14	0
Lean only, 3 oz	185	9	0

Rib Roast, roasted:

	C	F	Cb
Lean + fat, 3 oz	215	13	0
Lean only, 3 oz	180	9	0

Loin Roast, roasted:

	C	F	Cb
Lean + fat, 3 oz	190	10	0
Lean only, 3 oz	160	7	0

Pork (Cont)

	C	F	Cb
Sirloin Chop, broiled:			
Lean + fat, 3 oz	175	8	0
Lean only, 3 oz	165	6	0
Sirloin Roast, roasted:			
Lean + fat, 3 oz	175	8	0
Lean only, 3 oz	170	7	0
Tenderloin, roasted:			
Lean + fat, 3 oz	147	5	0
Lean only, 3 oz	140	4	0
Ground Pork			
Raw: Average, ¼ lb, 4 oz	300	24	0
Broiled, 3 oz	250	18	0
Pan-fried, drained, 3 oz	260	19	0

Bacon

	C	F	Cb
Raw: 1 med. slice (20 lb), ¾ oz	95	9	0
1 thick slice (12 lb), 1⅓ oz	175	17	0
(1 lb raw yields approx. 5 oz cooked)			
Broiled/Pan-Fried: 1 med. sl., 8 g	40	3	0
3 medium slices, 24g	125	10	0
2 thin slices, ½ oz	75	6	0
1 thick slice, 12g	65	5	0
Canadian-style: Cooked, 1 slice	35	1.5	0.5
As purchased, 1 slice, 1 oz	35	1.5	0.5
Bacon Bits, 1 Tbsp, ¼ oz	35	2.5	0
Breakfast Strips, Broil., 1 sl., 12 g	50	4	0

Ham

	C	F	Cb
Boneless Ham, cooked:			
Regular, (approx. 11% fat):			
Unheated (as purch.), 1 oz	50	2.5	0
Roasted, 3 oz	150	8	0
Extra Lean (5% fat):			
Unheated, 1 oz	45	2.5	0
Roasted, 3 oz	125	5	0
Whole Ham, cooked:			
Lean + fat (as purchased)			
Unheated, 1 oz	70	5	0
Roasted, 3 oz	210	15	0
Lean only, unheated, 1 oz	40	2	0
Roasted, 3 oz	135	5	0
Canned Ham: Similar to boneless ham			
Chopped, canned, 3 oz	200	16	0
Ham Patties, ckd, 1 pty, 2¼ oz	215	20	1
Ham Steak, extra lean, 2 oz	70	2.5	0
Luncheon Slices: See Deli Meats, Page 53			

Game & Other Meats

	C	F	Cb
Bison Steak,			
lean, 6 oz (raw)	205	4	0
Boar (wild), roasted, 3 oz	140	4	0
Buffalo Steak: New West Foods, 4 oz	70	3	0
Trader Joes, 1 patty	430	30	1
Caribou, roasted, 3 oz	140	4	0
Deer/Venison, roasted 3 oz	135	3	0
Goat (Capretto): Raw, 3 oz	95	2	0
Roasted, 3 oz	120	2.5	0
Ostrich: Blackwing Ostrich Meats,			
Sport Jerky, ½ oz pce	25	0	0
Sausage Patties (2) 2 oz	60	0.5	0
New West Foods:			
Ground Ostrich, 4 oz	165	7	0
Ostrich Steak, 4 oz steak	130	2.5	0
Rabbit: Roasted, 3 oz	165	7	0
Stewed, 1 cup, diced, 5 oz	290	12	0

Variety & Organ Meats

	C	F	Cb
Brains: Braised, 3 oz	130	9	0
Pan-fried, 3 oz	200	14	0
Chitterlings, pork, simmered, 3 oz	200	17	0
Ears, pork, simmered, 1 ear	185	12	0
Feet, pork: Simmered, 3 oz	200	14	0
Cured, pickled, 3 oz	170	14	0
Hormel, 2 oz	80	6	0
Head Cheese (Pork Snouts/Ears/Vinegar/Spices)			
1 oz slice	50	4	0
Heart: Average, braised, 3 oz	125	5	0
Jowl, pork, raw, 4 oz	750	80	0
Kidneys, simmered, 3 oz	135	4	0
Liver (beef): Raw, 4 oz	150	4	4
Braised, 3 oz	145	4	4
Pan-fried, 3 oz	160	4.5	4
Pancreas, pork, braised, 3 oz	185	8	0
Pork Cracklins, 0.5 oz	80	6	0
Pork Hocks, 1 piece, 6 oz	340	23	0
Scrapple, pork, 2 oz	120	8	8
Spleen, pork, braised, 3 oz	130	3	0
Stomach, pork, raw, 4 oz	185	12	0
Sweetbreads: Beef, ckd., 3 oz	125	9	0
Lamb, cooked, 3 oz	125	9	0
Tail, pork, simmered, 3 oz	340	31	0
Tongue, braised, 3 oz: Veal	170	9	0
Beef/Lamb/Pork, average, 3 oz	235	17	0
Tripe, beef, raw, 4 oz	95	4	0
Lean + fat, 3 oz	80	3.5	1.5

Sausages, Franks

Quick Guide

Franks & Weiners
Average All Brands

	C	F	Cb
Regular/Smoked: *Per Frank*			
Regular, 1.5oz (10/16oz pkg)	140	13	1
Jumbo, 2 oz (8/16 oz pkg)	170	16	0
Bun Length, 2 oz	180	17	2
Extra Long, 2.75 oz	240	21	2
Small/Cocktail (50/lb) each	30	3	0.5
Beef Franks: *Per Frank*			
Regular, 1.6 oz (10/16 oz pkg)	140	13	1
Jumbo, 2 oz (8/16 oz pkg)	170	15	2
Bun Length, 2 oz	180	16	1
¼ lb Dog, 4 oz	300	24	4

Brands

	C	F	Cb
Ball Park			
Reg./Smoked, Fat-Free (1), 1.76 oz	40	0	4
Beef: Fat-Free, 1.76 oz link	45	0	5
Reduced-Fa, 2 oz link	100	7	3
Turkey Frank, 1.76 oz link	45	0	5
Beef Kosher			
Beef: 2 oz link	180	14	4
2.6 oz link (6/16 oz)	230	19	6
Foster Farms			
Chicken Franks, 2 oz (8/16 oz)	140	12	1
Healthy Choice			
Turkey Franks, 1.76 oz link	70	2.5	6
Hebrew National			
Beef: 1.72 oz link	150	14	1
14 lb link, 4 oz	340	32	1
97% Fat-Free, 1.72 oz link	50	1.5	2
Jennie-O			
Turkey Franks: 1 oz link	70	5	1
2 oz link	120	10	2
Oscar Mayer			
Reg./Smoked, Fat-Free, 1.76 oz link	40	0	3
Beef, Reduced-Fat, 2 oz link	110	8	2
Cheese Frank, 1.6 oz link	140	13	1
Turkey Frank: 1.6 oz link	100	8	2
2 oz link	120	10	3
Shelton's			
Chicken Franks, 1.2 oz link	70	6	0
Turkey Franks, 1.2 oz link	60	4.5	1
Zacky Farms			
Chicken Frank, 2 oz link	160	12	1

Vegetarian Sausages

See Frozen/Canned & Packaged Meals

Quick Guide

Fresh Sausages
Pork/Beef: *Average All Types*

	C	F	Cb
Small: Raw, 4" link, 1 oz	85	7.5	0
Broiled/Pan-fried	80	7	0
Medium: Raw, 2 oz	170	15	0
Broiled/Pan-fried	165	14	0
Large: Raw, 3 oz	255	22	0
Broiled/Pan-fried	245	21	0
Italian: Raw, 3.2 oz	315	28	0.5
Cooked, 2.4 oz	230	18	3
Chorizo: Beef Chorizo, 2.5 oz pce	250	23	5
Pork Chorizo, 2 oz piece	250	23	5

Note: Fat is lost in broiling/pan frying.
(Cooked wt. = approx. 60-70% raw wt.)

Smoked Sausage

	C	F	Cb
Average All Brands: 2 oz link	170	15	0
3 oz link	255	22	0
Ball Park, Bun Size, 2 oz	180	17	2
Butterball (w. Turkey), 2 oz	100	6	4
Eckrich, 2 oz	180	16	2
Healthy Choice, Beef/Polska, 2 oz	80	2.5	6

Breakfast Sausages/Patties

	C	F	Cb
Armour Brown 'n Serve			
Pork/Turkey, 3 links, 2.1 oz	210	19	2
Lite Original, 3 links	120	8	3
Beef Sausage, 3 links, 2.3 oz	230	22	1
Butterball: Turkey Brkfast Pats (2)	120	7	2
Turkey Breakfast Links (3)	120	8	2
Healthy Choice, Patties/Links (3), 2 oz	70	3	3
Jennie-O, Italian Turkey Saus. (2)	160	10	0
Jimmy Dean: Pork Saus. Patties (3)	260	24	0
Pork Sausage Links: Original (3)	290	28	0
Country Maple (3)	230	20	3
Breakfast Sandwiches: See Page 47			
Jones/Golden Brown:			
Pork Sausage Patties: Original (1)	75	7	0.5
All Natural (1)	95	9	0
Sandwich Patties (1)	170	16	1
Pork Sausage Links: 2 links	180	18	2
Light, 2 links	110	8	1
Swanson 'Great Starts': See Page 47			

Vegetarian Patties:
Boca: *See Page 61*
Garden Burger: *See Page 62*

BAR B-Q
CHICKEN & RI...

Bagel, Corn & Hot Dogs

Hot Dogs, Ready-To-Go	C	F	Cb
(Includes Ketchup/Relish; no Mayo)			
Regular (1.5 oz frank, 1.5 oz bun)	260	15	22
Bun Length (2 oz frank, 1.5 oz bun)	290	18	21
Jumbo Dog (2 oz frank, 2 oz bun)	360	20	36
¼ lb Beef Dog (¼ lb dog, 2 oz bun)	480	15	36
Mile Long Dog (2.6 oz dog, 1.5 oz bun)	360	24	23

Weinerschnitzel: *See Fast-Foods*

Corn Dogs

Beef/Pork Frank: Average, 2.6 oz	170	10	16
Foster Farms Chicken Franks:			
1 dog, 2.6 oz (75g)	180	10	15
Chili Cheese, 1 dog, 2.6 oz (75g)	200	9	24
Mini Corn Dogs (4), 2.68 oz	210	12	18
Oscar Mayer Turkey & Pork, 3.2 oz	260	15	25
State Fair w. Ball Park Franks,			
Corn Dogs, 1 dog, 2.7 oz (76g)	210	12	23
Mini Corn Dogs (4)	230	13	22

Bagel Dogs

Best's Kosher: 1 dog, 1 oz	320	11	43
Mini, 1 piece, 0.8 oz	60	2	8
Vienna Beef: 1 piece, 1 oz	85	3.5	7

Hot Dog Toppings/Extras:

American Chse, 1 slice, 1 oz	110	9	1
Catsup, 1 Tbsp	16	0	4
Chili (w. Beans), ¼ cup	70	3.5	9
Mustard, 1 Tbsp	20	0	1
Pickle Relish, 1 Tbsp	20	0	5
Sauerkraut, ½ cup	20	0	5

> ## WILL-POWER TONIC
> ### ~ RECIPE ~
>
> - 1 Cup of Desire
> - 1 Quart of Determination
> - 1 Tbsp of Common Sense
> - 1 Tbsp of Stick-to-itiveness
> - 1 Tbsp of Foresight
> - 1 Cup of Energy

Deli & Luncheon Meats

Beef Jerky:	C	F	Cb
Bridgeford Beef Jerky, 1 oz	100	0.5	5
Beef Stick (5.5 oz stick), 1 oz	150	13	2
Beef Steak, 1 oz	70	0.5	2
Beef & Cheese (Giant Size),			
½ pkg, 1.5 oz	170	14	1
Pepperoni Sticks (2), 1 oz	160	13	2
Pepperoni (1" diam.), 1 oz	130	12	0
Teriyaki, 1 oz pkg	80	0.5	4
Original; Hot 'n Spicy	70	1	5
Berliner (pork/beef), 1 oz	65	5	1
Beerwurst (Beef):			
Small (2.75"diam), ⅛" slice	20	2	0
Large (4"diam), ⅛" slice	75	7	0.5
Beerwurst (Pork):			
Small (2.75"diam), ⅛" slice	15	1	0
Large (4"diam), ⅛" Slice	55	4	0.5
Bologna: 1 Slice, 1 oz	65	6	1
Fat-Free, 1 slice, 1 oz	20	0	2
Beef Bologna: 1 slice, 1 oz	90	8	1
Light, 1 slice, 1 oz	60	4	2
Light *(Oscar Mayer),* 1 sl., 1 oz	60	4	2
Red. Fat *(Hebrew Nat.),* 2 sl.,1 oz	40	2.5	0.5
Fat Free *(Osc. M.),* 2 sl., 1.6 oz	40	0	1
Healthy Choice, 1 oz	35	1	3
Weight Watchers, 2 sl., ¾ oz	35	2	0
Beef *(Tyson),* 1 slice	80	7	1
Ring *(Boar's Head),* 2 oz	145	13	0
Turkey, average, 1 oz	60	5	0.5
Blood Sausage, 1 oz	100	9	0.5
Bratwurst: Average, 1 oz	80	7	1
Boar's Head, cook., 1 wurst, 4 oz	300	25	0
Bob Evan's, Beer, 2.6 oz link	270	21	1
Braunschweiger (Pork/Liver/Sausage),			
Oscar Mayer, 1 oz slice	110	10	1
Chicken, *Average All Brands*			
1 thick or 2 thin slices, 1 oz	30	1	1
Chicken Roll, 1 slice, 2 oz	90	4	1.5
Corned Beef: Average, full fat, 1 oz	60	5	0.5
Healthy Choice, Hillshire Farm, 1oz	30	1	0
Hebrew National, 4 slices, 2 oz	90	4.5	0
Loaf, jellied, 1 oz	45	2	0
Hash, canned, average, 1 oz	50	3	3
Dutch Brand Loaf, average, 1 oz	70	5	1.5

Continued Next Page

Deli & Luncheon Meats

Ham, Luncheon:	C	F	Cb
Baked/Boiled, sliced, 1 oz	30	1	0.5
Chopped: *Eckrich* (97% FF), 1 oz	25	1	1
Armour: Canned, 1 oz	35	1.5	0.5
97% Fat Free, 1 oz	25	1	1.5
Healthy Choice, 2 sl., 2 oz	60	1.5	1
Hormel (Black Label), 1 oz	70	6	0
Oscar Mayer, 1 oz slice	60	2	0.5
Honey/Brown Sugar: Avg., 1 oz	30	1	1
Healthy Choice Deli Traditions:			
2 slices, 2 oz	60	1.5	2
Prosciutto, average, 1 oz	70	5	0
Ham & Cheese Loaf, avg., 1 oz	70	5	1
Head Cheese (Osc. Mayer), 1 oz sl.	50	4	0
Honey Loaf (Osc. Mayer), 1 oz sl.	35	1	2
Italian Sausage, 2.6 oz	250	20	3
Kielbasa (Polish Sausage), 1 oz	65	5	1
Scott Petersen, 3.4 oz link	320	27	4
Beef, 2 oz link	190	17	1
Boar's Head, 1 oz	60	5	0
Kippered Beefsteak:			
Hickory Farms, 3 slices, 0.75 oz	50	1	1
Knockwurst, 1 oz	90	8	0.5
Linguica (Gaspar's), 2 oz	180	8	1
Liverwurst, 1 oz	65	5	2
Liver Pate, fresh, average, 1 oz	90	8	1
Luncheon Loaf (Foods Co), 1 oz	65	5	2
Mortadella, 1 oz	105	9	0
Olive Loaf: Average, 1 oz	70	5	3
Oscar Mayer, 1 oz slice	75	6	2
Pastrami (Beef): Average, 1 oz	45	3	0.5
Healthy Deli, 1 oz	34	1	0.5
Hillshire (DeliSelect), 6 sl., 2 oz	60	1	0
Boar's Head, 2 oz	70	4	2
Peppered Beef, 1 oz slice	40	2	1
Pepperoni, 5 slices, 1 oz	140	13	0
Pickle Loaf, average, 1 oz	70	5	5
Pickle & Pimiento Loaf			
Oscar Mayer, 1 oz	75	6	3
Polish Sausage: See Kielbasa			
Proscuitto/Proscuitti: Avg., 1 oz	70	5	1
Hormel, 1 oz	90	7	1
Roast Beef: Lean, 1 oz	40	2	0
Healthy Choice, all types, 2 oz	60	1.5	4
Salami: Beef, average, 1 oz	80	7	1
Beer Salami, average, 1 oz	50	4	0.5
Cotto: *Oscar Mayer,* 1 slice, 1 oz	70	6	1
Dry: Hard, avg., 4 slices, 1 oz	110	10	3
Oscar Mayer, 2 slices, 1.6 oz	100	8	1

Salami (Cont):	C	F	Cb
Genoa: Average, 1 oz	120	9	1
Stick (Best's Kosher), 2, 1.75 oz	180	15	2
Italian (Bridgeford), 1 oz	120	11	0
Turkey, average, 1 oz	55	4	1
Spam (Hormel):			
Regular: ¼" slice, 1 oz	90	8	1
½" slice, 2 oz	180	16	2
Lite: ¼" slice, 1 oz	55	4	0
½" slice, 2 oz	110	8	1
Turkey: ¼" slice, 1 oz	40	2	1
½" slice, 2 oz	80	4	2
Singles: Classic, 3 oz pkg	210	16	2
Turkey, 3 oz pkg	110	4	3
Summer Sausage:			
Bridgeford, 1 oz	100	9	1
Oscar Mayer, 1 slice, 0.8 oz	70	7	0.5
Treet (Armour), canned, 1 oz	100	9	1.5
Turkey: Average, 1 oz slice	30	1	0.5
¾ oz slice	22	0.5	0.5
Turkey Breast:			
Butterball Fat Free, 3 sl., 2 oz	60	0	4
Deli Thin Smoked, 2 sl., 1 oz	50	0.5	2
Hillshire Deli Select, 6 sl., 2 oz	50	0.5	2
Louis Rich Carvery Board,			
2 slices, 1.8 oz (52g)	50	0	2
Free, 2 slices, 2 oz	50	0	2
Healthy Choice: Deli Thin: *Per 4 Slices, 52g (1.8 oz)*			
Oven-Roasted	60	1.5	2
Smoked/Rotisserie Seasoned	60	1.5	3
Honey Roasted & Smoked	60	1.5	4
Hearty Deli Sliced:			
Oven Rstd Turkey Brst 1 sl., 1 oz	30	1	1
Turkey Ham, 1 slice, 1 oz	35	1.5	0.5
Turkey Pastrami, 1 oz	35	1.5	1
Turkey Roll, 1 oz	40	2	0.5
Turkey Loaf, 1 oz	30	1	0.5
Vegetarian Deli (Worthington, Yves): See Page 76			

Meat Spreads

	C	F	Cb
Average All Brands: *Per ¼ Cup (2 oz)*			
Chicken	90	10	2
Ham, deviled	140	11	0
Liverwurst	190	16	2
Roast Beef	130	10	2
Sandwich Spread	140	10	9
Turkey	110	7	2

Paté	C	F	Cb
Canned: *Average All Brands*			
Chicken Liver, 2 Tbsp, 1 oz	**60**	4	2
Paté de Foie Gras, goose liver, 1 oz	**130**	12	2
Fresh (Refrigerated):			
Average all types, 1 oz	**110**	10	1
Boar's Head Liverwurst Pate, 2 oz	**145**	12	0
Marcel Henri			
Pate de Champagne	**210**	18	2
Chicken Liver w. Port Wine, 2 oz	**210**	18	2
Duck Truffle w. Port Wine, 2 oz	**240**	24	2
Old Wisconsin Pate			
All types, 1 oz	**105**	9	1.5
Vegetable Pate; Spin/Mushr., 2 oz	**105**	7	10
Trois Petit Cochons			
Mediterranean, 2 oz	**130**	11	3
Smoked Salmon, 2 oz	**115**	9	2
Wegmans			
Alexian Wild, 2 oz	**270**	27	1
Cognac; Black Peppercorn, 2 oz	**160**	17	4

Lunch Packs	C	F	Cb
Lunchables (*Oscar Mayer*): Per Package			
Cracker Stackers Ham & Cheddar	**420**	23	37
Nachos Cheese & Salsa, 4.4 oz	**380**	21	39
Pizza varieties, avg., 4.5 oz	**300**	13	28
Taco Bell Beef Tacos, 5.35 oz	**310**	11	34
Fun Fuel: Ham Bagels, 5.6 oz	**410**	10	64
Chicken/Ham Wraps, 5.5 oz	**435**	13	64
Peanut Butter Soft White Bread	**600**	19	85
Turkey Bagels, 5.6 oz	**420**	10	64
Pizza Dunks Soft Breadsticks	**500**	13	84
Beef Taco, 5.7 oz	**495**	15	69
Waffles & Sausage, 4.8 oz	**460**	16	66
Fun Snacks: Chips Ahoy!, 3.1 oz	**200**	9	30
Fudge Brownie, 4.3 oz	**260**	9	42
Oreo Cookies 'N Frosting, 3.7 oz	**230**	9	37
S'Mores, 3.4 oz	**200**	6	35
Star Cookies 'N Frosting, 3.6 oz	**230**	10	34
Mega Pack: Combo Ham & Ched.	**765**	32	101
Combo Turkey & Cheddar, 5.4 oz	**750**	31	101
Pizza: Pepperoni, 6.85 oz	**760**	28	105
Extra Cheesy, 6.8 oz	**700**	25	104
Pizza Stix, 7.15 oz	**680**	16	118
Ultimate Nachos Cheese & Salsa	**780**	32	113
Lunch Bucket (*Armour*)			
Beans 'n Weiners, 7.5 oz	**290**	10	37
Chili w. Beans, 7.5 oz	**235**	9	35
Hearty Beef Stew, 7.5 oz	**155**	8	15
Rings 'n Franks, 7.5 oz	**225**	9	30
Lunchmakers (*Armour*)			
Loco Nachos	**370**	13	59
Cheese Pizza	**310**	13	36
Smuckers			
Snackers, 3.3 oz pkg	**410**	20	47
Uncrustables, 1 sandwich	**210**	8	26
South Beach Diet (*Kraft*)			
Wraps: *Per Package*			
Deli Ham & Turkey, 1 pkg	**220**	10	24
Grilled Chicken Caesar, 1 pkg	**230**	10	24
Southwestern Style Chicken	**240**	10	26
Turkey & Bacon Club, 1 pkg	**250**	12	25

Full Nutritional Data
~ See Author's Website
www.CalorieKing.com

Chicken

Chicken	C	F	Cb
From 3lb ready-to-cook chicken			
Breast/Wing Quarter			
Roasted: With skin	300	15	0
Without skin	185	5	0
Fried, batter dipped	530	30	17
Leg Quarter: Thigh & Drumstick			
Roasted: With skin	270	16	0
Without skin	185	8	0
Fried, batter dipped	435	25	15

KFC: See Fast-Foods Section

Average - All Meats

	C	F	Cb
Average of Light Meat: *Per 4 oz (no bone)*			
Roasted: with skin	250	12	0
without skin	190	5	0
Stewed: with skin	225	12	0
without skin	180	4.5	0
Fried: Batter-dipped, 4 oz	310	17	0
Flour coated, 4 oz	275	14	2
Average of Dark Meat: *Per 4 oz (no bone)*			
Roasted: with skin	285	18	0
without skin	230	12	0
Stewed: with skin	260	16	0
without skin	215	10	0
Fried: Batter-dipped, 4 oz	330	21	12
Flour coated, 4 oz	320	20	5

Chicken Parts

Broilers or Fryers: Edible Weights (no bone)

Breast: *Per ½ Breast*	C	F	Cb
Raw: With skin, 5 oz	240	13	0
Without skin, 4¼ oz	130	1.5	0
Roasted: With skin, 3½ oz	195	8	0
Without skin, 3 oz	140	3	0
Stewed: With skin, 4 oz	210	8	0
Without skin, 3¼ oz	145	3	0
Fried: Batter-dipped, 5 oz	365	19	12
Flour coated, w. skin, 3½ oz	220	9	7
Drumstick: *Per Drumstick*			
Roasted: With skin, 2 oz	115	6	0
Without skin, 1½ oz	75	2.5	0
Fried: Batter-dipped, 2½ oz	195	11	7
Flour coated, 1¾ oz	120	7	1
Stewed: With skin, 2 oz	115	6	0
Without skin, 1½ oz	80	3	0

Thigh Portion: Edible Wt. (no bone)	C	F	Cb
Raw: With skin, 3.3 oz			
(4¼ oz with bone)	200	14	0
Without skin, 2.4 oz	80	3	0
Roasted: With skin, 2¼ oz	155	10	0
Without skin, 2 oz	110	6	0
Stewed: With skin, 2½ oz	160	10	0
Without skin, 2 oz	105	5	0
Fried: Batter-dipped, 3 oz	240	14	8
Flour coated, 2¼ oz	165	9	2
Wing: *Per Wing*			
Raw Weight 3.2 oz (with bone)			
Raw: With skin	110	8	0
Without skin	35	1	0
Roasted: With skin	100	7	0
Without skin	45	2	0
Fried: Batter-dipped	160	11	5
Flour coated	105	7	1
Stewed: With skin, 4 oz	100	7	0
Buffalo Wings: *See Fast-Foods Section*			
Neck: Simmered, with skin	95	7	0
Without skin	30	2	0
Skin Only: *Skin from ½ Chicken*			
Raw skin, 2¾ oz	275	26	0
Roasted skin, 2 oz	255	23	0
Stewed skin, 2½ oz	260	24	0
Fried, Flour coated, 2 oz	280	24	5
Fried, Batter-dipped, 6¾ oz	750	55	45
Roasters			
Average of Light & Dark Meat:			
Roasted: With skin, 4 oz	250	15	0
Without skin, 4 oz	190	8	0
Light Meat: Without skin, roasted	175	5	0
Dark Meat: Without skin, roasted	200	10	0
Stewing Chicken			
Average of Light & Dark Meat: *Per 4 oz Stewed*			
With skin	320	21	0
Without skin	265	14	0
Light Meat: Without skin	240	9	0
Dark Meat: Without skin	290	17	0
Capon Chicken			
Roasted: With skin, 4 oz	260	13	0
½ Chicken, with skin	1460	74	0

Chicken Offal & Stuffing	C	F	Cb
Giblets: Simmered, 1 cup	230	7	0.5
Fried, flour-coated, 1 cup	400	20	6
Gizzard, simmered, 1 cup	225	4	0
Heart, simmered, 1 cup	270	12	0.2
Liver: Raw, 4 oz	135	5.5	1
Simmered, 1 cup	215	8.5	1
Liver Pate Fresh, 1 Tbsp, ½ oz	30	2	1
Stuffing: Average, ½ cup	180	9	22

Chicken Products | C | F | Cb

Shop Stop

	C	F	Cb
Blazing Chicken Wings, 3 oz	200	12	1
Breaded Tenderloins (3), 4 oz	240	12	15
Boneless Skinless Breasts (1), 8 oz	210	5	3

Stove Top

	C	F	Cb
Chicken Stuffing Mix: 1 oz	110	1	20
½ cup prepared	170	9	20
Tyson: Breaded Nuggets (5)	280	18	16
Breast Nuggets (5)	280	16	21
Southern Fried Nuggets (6)	270	21	11
Breast Patties: Regular, each	180	11	12
Southern Fried, each	240	18	10
Wings: Flavored, average (3)	220	15	1
BBQ Style (3)	230	13	15
Stir Fry Kit: Chicken, 2¾ c. froz.	430	4.5	73

Duck, Goose, Quail

	C	F	Cb
Duck: Roasted, with skin, 3 oz	285	24	0
Without skin, 3 oz	170	10	0
½ whole duck, with skin	1290	108	0
Goose: Roast, with skin, 3 oz	260	19	0
Without skin, 3 oz	200	11	0
Pheasant: ½ bird, raw	725	37	0
Quail: 1 whole, raw	210	13	0

Turkey

Fryer-Roasters: Per 3 oz Serving

	C	F	Cb
Roasted: Light Meat, with skin	140	4	0
without skin	120	1	0
Dark Meat: with skin	155	6	0
without skin	140	4	0

½ of Whole Turkey: (Approx. 3¼ lbs raw wt. w/out neck and giblets; 1.8 lbs cooked wt.)

	C	F	Cb
Roasted: With skin	1400	46	0
Without skin	1030	18	0

Ground Turkey, Raw: (4 oz raw wt. = 3 oz ckd wt.)

	C	F	Cb
Regular (85% lean), 4 oz	170	10	0
Lean (90% lean), 4 oz	160	8	0
Foster Farms (94% lean), 4 oz	150	7	0
Jennie-O (93% lean), 4 oz	160	8	0
Breast, no skin, 4 oz	115	1	0
Patties: Small, 3 oz	110	6.5	0
Medium, 4 oz	160	9	0
Large, 5.3 oz	175	10	0

Turkey Parts | C | F | Cb

Roasted, Edible Weights (no bone)

Breast (½): (from 17¼ oz raw wt. w/bone)

	C	F	Cb
With skin, 12 oz (no bone)	525	11	0
Without skin, 10¾ oz	415	2	0

Back (½): With skin, 4½ oz

	C	F	Cb
With skin, 4½ oz	305	18	0
Without skin, 3½ oz	165	6	0

Leg (Thigh & Drumstick): (from 1 lb raw wt. w/bone)

	C	F	Cb
With skin, 8½ oz (no bone)	345	16	0
Without skin, 7¾ oz	235	5	0

Wing: (from 7¼ oz raw wt. w/bone)

	C	F	Cb
With skin, 3 oz (no bone)	185	9	0
Without skin, 2 oz	100	2	0

Neck: Simmered, 1 neck, (9 oz w. bone)

	C	F	Cb
Neck: Simmered, 1 neck, (9 oz w. bone)	275	11	0
Giblets, simm., 1 cup, 5 oz	240	7	3

Young Hens (Roasted) | C | F | Cb

	C	F	Cb
Light Meat: With skin, 3 oz	175	8	0
Without skin, 3 oz	135	3	0
Dark Meat: With skin, 3 oz	200	11	0
Without skin., 3 oz	165	7	0

Young Toms – Similar to Young Hens

Turkey Products

Banquet: *See Frozen Meals, Page 61*

	C	F	Cb
Circle L: Boneless Bacon, 3 oz	120	9	1

Hormel: Turkey Ham & Chunks (canned), ckd:

	C	F	Cb
Breast & White Turkey, 2 oz	60	1	2
Turkey Ham/Pastrami, 2 oz	70	3	1
Turkey Salami, 2 oz	100	8	0

Jennie-O: Turkey Bacon, 2 slice

	C	F	Cb
Turkey Bacon, 2 slice	40	1	0
Turkey in BBQ Sauce, ½ cup	125	3.5	3

Louis Rich: Fat Free Breast of Turkey

	C	F	Cb
Rotiss'd/Smoked/Rstd, 2 oz	60	0	1

Luncheon Slices: *See Deli Meats, Page 54*

	C	F	Cb
Franks: Medium, 1½ oz	90	8	1
Large, 2 oz	120	10	2
Smoked Sausage/Kielbasa, 1 oz	40	2	3
Turkey Bacon, 1 oz	50	5	0
Turkey Nuggets/Sticks, ckd, ea.	75	5	4.5
Turkey Patties, cooked, each	220	13	13

Swanson: *Frozen Meals, Page 67*

Turkey Store (Jennie-O)

	C	F	Cb
Lean Burger Patties, 1 patty	160	8	0
Lean Italian Sausage, 1 link	160	10	0

Fish ~ Fresh & Canned

Quick Guide

Fresh Fish C F Cb

Low Oil (Less than 2.5% fat)
White/pale colored flesh. Examples:
Cod, Flounder, Haddock, Halibut, Mahi Mahi
Perch, Pike, Pollock, Snapper, Sole, Whiting.

Per 4 oz Edible Portion

Raw, 4 oz (no bones)	90	1	0
Steamed, Broiled, Baked	130	1	0
Fried: Lightly Floured	210	8	3.5
Breaded	260	12	8
In Batter	320	16	27

Medium Oil (2.5-5% fat)
Pale colored flesh. Examples: C F Cb
Bluefin Tuna, Catfish, Kingfish, Orange Roughy,
Salmon (Pink), Swordfish, Rainbow Trout, Yellowtail.

Raw, 4 oz (no bones)	140	5	0
Baked, Broiled, 4 oz	175	6	0
Fried, 4 oz	230	11	8

High Oil (Over 5% fat) C F Cb
Darker colored flesh. Examples:
Albacore Tuna, Bluefish, Herring, Mackerel,
Salmon (Atl./Chinook/Sockeye), Sardines, Trout,
Whitefish.

Raw, 4 oz (no bones)	230	16	0
Baked, Broiled, 4 oz	275	17	0
Fried, 4 oz	340	23	12

Cooking Yields (Fin Fish):
4 oz Raw wt. = 3 ½ oz Cooked wt.
4 oz Cooked wt. = 5 oz Raw wt.

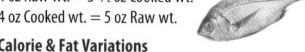

Calorie & Fat Variations
The amount of fat/oil in fish varies with the species,
season and locality. Within the same fish, fat/oil content
is generally higher towards the head.

Fish & Shellfish C F Cb

Edible Weights: (no bones/shell)

	C	F	Cb
Abalone, Raw, 4 oz	120	1	7
Ahi Tuna, grilled, 6 oz fillet (no fat)	220	2	0
Anchovy: Paste, 1 Tbsp, ¼ oz	15	1	0.5
Cnd. in oil, drnd., 5 only, ¾ oz	40	2	0
Pickled, 1 oz	50	3	0
Barracuda (Pacific), raw, 4 oz	130	3	0
Bass: Black, raw, 4 oz	105	1	0
Striped: Raw, 1 fillet, 5½ oz	150	4	0
Baked, 3 oz	105	3	0
Blue Fish: Raw, 1 fillet, 5¼ oz	185	6	0
Baked, 3 oz	130	5	0
Butterfish, raw, 4 oz	165	9	0
Cajun & Creole Dishes: *See Page 176*			
Calamari, breaded/fried, 1 serve	360	21	10
Carp, raw, 4 oz	145	6	0
Catfish: Raw Frozen, 4 oz	150	9	0
Fried, breaded, 1 fillet, 3 oz	200	12	7
Baked, 3 oz	120	5	0
Caviar, black/red, 1 Tbsp, 16g	40	3	0.5
Clams: Raw, 3 oz (4 lge/9 small)	65	1	2
Fried, breaded, ¾ cup, 4 oz	450	26	39
Canned *(Snow's)* in clam jce 2 oz	25	0	2
Minced, ¼ cup, 2 oz	25	0	0.5
Clam Juice: *(Snow's)* 1 Tbsp	0	0	0
Cod, Atlantic/Pacific: Raw, 4 oz	95	1	0
Baked/Broiled, 1 fillet, 6¼ oz	135	2	0
Canned, 3 oz	90	1	0
Minced, ¼ cup, 2 oz	25	0	0
Smoked, 3 oz	95	1	0
Crab: Alaska King, raw, 4 oz	95	1	0
1 leg, cooked, 4¾ oz	130	2	0
Blue: Raw, 1 crab			
(⅓ lb whole crab, ¾ oz flesh)	18	0.5	0
Steamed, 3 oz	85	1	0
Canned, ½ cup, 2½ oz	65	0.5	0
Dungeness, 1 crab, 5¾ oz edible			
(from 1½ lb whole crab)	140	2	2
Imitation Crab Legs/Stix, 3oz	80	1	8.5
Crab Cakes (Low-fat), (1), 2 oz	100	4	12
Regular (1), 3 oz	190	12	16
Crab Legs, restaurant-style	130	2	0
Crayfish, raw, 4 oz (edible)	100	1	0
Croaker, raw, 4 oz	120	3	0
Cuttlefish, raw, 3 oz	70	1	1
Dolphinfish, raw, 4 oz	95	1	0
Eel: Raw, 4 oz	210	13	0
Smoked, 2 oz	190	16	0
Fish & Chips: *Arthur Treachers*	1540	101	132
Denny's	960	54	83
Fish S'wich, w. Tartar Sce, 5½ oz	430	23	41
Fish Sticks, frozen, breaded, ½ oz	35	2	3

Fish & Shellfish (Cont)

Edible Weights: (no bones/shell)	C	F	Cb
Fish Oil, 1 Tbsp, ½ oz	125	14	0
Flounder/Sole: Raw, 4 oz	120	0.5	0
Baked, 3 oz	90	1	0
Frozen Fish & Entrees: *See Page 60*			
Gefilte Fish: *See Kosher/Deli Foods, Page 179*			
Grouper, raw, 4 oz	105	1	0
Haddock: Raw, 4 oz	100	0.5	0
Broiled, 1 fillet, 5¼ oz	170	1	0
Smoked, 2 oz	22	0.5	0
Baked, 3 oz	90	1	0
Halibut: Raw, 4 oz	125	3	0
Baked, 3 oz	105	2	0
Herring: Atlantic, raw, 4 oz	180	10	0
Pickled, 2 pieces, 1 oz	60	4	2
In Sour Cream, 1 oz	75	5	1
Party Snacks, ¼ cup, dr., 2 oz	120	5	0
Rollmops, 1½ oz	110	8	6
Canned: Plain w. liq., 4 oz	235	15	0
in Tomato Sauce, 4 oz	200	12	1
Smoked, kippered, 4 oz	245	14	0
Jellyfish: Raw, 4 oz	30	0	0
Dried, Salted, 1 cup, 2 oz	20	1	0
Kingfish, raw, 4 oz	120	3.5	0
Ling, raw, 4 oz	100	0.5	0
Lobster: Northern: Raw, 4 oz	105	1	0.5
1 Lobster, 6¼ oz			
(from 1½ lb whole lobster)	135	1.5	0.5
Cooked, 1 cup, 5 oz	140	1	2
Lobster Newberg, ¾ cup	360	20	9
Lobster Thermidor, 1 serving	370	22	15
Lobster Salads, ½ cup	220	13	5
Lobster Tail, restaurant-style	105	5	2
Lomi Salmon, ¼ cup, 4 oz	20	1	3
Lox, Regular/Nova, 2 oz	65	2.5	0
Mackerel: Atlantic, raw, 4 oz	235	16	0
Broiled, 3 oz	190	12	0
Jack, canned, ½ c., 3⅓ oz	150	6	0
King, raw, 4 oz	120	2	0
Pacific/Jack: Raw, 4 oz	180	9	0
Broiled, 3 oz	190	12	0
Spanish, raw, 4 oz	160	7	0
Mahi-Mahi, raw, 4 oz fillet	100	1	1
Milkfish, raw, 4 oz	165	7.5	0
Monkfish: Raw, 4 oz	75	1	0
Baked, 3 oz	80	2	0
Mullet, striped, raw	135	4	0
Mussels: Raw, 4 oz (edible wt.)	100	2	4
1 cup, 5¼ oz (edible wt.)	130	3	5
Cooked, moist heat, 3 oz	150	4	6

	C	F	Cb
Ocean Perch: Raw, 4 oz	90	1.5	0
Baked, 3 oz	100	20	0
Octopus, common, raw, 4 oz	95	1	2
Orange Roughy, raw, 4 oz	145	9	0
Oysters: Common, raw, 3 oz	70	1	3.5
Eastern raw: 6 medium, 3 oz	60	2	3
1 cup, 8¾ oz	170	6	8.5
Fried/breaded, 6 med., 3 oz	170	11	10
Pacific, raw, 1 med., 1¾ oz	40	1	2
Oysters Rockerfeller, 3 oysters	220	13	12
Perch, average, raw, 4 oz	105	2	0
Pike: Northern, raw, 4 oz	100	1	0
Walleye, raw, 4 oz	105	2.5	0
Pollock, raw, 4 oz	100	1	0
Pout, (Ocean), raw, 4 oz	90	1	0
Pompano, Florida, raw, 4 oz	190	10	0
Porgy/Scup, raw, 4 oz	130	4	0
Quahogs ~ See Clams			
Red-Snapper, raw, 4 oz	115	1.5	0
Rockfish, Pacific, raw, 4 oz	110	2	0
Roe, raw, 2 Tbsp, 1 oz	40	2	0.5
Sablefish: Raw, 4 oz	220	17	0
Smoked, 3 oz	220	17	0
Salmon:			
Raw: Chinook, 4 oz	205	7	0
Atlantic; Coho/Silver, 4 oz	160	7	0
Chum; Pink, 4 oz	135	4	0
Red/Sockeye, 4 oz	190	10	0
Baked: Atlantic/Coho, 3 oz	150	7	0
Smoked Salmon: Chinook, 3 oz	100	4	0
Pacific Supreme, 2 oz	100	4	0
Wild Oats, Pastrami Style, 2 oz	130	9	0
Canned Salmon: *Average All Brands*			
Pink: 1 oz	40	2	0
¼ cup, 63g (2.2 oz)	90	5	0
3¾ oz can, whole	155	8.5	0
7½ oz can, whole	300	17	0
Skinless/boneless, ¼ c., 2 oz	70	2	0
Red Sockeye: 1 oz	50	3	0
¼ cup, 63g (2.2 oz)	110	7	0
3¾ oz can, whole	190	12	0
Atlantic, ½ cup, 3½ oz	230	14	0
Chinook/King, ½ cup	210	14	0
Chum, ½ cup, 3½ oz	140	5	0
Coho/Silver, ½ cup	155	5	0
Atlantic Steaks: Small, 8 oz	320	14	0
Medium, 12 oz	480	21	0
Large, 16 oz	640	28	0
Salmon Cake, take-out, 3 oz	240	15	6

Fish ~ Fresh & Canned (Cont)

Fish (Cont)

	C	F	Cb
Sardines (Canned): *Average All Brands*			
In Oil, undrained, 1 oz	85	7	0
Drained of oil, 1 oz	60	3	0
3¾ oz can, drained, (3¼ oz)	190	11	0
1 lrg/2 med. ³/₅" small, 0.8 oz	50	3	0
In Tom./ Mustard Sce, 1 oz	45	3	0
3¾ oz can (8 sardines)	170	11	0
Sashimi: *See Japanese Foods, Page 178*			
Scallop: Raw, 6 lge/10 small, 3 oz	75	0.5	2
Breaded/fried, 6 pces, 5 oz	380	19	38
Seabass, raw, 4 oz	110	2	0
Seafood Salad, 1 scoop (#16)	140	10	8
Shark: raw, 4 oz	150	6	0
Batter-dipped, fried, 4 oz	260	16	7
Baked, 3 oz	135	5	0
Shark Fin, dried, 1 oz	30	0	0
Shrimp: Raw, in shell, ½ lb	140	2	1.5
Raw, shelled, 3 oz (12 lge)	90	1.5	0.5
Breaded/fried, 3 oz (11 lge)	210	11	10
Canned, 2 oz	45	0.5	0.5
Tiger, cooked, 1 shrimp, ½ oz	15	0.5	0
Battered, fried, 1 shrimp	60	4	3
Shrimp Cocktail, restaurant-style	140	2	1
Smelt, Rainbow, raw, 4 oz	115	3	0
Snapper, raw, 3 oz	85	1	0
Cooked, 1 fillet, 6 oz	215	3	0
Sole, Lemon, raw, 4 oz	90	1	0
Squid: Raw, 4 oz	105	1	3.5
Fried, 3 oz	140	6	7
Surimi (Imitation Crab), 4 oz	110	1	7.5
Sweet & Sour Fish, ½ dish, 10 oz	580	29	53
Swordfish raw:			
Small Steak, 4 oz	135	4.5	0
Medium Steak, 6 oz	200	7	0
Tilapia, Rain Forest Fillets, 4 oz	95	1	0
Trout, Rainbow: Raw, 4 oz	135	4	0
Broiled, 3 oz	125	4	0
Smoked, 2 oz	110	6	0
Tuna: *Average All Brands*			
Raw: Albacore, 4 oz	190	8	0
Bluefin, 4 oz	160	5.5	0
Skipjack, Yellowfin, 4 oz	120	1	0
Broiled, 3 oz	110	1	0
Canned:			
In Water, drained:			
Chunk/Solid, 2 oz can	60	0.5	0
3 oz can	90	1	0
6 oz can	150	1.5	0
In Oil, drained:			
Chunk Light, 2 oz	110	5.5	0
6 oz can, drained	275	14	0

Tuna (Cont)	C	F	Cb
Solid White, 2 oz	90	2.5	0
6 oz can, drained	225	6.5	0
Tuna Salad: Deli Style, ½ c., 4oz	300	24	15
Lower fat, 4 oz	210	10	11
Whitefish: Raw, 4 oz	150	6.5	0
Baked, 3 oz	140	6	1
Smoked, 3 oz	90	1	0
Whiting: Raw, 4 oz	100	1.5	0
Baked, 3 oz	85	1	0
Yellowtail: Raw, 3 oz	125	4.5	0
Grilled, 3 oz (from 4 oz raw)	160	6	0

Other Canned/Packaged Fish

	C	F	Cb
Bumble Bee: *Incl. Mayo & Crackers*			
Tuna Salad Kit	420	22	24
Fat-Free Kit	150	2	24
Albacore Entrees:			
Ginger & Soy, 4 oz	170	2.5	3
Other varieties, avg., 4 oz	155	1	0
Chicken of the Sea			
Smoked Pacific Salmon, 1 pouch	120	3.5	1
Tuna Salad Kits: *Per 5 oz*			
Light Tuna: in Mayo/Onion	365	23	18
w. Sweet Pickle Relish	315	17	19
Libby's: Crab Delights, 2 oz	30	0	5
Shrimp/Lobster Delight, 2 oz	35	0	4
Starkist			
Pouch: *Per 3 oz*			
Tuna Chunk Light, in water	90	1	0
Albacore Tuna, in water	105	1.5	0
Lunch-To-Go: Chunk Light Tuna			
w. Mayo/Crackers, 4.5 oz	210	9	27
Tuna Creations: Chunk Light Tuna			
w. Mayo/Crackers, 4.5 oz	210	9	27
Hickory Smoked (Tuna only), 2 oz	60	0	0

Frozen Fish Products

Gorton's: See Page 63
Kroger: See Page 64
SeaPak: See Page 66
Van De Kamp's: See Page 68
Fast-Foods & Restaurant Chains: See Page 183
Captain D's Seafood: See Fast-Food Section
Long John Silvers: See Fast-Food Section
Shoney's: See Fast-Food Section

Amy's (Vegetarian)

	C	F	Cb
Per Serving			
Bowls: Brown Rice & Vegs, 10 oz	250	8	36
Santa Fe Enchilada, 10 oz	350	11	47
Other varieties, average	300	12	45
Asian Meals: Thai Stir Fry, 9.5 oz	310	11	45
Asian Noodle Stir Fry, 10 oz	240	4.5	41
Entrees: Chse Enchilada, 4.5 oz	220	12	18
Cheese Lasagna, 10.3 oz	380	14	44
Macaroni & Cheese, 9 oz	410	16	47
Macaroni & Soy Cheeze, 9 oz	370	15	42
Whole Meals: Chse Enchilada, 9 oz	330	14	38
Black Bean Enchilada, 10 oz	320	8	55
Veggie Loaf, 10 oz	280	7	47
Pot Pies: Country Vege, 7½ oz	370	16	47
Mex. Tamale; Shepherd's Pie, avg.	160	4	27
Vegetable (Non Dairy), 7½ oz	360	13	50
Burgers: Californian, 2½ oz	130	5	19
Other varieties, avg., 2½ oz	120	2.5	14
Burritos: Bean & Rice, 6 oz	280	6	48
Breakfast Burrito, 6 oz	230	6	38
Non Dairy, 6 oz	280	6	48
Snacks: Tofu Scramble, 4 oz	180	6	23
Vege Pie, 5 oz	300	9	45

Banquet

	C	F	Cb
Pot Pies: Beef, 7 oz	430	25	38
Chicken, 7 oz	400	23	37
Turkey, 7 oz	390	21	38
Chicken: Breast Patties (1)	260	19	13
Chicken Breast Tenders (5)	280	19	14
Chicken Breast Nuggets (5)	280	20	14
Fried Chicken Breasts, 1 piece	230	17	10
Crispy Chicken, Skinless, 3 oz	370	23	14
Buffalo Style Jumbo Wings, 3 oz	170	10	0.5
Popcorn Chicken, 11 pieces	190	9	18
Original Chicken: Nuggets. 5 pce	280	20	14
Crispy Chicken, 3 oz	380	25	13
Crispy Chicken, Country, 3 oz	360	23	15
Buffalo Style Tenders, 3 oz	270	18	14
Wings: Hot & Spicy, 3 oz	280	19	7
Honey Barbecue, 3 oz	290	20	10
Crock Pot Classics: *Per Cup*			
Beef Stew	210	5	23
Chicken & Dumplings	310	14	27
Chicken & Red Potatoes	240	11	21
Creamy Chicken & Pasta	430	20	39
Herb Chicken & Rice, 1 cup	310	3.5	51
Stroganoff Beef & Noodles	350	12	38

Banquet (Cont)

	C	F	Cb
Meals: BBQ Beef Patty, 9.5 oz	370	18	35
BBQ Chicken Meal	310	11	37
Chicken & Pasta Marinara, 9.5 oz	420	22	40
Chicken & Stuffing Bake, 9.5 oz	280	9	37
Chicken Fingers, 7.1 oz	570	30	57
Country Fried Pork	430	24	40
Fettuccine Alfredo	450	20	53
Fried Chicken, 9 oz	390	20	30
Fried Rice w. Chicken & Egg Roll	320	9	46
Homestyle Noodles & Chicken	450	20	47
Lasagna w. Meat Sauce, 11 oz	340	10	46
Mac & Cheese, 6.5 oz	210	5	34
Meatloaf Meal, 9.5 oz	280	16	18
Mexican Style Enchilada Combo	410	16	27
Our Original Fried Chicken	470	27	35
Pepperoni Pizza, 6.75	470	20	60
Salisbury Steak Meal, 9.5 oz	340	20	26
Spaghetti & Meatballs, 10.5 oz	440	20	43
Swedish Meatballs, 10.25 oz	400	19	33
Turkey Mostly White Meat	290	13	28
Hearty One Dinners: Turkey, 16 oz	520	22	48
Boneless Pork Rib, 16 oz	650	34	55
Chicken Fried Beef Steak, 16 oz	790	47	65
Fried Chicken, 16 oz	750	33	70
Salisbury, 16 oz	630	40	44

Birds Eye – Voila!

	C	F	Cb
Per Cup, Cooked (2 Cups Frozen)			
Chicken Voila!: Garlic Chicken	240	8	21
Other varieties, average	240	9	24
Steak Voila! Beef Sirloin/Potato	190	7	22
Reduced Carb Voila: *Per 1 cup Cooked*			
Chicken & Sausage Tuscano	170	8	10
Chicken Teriaki & Vegetables	150	2.5	15
Down Home Chicken and Vegetables	180	5	17
Roasted Garlic Chicken & Vege.	120	2.5	13
Teriaki Beef & Vegetables	160	4	15

Boca (Vegetarian)

	C	F	Cb
Burger: Cheeseburger, 1 patty	100	5	5
All American Flame Grilled (1)	90	4	5
Vegan, Original, 1 patty	70	1	6
Organic Burgers: Vegan, Orig. (1)	100	2	9
Roasted Garlic/Onion, 1 patty	130	3	10
Chik'n: Nuggets (4), 3 oz	180	6	17
Hot & Spicy Buffalo Wings (4)	160	7	14
Patties (1), 2.5 oz	160	6	15
Sausages: Bratwurst (1), 2.5 oz	140	7	6
Italian, 2.5 oz	130	6	6
Organic Pizza, ⅓ Pizza	260	8	36

Budget Gourmet (Michelina's)

	C	F	Cb
Classics: Per Container (8 oz)			
Escalloped Noodles & White Turkey	290	12	37
Fettuccini Alfredo w. 4 Cheeses	310	10	42
Lasagna Alfredo w. Broccoli	290	10	38
Pizza Snacks, 5 oz	420	24	38
Spicy Szechwan Vege w. Chicken	310	6	51
Stir Fry Rice & Vegetables	380	11	62
Other varieties, average	270	7	45
Premium: Beef Stroganoff, 8 oz	270	7	37
Beef Pepper Steak w. Rice, 8 oz	260	4.5	43
Chicken and Pasta, 8.5 oz	340	14	34
Orange Glazed Chicken, 8.5 oz	300	3	56
Swedish Meatballs, 10 oz	500	22	52
Bistro Bowls: Spicy Beef & Broccoli	300	2	49
Shrimp & Vegetables	240	8	32
Other varieties, average	300	4.5	55
Lean Gourmet: Cheese Lasagna	230	6	35
Salisbury Steak w. Pot. & Gravy	210	7	26
Santa Fe Style Rice & Beans	350	9	59
Shrimp w. Pasta & Veges, 8 oz	260	6	37
Swedish Meatballs, 9 oz	300	8	40

Cedarlane (Vegetarian)

	C	F	Cb
Burrito, Beans, Rice, Chse (1), 6 oz	260	1	48
Eggplant Parmesan, ½ pkg, 5 oz	165	8	16
Carb Buster: 4 Cheese Quiche, 6 oz	500	38	5
Chili Relleno Pie, 9.5 oz	520	40	9
Spinach Enchilada, 9 oz	490	37	11
Enchilada: Garden Vege (1), 4.8 oz	140	3	20
Three-Layer Pie, ½ pkg, 5.5 oz	315	7	27
Lasagne: Cheese, ½ ctn, 5 oz	190	6	22
Garden Vege, ½ ctn, 5 oz	180	3	26

Claim Jumper

	C	F	Cb
Meals: Baby Back Pork Ribs (3)	210	14	8
Beef Pot Pie	550	39	37
Beef Pot Roast	500	18	50
Buffalo Wings (2)	160	9	5
Chicken Fried Beef Steak	630	30	72
Chicken Pot Pie, ½ pie, 8 oz	550	39	38
Chicken Tenderloins, 2 pieces	210	8	20
Country Fried Beef Steak (1)	945	58	80
Country Fried Chicken, 19 oz	660	24	81
Lasagna w. Meat Sauce, 8 oz	280	13	22
Meatloaf Dinner	640	40	42
Rst Turkey Brst w. Gravy & Dressing	550	23	51
Salisbury Steak	630	35	40
Spicy Chicken Tenderloins, 3 oz	180	7	17
Turkey Pot Pie, ½ pie, 8 oz	575	41	35
Sauce: Hot Sauce, ½ Tbsp	0	0	0
Original Barbecue, 4 Tbsp	70	0.5	17

Croissant Pockets

	C	F	Cb
Egg, Sausage & Cheese	360	20	37
Five Cheese Pizza (1)	390	20	40
Ham & Cheddar	340	16	36
Pepperoni Pizza	390	20	42
Philly Steak & Cheese	360	19	36
Other varieties, average	320	15	35

El Monterey

	C	F	Cb
Shredded Beef Tamales (1)	200	9	24
Soft Taco: Beef & Cheese (1)	440	22	42
Spicy Beef & Cheese (1)	420	22	40
Spicy Chicken & cheese (1)	340	11	44
Sausage Egg & Cheese (1)	370	23	29
Quesadilla: Gr. Chkn & 3 Chse (1)	260	14	20
Char Broiled Chicken & Chse (1)	230	10	20
Taquitos: Fiesta Appetizers Pack	370	23	29
Fiesta Minis Pack	260	12	27

Essensia (Albertson's)

	C	F	Cb
Entrees: Corn Souffle, 1 cup	300	19	17
Eggplant Parmesan, 1 cup	340	17	35
Herbed Chicken, ⅓ pkg	180	4.5	17
Jambalaya, 1 cup	220	4.5	26
Mac & Cheese, 1 cup	330	16	32
2 Meat Lasagna, 1 cup	340	17	26
Pork & Vege Spring Roll (1)	210	10	23
Roast Garlic Mash Potatoes, 5 oz	190	9	26
6 Cheese Cannelloni	190	6	22
7 Cheese Lasagna, 5 oz	160	8	16
Striped Ravioli, 1 cup	340	20	31
Vegetable Lasagna, 1 cup	220	7	29

GardenBurger (Vegetarian)

	C	F	Cb
Meals: BBQ Chicken, 1 patty/sce	250	8	30
Citrus Glazed Chicken w. Rice	220	2	29
Herb Crusted Chicken Patty (1)	170	9	12
Flame Grilled Chicken, 1 patty	100	2.5	5
Herb Grilled Chicken w. Vege.	220	5	16
Meatballs (Soy), 6 balls, 3 oz	110	4.5	8
Meatballs w. Penne Marinara	300	4.5	31
Meatloaf, 1 slice w. gravy	130	3.5	12
Meatloaf w. Broc. & Red Peppers	180	4.5	19
Riblets, 1 riblet + sauce	160	5	11
Southwestern Chicken w. Vege.	210	1.5	26
Burgers: Per 2½ oz Patty			
Original Burger; Black Bean, avg	90	2	6
Flame Grilled, Homestyle Classic, avg.	110	5	6
Garden Vegan	100	1	12
Other varieties, average	100	3	1

Gorton's

	C	F	Cb
Fish Fillets: Beer Batter (1)	115	7	9
Crispy Battered (1)	130	8.5	8.5
Crunchy Golden (Breaded) (1)	120	6	12
Grilled, average all flavors (1)	100	3	1
Grilled Salmon, average (1)	100	3.5	1
Fish Sticks, Breaded, 6, 3 oz	250	14	20
Grilled Fillet Meal: Alfredo	160	3	14
Lemon & Herb Butter	240	3.5	34
Popcorn Shrimp, 20 shrimp, 3 oz	240	12	24
Shrimp Bowl: Alfredo, 1 bowl	250	5	39
Fried Rice, 1 bowl	350	2.5	68
Garlic Butter, 1 bowl	260	6	38
Primavera, 1 bowl	270	6	41
Teriyaki, 1 bowl	320	6	57
Tenders: Extra Crunchy, 3½ pcs	260	12	29
Original, 3½ pieces, 4 oz	270	15	25

Green Giant

Create A Meal: *Prepared with Meat & Oil (Prepared Wt. ~ Approx 10 oz)*

	C	F	Cb
Oven Rstd: Garlic Chkn, 1¾ cup	350	9	35
Parmesan Herb Chicken, 1¾ c.	340	11	29
Stir Fry: Lo Mein, 1¼ cup	330	9	34
Szechuan, 1¼ cup	330	5	15
Teriyaki, 1¼ cup	210	9	12

Complete Skillet: *Per 1¼ Cup (Prep.)*

	C	F	Cb
Beef Stew	180	3.5	27
Chicken Alfredo/& Cheesy Pasta	270	7	39
Chicken Lo Mein	200	2.5	30
Chicken Noodle, 1¼ cups	320	6	45
Chicken Teriyaki, 1½ cups	250	1.5	45
Garlic Chicken & Pasta, 1 cup	260	7	31
Steak Teriyaki, 1½ cups	300	3.5	53

Pasta Accents: *Per Serving (Cooked)*

	C	F	Cb
Broccoli & Alfredo Sce, 2½ cups	210	4	34
Creamy Cheddar, 1 cup	250	11	33
Garlic, 1 cup	240	10	31
Pasta Broccoli Carrots, avg., 1 cup	210	5	34

Healthy Choice

Mixed Grills: *Per Serving*

	C	F	Cb
Chicken: w. BBQ/Honey Mustard	360	5	49
w. Roasted Garlic Tomato Sce	410	9	47
Steak: w. Teriyaki Dipping Sce	490	10	74
w. Zesty Dipping Sce	340	10	37

Entrees/Familiar Favorites: *Per Meal*

	C	F	Cb
Cheesy Rice & Chicken	230	4	33
Chicken Enchilada	360	7	59
Lasagna Bake	270	6	36
Macaroni & Cheese	270	6	40
Roast Turkey Breast	230	6	25

Healthy Choice (Cont)

	C	F	Cb
Dinners: Beef Pot Roast	320	9	39
Beef Tips Portabello	280	8	28
Chicken Enchilada; Meatloaf	310	2.5	46
Chicken Parmigiana	320	9	40
Chicken Teriyaki w. Rice	270	6	37
Lemon Pepper Fish	280	5	49
Roasted Chicken Breast	280	8	32
Salisbury Steak	360	9	45
Sweet & Sour Chicken	340	7	54
Flavor Adventures: Beef Merlot	240	8	26
Chicken Tuscany	330	9	42
Grilled Chicken Caesar	240	7	42
Oriental Style Beef	300	9	27

Home Bistro

Meals (Low Carb): *Per Package*

	C	F	Cb
Beef Stir Fry	400	17	15
Blackened Chkn in Champagne Sce	560	32	8
Chicken Stir Fry	310	7	15
Filet Mignon w. Bearnise Sauce	870	73	14
French Toast Breakfast	720	59	28
Grilled Chkn Brst in Caper Parmesan	480	31	7
Grilled Chicken Satay	640	40	20
Poached Salmon Fillet in Sauce	580	44	10
Pork Lion in Red Curry Sauce	580	39	13
Roasted Crab Cakes w. Sauce	540	43	10
Roasted Rack of Lamb w. Sauce	700	41	16
Roasted Turkey Breast w. Stuffing	440	20	19
Sea Scallops in Chili Hollandaise Sce	590	31	51
Shrimp Scampi	710	44	49
Szechuan Beef	390	21	8
Western Omelette w. Sausage	660	57	9

Hot Pockets

	C	F	Cb
Breakfast Pastries: Ham, Egg & Chse	150	7	17
Sausage, Egg & Cheese	170	9	18
Fruit Pastries: Apple/Strawb., avg.	250	9	39
Cream Cheese & Strawb. w. Icing	240	10	34
Pizza Mini's, avg., 5 pces, 3 oz	240	12	29

Sandwiches: *Per Serving (4.5 oz)*

	C	F	Cb
Barbecue Sce with Beef; Italian	340	12	47
Chicken Melt with Bacon	350	17	39
Four Cheese Pizza (no meat)	390	20	44
Pepperoni Pizza	360	17	44
Steak Fajita	260	7	39
Other varieties, average	310	13	36

Hot Pocket Subs: *Per Sub (5.6 oz)*

	C	F	Cb
Ham & Cheese	360	10	49
Meatballs & Mozzarella	390	14	45
Other varieties, average	410	16	49
Pot Pie Express: Turkey, 1 pce	340	18	35
Other varieties, average, 1 pce	350	17	40

Impromptu Gourmet (Schwan's)

Entrees:	C	F	Cb
Choice Beef Filet Mignon	620	50	0
Choice Beef Rib Eye Steak, 10 oz	360	31	0
French Cut Rack of Pork, 4 oz	150	9	1
Fully Cooked Cajun Turkey, 3 oz	140	7	2
Gourmet Chkn Wellington, 8 oz	420	18	13
New York Strip, 10 oz	660	48	0
Orange Ginger Mahi Mahi, 7 oz	240	6	9
Prime Rib Roast, 12 oz	840	68	2
Spiral Sliced Ham, 3 oz	150	7	7
Stuffed Chkn Breast Saltimbocca	330	14	3
T-Bone Steak, 16 oz	250	18	0

José Olé

Breakfast Burrito	C	F	Cb
Egg, Sausage & Cheese, 4 oz	270	11	34
Egg, Ham & Cheese, 4 oz	260	9	34
Taquitos: Chicken in Corn, 3 pces	190	9	21
Shredded Beef, 3 pces	180	9	20
Mexi-Minis: Beef & Chse Tacos (4)	200	11	18
Chimichangas, 3 pces	230	11	25
Taquitos, 4 pces	190	9	20
Quesadillas, 3 pces	220	8	28
Burrito: Beef & Cheese (1)	300	10	39
Chicken Monterey (1)	300	7	46
Chimichanga: Beef, 1 pce	380	17	42
Chicken , 1 pce	340	12	45

Kid Cuisine

	C	F	Cb
Cheese Pizza Painter	320	6	53
Chicken Nuggets	500	18	66
Fun Nuggets	400	16	51
Macaroni & Cheese	420	15	58
Pepperoni Pizza	460	20	57
Taco Roll-Up, 7.35 oz	380	13	51

Kroger

	C	F	Cb
Rice Bowls: Alfredo, 10.5 oz	320	7	41
Teriyaki, 10.5 oz	320	2	59
Garlic Butter, 10.5 oz	330	8	47
Stir Fry: Beef Stir Fry, 1¾ cup	180	4	26
Calamari Rings (13)	230	14	18
Chicken Stir Fry, 1½ cup	200	2	30
Chicken Alfredo, 1¾ cup	270	9	30
Coconut Shrimps (5) w. Sauce	360	22	30
Fish Sticks (5)	270	14	26
Garlic Herb & Shrimp Scampi, 1 c.	80	2.5	2
Grilled Fillet varieties, avg., 1 pce	100	3	1
Jumbo Butterfly Shrimp (4)	210	10	22
Popcorn Shrimp (19)	200	11	16
Salmon Cakes, 1 cake/patty	140	6	7
Swedish Style Meatballs (6)	250	18	7

Lean Cuisine

Cafe Classics Bowls: Per Bowl	C	F	Cb
Beef Portabello	260	4	38
Bow Tie Pasta & Chicken	240	4.5	33
Chicken Teriyaki	320	3	58
Garlic Beef & Broccoli	170	6	16
Grilled Chicken Caesar	270	7	32
Sweet & Sour Chicken	290	2.5	51
Thai Style Chicken	230	4	30
Three Cheese Stuffed Rigatoni	260	7	38
Comfort Classics: Per Bowl			
Baked Chicken	230	4.5	32
Cheese Lasagna w. Chicken	285	8	36
Honey Roasted Pork	230	9	18
Meatloaf & Whipped Potato	280	9	29
Roasted Turkey Breast	270	2.5	51
Salisbury Steak	280	8	26
Dinnertime Selects: Per Meal			
Beef Steak Tips Dijon	330	8	44
Grilled Chicken & Penne Pasta	320	4.5	52
Salisbury Steak	270	8	27
One Dish Favorites: Rstd Chicken	250	6	32
Angel Hair Pasta	260	4	48
Chicken Enchilada	280	5	49
Lasagna w. Meat Sauce	310	7	43
Macaroni & Cheese	300	7	43
Santa Fe Rice & Beans	390	5	50
Stuffed Cabbage	200	6	26
Swedish Meatballs	290	8	33
Teriyaki Stir-Fry	300	4.5	49
Skillets: Chkn Alfredo	180	4	25
Chicken Primavera	180	2.5	28
Garlic Chicken	240	4	40
Herb Chicken & Roasted Potatoes	170	3	24
Spa Cuisine: Chicken Pecan	260	6	34
Pork w. Cherry Sauce	260	5	38
Salmon w. Basil	260	8	31

Lean Pockets

Per Piece	C	F	Cb
BBQ Sauce w. Beef	290	7	47
Cheeseburger; Chicken Parmigiana	280	7	43
Ham & Cheddar, 1 pce	280	7	40
Meatballs & Mozzarella	280	7	43
Pepperoni/Saus. & Pepperoni Pizza	280	7	42
Philly Steak & Cheese, 1 pce	280	7	40
Steak Fajita	240	7	22
Turkey/Broccoli/Cheese	270	7	39
Lean Pockets Subs, average	310	7	44
Lean Pockets Ultra, 4 oz	200	6	19

Marie Callender's

	C	F	Cb
Complete Dinners: *Per Serving*			
Beef Stroganoff	410	16	39
Beef Tips in Mushroom Sce, 13.6 oz	360	12	35
Chicken Cordon Bleu, 1 dinner	520	24	40
Chicken Fried Beef Steak	640	38	55
Chicken Parmigiana, 1 dinner	670	34	60
Country Fried Chick. & Gvy, 1 din.	670	37	58
Fish w. Mac & Cheese	450	18	44
Grilled Chkn & Mashed Pot., 15 oz	480	26	28
Ham Steak w. Macar. & Chse, 1 din.	410	13	43
Herb Rstd Chicken & Mashed Pot.	530	35	20
Meatloaf & Gravy w. Mashed Pot.	560	31	39
Pork Chop, 1 dinner	590	33	50
Roast Beef w. Mashed Potato	430	22	31
Salisbury Steak & Gravy, 14 oz	490	23	40
Sweet & Sour Chicken, 1 dinner	620	20	90
Pot Pies: Beef	510	32	40
Chicken Au Gratin, 1 cup	510	31	43
Turkey, 1 cup	510	31	43
One Dish Classics: Cheese Ravioli	590	20	80
Cheesy Chicken Breast & Rice	480	18	47
Chicken and Rice w. Broccolo	440	14	47
Chili Cornbread, 16 oz	495	21	49
Country Beef Stew w. Cornbread	440	16	52
Fettucini Alfredo, 14 oz	880	51	82
Grilled Chicken Breast w. Pasta	570	25	55
Macaroni & Cheese, 8 oz	370	18	36
Meat Lasagna, 8 oz	240	9	24
Swedish Meatballs, 14 oz	580	30	48
Tuna & Noodles, 14 oz	605	35	46
Turkey Breast Medallions w. Pasta	630	32	58

Michael Angelos

	C	F	Cb
Entrees: Chicken Parmesan	260	10	25
Eggplant Parmesan, 6 oz	285	19	23
Fettuccine Alfredo	280	8	40
Manicotti w. Sauce	230	12	11
Saus. & Pepper & Onion	490	16	64
Spaghetti & Meatballs, 15.25 oz	500	15	67
Bowls: Angel Hair & Shrimp, 6 oz	200	6	28
Angel Hair Pasta Pomodoro, 7 oz	200	5	34
Chicken Milano Pasta, 6 oz	290	11	30
Chkn Rosemary Pasta; Saus., 6 oz	250	8	30
Lasagna: Chicken, 8 oz	290	7	37
Four Cheese, 8 oz	400	22	28
Meat Lasagna/Sausage, 8 oz	440	25	24
Vegetable, 8 oz	230	7	23
Snacks: Four Chse Calzone (1)	360	13	50
Meatball Calzone (1), 5 oz	390	15	45
Mini Calzone (1), avg. 0.7 oz	60	2.5	8

Morningstar Farms

	C	F	Cb
Breakfast Pattie, 1 patty	80	3	4
Burgers: *Made with Organic Soy*			
Classic Burger	150	7	10
Tex Mex Burger	120	1.5	17
Vegan Burger	100	3	8
Veggie Medley	120	4	11
Zesty Tomato Bassil Burger	130	6	7
Thai Burger	100	3.5	7
Poultry: *Made with Organic Soy*			
Okara Pattie	120	5	6
Roasted Herb Chicken	110	2.5	9
Veggie Corn Dogs (1)	170	6	22
Entrees: Lentil Rice Loaf, 1" slice	160	7	16
Nine Bean Loaf, 1" slice	150	7	15

Ore-Ida

	C	F	Cb
Bagel Bites: *Per 4 Pieces (3 oz)*			
Three Cheese, 4 pieces	200	6	28
Cheese, Sausage, Pepperoni	200	6	29
Spicy Nacho; Nacho Cheese	240	10	26

Quorn (Vegetarian)

	C	F	Cb
Turkey Style Roast, 3 oz	90	2.5	8
Garlic & Herb Ckn-Style Cutlets (1)	200	8	20
Nuggets, 3-4 pieces, 3 oz	180	8	18
Patties (1), 2.6 oz	160	7	12
Tenders, 1 cup, 3 oz	90	2	8
Meat-free Dogs (1), 1.5 oz	70	4	3
Meat-free Links (2), 1.6 oz	70	3	2
Meat-free Meatballs (4), 2.4 oz	110	3	7
Naked Cutlets (1), 2.4 oz	80	2.5	5

Rosina/Celentano

	C	F	Cb
Entree: *Per Serving*			
Cheese Ravioli, 4 pces	260	6	40
Eggplant Parmigiana, 10 oz	390	28	24
Eggplant Rolletts, 10 oz	340	17	36
Manicotti, 7 oz	350	11	43
Ravioli Stuffed Cheese, Mini, 4 oz	200	3.5	31
Stuffed Shell: 6.5 oz	320	12	36
Light Broccoli, 10 oz	250	4	39

Frozen Entrees & Meals (Cont)

Safeway Select

	C	F	Cb
Gourmet Club Meals: *Per Serving*			
Enchiladas	180	12	13
Chicken Nuggets, 6 pces	210	12	10
Chicken Strips	230	13	11
Low Fat Turkey Lasagna	300	3	48
Macaroni & Cheese	350	18	30
Meat Lasagna, 10.5 oz	400	14	43
Meatloaf	180	9	9
Mexican Style Lasagna	390	22	26
Scalloped Potatoes, ²/₃ cup	250	16	20
Tamale Bake, 1 cup	290	16	25
6 Vegetable Lasagna, 1 cup	310	17	27
Stir Fry: Chicken Fajita	130	3	14
Shrimp & Vegetable	120	0	20
Teriyaki Beef	170	4	24
Gourmet Club Eating Right: *Per ½ Package*			
Burgundy Beef Stew	250	9	38
Chicken Penne Pasta	280	8	34
Chicken Tamales Verde	220	9	25
Creamy Broccoli Beef	290	7	40
Ginger Chicken	350	6	49
Meatloaf Dinner	230	6	31
Orange Glazed Chicken	350	5	56

SeaPak

	C	F	Cb
Coconut Shrimp, 4 pces	270	17	19
Jumbo Butterfly Shrimp, 4 pces	200	9	20
Popcorn Shrimp, 15 pces, 3 oz	240	11	25
Shrimp Scampi, 8 pces	350	32	4

Seeds of Change

Per Bowl (11 oz)

	C	F	Cb
Bowtie Primavera	380	12	51
Creamy Spinach Lasagna	370	16	36
Macaroni & Cheese	420	16	52
Mushroom Wild Pilaf	350	16	40
Penne Marinara	290	7	44
Seven Grain Pilaf	390	14	52
Spicy Peanut Noodles	370	12	53
Teriyaki Stir-Fried Rice	340	8	56

Stouffer's

	C	F	Cb
Entrees: Stroganoff, 9.75 oz	380	17	34
Creamed Chipped Beef	140	8	9
Grilled Teriyaki Chicken	300	3.5	45
Chicken a la King	370	12	45
Cheesy Spaghetti Bake	500	25	45
Lasagna w. Meat Sce, 10½ oz	350	11	38
Macaroni & Beef w. Tomatoes	360	13	39
Macaroni & Cheese, 1 cup, 8 oz	320	15	32
Maxaroni, Macaroni & Cheese	395	17	44
Spaghetti w. Meat Sauce	340	12	44
Stuffed Pepper, 10 oz	230	9	25
Swedish Meatballs w. Pasta	570	33	39
Tuna Noodle Casserole	370	17	35
Turkey Tetrazzini	370	18	32
Family Style Recipes: *Per Serving*			
Grandma's Chkn & Vege Bake	360	15	36
Lasagna w. Meat Sce, ¹/₁₂ pkg	310	13	27
Macaroni & Cheese, 1 cup	320	15	32
Italian Style: 3 Cheese Manicotti	335	13	39
Cheese Stuffed Rigatoni, 8.2 oz	460	20	52
Italian Sausage Stuffed Rigatoni	380	14	46
Roasted Chicken Ravioli, 8.2 oz	370	14	42
Homestyle Dinners: *Per Serving*			
Chicken Fettucini, 16.75 oz	620	24	69
Country Fried Beef Steak, 16 oz	520	33	52
Grilled Lime Chicken, 14 oz	490	14	66
Meatloaf, 17 oz	590	32	43
Monterey Chicken, 14.25 oz	570	20	70
Roast Turkey Breast, 16 oz	440	16	52
Salisbury Steak, 16 oz	470	16	49
Homestyle Dinners: *Per Serving*			
Breaded Boneless Pork Cutlet	370	20	33
Fish Fillet w. Mac Cheese, 9 oz	430	18	47
Roasted Pork, 9.5 oz	400	18	46
Skillets: *Per Bowl*			
Homestyle Beef	360	14	37
Teriyaki Chicken, 12.5 oz	310	4.5	44

 For full nutritional data and product updates check the food database of the author's website www.CalorieKing.com

Swanson

	C	F	Cb
Standard Meal: Salisbury Steak	380	20	24
Boneless White Meat Fr. Chkn	520	22	75
Breaded Fish fillet, 10 oz	400	15	51
Chicken Strips w. Fries	610	28	75
Chicken Teriyaki (Standard)	340	7	49
Classic Fried Chicken, 11½ oz	720	37	72
Grilled Glazed Turkey Medallions	380	11	45
Macaroni & Cheese: Alfredo, 6 oz	210	3	39
Traditional Cheddar, 6 oz	200	7	25
White Cheddar, 6 oz	210	3.5	38
Turkey Breast w. Stuffing & Gravy	430	17	50
White Meat Chicken w. Penne	310	11	31
Hungry Man Dinners: Mexican	690	27	87
Boneless Pork Rib	840	39	99
Boneless White Meat Fried Chkn	710	29	86
Buffalo Chicken Strips	870	28	106
Classic Fried Chicken	790	40	75
Grilled Chicken w. Cheese Sauce	590	24	56
Hearty Breakfast	450	27	35
Hearty Meatball Lasagne Bake	530	26	49
Meatloaf Angus Beef	850	43	87
Mexican Style Fiesta	780	33	96
Rotisserie Chicken	440	16	38
Salisbury Steak	490	18	54
Turkey Breast	520	15	66
Hungry Man XXL: Backyard BBQ	1160	48	110
Roasted Carved Turkey Dinner	820	36	84
Southern Fried Boneless Chicken	760	16	84
Sports Grill: American Classic	1110	66	93
Beer Battered Chicken & Fries	660	26	64
Chicken Quesadilla & Potato Skins	765	35	72
Pulled Pork w. BBQ Sauce			
in Flatbrd & Cheese Fries, 16 oz	810	44	90
Beer Battered Chicken & Chse Fries	790	40	60
Popcorn Fish & Chips	910	50	96
Steak House: *Per Serving (20 oz)*			
Grilled: BBQ Chicken	600	23	80
Beef Steak Strips	460	25	16
Smothered Chicken	595	24	56
Pot Pies: Flaky Crust Chicken/Turkey	320	17	31

Trader Joe's

	C	F	Cb
Quiche: Broccoli & Cheddar, 6 oz	490	33	33
Mexicaine, 6 oz	510	36	29
Spinach & Mushroom, 6 oz	470	30	32

For Complete Nutritional Data ~ see CalorieKing.com

TGI Friday's

	C	F	Cb
Buffalo Wings (3)	175	13	2
Honey BBQ Wings (3)	190	12	5
Mozzarella Sticks & Sce, 1 Serve	130	6	10
Popcorn Chicken, 3 pces, 2.6 oz	160	6	17
Potato Skins, Ched. & Bacon, 3 pces	210	12	20
Snack Chips, average, 16 pces, 1 oz	150	9	16
Quesadilla Rolls: Chicken (2)	260	12	27
Steak (2)	200	8	23
Sides: Spinach Dip, , 2 Tbsp (1 oz)	50	3.5	2

Tyson

	C	F	Cb
Buffalo Hot Wings, 4 pieces	220	15	1
Chicken Bites, 13 pieces	270	18	15
Chicken Breast Fillets, breaded (1)	240	9	20
Chicken Breast Nuggets, 5 pieces	280	16	21
Chicken Breast Strips, 3 oz	120	3.5	1
Chicken Breast Tenderloins, 1 pces	150	7	12
Country Fried Steak, 1 piece	310	23	15
Crispy Chicken Strips, 2 pces	200	10	13
Fajita Style Chicken Strips, 3 oz	110	4	1
Honey Barbecue Wings, 3 pces	250	13	15
Honey Chicken Brst Tenders, 5 pces	220	13	13
Popcorn Chicken, 9 pces	230	11	21
Pork Pattie Fritters, 1 piece	260	16	17
Southern Style Chkn Brst Patties (1)	240	18	10
Southern Style Chkn Brst Strips, 3 oz	110	3	2
Steak Fingers, 2 pces	250	18	14
Meal Kits: Beef/Chicken Fajita (1)	140	4	17
Chicken Fajita (1)	130	3.5	17
Chicken Fried Rice, 2½ cups	440	6	69
Chicken Quesadilla (1)	250	10	26
Chicken Stir Fry, 2¾ cups	430	4.5	73

Uncle Ben's

	C	F	Cb
Pasta Bowls: *Per Bowl (12 oz)*			
4-Cheese Lasagna	330	7	41
Chicken Fettuccini Alfredo	350	7	47
Parmesan Shrimp Penne, 12 oz	380	7	58
Savory Portabhole Mushroom	280	4.5	43
Thai Style Chicken	400	8	60
Rice Bowls: Roasted Chicken Vege	360	4.5	56
Broccoli, Cheese & Ham	420	12	56
Chicken Fried Rice	410	7	65
Chicken Stir Fry	360	4	58
Spicy Beef & Broccoli	370	4.5	62
Sweet & Sour Chicken	360	3	65
Teriyaki Chicken	400	3.5	66
Teriyaki Stir Fry Vegetable	355	3	74

Frozen Entrees & Meals (Cont)

Van De Kamp's

	C	F	Cb
Butterfly Shrimp, 7 pces, 4 oz	300	15	30
Crispy Battered Halibut, 3 fillets	240	12	22
Crispy Fish Tenders, 4 pces, 4 oz	260	14	23
Crispy Fish Portions, 1 pce	150	8	14
Popcorn Shrimp, 20 pces, 4 oz	270	12	30
Fish Sticks, Breaded, 6 stix, 4 oz	240	12	20
Battered Fillets, 2.6 oz fillet	130	6	11
Crispy Fish Fillets, 1 pce, 2.6 oz	130	7	10
Crisp & Healthy, Breaded (2), 1.8 oz	170	2.5	25

Weight Watchers

Smart Ones: *Per Meal*

	C	F	Cb
3 Cheese Ziti Marinara	290	7	47
Fettucini Alfredo w. Broc., 9.25 oz	270	6	39
Fiesta Chicken, 8.5 oz	210	2	35
Lasagna Bolognese	240	2.5	43
Lasagna Florentine, 10.5 oz	290	8	36
Lemon Herb Chicken Piccata	250	5	36
Mac & Cheese	240	2.5	45
Radiatore Romano	280	8	40
Ravioli Florentine, 8.5 oz	220	5	34
Salisbury Steak	260	6	25
Santa Fe Style Rice & Beans, 10 oz	300	8	49
Southwestern Style Chkn Bowl	230	3.5	32
Spaghetti Bolognese	280	5	43
Spaghetti Marinara, 9 oz	280	7	46
Spicy Szechuan Veg. & Chicken	220	5	34
Swedish Meatballs, 9 oz	280	7	34
Three Cheese Macaroni	290	7	45
Tuna Noodle Gratin	270	7	38
Smartwiches: Avg., all varieties	270	7	38

Smart Ones Bistro Selections:

	C	F	Cb
Basil Chicken	270	6	34
Chicken Parmesan	300	5	32
Chicken Tenderloins w. BBQ Sce	300	8	30
Fire-Grilled Chkn & Vegetables	280	3.5	45
Golden Baked Garlic Chicken	270	5	42
Meat Loaf w. Gravy & Potatoes	260	8	22
Peppercorn Beef Fillet	230	8	24
Roast Beef w. Gravy	220	7	19
Roast Chicken w. Sour Crm & Chives	190	3.5	23
Slow Roasted Turkey Breast	220	8	18
Thai Style Chkn & Rice Noodles	290	4	39

Weight Watchers (Cont)

	C	F	Cb
Truth About Carbs: *Per Package (9 oz)*			
Chicken Marsala w. Broccoli	180	7	12
Creamy Chicken Tuscan	180	8	9
Creamy Parmesan Chicken	210	8	12
Grilled Chicken in Garlic Sce	190	8	9
Sirloin Beef & Asian Style Vege	160	4	11
Turkey Medallions w. Gravy	200	4	10
For Complete Nutritional Data ~ see CalorieKing.com			

White Castle

	C	F	Cb
Cheese Burger, Microwaveable, 1 pkg, 3.7 oz	310	17	23
Hamburgers, 1 pkg (2 s'wiches)	270	14	23

Worthington/Loma Linda

	C	F	Cb
Bolono, 3 slices, 2 oz	80	3	3
Chik-Nuggets, 5 pieces	250	15	14
Chicken Roll, 3/8 slices, 1.9 oz	90	4.5	2
Chicken Slices, 3 slices, 2 oz	90	4.5	2
ChikSticks, 1 pce, 1.6 oz	100	6	4
Corn Dogs (1)	150	4	22
Corned Beef Slices, 3 slices, 2 oz	140	9	5
Crispy Chik Patties (1), 2.5 oz pattie	150	6	16
Dinner Roast ¾" slice	180	11	6
Fillets, 2 pieces, 2.9 oz	180	9	8
Fried Chik'n w. Gravy, 2 pieces	150	10	5
FriPats, 1 pattie, 2.25 oz	130	6	5
Golden Croquettes, 4 pieces, 2.9 oz	210	11	14
Leanies, 1 link, 1.4 oz	100	7	2
Meatless Smoked Beef, 3 slices	130	7	7
Prosage: Links, 2 links, 1.6 oz	80	3	3
Patties, 1.3 oz Pattie	80	3	3
Salami, 3 slices, 2 oz	120	7	3
Smkd Turkey Slices, 3 slices	140	9	4
Stakelets, 2.5 oz piece	150	7	7
Stripples, 2 slices	60	4.5	2
Swiss Steak, 1 piece	130	6	9
Tuno tuna substitute ½ cup	90	6	3
Wham Vege Slices, 2 slices	110	7	3

Zatarain's

	C	F	Cb
Blackened Chicken Alfredo, 10.5 oz	535	30	44
Jambalaya seasoned w. Chicken w. Sausage	360	8	53
	390	12	58
Red Beans & Rice w. Sausage	565	19	76

Frozen Pizzas	C	F	Cb
Amy's: *Per ⅓ Pizza*			
Cheese; Spinach; Pesto, avg.	310	12	38
Cheese Pesto (Whole Wheat Crust)	360	18	37
Cheese Pizza (Rice Crust) ½ pizza	300	14	31
Mushroom & Olive	250	9	33
Roasted Vegetable	260	9	42
California Pizza Kitchen			
Large: Five Cheese & Tomato, ⅙	320	15	29
BBQ Chicken, ⅛ pizza	290	9	33
Small: BBQ/Jamaican/Thai Chkn, ⅓	290	10	33
Five Cheese & Tomato , ⅓	320	15	29
Chse & Pesto (Wheat Crust), ⅓	360	18	37
Celeste			
Pizza For One: Cheese, 1 pizza	360	14	42
Deluxe; Pepperoni	410	21	42
Original Four Cheese	400	18	41
Sausage & Pepperoni; Suprema	470	26	44
Zesty Chicken Supreme	340	15	39
Di Giorno			
Rising Crust (Large): *Per ⅙ Pizza*			
Four Cheese	320	11	39
Pepperoni; 3 Meat	360	15	40
Spicy Chicken Supreme	310	10	40
Spinach, Mushr. & Garlic; Vege	300	9	41
Supreme	360	15	41
Rising Crust (Small): *Per ⅓ Pizza*			
Four Cheese; Spicy Chkn Supreme	270	9	34
Saus. & Pepperoni; 3 Meat, avg.	320	14	35
Spinach, Mushr. & Garlic; Vege	260	8	36
Supreme	320	14	36
Deep Dish: Three Meat, ⅛ pizza	300	16	25
Supreme, ⅙ pizza	320	15	33
Pepperoni, ⅙ pizza	340	18	32
Cheese Stuffed Crust: Supreme, ⅛	300	14	30
Pepperoni, ⅓ pizza	370	16	40
Half & Half: *Per ⅙ Large Pizza*			
Supreme/Pepperoni: Supreme	360	15	40
Pepperoni	370	16	41
Supreme/Cheese: Supreme	390	18	41
Cheese	320	11	41
Pepperoni/Cheese: Pepperoni	390	18	40
Cheese	310	11	40
Microwave: 3 Meat, ½ pizza	420	19	44
4 Cheese, ½ pizza	340	12	43
Pepperoni; Supreme, avg., ½	375	16	44
Thin Crispy Crust: *Per ⅓ Large Pizza*			
Four Meat	310	13	32
Pepperoni; Supreme, avg.	340	14	38
Four Cheese	300	11	34

	C	F	Cb
Essensia (Albertson's):			
Cheese, ⅙ pizza	320	11	42
3 Meat; Pepperoni, ⅙ pizza	360	15	40
Supreme, ⅙ pizza	210	11	31
Freschetta			
Bake & Rise (Large): 4 Cheese, ⅕	370	13	44
4 Meat, ⅙ pizza	350	15	40
Pepperoni, ⅙ pizza	350	15	37
Special Delux, ⅙ pizza	370	16	40
Supreme, ⅙ pizza	350	15	38
Vegetable Primavera, ⅙ pizza	310	11	40
Brick Oven 8": BBQ Chicken, ⅓ pizza	290	13	30
Ham & Mushroom, ½ pizza	325	11	39
Potato, Bacon & Cheese, ½ pizza	395	17	43
Thai Chicken, ⅓ pizza	300	14	27
Italian Style Pepperoni, ¼ pizza	400	20	36
Sauce Stuffed Crust: 4 Chse, ⅕ pizza	340	12	43
Sausage & Pepperoni, ⅕ pizza	370	16	43
Supreme, ⅕ pizza	360	15	42
Grilled Vege, ⅙ pizza	330	13	37
Small Pizzas: Pepperoni, ½ pizza	460	19	56
Rstd Garlic Chicken, ½ pizza	370	12	49
Mozzarella & Basil, ½ pizza	370	15	46
Southwest Chkn Supreme, ½ pizza	350	12	47
Healthy Choice: *Per Pizza*			
French Bread Pizza: Cheese	360	5	57
Pepperoni	360	5	56
Supreme	330	5	51
Vegetable	320	5	50
Jeno's: *Per Pizza*			
Crispy & Tasty: Cheese	460	21	51
Pepperoni; Supreme; Comb.	520	28	50
Three Meat	490	25	49
Heaven's Bistro: *Per ⅓ Pizza*			
Chicken w. BBQ Sauce	270	2	48
Grilled Vegetable	230	1	42
Other varieties, avg.	240	2	42

Frozen Pizzas (Cont)

Lean Cuisine	C	F	Cb
French Bread Pizza: Cheese, 6 oz	320	7	47
Deluxe, 6 oz	310	9	44
Pepperoni, 6 oz	300	7	44
Casual Eating: Deluxe, 6 oz	370	9	55
Four Cheese, 6 oz	400	9	59
Margharita, 6 oz	320	9	48
Roasted Vegetable, 6 oz	330	5	58
Pizza Fit 'n Free			
7" Pizza, 6 oz	210	0	28
Ralph's			
Pizza Pals: Taco Supreme, 5 oz	380	12	47
Cheeseburger, 6.1 oz	450	16	57
Hamburger, 6.5 oz	410	12	57
Small: Cheese, 1 pizza	410	11	58
Combination, 1 pizza	460	17	58
Pepperoni, 1 pizza	460	17	58
Red Baron			
Classic (Large): 4 Cheese, ¼ pizza	410	19	40
Pepperoni, ⅕ pizza	340	18	32
Sausage & Pepperoni, ⅕ pizza	360	21	29
Supreme, Special Deluxe, ⅕ pizza	350	18	32
Deep Dish Pan Style:			
4 Cheese, ⅓ pizza	370	17	39
Pepperoni; Meat Trio, avg., ⅓ pizza	400	20	41
Supreme, ⅓ pizza	420	21	41
Deep Dish Singles: 4 Cheese, 1	450	21	50
Pepperoni, 1 pizza	450	21	48
Cheese; Meat Trio, avg., 1 pizza	420	21	42
Special Deluxe, 1 pizza	430	24	40
Supreme, 1 pizza	410	18	49
French Bread Pizzas: Supreme (1)	370	15	43
5 Cheese & Garlic (1)	420	23	39
Pepperoni	360	15	40
Pizzeria Style, average, ⅓ pizza	380	16	40
Thin Crust: *Per ¼ Pizza*			
Mozzarella Tomato Basil	270	13	27
Five Cheese; Meat Trio, avg.	310	16	27
Pepperoni varieties, average	355	20	27
Reggio's			
Family Size: Cheese, ⅙ pizza	320	12	38
Sausage , ⅙ pizza	330	12	38
Dinner Size: Cheese, ¼ pizza	330	12	41
Pepperoni & Sausage, ¼ pizza	400	18	41
Sausage; Supreme, ¼, avg.	380	16	41
Stop & Shop			
Single Serving, Cheese, 1	390	19	42
9 Slices, Cheese, 2 slices	350	10	49

Stouffer's	C	F	Cb
French Bread Pizzas: Deluxe, 1 pce	420	19	49
Cheese, 1 piece (½ pkg)	380	16	43
Extra Cheese, 1 piece	400	16	49
Pepperoni, 1 piece	430	21	44
Tombstone			
Original Pizza, 12 inch: *Per Serving*			
BBQ Chicken, ¼ pizza	320	12	38
Extra Cheese, ¼ pizza	340	15	37
4-Meat, ⅕ pizza	310	15	30
Pepperoni, ⅕ pizza	380	19	36
Sausage & Pepperoni, ⅕ pizza	320	16	29
Supreme, ⅕ pizza	300	14	30
Half & Half Pepperoni & Cheese:			
Pepperoni, ¼ pizza	420	22	37
Cheese, ¼ pizza	340	15	37
Deep Dish: *Per ⅙ Package*			
Cheese; Pepperoni; Supreme, avg.	500	25	51
Brick Oven Style: Cheese, ⅓ pizza	350	15	38
Other varieties, average, ¼	315	16	30
Tony's			
Original: Cheese, ⅓ pizza	380	16	41
Pepperoni, ⅓ pizza	420	22	40
Sausage & Pepperoni, ⅓ pizza	440	22	42
Supreme, ⅓ pizza	420	22	39
Thin Crust: Cheese, ⅓ pizza	340	15	36
Sausage &/Pepperoni, ⅓ pizza	390	19	34
Supreme, ⅓ pizza	360	19	34
Deep Dish (Individual)**:** Cheese (1)	380	16	45
Pepperoni (1)	480	25	47
Totino's			
Crisp Crust Party Pizza: *Per ½ Pizza*			
Cheese	320	15	34
Pepperoni; Supreme	380	22	34
Verdi (Safeway Select)			
Self-Rising Crust (Large): *Per ⅙ Pizza*			
Meat Magnifico	350	15	41
4 Cheese	310	11	41
Other varieties, average	365	16	41
Self-Rising Crust (Small): *Per Serving*			
Margherita, ½ pizza	360	12	48
Primo Pepperoni, ⅓ pizza	300	13	32
Other varieties, average	240	7	34
Weight Watchers (Smart Ones): *Per Pizza*			
Deluxe, 6.6 oz	360	10	47
Four Cheese, 6.5 oz	330	8	49
Pepperoni, 7 oz	350	9	49
Spicy Sausage	350	9	48
Veggie Ultimate, 7.7 oz	340	7	50

Canned & Packaged Meals	C	F	Cb
Annies Homegrown: *Per Cup (Prepared)*			
Alfredo Chicken, 1 cup	330	8	30
Arthur Mac & Cheese	370	14	50
Beef Stroganoff	320	13	24
Cheeseburger Macaroni	350	13	27
Fettuccine Alfredo	270	8	43
Roasted Garlic & Herb Pasta	270	9	39
Shells & Cheddar	290	5	49
B & M: *Per ½ Cup (4½ oz)*			
Baked Beans: Original	170	2	30
Barbeque	210	1	42
Brown Raisin Bread, ½" slice, 2 oz	130	0.5	29
Banquet			
Homestyle Bakes: *Per Serving (Prepared)*			
Beef Stew & Biscuits, ⅔ cup	300	10	44
Cheesy Ham & Hashbrowns	290	15	30
Chicken & Dumplings, 7.8 oz	260	8	33
Chicken Alfredo w. Italian Bread	350	17	36
Country Chicken, Potato, Biscuits	370	15	50
Creamy Chkn & Biscuits, 7.4 oz	340	16	40
Tuna Mac & Cheese, 7.7 oz	420	20	44
Meal Toppers, Chicken flavor, ½ cup	50	1	8
Betty Crocker			
Casserole Potatoes, prep., avg.	150	5	22
Complete Meals: *Per Serving (⅕ Pkg)*			
Chicken & Buttermilk Biscuits	320	13	41
Chicken Fettuccini Alfredo	310	11	38
Ham & Au Gratin Potatoes	300	13	37
Homestyle Chkn & Dumplings	250	9	33
Italian Sausage	310	11	42
Stroganoff	230	5	34
Hamburger Helper: *Per Cup (Prep. As Directed)*			
Bacon Cheeseburger	380	18	33
Cheeseburger Macaroni; Taco	350	16	31
Cheesy Enchilada; Quesadilla	370	15	38
Cheesy Hashbrown	410	20	39
Chili Macaroni	290	11	28
Other varieties, average	320	15	27
Tuna Helper: *Per Serving (Prep. As Directed)*			
Creamy Parmesan	260	9	31
Other varieties, average	300	13	33
Chicken Helper: *Per Cup (Prep. As Directed)*			
Cheesy Chicken Enchilada	340	9	40
Chicken Fried Rice	250	9	23
Fettuccine Alfredo	270	8	27
Chicken Teriyaki	290	6	35
Mashed Potatoes: *Per Serving (Prepared)*			
Potato Buds, ⅓ cup	160	18	19
Other varieties, average, ½ cup	160	7	22

Betty Crocker (Cont)	C	F	Cb
Side Dishes/Caseroles: *Per Serving (Prepared)*			
Au Gratin; Cheesy Scalloped, ½ cup	150	6	21
Scalloped Potatoes, ⅔ cup	130	4	22
Three Cheese Potatoes, ½ cup	130	4	22
Deluxe Potatoes: *Per ½ Cup (Prepared)*			
Cheesy Cheddar Au Gratin	180	9	22
Loaded Au Gratin	140	4.5	23
Three Cheese Mashed Pot. Bake	190	10	24
Slow Cooker Helper: *Per Cup (Prepared)*			
Beef Stew, 1 cup	200	5	24
Beef Stroganoff	250	8	28
Pot Roast	290	12	27
Chicken & Dumpling	240	6	26
Suddenly Salad: *Prepared As Directred*			
Caesar, ½ cup dry	170	1	34
Classic, ⅔ cup	240	8	37
Ranch & Bacon, ¾ cup	330	20	31
Rstd Garlic & Parmesan, ¾ cup	260	11	33
Bowl Appetit: *Per Bowl*			
Pasta Alfredo	360	12	52
Three Cheese Rotini	360	10	56
Cheddar Broccoli Rice	290	7	51
Bush's Best: *Per ½ Cup*			
Chili Beans	120	1	20
Dark Red Kidney Beans, ½ cup	130	1	21
Frijoles Negras, ½ cup	100	0.5	20
Frijoles Pintos, ½ cup	110	0	19
Garbanzo Beans/Chick Peas, ½ c.	130	2	22
Refried Beans: Traditional	150	3	24
Fat Free	130	0	24
Baked Beans: Vegetarian	130	0	24
Other flavors, average	160	1	30
Campbell's: *Per Cup (8 fl.oz)*			
Chunky Chili: Roadhouse; Firehouse	220	8	25
Tantalizin Turkey	190	2	27
Pork & Beans in Tomato Sauce	140	1	27
Spaghetti O's Original	180	1	37
Spaghetti O's Meatballs	240	8	32
Sliced Franks	230	10	27
Supper Bakes: *Per ⅙ Box (Prepared As Directed)*			
Cheesy Chicken	180	4	28
Creamy Stroganoff	190	4	31
Garlic Chicken w. Pasta	230	1	44
Herb Chicken w. Rice	190	1	40
Lemon Chicken w. Rice	200	1	43
Savory Pork Chops	160	1	31
Southwestern Style Chicken	150	1	32
Trad. Roast Chicken w. Stuffing	160	3	29
CarbSense: *Per Package*			
Simple Suppers: Kathmandu Curry	210	12	15
Texas Style Chili	150	4	16

Canned & Packaged Meals (Cont)

Chef Boyardee	C	F	Cb
Beefaroni, all types, 1 cup	260	10	33
Deep Dish Meals: Per ⅙ Package			
Cheese Lover's Lasagna	370	16	47
5 Chse Ravioli; Cheesy Burger Mac	340	13	48
Pepperoni & Sausage Rotini	330	13	43
Mini Bites (14.5 oz Can): Per Cup			
Mini Beef Ravioli w. Meatballs	290	13	34
Mini Pasta Shells w. Meatballs	260	10	32
Mini Spaghetti w. Meatballs	270	10	32
Jumbo (15 oz Can): Per Cup			
99% Fat Free: Beef Ravioli	190	1.5	37
Cheese Ravioli	240	2.5	45
Lasagna	270	10	36
Mini Ravioli	240	7	35
Spaghetti w. Jumbo Meatballs	280	12	30
Overstuffed Ital. Sausage Ravioli	280	4	50
Microwaveable Bowls: Per Bowl			
Beef Ravioli	190	5	31
Macaroni & Cheese	190	6	28
Mini Bites Spaghetti Rings	220	8	29
Spaghetti & Meatballs	200	8	23
Rice w. Chicken/Vegetables	220	7	32
Twistaroni: Cheesy Nacho, 1 cup	230	6	36
Chili Cheese Dog, 1 cup	220	7	30
Tomato & Beef, 1 cup	250	6	40
Dennison's Chili (15 oz Can): Per Cup			
Chili Con Carne With Beans:			
Original; Hot, 1 cup	360	14	38
Chunky	300	10	32
99% Fat Free: Beef Chili w. Beans	210	2	29
Turkey Chili w. Beans	210	3	29
Dinty Moore (Hormel Foods)			
1½ lb Can: Beef Stew, 1 cup	180	8	17
7½ oz Can: Beef Stew, 1 cup	180	8	17
American Classics: Per Microwave Bowl (10 oz)			
Beef Stew	250	11	22
Noodles & Chicken	250	8	28
Microwave Cup: Beef Stew, 1 cup	160	7	16
Chicken & Dumplings	190	6	24
Other varieties, average	240	13	19
Dr. McDougall's: Per 10 oz			
Ramen Noodles	150	0.5	29
Rice & Pasta Pilaf	190	1	41
Eden Soy (Vegetarian): Per ½ Cup (4½ oz)			
Baked Beans w. Sorghum, Mustard	150	0	27
Black Eyed Peas	90	1	16
Black Soybeans	120	6	8
Refried Black/Pinto/Kid. Beans, avg.	90	2	15
Other varieties, average	125	0	21

Fantastic: Per Cup	C	F	Cb
3-Bean Chili	180	4	28
Spanish Paella	280	5	55
Tuscan Mushroom Risotto	210	1.5	50
Cup Meals: Cajun w. Red Beans	185	1.5	35
Bombay Curry w. Lentils	200	1.5	39
Broccoli & Cheddar	130	25	21
Spicy Jamaican w. Beans	195	1	39
Tex Mex w. Pinto	185	3	34
Rice Noodles: Pad Thai, 7.8 oz	400	11	59
Ginger Shiitake, 7.8 oz	340	10	58
Carb 'Tastic: Penne Alfredo	280	15	25
Vegetarian Chili Mac	290	18	19
Vegetarian Teriyaki	220	10	29
Other varieties, avg.	295	14	22
Farmhouse			
Pasta: Per ¾ Cup			
Chicken Pasta	400	15	54
Four Cheese Pasta	420	20	48
White Cheddar Pasta	370	13	52
Other varieties, average	450	21	53
Rice: Per ⅓ Cup			
Broccoli Au Gratin	200	2.5	40
Long Grain & Wild Herb Butter	200	2	42
Other varieties, average	190	1	41
French's Fried Onions			
Regular or Cheese:			
2 Tbsp, ¼ oz	45	3.5	3
¼ cup, ½ oz	90	7	6
1 cup, 2 oz	360	28	24
Health Valley (Vegetarian)			
Fat-Free Beans & Chili:			
Chili in a Cup, all types, ⅓ cup	120	1	21
Vegetarian/Chili, 1 cup	160	1	30
Turkey w. Chili Beans, 1 cup	220	3	34
Other varieties, ½ cup	80	0	15
Meal Cups, average all varieties	140	1	27
Heinz			
Vegetarian Beans, ½ cup	140	0.5	27

Eat at least
5 servings of fruit
and vegetables
every day . . . and
Enjoy Better Health!

Hormel: Per Cup	C	F	Cb
Kid's Kitchen: Beans & Wieners	320	13	37
Cheesy Mac 'N Cheese	270	11	32
Mini Beef Ravioli	240	7	34
Noodle Rings & Chicken	140	4	18
Chili (15 oz Can): Per Cup			
With Beans: Homestyle Chili	350	20	28
Reg./Hot/Chunky	270	7	34
Turkey (99% Fat Free)	200	3	26
Vegetarian (99% Fat Free)	200	1	38
Less Sodium Without Beans:			
Hot/Chili, 1 cup	210	9	17
Chunky No Beans	210	6	22
Turkey No Beans	190	3	17
Tamales (15 oz Can), 2 Tamales	140	7	15

Hungry Jack Potatoes
	C	F	Cb
Instant Potato Flakes, 1/3 cup	80	0	18

Hunt's
	C	F	Cb
Chilli Beans, 1/2 cup	90	1	17
Manwich Sloppy Joe, 1/4 cup	30	0	6

Ken & Robert's (Vegetarian)
	C	F	Cb
Veggie Burger	130	1	26
Veggie Pockets, average, 4.5 oz	250	8	39
Keto: Ketatoes Mix, all types,			
1/4 cup dry (makes 1/2 cup)	95	2	11

Kraft
	C	F	Cb
Minute White Rice, 3/4 cup	160	0	36
It's Pasta Anytime Meals: Per Package			
Fettuccine w. Classic Alfredo Sce	580	22	74
Dinners: Per Serving (Prepared As Directed)			
Macaroni & Cheese: Orig., 1/3 box	380	16	49
Scooby-Doo Spirals	390	20	47
Mac & Chse: Crazy Noodles, 1/2 box	390	18	49
Thick'n Creamy, 1/2 box	380	15	52
Easy Mac, avg. all varieties., 1 pch	240	6	40
Deluxe: Orig.; Sharp Chedd., 1/4 box	320	9	47
Rotini White Cheese Sce, 1/2 box	390	15	48
Velveeta Shells & Cheese, 1/3 box	360	12	49
Cheesy Potatoes: Per 1/2 Cup (Prep. As Directed)			
Au Gratin Potatoes	180	6	26
Bacon Scalloped Potatoes	190	7	26
Mashed Potatoes	200	12	20

La Choy
	C	F	Cb
Beef Chow Mein, 1 cup	80	1.5	10
Chicken Chow Mein, 1 cup	100	3	10
Beef Pepper Oriental, 1 cup	100	2	12
Chop Suey Vegetables, 1/2 cup	15	0	3
Chow Mein Noodles, 1/2 cup	140	6	19

Lipton Packet Meals	C	F	Cb
Asian Sides: Per Cup (Prepared As Directed)			
Beef Lo Mein; Thai Ses. Noodles	220	3.5	44
Teriyaki/Swt & Sour Noodles, avg.	260	2	50
Cajun Sides: Per Cup (Prepared)			
Garlic Butter Rice	310	9	49
New Orleans Style Chicken	290	9	51
Dirty Rice	300	6.5	50
Red Beans & Rice	340	6.5	62
Fiesta Sides: Per Cup (Prepared As Directed)			
Taco Rice	300	6	51
Smoked Chipotle Rice	310	7.5	55
Nacho Pasta	320	10	44
Pasta Sides: Per Cup (Prepared As Directed)			
Alfredo; Parmesan	320	12	43
Butter; Stroganoff	290	9	43
Rice Sides: Per Cup (Prepared)			
Cheddar Broccoli	310	7.5	50
Creamy Chicken	320	10	49
Herb & Butter	300	9	48
Other varieties, average	290	6	48

Maruchan
	C	F	Cb
Ramen Noodles: Per Serving			
Beef/Chicken/Shrimp Flavors,			
1/2 block, 1 1/2 oz	190	8	26
Noodles: Fat Fried Shrimp, 1 1/2 oz	170	6	26
Other Flavors, 1 1/2 oz	160	6	26
Fried Cup Beef, 1 packet, 2.2 oz	300	13	38
Low-Fat varieties, average, 2 oz	215	1.5	45

Morningstar Farms
	C	F	Cb
Kaffree Roma, 1 rounded tsp, 2g	10	0	2
Vegetarian Tuno, 1/3 cup, dr., 2 oz	80	2	2
Vegetarian Chili, 1 cup, 8 oz	180	1.5	25

Near East
	C	F	Cb
Couscous: Per Cup (Prepared)			
Original Plain	230	2	46
Parmesan; Rst Garlic & Oil	240	4	41
Pasta Garlic & Olive Oil Vermicelli	310	9	48
Toasted Pine Nut	230	6	40
Other varieties, avg.	220	3.5	42
Creative Grains: Per 1/3 Cup (Prepared)			
Chicken & Herbs w. Brown Rice	270	6	51
Creamy Parmesan w. White Rice	280	8	43
Roasted Garlic w. Brown Rice	220	5	41
Roasted Pecan & Garlic w. Brown	240	9	37
Pasta, all types	310	9	48
Falafels, 1/4 cup, (2 1/2 patties)	230	15	18
Rice Pilaf: Per Cup (Prepared)			
Spanish Mix	310	8	54
Tabouli Mix, Wheat Salad	110	0	21
Toasted Almond Mix	230	6	40
Wheat Mix; Brown Rice Mix	220	4	40
Other varieties, average	200	0.5	44

Canned & Packaged Meals (Cont)

New Menu (Vitasoy) Vegetarian	C	F	Cb
Tofumate (Seasoning Mixes), ¼ pkt	25	0	6
Noodles, all varieties, 1 cup	210	0.5	43
Nile Spice: *Per Cup*			
Couscous: Almondine	200	2.5	37
Lentil Curry	200	1.5	36
Minestrone	140	1	3
Parmesan	200	3	34
Nissan: Cup Noodles, all types, avg.	300	14	38
Chow Mein: Garlic Shrimp, ½ pkg	280	14	32
Chicken Flavor, ½ pkg	240	9	34
Souper Meal, average, ½ pkg	275	11	37
Noodle Chef			
Delecta Bowl: *Per Bowl*			
Tomato Penne	380	4	74
Pizza Mac & Cheese	370	4	70
Mac & Cheese	380	5	70
Nutritious Living: *Per Tray*			
Hi Low: Beef Stew	200	7	14
Turkey Chili w. Beans	170	5	8
Other varieties, average	170	5	13
Old El Paso			
Dinner Kits: *Per Serving (Prepared)*			
Soft Taco, 82g	380	12	33
Burrito (1), 57g	180	4.5	33
Hard & Soft Taco (2)	360	16	32
Shells, Taco Sce, Seasoning (2)	310	18	19
Fajita (2), 84g	310	9	35
Taco Dinner (2)	300	11	19
Side Dishes: Chili Beans, 1 cup	240	11	19
Mexe/Pinto Beans, ½ cup	110	0.5	19
Boxed: Chsy Mexican Rice ⅓ pkt	250	2	55
Spanish Rice, ⅓ pkt	280	4.5	55
Refried Beans: Regular, ½ cup	100	0.5	17
w. Green Chilies, ½ cup	100	0.5	19
w. Sausage, ½ cup	200	13	14
Fat Free varieties, ½ cup	100	0	18

Pasta-Roni: *Per Cup (Prepared)*	C	F	Cb
Angel Hair Pasta varieties, avg.	320	13	42
Fettuccine Alfredo	460	25	48
Chicken (flavor)	310	13	41
Chicken, Shells & White Cheddar	300	13	39
Chicken & Broccoli	370	16	49
Homestyle Deluxe: Creamy Garlic	350	17	40
Four Cheese; Parmesano	390	17	50
Homestyle Chicken	310	13	31
World Flavors: *Per Cup (Prepared)*			
Asian Garlic Chicken	280	11	39
Butter Herb Italiana	350	16	41
Chicken Quesadilla	310	13	40
Ragu			
Express! Pasta Snacks: *Per ⅙ Box (4.2 oz)*			
Classic Meat Flavor; Tomato, avg.	200	3	37
Sweet Tomato & Garlic	200	2.5	39
Rice Pride			
Rice Bowls: Spicy Shrimp	230	0.5	48
Teriyaki Beef	260	1	56
Tex Mex Beef	250	2	52
Rice-A-Roni: *Per Cup (Prepared)*			
Beef; Herb & Butter; Rice Pilaf	310	9	53
Broccoli Au Gratin	360	17	46
⅓ Less Salt	320	11	50
Chicken	310	9	51
⅓ Less Salt	280	5	52
Low-fat	210	3	41
Chicken & Broccoli	230	5	41
Chicken & Garlic; Chkn Teriyaki	260	8	41
Fried Rice	320	11	50
Spanish Rice	300	8	51
(Reduced Fat Recipe: If only 1 Tbsp fat is used instead of 2 Tbsp, deduct 35 calories and 4g fat.)			
Express: *Per Cup (prepared)*			
Asian Fried Rice	280	6	51
Golden Chicken	270	6	51
Other varieties, average	270	6	50
Rosarita			
Refried Beans: *Per ½ Cup*			
Traditional; Vegetarian; Spicy	100	2	18
Low-Fat Black Bean	90	0.5	18
Fat-Free varieties	90	0	17

Confucious say:
"Man who eat with one chopstick never have problem with obesity"

Shedd's	C	F	Cb
Country Crock Side Dishes			
Mashed Potatoes: Homestyle, ⅔ cup	190	9	23
Garlic, ⅔ cup, 5 oz	170	7	23
Chicken Rice w. Herbs, 1 cup	210	3.5	42
Elbow Macaroni & Cheese, 1 cup	380	17	40
Stagg Chili			
14.3 oz Box: *Per Cup (8.7 oz)*			
Chili w. Beans: Classic/Dynamite	330	16	30
Country/Laredo	320	15	27
Fiesta Grille	240	9	25
Ranch House Chicken	290	9	32
Rio Blanco Chicken	250	12	19
No Beans: Steakhouse/Double	330	21	16
99% Fat Free: Veg. Gdn/4 Bean	200	1	37
Turkey Ranchers/Silverado Beef	230	3	33
S & W: *Per ½ Cup*			
Baked Beans, avg. all types	145	0.5	28
Caribbean Black Beans	90	0	18
Kidney Beans	100	0.5	23
Red Beans Louisiana Style	80	0	20
San Antonio; Santa Fe Beans	90	0.5	21
White Beans	80	0.5	19
Sun Bird: *Noodle/Rice Mix (Prepared)*			
Chow Mein; Hunan Beef, ¼ cup	110	1	24
Kung Pao Chicken, ¼ cup	130	2	28
Mongolian Beef, ¼ cup	120	0.5	28
Teriyaki Beef; Sweet & Sour, ¼ cup	160	0	39
Thai Beef, ¼ cup	140	1.5	28
Sesame Chicken, ¼ cup	150	0	34
Taco Bell: *Per ½ Cup*			
Home Originals: Refried Beans	120	1	20
Fat Free Beans w. Green Chilles	100	0	18
Tasty Bite			
Ready Meals: *Per Package (w. Rice)*			
Peas Paneer	425	15	54
Spinach Dahl	370	9	62
Vegetable Supreme	315	6	55
Vegetarian Entrees: *Per ½ Package*			
Agra Peas & Greens	140	10	9
Bengal Lentils	160	8	16
Bombay Potatoes	105	4	13
Jaipur Vegetables	170	11	10
Jodhpur Lentils	105	4	12
Kashmir Spinach	115	8	8
Madras Lentils	125	5	14
Punjab Eggplant	110	9	13
Chicken Entrees: *Per Package*			
Chicken Moglai	320	15	29
Chicken Roganjosh	300	16	28
Chicken Vindaloo	350	17	29

Thai Kitchen	C	F	Cb
Bowls, avg. all types, 1.7 oz	120	2	24
Rice Noodles: *Per Serving*			
Curry Stir Fry, 1 cup	290	4	59
Lemongrass & Chili Stir Fry, 1 cup	285	3	60
Pad Thai varieties, ½ package	400	1	93
Savory Garlic, ½ package	220	3	46
Thai Peanut, ½ package	310	7	55
Thin/Stir Fry/Wide, 2 oz	195	0	46
Toasted Sesame Stir Fry, 1 cup	280	5	54
The Spice Hunter: *Per Package*			
Risotto: Wild Mushroom	230	1	47
Three Cheese; Spinach, avg.	245	2.5	46
Stuffed Potato: Creamy Butter	140	3	25
Bacon & White Cheddar	160	3	29
Sour Cream & Chives	160	2	31
Quick Hot Pasta: *Per Cup (Prepared)*			
Primavera Pasta	250	3	45
Roasted Peppers & Garlic	225	3	40
Tomato & Basil	220	1	42
Quick & Natural: Potato Leek, 1 pkg.	150	3	25
Creamy Thai Noodle, 1 bowl	180	4.5	29
Tofurky			
Deli Slices, average all	105	3	8
Holiday: Dumplings (2), 4 oz	215	1	45
Tofurky Roast, 4 oz	190	5	10
Tofurky Wild Rice Stuffing, ½ cup	140	5	21
Tofurky Wishstix, ½ piece	10	0	1
Jurky, 4 pieces	100	2	9
Sausages: Beer Brats (1), 3.5 oz	245	11	8
Kielbasa (1), 3.5 oz	245	12	8
Sweet Italian Sausages (1), 3.5 oz	280	13	12
Trader Joe's			
Bean Medley, ½ cup	150	1	26
Beef/Turkey Chili w. Beans, 1 cup	230	3	33
Black Bean Chili, 1 cup	230	1.5	37
Chicken Chili w. Beans, 1 cup	290	9	32
Pasta, Shells & White Cheddar, 1 cup	280	4.5	47
Refried Beans, avg., ½ cup	110	0	20
Organic Beans, avg., ½ cup	140	0	29
Black Beans: Regular, ½ cup	110	0	19
Cuban Style, ½ cup	120	2	20
Potatoes: Mashed Potatoes, ⅔ cup	120	4.5	20
Garlic Mashed Potatoes, ½ cup	150	7	19
Cheddar Cheese Au Gratin, ½ cup	140	4.5	21
Premium: Beef Stew, 1 cup	240	11	21
Chicken Stew, 1 cup	230	14	16
Tuna Helper: *See Betty Crocker, Page 71*			

Canned & Packaged Meals (Cont)

Uncle Ben's	C	F	Cb
Flavorful Rice: *Per Cup (Prepared w. Margarine)*			
Average all varieties	295	12	42
Country Inn: *Per Cup (Prepared w/out Margarine)*			
Broccoli Rice Au Gratin	200	2	43
Three Cheese Rice	200	2	40
Other varieties, avg.	200	1	43
Ready Rice: *Per ½ Pouch (Prepared)*			
Spanish Style	240	3.5	44
Other varieties, average	270	4	43

Valley Fresh	C	F	Cb
Chicken: *Per 2 oz*			
White & Dark Chunk	80	2	0
Premium Chunk White	70	1	0
Turkey, Premium Chunk White, ¼ can	80	1.5	0

Van Camps	C	F	Cb
Pork & Beans, ½ cup	110	1	23
Original Baked Beans, ½ cup	140	1	30
Beanie Weanie Original, 7¾ oz	220	8	29
Baked Beans: w. Hot Dog, 1 cup	340	6	47
w. Ground Beef, 1 cup	370	7	57
w. Chicken, 1 cup	360	2	62
Spanish Rice, 1 cup	180	3	37

White Wave (Vegetarian)	C	F	Cb
Seitan: Chicken w. Broth, 5 oz	130	0	12
Traditional, 3 oz	140	1	3
Tofu: Baked, all flavors, 2 oz	90	5	2
Organic, Soft/Firm, ⅕ pkg, 3.2 oz	110	6	4
Fat-Reduced, ⅕ pkg, 3.2 oz	90	4	1
Extra Firm, ¼ pkg, 3 oz	110	6	4
Soy Milks & Yogurts: See Pages 27, 30			

Wolf	C	F	Cb
Chili w. Beans: 227g Can	300	16	27
1 cup, 254g	330	18	30
Chili No Beans: 227g Can	390	27	18
1 cup, 248g	420	30	20
Chunky Beef w. Beans:			
1 cup, 254g	300	15	28
No Beans, 1 cup, 246g	330	22	18

Worthington/Loma Linda (Vegetarian)	C	F	Cb
Big Franks: 1 link, 1.8 oz	110	6	3
Low-fat, 1 link, 1.8 oz	80	2.5	3
Chili, 1 cup, 8 oz	280	10	25
Choplets, 2 slices, 3.2 oz	90	1	4
Dinner Cuts, 2 slices, 3.2 oz	90	1	4
FriChik, 2 pces, 3.1 oz	140	8	3
Linketts, (1), 1¼ oz	70	4	1
Little Links, 2 links, 1.6 oz	90	5	8
Low-Fat Vege-Links (1), 1 oz	45	1.5	3

Worthington/Loma Linda (Cont)	C	F	Cb
Multigrain Cutlets, 2 sl., 2¾ oz	100	1	5
Prime Stakes (1) 3.2 oz	120	8	7
Redi-Burger, ⅝" slice, 3 oz	120	2.5	7
Saucettes, 4 pces, 3 oz	90	6	1
Savory Slices, 3 sl., 2.9 oz	140	8	7
Sliced Chik, 3 sl., 3.1 oz	80	0.5	3
Sloppy Joe, ½ cup, 4.9 oz	140	1	23
Super Links (1) 1.6 oz	110	8	2
Tender Bits, 6 pieces, 3 oz	120	4	7
Tender Rounds, 8 pieces, 2¾ oz	120	4.5	6
Turkee Slices, 3 sl., 3.3 oz	180	12	5
Vege-Burger, ¼ cup, 2 oz	60	0.5	2
Vege-Links (1), 1 oz	50	3	1
Vegetable Skallops, ½ cup, 3 oz	90	1	4
Vegetarian Burger, ¼ cup, 1.9 oz	70	1.5	3

Yves Veggie Cuisine (Vegetarian)	C	F	Cb
Santa Fe Veggie Beef Bowl	360	9	57
Mac'n Soy Cheese	350	9	52
Breakfast: Brkfast Links (2) 1.8 oz	70	2	3
Breakfast Patties (1) 2 oz	80	2	4
Canadian Veg. Bacon, 3 slices	80	0.5	1
Burgers: Veggie (1) 2.6 oz	120	4.5	9
Garden Vege Patties (1) 3 oz	90	0	11
Savory Veggie (1)	150	6	18
Veggie Chick'n Burger (1) 2.6 oz	100	2.5	5
Dogs: Jumbo Veggie Dog (1) 2.6 oz	100	1.5	7
Hot & Spicy Chili/Good (1) 1.8 oz	70	1	3
Veggie/Tofu Dog, avg. (1)	60	0	1
Veggie Ground Round: Orig., Ital.	60	0.5	5
Meatballs (5), 2.6 oz	110	2.5	7
Mexican, ⅓ cup, 1.93 oz	90	2.5	5
The Good Deli: Bologna, 2 oz	80	1	4
Pizza Pepperoni, 1.7 oz (48g)	70	0	4
Veggie Ham/Salami, avg., 2 oz	85	0	6
Veggie Turkey, 2 oz (62g)	90	2	4
Veggie Entrees: Chili, 10.5 oz	230	1	37
Lasagne, 10.5 oz	300	3	51
Thai Lemongrass & Veggie Chkn	320	9	49
Veggie Penne, 300g pkg	220	1.5	36

Zatarain's: *Pasta Dinner Mix (Prepared)*	C	F	Cb
Alfredeaux, 1 cup	140	3.5	22
Gumbo, 1 cup	110	1	23
Jumbalaya, 1 cup	130	1	27
Scampi, 1 cup	100	1	27

Soybean Products	C	F	Cb
Cheeses (Soy): *See Page 44*			
Miso Paste, average, 1 Tbsp, ¼ oz	35	1	5
Miso Soup (dry mix), average			
1 Tbsp., dry mix	30	1	3
1 cup, prepared	30	1	3
Natto, ½ cup, 3 oz	190	10	13
Okara (Tofu fiber residue), ½ c., 2 oz	47	1	8
Tempeh: 1 piece, 3 oz	170	6	14
Fried, 3 oz	250	14	14
Seitan *(White Wave)*, Trad., 3 oz	140	1	3
Soybean Protein (TVP), 1 oz	100	0.5	9
Soy Bean Paste, 1 tsp	10	0	2
Soy Beans: *See Page 149*			
Soy Drinks: *See Page 27*			
White Wave: *See Page 76*			

Tofu ~ Packaged	C	F	Cb
Tofu Stir Fried, average all, 4 oz	120	8	3
Azumaya Tofu:			
Soft (Silken), 3 oz	45	2	4
Soft, Light (Silken), 3 oz	40	1	3
Firm, 3 oz	70	4	2
Extra Firm, 3 oz	70	4	2
Light Extra Firm, 3 oz	60	2	3
Seasoned Tofu, 3 oz	90	5	3

Tofu ~ Packaged (Cont)	C	F	Cb
Hinoichu Tofu:			
Soft, 3 oz, 1" slice	50	2.5	2
Reg. (Japanese), 3 oz, 1" slice	60	3	1
Firm (Chinese), 3 oz, 1" slice	70	3.5	2
Extra Firm, 3 oz	80	4	1
Mori-Nu Tofu (Silken):			
Soft, 3 oz, 1" slice	45	2.5	2
Firm, 3 oz, 1" slice	55	2.5	2
Extra Firm, 3 oz, 1" slice	45	1.5	2
Enriched, 3 oz, 1" slice	70	2.5	6
Organic, 3 oz, 1" slice	60	2.5	2
Lite: Firm, 3 oz	30	0.5	1
Extra Firm, 3 oz	35	0.5	1
Nasoya Tofu: Soft, 3 oz	60	3	1
Silken, 3 oz	45	2.5	2
Firm, 3 oz	70	3	2
Extra Firm, 3 oz	80	4	2
Chinese 5 Spice Tofu, 3 oz	90	5	3
Pulmuone Tofu: Soft, 3 oz	70	3	1
Firm, 3 oz	70	3	1
White Wave: Baked Tofu, 1 square	90	5	2
Soft/Firm Tofu, ⅕ block	110	6	4
Reduced Fat, ⅕ block	90	4	1
Firm, 3 oz	70	3	1

Soups

Homemade & Restaurant

Restaurant & Take-Out
Per 8 fl.oz

	C	F	Cb
Bean Medley	200	3	34
Beef Consomme	30	1	2
Borscht (w. Cream)	130	8	14
Bouillabaisse	400	15	10
Chicken & Corn	290	14	20
Chicken & Wild Rice	80	4	9
Chicken Consomme	50	0	2
Chicken Curry	180	8	18
Chicken Jambalaya	160	7	8
Chicken Noodle	80	2	12
w. Chicken	160	4	12
Chicken Soup	80	2	6
Chili with Beans	250	12	25
Clam Chowder	240	15	17
Corn & Crab	120	3	18
Corn Chowder	150	8	16
Cream of Broccoli	200	12	20
Cream of Potato	220	12	20
Cream of Mushroom	290	21	20
Creamy Pumpkin	210	10	26
Fish Chowder	220	15	6
French Onion	420	15	25
Gazpacho	60	0	13
Lentil Soup	250	9	28
Lobster Bisque	320	15	10
Matzo Ball (w. 1 large ball)	180	7	24
Minestrone	140	2	14
Mulligatawny	300	15	8
Pea & Ham	240	10	25
Potato & Bacon	170	7	19
Shark Fin Soup	220	6	4
Spicy Shrimp Soup, 1 bowl	160	7	10
Split Pea Soup	150	6	18
Vegetable (Fat Free)	75	0	18
Vegetable Beef	80	2	10
Vichyssoise	200	9	13
Watercress	90	4	13

Other Soups: *See International & Fast-Foods Sections*

(Arby's, Au Bon Pain, Boston Market, Dunkin' Donuts, Denny's, Schlotzsky's, Sizzler, Souplantation, Sweet Tomatoes, Zoup!)

Homemade Soups: Calculate calories, fat and carbohydrates from ingredients.

Bouillon Cubes & Powders

	C	F	Cb
Bouillon Cubes: *Average all Types*			
Regular, 1 cube	8	0	1
Low Sodium (LiteLine)	12	0	1
Powders: Average, 1 tsp	8	0	1
Herb-Ox: *Instant Broth & Seasoning,*			
Beef, 1 envelope	10	0	2
Chicken; Vegetarian	10	0	2
Herbs, Spices: 1 tsp	5	0	1
Soup Oyster Crackers			
40 small/3 large, ½ oz	60	2	8

Amy's
Per Cup (½ Can)

	C	F	Cb
Alphabet Soup	80	0.5	16
Black Bean Vegetable	130	1.5	25
Butternut Squash	100	2.5	20
Chunky Tomato Bisque	120	3.5	21
Cream of Mushroom, ¾ cup	140	9	13
Lentil Vegetable	150	4.5	19
Minestrone	90	1.5	17
Pasta & 3 Bean	130	5	19
Vegetable Barley	70	1	13

Andersen's
Per Cup

	C	F	Cb
Split Pea	130	0	24
Split Pea w. Bacon	135	1	22
Tomato	130	3	24

Bean Cuisine
Per Cup (Made as Directed)

	C	F	Cb
Barcelona Red Beans & Radiatore	155	1	29
Country French Beans w. Gemelli	0	0	0
Florentine Beans w. Bow Ties	0	0	0
Mediterranean Blk Beans & Fusilli	210	1	30
Island Black Bean	90	0	17
Soup Mix: *Dry Mix Only*			
Mesa Maize, 1 oz	95	0	18
White Bean Provencal, 1 oz	250	1	32

Campbell's

	C	**F**	**Cb**
Classic Red & White: *Per ½ Cup*			
Bean w. Bacon	170	4	25
Beef Noodle	75	2.5	9
Beef w. Vegetables & Barley	95	1.5	15
Black Bean	115	2	19
Cheddar Cheese	100	4.5	12
Chicken & Dumplings	80	3	10
Chicken Won Ton	60	1	8
Classic Chicken Noodle	100	2.5	16
Cream of Asparagus	110	7	10
Cream of Broccoli	90	3.5	12
Cream of Chicken & Brocc./Mushr.	80	6	7
Cream of Mushroom	105	7	9
Cream of Onion	100	5	12
Cream of Potato	95	3	15
Cream of Shrimp	90	6	8
Creamy Chicken Noodle	120	7	13
Fiesta Chili Beef	175	5	25
French Onion	45	1.5	6
Green Pea	175	3	28
Hearty Vegetable w. Pasta	95	0.5	19
Manhattan Clam Chowder	70	0.5	12
Minestrone	95	1	17
New England Clam Chowder	90	2.5	13
Old Fashioned Vegetable	80	1.5	14
Split Pea w. Ham & Bacon	180	2.5	27
Tomato	90	0	20
Tomato Bisque	130	3.5	23
Tomato w. Rstd Garlic & Herbs	95	0	23
Turkey Vegetable	75	2	11
Vegetable	100	0.5	20
Chunky: *Per Cup*			
Baked Potatoes w. Bacon Bits	160	5	21
Clam Chowder Manhattan	120	3.5	19
Grilled Chicken & Sausage Gumbo	140	2.5	21
Hearty Veges w. Pasta	120	2	23
Tomato Cheese Ravioli	140	3.5	27
Healthy Request: *Per ½ Cup*			
Chicken Rice	70	2	13
Vegetable Beef	90	1	15
Other varieties, average	90	1.5	18
98% Fat Free, prep., avg., ½ cup	70	2	10
Carb Request: *Per Cup*			
Chicken Broccoli; Cheese	130	7	8
Mediterranean Style Meatball	90	4.5	5
Roasted Chicken w. Veges	70	1	7
Savory Beef & Mushroom	70	2	7
Spicy Sausage w. Chicken	90	4	7

	C	**F**	**Cb**
Select: *Per Cup (8 fl.oz)*			
Bean & Ham	165	1	30
Beef w. Portabello Mushr. & Rice	105	1.5	15
Beef w. Roasted Barley	145	1.5	24
Chicken & Pasta w. Roasted Garlic	105	1.5	16
Chicken Rice	100	1	17
Chicken Vegetable	105	0.5	18
Chicken w. Egg Noodles	105	1.5	14
Creamy Chicken Alfredo	220	12	16
Creamy Potato w. Roasted Garlic	175	9	20
Fiesta Vegetable	115	0.5	24
Grilled Chicken w. Sundried Tom.	110	1	17
Herbed Chicken w. Rstd Vegetable	100	0.5	14
Honey Roasted Chkn w. Potatoes	110	1	16
Italian Style Wedding	110	2.5	16
Minestrone	100	0	20
New England Clam Chowder	220	14	16
Roasted Chicken w. Wild Rice	95	0.5	17
Rstd Chkn w. Rotini & Penne	100	1	16
Rosemary Chkn w. Rstd Potatoes	105	0.5	18
Savory Lentil	145	0.5	27
Split Pea w. Ham	165	1	29
Tomato Garden; Vegetable	100	0.5	21
Vegetable Beef	115	2	16
Soup at Hand: *Per Container*			
Chicken varieties, average	75	1.5	12
Creamy Mushroom	120	8	8
Creamy Tomato	180	4	34
Mexican Style Fiesta	150	5	22
New England Clam Chowder	120	6	12
Pizza Soup	140	0.5	27
Vegetable Beef	60	1	10
Velvety Potato	160	6	21
Soup & Recipe Mixes (Dry): *Per Tablespoon*			
Chicken Noodle/w. Broth	30	0.5	5
Onion	20	0	5

Soup is an excellent filler as part of a meal, or as a snack.

- *Add lots of veges, and beans (for extra protein & fiber)*
- *Avoid Noodle Cups (high in fat)*
- *If using low-fat soup mixes, add extra microwaved veges, tofu or canned beans*

Soups (Cont)

CarbSense

	C	F	Cb
Per Cup (Prepared)			
Miso	35	1	5
Thai Coconut Cream	100	6	9
Szechuan Beef	25	0.5	4

Dr McDougall's

	C	F	Cb
Per Serving (Mix)			
Split Pea w. Barley, 1.5 oz	150	2	28
Tortilla Soup w. Baked Chips. 1 oz	80	0.5	16
Vegetarian Vegetable, 1 oz	80	0.5	16

Fantastic Cup Soups

	C	F	Cb
Per Container (Mix):			
Split Pea	160	1	28
Cha Cha Chili	220	2	37
Corn & Potato Chowder	130	1	26
Couscous w. Lentils	170	1	35
Split Pea	220	1	38
Creamy Soups, average	150	2.5	27
Hearty Soup Cups: *Per ½ Ctn*			
Country Lentil; Five Bean	180	1.5	32
Jumpin' Black Bean	230	1.5	41
Minestrone	140	1.5	27
Vegetable Barley	120	0.5	27
Big Soup: *Per Cup*			
Hot & Sour	130	2	22
Italian Tomato Noodle	130	1	26
Mandarin Broccoli	110	0	20
Spring Vege; Vege Beef Noodle	100	0	20
Spicy Thai	110	1	22
Sesame Miso	90	1	17
Vegetarian Chicken Noodle	90	0.5	19
Carbtastic: Hot & Sour, 1 pkg	70	2.5	7
Vegetarian Beef w. Barley, 1 pkg	90	1	14
Broccoli Cheddar, 1 pkg	110	3	12

Healthy Choice

	C	F	Cb
Per Cup			
Bean & Ham	170	2.5	29
Beef and Potato; Chicken w. Pasta	110	1	19
Chicken & Dumplings; Vege Beef	140	2	22
Chicken w. Rice Soup	90	3	12
Country Vegetable	100	0.5	22
Creamy Tomato	100	1.5	18
Fiesta Chicken	100	2	17
Garden Vegetable	120	1	25
Hearty Chicken	120	2	20
New England Clam Chowder	110	1.5	21
Roasted Italian Chicken/ w. Garlic	120	2	18
Split Pea and Ham	170	2.5	30
Zesty Gumbo	90	1.5	16

Health Valley

	C	F	Cb
Per Cup			
Bean Vegetable	140	0	32
Beef Broth	10	0	0
Carotene varieties, average	70	0	16
Chicken Broth, Low-fat	35	1.5	0
Chicken Noodle/Rice	130	2	20
Corn & Vege; Super Broccoli	70	0	17
Garden/Tomato Vegetable	80	0	17
Italian Minestrone; Lentil & Carrots	100	0	20
Mushroom Broth	10	0	2
Real Minestrone; Italian Plus; Vege	80	0	20
Split Pea	110	0	17
Pasta Soups, avg. all varieties	115	0	24
Organic: Black Bean; Split Pea	130	0	25
Mushroom Barley; Potato Leek	70	0	16
Lentil; Tomato; Minestrone	100	0	21
Dry Soups: ⅓ cup, average	120	0	24
Soup Cups: *Per Cup*			
Chicken Broth	25	0	0
Corn Chowder w. Tomato	105	0	21
Creamy Potato w. Broccoli	80	0	17
Garden Split Pea; Zesty Blk Bean	115	0	22
Lentil w. Couscous	130	0	28
Pasta Marianara/Parmesan	100	0	20
Spicy Black Bean w. Couscous	130	0	29

Feedback Welcome
Please send comments and suggestions to the author.
Email: feedback@calorieking.com

80

Imagine

Per Cup

	C	F	Cb
No Chicken/Vegetable Broth	30	0.5	5
Free Range Chicken Broth	20	0.5	2
Organic Creamy: Broccoli	70	1.5	10
Butternut Squash	120	2	23
Portobello Mushroom	80	3	10
Potato Leek; Sweet Corn, avg.	100	3	15
Tomato	90	1.5	17

Knorr

	C	F	Cb
Recipe Classics: *Dry Mix*			
Cream of Spinach, 2 Tbsp	70	2.5	10
French Onion, 2 Tbsp	35	1	6
Hot & Sour, 2 Tbsp	45	1.5	8
Leek Soup, 2 Tbsp	70	2.5	10
Spring Vegetable, 2 Tbsp, 0.3 oz	25	0	5
Tomato w. Basil, 3 Tbsp, 0.7 oz	85	2.5	13
Vegetable, 2 Tbsp, 0.6 oz	60	1.5	10
Bouillon Cubes: *Per ½ Cube (1 Cup, Prepared)*			
Beef; Chicken, average	20	1.5	0.5

Lipton

	C	F	Cb
Cup-a-Soup: *Per Envelope*			
Cream of Chicken	70	2	12
Chicken Noodle	50	1	8
Carb Options: Cream of Chicken	35	1	6
Chicken Noodle	25	0	4
Recipe Secrets: *Per Serving (Dry Mix)*			
Beefy Onion, 1 Tbsp	25	0.5	5
Onion, 1 Tbsp	20	0	4
Onion Mushroom, 1⅔ Tbsp	35	0	7
Savory Herb w. Garlic, 1 Tbsp	25	0	6
Soup Secrets: *Per Cup (Prepared)*			
Noodle Soup	60	1.5	9
Chicken Noodle	80	2	12

Manischewitz

	C	F	Cb
Condensed: *Per ½ Cup (Unprepared)*			
Chicken	15	0.5	2
Chicken w. Kieplach	35	1	5
Chicken w. Matzo Balls	80	4	9
Quart Jars: *Per 8 fl.oz (Prepared)*			
Borscht w. Beets	90	0	21
Borscht Low Calorie	25	0	6
Ready To Serve: Matzo Ball Soup	110	5	13
Matzo Balls in Broth	215	9	27
Whitefish & Pike in Broth	50	1.5	3
Dry Mixes: *Per Cup*			
Matzo Ball & Soup Mix	40	0.5	9
Split Pea Cello	140	0	25
Vegetable Soup Cello	120	0	22

Maruchan - *Per Cup*

	C	F	Cb
Instant Lunch, avg. all flavors	290	12	37
Ramen flavors, ½ pkt, 1½ oz	190	8	26

Miso Cup

	C	F	Cb
Original; Golden Seaweed, 1 cup	30	1	3
Traditional, 1 pkg	35	1	4
Reduced Sodium, 1 pkg	25	1	3

Nile Spice

Per Cup:

	C	F	Cb
Black Bean; Lentil	170	1.5	36
Cheddar Broccoli	130	3	20
Chicken Flavored Vegetable	110	1.5	21
Country Mushroom	140	2.5	26
Minestrone	140	1	30
Red Beans & Rice	170	1	35
Split Pea	200	1	35
Couscous: Parmesan	200	3	34
Other varieties, average	190	2	36

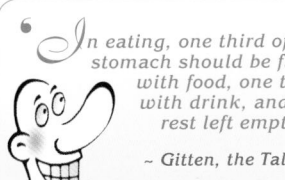

> *In eating, one third of the stomach should be filled with food, one third with drink, and the rest left empty.*
>
> ~ Gitten, the Talmud

Eat it Today...
Wear it Tomorrow!

Soups (Cont)

Pacific Foods

	C	F	Cb
Per Cup			
Chicken Broth	10	0	1
Natural, Beef Broth	20	0	1
Organic: French Onion	35	0	6
Creamy Butternut Squash	90	2	17
Creamy Tomato	100	2	16
Roasted Red Pepper & Tomato	100	2	16
Vegetable Broth	15	0	3

Pritikin

Per Cup			
Chicken Pasta	80	0	15
Fat Free Chicken Broth	10	0	0.5
Hearty Vegetable	90	0.5	16
Minestrone	90	0.5	18
Split Pea	180	0.5	32
Three Bean Chili	230	1	39
Vegetarian Vegetable	100	0	21

Progresso *- Per Cup*

Beef Barley; Chickarina, avg.	130	4	13
Beef & Vegetable	110	1.5	15
Broccoli Cheese Chowder	220	13	19
Chicken & Herb Dumplings	120	2.5	15
Chicken with Wild Rice/Barley	90	1.5	14
Creamy Mushroom	130	10	9
Green Split Pea	170	3	28
Grilled Chicken Italiano	110	2.5	14
Grilled Steak w. Veg. Penne	120	3.5	13
Hearty Black Bean	160	1.5	30
Hearty Tomato	110	2	23
Hearty Penne in Chicken Broth	80	1	14
Home Style Chicken; Turkey Noodle	110	1.5	11
Macaroni & Bean	160	4	23
Minestrone; Turkey Rice	110	1.5	19
New England Clam Chowder	190	13	23
Roasted Chicken varieties, avg.	80	1.5	10
Southwestern Style Chicken	120	2	19
Southwestern Style Corn Chowder	190	7	29
Split Pea w. Ham	140	4	20
Steak & Baked Potato	130	2.5	18
Steak & Mushrooms/Vegetables	130	2	20
Tomato; Tomato Basil; Lentil	160	2	30
Tomato Rotini	140	5	30
Other varieties, average	100	2	19

Progresso (Cont)

	C	F	Cb
Rich & Hearty: Chicken Pot Pie	170	6	20
Beef Pot Roast w. Veges	130	1.5	17
Creamy Chicken w. Rice	150	8	13
Other varieties, avg.	120	1	17
99% Fat Free: Chicken Noodle	90	1.5	13
Beef Barley; Lentil; Minestrone	130	2	20
New England Clam Chowder	120	1.5	18
White Cheddar Potato	100	1.5	20
Carb Monitor: *Per Cup*			
Beef Vegetable	60	1.5	6
Chicken Cheese Enchilada	190	13	7
Chicken Vegetable	70	2	7

Safeway Select

Signature Soups: *Per Cup (8.6 oz)*			
Broccoli & Cheesy Cheddar	280	21	14
Chunky Chicken Noodle	130	3.5	13
Clam Chowder	250	15	19
Craving Crab	410	33	18
Fajita Chicken & Corn Chowder	350	23	25
Hearty Pot Roast	140	5	12
Mediterranean Vegetable	70	2	11
Pacific Coast Clam Chowder	330	24	19
Savory Chicken & Wild Rice	170	6	20
Stompin' Steakhouse Chili	260	8	23
Tuscan Tomato & Basil Bisque	310	26	17

Schwan's

Soups: *Per Bowl (10 oz)*			
Cheesy Broccoli	360	27	18
Chicken Noodle	175	6	18
Chili w. Beans	385	19	33

Swanson

Per Cup			
100% Fat Free Chicken Broth	15	0	1
Beef Broth	15	0.5	0
Chicken Broth	10	0.5	1
Vegetable Broth	15	0	3

Tabatchnick

	C	F	Cb
Per ½ Container			
Barley Mushroom	80	1	17
Black Bean	230	2.5	39
Broccoli & Cheese	200	12	15
Cabbage	90	1	21
Chicken w. Dumplings	150	6	19
Corn Chowder	130	4.5	21
Cream of Broccoli	130	5	18
Cream of Mushroom	100	5	11
Cream of Spinach	90	5	10
Creamed Spinach	40	1	7
Lentil	160	0	29
Macaroni & Cheese	250	8	34
Minestrone	100	1.5	18
New England Potato	110	5	17
New York Chicken	70	1	13
Old Fashioned Potato	100	1.5	21
Onion	60	1.5	11
Pea	140	0	34
Salmon Chowder	80	1.5	15
Seafood Chowder	130	6	15
Southwest Bean	220	5	35
Tomato Rice	110	3.5	18
Vegetable	90	1.5	17
Yankee Bean	180	1.5	33
Vegetarian Chili	180	3.5	28
Wild Rice	80	0.5	16
No Salt: Mushroom	80	1	17
Pea	140	0	34
Vegetable	90	1.5	17

Thai Kitchen

	C	F	Cb
7 oz Can: *Per Serving*			
Coconut Ginger	190	15	11
Hot & Sour	40	0.5	7
Instant Rice Noodle: *½ Package (Prep. As Directed)*			
Bangkok Curry	90	3	16
Garlic & Vegetable	80	1.5	17
Lemongrass & Chili	80	1.5	17
Spring Onion, 1.6 oz	90	1.5	16
Thai Ginger	80	12	16
Other varieties	120	1.5	25
Rice Noodle Soup Bowls: *Per Serving*			
Curry, ½ pkg., 2.5 oz	290	6	55
Hot & Sour, ½ pkg., 2 oz	115	0.5	26
Lemongrass & Chili, ½ pkg., 2.5 oz	115	0.5	24

Trader Joe's

	C	F	Cb
Per Cup			
Barley w. Vegetables; Rich Onion	95	1	19
Chicken Broth	15	0.5	0
Chicken Noodle	90	1	14
Chunky Minestrone	100	2	16
Creamy Corn Chowder	165	7	23
Lentil w. Vegetables	175	1.5	30
Mixed Vegetable	105	6	10
Mostly Unsplit Pea	175	0.5	32
Spicy Bean	200	5	30
Spicy Black Bean	230	3	41
Split Pea, Low Fat	145	1	26
Condensed: Clam Chowder	150	4	22
Crab Bisque	150	6	18

Walnut Acres

	C	F	Cb
Per Cup (250g)			
Autumn Harvest	100	2	19
Country Corn Chowder	150	3	28
Cuban Black Bean; Four Bean Chili	150	1	30
Ginger Carrot	100	1	22
Classic Minestrone	100	0	22
Mediterranean Lentil	130	0	26
Savory Tomato	120	2	23

Westbrae

	C	F	Cb
Canned: *Per Cup (240g) Unless Indicated*			
Alabama; Mediterranean Lentil	140	0	24
New York UnChicken Noodle	60	1	10
Old World Split Pea	150	0	28
Santa Fe Vegetable	160	0	31
Other varieties, average	125	0	25
Condensed: *Per ¾ Cup, Prepared*			
California UnChicken Broth, 180g	15	0.5	2
Monte Carlo Crmy Mushr., 180g	70	3	10
Tuscany Tomato, 180g	70	0	16

Wylers

	C	F	Cb
Dry Mix: Mrs Grass Onion, 10g	30	0	6
Homestyle Vegetable, 12g	35	0	7
Soup Starter: *Per Cup*			
Chicken Noodle	70	1	13
Beef Vegetable	90	0.5	18

Herbs & Spices

Herbs & Spices

	C	F	Cb
Per Teaspoon: Average all types	5	0	1
Allspice, ground	5	0	1
Chili Powder	8	0	1
Cinnamon, ground	6	0	2
Curry Powder	6	0	1
Garlic Powder	9	0	1
Nutmeg, ground	12	0	1
Onion Powder	7	0	1
Parsley, dried	4	0	1
Pepper, black/red/white, avg.	6	0	1
Saffron	2	0	0
Tumeric, ground	8	0	1
Seeds: Fenugreek	12	1	2
Mustard, Poppyseed	15	1	1
Other types, average	7	0	1
Parsley Patch: Sesame, 1 tsp	16	1	1
Salt-free blends, average	10	1	2
All-purpose, 1 tsp	6	0	1

Seasonings & Flavorings

	C	F	Cb
Accent Flavor Enhancer, 1 tsp	10	0	0
Angostura Bitters, 1 tsp	12	0	3
Bacon Bits, average, 1 Tbsp	30	1	0
Bacon Chips *(Durkee)*, 1 Tbsp	45	1	0
Best O'Butter, 1 tsp	10	0.5	2
Bragg Liquid Aminos, 1 tsp	5	0	0
Butter Buds, 1 tsp	8	0.5	2
Garlic Bread Sprinkle, 1 tsp	8	0.5	1
Garlic Salt, 1 tsp	2	0	0
Italian Seasoning, 1 tsp	4	0	1
Lemon Pepper Seasoning, 1 tsp	7	0	1
Meat Tenderizer, avg., 1 tsp	7	0	1
Molly McButter, 1 tsp	5	1	1
Mrs Dash Blends, 1 tsp	0	0	1
Perc Salt-free Seasoning, 1 tsp	8	0	2
Potato Toppings *(Knudsen)*, 1 Tbsp	30	2.5	1
Salad Sprinkles *(Lawry's)*, 1 tsp	16	0.5	2
Salad Supreme *(McCormick)*, 1 tsp	10	0.5	2
Salt: Regular, Sea Salt, Lite Salt	0	0	0
Seasoning Mixes, avg., ¼ pkg	70	1	9
Taco Seasoning, avg., ¼ pkg	30	0.5	4
Old El Paso: Chili Season. Mix, 1 T.	15	0.5	3
Cheesy Taco Season. Mix, 1 T.	15	0.5	3
Taco/Burrito Seasoning Mix, 2 tsp	15	0	3
Enchilada Seasoning Mix, 2 tsp	10	0	2
Fajita Seasoning Mix, 2 tsp	10	0	3
Vegit Seasoning Mix, 1 tsp	5	0	1

Condiments, Sauces

	C	F	Cb
Average of Brands & Homemade			
Apple Sauce: *Also see Page 146*			
Sweetened, ¼ cup, 2¼ oz	45	0	11
Unsweetened, ¼ cup, 2 oz	27	0	6.5
Bac O's *(Betty Crocker)*, 1 tsp, ½ oz	60	3	4
Barbecue, average	25	0	6
Bearnaise Sce, ¼ cup, 2½ oz	190	19	5
Buffalo Wing Sce: Honey Mustard, 1 T.	40	3	3
Average other varieties, I Tbsp	25	2	2
Catsup (Ketchup): Reg., 1 Tbsp	15	0	4
Cheese, h/made, ¼ cup, 2½ oz	150	10	12
Chili Sauce: *Heinz*, 1 Tbsp	15	0	4
Del Monte, 1 Tbsp	20	0	5
Wolf Hot Dog, 1 Tbsp	15	1	2
Cocktail Sauce, ¼ cup	110	0	15
Cranberry, all types, ¼ c., 2½ oz	110	0	27
Escoffier Sauces, 1 Tbsp	20	0	4
Honey Mustard *(French's)* 1 tsp	5	0	1
Horseradish: 1 tsp	2	0	0
Sauceworks Sauce, 1 tsp	20	2	0
Ketchup: Regular, 1 Tbsp	16	0	4
Heinz Lite, 1 Tbsp	8	0	2
Heinz Kick'rs, 1 Tbsp	20	0	4
Mushroom Sauce, ½ cup, 2 oz	50	2	5
Mustard, average, 1 tsp	5	0	0.5
Pesto, ¼ cup, 2 oz	35	3	2
Pizza Sauce, cnd., ¼ cup, 2 oz	25	0	5
Seafood Cocktail Sce, ¼ cup	60	0	14
Soy Sauce, all types, avg., 1 Tbsp	10	0	1
Sour Cream Sce, ½ cup	250	15	22
Spaghetti Sce, ½ cup, 4½ oz	135	6	19
Steak Sauce: *Heinz*, 1 Tbsp	15	0	3
Lea & Perrins, 1 Tbsp	25	0	6
Lawry's Low Carb, 1 Tbsp	5	0	1
Str'berry Puree Sce: Unsweet., 2 T.	9	0	2
Sweet & Sour Sauce:			
Contadina, 2 Tbsp	40	1	8
Kikkoman Lite Soy, 1 Tbsp	10	0	1
La Choy, 2 Tbsp, 34g	60	0	14
Tabasco Sauce, 1 Tbsp	2	0	0
Taco Sauce, average, 1 Tbsp	10	0	1
Tartar Sauce: *Heinz,* 2 Tbsp, 30g	140	14	4
America's Choice, 2 Tbsp, 27g	160	17	1
Hellman's: Regular, 2 Tbsp, 30g	80	7	3
Low-fat, 2 Tbsp, 30g	40	1.5	7
Teriyaki Sauce, *Kikkoman,* 1 Tbsp	15	0	2
Vinegar, White or wine, 1 fl.oz	4	0	1
White Sauce, ½ cup, 5 oz	130	7	12
Worcestershire Sauce, 1 tsp	5	0	1

Pickles & Relish

	C	F	Cb
Average All Brands			
Bread & Butter Pickles, 4 sl., 1 oz	20	0	5
Chutney, 2 Tbsp, 1¼ oz	40	0	12
Dill Pickle:			
Slices, 4 slices, 1 oz	3	0	0.5
1 large,			
(3¾"x 1¼ diam.), 2¼ oz	12	0	3
Extra lrg (4"x 1¾ diam.), 5 oz	30	0	6
Halves: Small, 1 oz	3	0	0.5
Large, 2½ oz	8	0	2
Sweet, small, ½ oz	22	0	6
Gherkins, sweet, 1 med., 1 oz	15	0	7
Green Chilies, chopped, 2 Tbsp	5	0	1
Horseradish, 1 Tbsp	10	0	2
Jalapenos, pickled, 2 whole	5	0	1
Jalapeno Relish, 1 Tbsp, ½ oz	5	0	1
Mustard, avg. all brands, 1 tsp	5	0	0.5
Peppers: Hot/Mild, 1 oz	8	0	2
Pickled: Beets, ½ cup, 4 oz	75	0	19
Onions, 1 medium, ¾ oz	10	0	2
Cocktail Onion, 1 onion	2	0	0
Red Cabbage, ½ cup, 3 oz	60	0	13
Pickles: Sweet, 2 Tbsp, 1 oz	35	0	0
Large (3"x ¾ diam.), 1¼ oz	40	0	10
Pickle in a Pouch, 1 large	12	0	3
Relishes: Sandwich Spread, 1 tsp	20	1	5
Cranberry-Orange, 1 Tbsp	30	0	7
Hot Dog (*Heinz*), 1 Tbsp	17	0	28
Sweet Pickle, 1 Tbsp	20	0	5
Sauerkraut, ½ cup, 3½ oz	25	0	5
Sweet Cauliflower	35	0	8

Salsa

	C	F	Cb
Average all Types: *Per 2 Tablespoons*			
Regular, no oil, 2 Tbsp	15	0	3.5
Homemade w. Oil, 2 Tbsp	40	3	8
Chef's Kitchen, 2 Tbsp	10	0	2
Del Monte, all flavors, 2 Tbsp	10	0	2
Kaukauma, 2 Tbsp	15	0	3
La Victoria, 2 Tbsp	10	0	2
Wild Oats, 2 Tbsp, 1 oz	10	0	2

Gravy

	C	F	Cb
Homemade Gravy:			
Thin, little fat, 2 Tbsp, 1 oz	20	1	3
Thick, 2 Tbsp, 1¼ oz	50	2	9
¼ cup, 2½ oz	100	4	18
Franco-American (Canned)			
Au Jus Gravy, ¼ cup, 2 oz	10	0	2
Beef; Turkey Gravy, 2 oz	25	0.5	3
Chicken Gravy, ¼ cup, 2 oz	40	4	4
Franco-American (In Jars)			
99% Fat Free, ¼ cup, 2 oz	25	0.5	4
Pillsbury (Gravy Mixes)			
Brown; Homestyle, ¼ cup, 2 oz	15	0	3
Chicken, as prep., ¼ cup, 2 oz	20	0	4

Gravy-In-Jars-Homestyle

Boston Market, ¼ cup, 2 oz	25	1	3
Heinz, reg., all types, ¼ c., 2 oz	25	1	3
Fat Free Rst. Turkey, ¼ c., 2 oz	10	0	2
Vons, all types, ¼ c., 2 oz	20	0.5	4

Tomato Products

	C	F	Cb
Whole/Chopped/Crushed/Diced			
1 cup, 8½ oz	50	0	10
In Aspic, ½ cup	50	0	12
w. Green Chili, 1 cup, 8½ oz	45	0.5	11
Stewed, ½ cup	40	2.5	9
Wedges in Tom Juice, 1 cup	70	0.5	15
Salsa, average, 1 Tbsp	15	0	3.5
Tomato Ketchup:			
Regular, 1 Tbsp	16	0	4
Green (*Heinz*), 1 Tbsp	20	0	5
Tomato Paste, 2 Tbsp	25	0	5
Regular, 6 oz, ¾ cup	150	0	34
Tomato Puree, ½ cup	50	0	10
Tomato Sauce:			
Regular, ½ cup	40	0	9
Spanish Style, ½ cup	40	0	9
w. Mushrooms, ½ cup	40	0	9
w. Onions, ½ cup	50	0	11
Tomato Seasoning, 3 tsp	20	0	4
Sundried Tomatoes:			
Natural, 5-6 pces, 0.4 oz	22	0	5
In Oil, drained, 6 pces, ½ oz	60	4	5

Sauces ~ Pasta, Cooking

Brands

	C	F	Cb
A-1			
Steak & Marinades Sauce: *Per Tablespoon (½ oz)*			
Bold & Spicy; Teriyaki	20	0	5
Carb Wel	5	0	1
Chicago	21	1	2
Jamaican Jerk	25	0.5	5
New Orleans Cajun	25	0	5
New York Steakhouse	20	0	5
Roasted Garlic	20	0	5
Steak Sauce	15	0	3
Barilla: *Per ½ Cup*			
Marinara; Sweet Peppers & Garlic	90	3	11
Roasted Garlic & Onion	80	3.5	11
Tomato & Basil	70	2.5	12
Bertolli/Five Brothers: *Per ½ Cup*			
Alfredo w. Mushrooms	160	12	6
Creamy Alfredo	220	20	4
Grilled Summer Vegetable	80	5	12
Marinara w. Burgundy Wine	80	3	12
Mushroom & Garlic	90	3	13
Olive Oil & Garlic	90	4	9
Olive w. Sundried Tomato	100	4	13
Oven Roasted Garlic & Onion	70	1.5	10
Roasted Red Pepper	80	3	13
Tomato Basil	80	2	10
Best Foods			
Dippin' Sauce: *Per Tablespoon*			
Honey Mustard Madness	30	1	5
Rockin' Ranch	45	3	4
Totally BBQ	55	6	0.5
Bookbinders: *Per ½ Cup*			
White Clam Sauce	300	30	4
Buitoni			
Pasta Sauce: *Per ½ Cup*			
Alfredo	140	12	5
Light Alfredo	80	5	5
Marinara	80	3	11
Roasted Garlic Marinara	60	1.5	9
Tomato Herb Parmesan	120	8	9
Bullseye			
BBQ Sauce: *Per 2 Tbsp*			
Grilled Onion w. Garlic, 1.3 oz	60	0	14
Sweet Hickory Smoke, 1.3 oz	65	0	15
Avg., other flavors	50	0	13

	C	F	Cb
Carb Options: *Per Serving*			
Alfredo, ¼ cup	110	10	2
Barbeque varieties, 2 Tbsp	10	0	3
Double Cheddar, ¼ cup	90	8	2
Garden Style, ½ cup	75	4.5	7
Hickory Barbeque, 2 Tbsp	10	0	3
Marinades: Italian Garlic, 1 Tbsp	0	0	0
Steak, 1 Tbsp	5	0	1
Catelli			
Meat Sauce, ½ cup	85	2.5	11
Garden Select 6, avg, ½ cup	80	2	14
Garden Select Pizza Sauce, 1 oz	15	0.5	2.5
Thick & Chunky Pasta Sauce, avg. all types, ½ cup	70	1.5	12
Cento: *Per Serving (½ Cup)*			
Sauces: Passata Tomatoes	40	0	8
Pasta, all natural	50	3	3
Pizza, fully prepared	25	0	5
Tomato: Arrabbiata; Vodka	70	3	6
Marinara; Puttanesca	115	9	6
White Clam	165	13	5
Classico: *Per ½ Cup Unless Indicated*			
Alfredo, ¼ cup	120	11	3
Florentine Spinach & Cheese	80	5	6
Four Cheese	95	5	10
Italian Sausage w. Peppers	90	2	13
Roasted Garlic Alfredo, ¼ cup	100	9	3
Spicy Red Pepper	50	1.5	7
Spicy Tomato & Pesto	90	4	11
Sundried Tomato	80	3	11
Sundried Tomato Alfredo, ¼ cup	120	10	4
Traditional Basil Pesto, ¼ cup	230	21	6
Other varieties, avg.	60	1	11
Contadina			
Tomato Sauce: *Per ¼ Cup (2.1 oz)*			
Regular	15	0	3
Garlic & Onion	20	0	4
Italian Style	15	0	3
Extra Thick & Zesty	20	0	3
Del Monte			
Pasta Sauces: *Per ½ Cup*			
Chunky Sce, average all varieties	60	1.5	11
D'Italia Pasta: Four Cheese	70	2	14
Other varieties	50	1.5	9
Spaghetti Sauce: Traditional	60	0.5	15
Garlic & Onion	80	1.5	16
w. Mushroom/Meat	70	1.5	14
Sloppy Joe Sauce, ¼ cup, 67g	50	0	11

Brands (Cont)

	C	F	Cb
Dominick's: *Per ½ Cup*			
All Natural: Garl. & Onion; Marinara	80	4	10
Mushr. & Olive; Tomato & Basil	80	1	8
Italian Classics: Four Cheese	80	2.5	12
Portabella Mushroom	60	2	9
Puttanesca	70	3	8
Spicy Roasted Garlic	70	2	10
Sun Ripened Tomatoes	80	4	8
Tomato Basil	50	1	8
Enrico's			
Tomato Basil, 3.5 oz	65	2	10
Traditional Italian Style, 3.5 oz	55	0.5	11
Mushroom Onion, ½ cup, 125g	70	1	12
Other varieties, ½ cup, 125g	70	2	12
Emiril's: *Per ½ Cup (123g)*			
Puttanesca	80	5	9
Roasted Red Pepper	60	3	7
Vodka Sauce	130	8	13
French's Grill & Glaze			
Honey Mustard, 2 Tbsp	90	1	18
Teriyaki, 2 Tbsp	60	0	13
Green Giant			
Sloppy Joe S'wich Sce, ¼ c., 2.5 oz	50	0	11
Sloppy Joe Sauce & Meat	200	11	11
Healthy Choice: *Per Serving*			
Garlic & Herbs, ½ cup	50	0	13
Traditional Pasta Sauce, ½ cup	50	0	13
Super Chunky: Vege Primavera, ½ c.	60	0	13
Tomato, Mushroom Garlic, ½ c.	50	0	10

Heinz: *Per 1 Tbsp (Approx. ½ oz)*	C	F	Cb
Barbecue Sauces, all flavors	35	0	9
Chili Sauce, 1 Tbsp	15	0	4
Horseradish Sauce	70	7	2
Mustard: Pourable/Mild, 1 Tbsp	10	0.5	0
Spicy Brown	15	1	1
Seafood Cocktail Sauce	20	0	3
Steak Sauce 57	15	0	4
Tartar Sauce, 1 Tbsp	70	7	2
Tomato Ketchup	15	0	4
Worcestershire Sauce, 1 Tbsp	10	0	1
Sloppy Joe Sauce, ½ cup, 125g	70	0.5	14
Hunt's			
BBQ Sauce: Original, 2 Tbsp	50	0	13
Hickory & Brown Sugar, 2 T.	70	0	18
Manwich Sloppy Joe Sce, ¼ cup	30	0	6
KC Masterpiece: *Per Tablespoon*			
Marinades: Garlic & Herb	30	1.5	4
Honey & Teriyaki	35	0.5	7
Original BBQ	40	1.5	7
Knorr			
Classic Sauce: *Per 2 Tbsp (Prepared)*			
Bernaise	20	0	4
Hollandaise	20	0	4
Classic Gravy, avg., ¼ cup, prepared	25	0	4
Knudsen: Potato Toppings, 2 Tbsp	50	4.5	2
Kraft			
CarbWell Sauce, 2 Tbsp	15	0	3
Sauceworks: Cocktail, 2 Tbsp	30	0.3	6
Horseradish, 1 tsp	20	1.5	0
Sweet 'n Sour, 1 Tbsp	30	0	7
Tartar: 1 Tbsp	50	5	2
Lemon & Herb, 1 Tbsp	75	8	0
Nonfat Tartar, 1 Tbsp	12	0	5
Barbecue Sauces: Average, 2 T.	50	0.5	9
Other Sauces: Mustard, 1 Tbsp	10	0	0
Horseradish, Reg./Crm Style, 1 T.	10	0	0
Sandwich Spread & Burger, 1 T.	75	7	2
Sweet 'n Sour, 1 Tbsp	40	0.5	9
Las Palmas			
Red Chile Sauce, ¼ cup, 2 oz	15	0.5	2
Enchilada Sauces: Green Chile	25	1.5	3
Hot/Original, ¼ cup, 2 oz	15	0.5	3
Salsa: Mexicana. Mild, 2 Tbsp, 1 oz	5	0	1
Mexicana Hot/Medium, 2 Tbsp	10	0	2

Sauces ~ Pasta, Cooking (Cont)

Brands (Cont)

	C	F	Cb
Lawry's 30 Minute Marinade: *Per Tbsp*			
Caribbean Jerk	25	0	5
Lemon Pepper	10	0	2
Mesquite	5	0	1
Thai Ginger; Herb & Garlic	10	0	2
Other varieties, average	20	0	3.5
Packet Seasonings: *Per Tablespoon (Dry)*			
Fajitas; Taco, 2 tsp., average	30	0	6
Average other flavors, 1 Tbsp	40	0	8
Libby's			
Sloppy Joe Sauce, ⅓ cup, 78g	45	0	10
McCormick Sauce Mixes			
Grillmates: Marinade, avg., 2 Tbsp	60	5	15
Sauce Blend Seasoning Mixes:			
Lemon Garlic Chicken, 1 Tbsp	30	0	5
Stir Fry Chicken, 2 tsp	20	0	4
Chicken Teriyaki, 1⅓ Tbsp	40	1	5
Mr Yoshida's			
Original Gourmet, 2 Tbsp, 30ml	90	0	20
Hawaiian Sweet & Sour, 2 Tbsp	35	0	9
Muir Glen: *Per ½ Cup (125g)*			
Organic Pasta Sauce:			
Mushr. Marinara; Portobello Mushr.	50	0	11
Other varieties, average	50	1	11
Newman's Own: *Per ½ Cup*			
Bombolina (Tomato & Basil)	100	4	13
Five Cheese	90	3	10
Fra Diavlo	70	3	10
Marinara; Sockarooni	60	2	12
Roasted Garlic & Peppers	70	2.5	11
Vodka	110	5	11
Old El Paso			
Salsa: Thick 'n Chunky, 2 T., 1 oz	10	0	2
Homestyle; Green Chili; Verde 2 Tbsp, 1 oz	10	0	2
Taco Sce, all varieties, 2 Tbsp, 1 oz	10	0	2
Enchilada Sce, all types, ¼ c., 2 oz	20	1	3
Grilling Sauces, all types, 2 Tbsp	60	0	14
Tom. & Gr. Chiles/Jalapenos, ¼ c., 2 oz	10	0	2
Pace: *Per 2 Tbsp*			
Picante Sauce	10	0	2
Chunky Salsa, average all types	10	0	2
Salsa Con Queso	90	6	6
Prego: *Per ½ Cup*			
Extra Chunky: Garden Comb.	90	1.5	16
Mushroom & Green Pepper	120	3.5	17
Mushroom Supreme	120	4	19
Three Meat Supreme	170	10	13
Tomato, Onion & Garlic	110	3.5	17
Pizza Sauce, ¼ cup	30	1	4

	C	F	Cb
Premier Japan (Organic)			
Garlic/Ginger/Wasabi Tamari, 1 T.	10	0	2
Thai Soynut, 1 Tbsp	25	2	2
Ragu: *Per ½ Cup*			
Sauces: *Per ½ Cup*			
Meat Flavored Sauce	80	3	10
Pizza Sauce	60	2	4
Traditional	70	3	8
Cheese Creations: *Per ¼ Cup*			
Classic Alfredo	110	10	3
Double Cheddar	100	9	3
Light Parmesan Alfredo	80	6	3
Parmesan & Mozzarella	60	4.5	3
Chunky Garden Style: *Per ½ Cup*			
Tomato, Basil & Italian Cheese	110	2.5	19
Super Chunky Mushroom	120	3	21
Other varieties, average	110	3	20
Rich & Meaty: *Per ½ Cup*			
Classic Italian Style	130	8	10
Beef, Onion & Garlic	110	5	11
Mama's Meat Sauce	110	5	10
Robusto!: *Per ½ Cup*			
Six Cheese	90	3.5	12
Italian Sausage & Cheese	100	4.5	12
Sauteed Onion & Mushr./Garlic	90	4	11
Tomato, Olive Oil, Garlic	90	4.5	12
Organic: *Per ½ Cup*			
Traditional; Cheese	80	3	11
Garden Vegetables	80	2.5	11
Pizza Quick: *Per ¼ Cup*			
Traditional	45	2	6
Chunky Mushroom	40	1.5	6
Chunky Tomato	50	1.5	7
Rainforest Organic			
Ginger Curry, 1 Tbsp	15	1.5	1
Papaya Pepper, 1 Tbsp	5	0	1
Rinaldi: *Per ½ Cup*			
3-Cheese	90	4	15
Original; Meat/Mushroom, avg.	80	3	12
Other varieties, average	70	2.5	12
Roberto's			
Salsa: Peach, 1 Tbsp, 15g	10	0	2
Black Bean & Corn, 2 Tbsp, 32g	10	0	2
Burrito Sce, ¼ cup, 60g	60	4	3
Enchilada Sauce, ¼ cup, 65g	90	5	10
Green Chile, Hot/Mild, 1 Tbsp, 15g	5	0	0

Brands (Cont) C F Cb

S & W: *Per Tablespoon*

	C	F	Cb
Teriyaki, Light/Marinade	25	0	5

Seeds of Change: *Per ½ Cup* 50 0.5 9

Steel's Gourmet Sauce

	C	F	Cb
Barbeque Sce, Sweet & Spicy, 2 Tbsp	15	0	2
Cocktail Sce w. Dill & Lemon, 4 Tbsp	36	0	1
Rocky Mountain Ketchup, 1 oz	10	0	0
Spiced Cranberry Sce, 4 Tbsp	16	0	4

The Wizard's (Organic)

	C	F	Cb
Hot Stuff, 1 Teaspoon	0	0	0
Vegetarian Worcestershire, 1 Tbsp	10	0	2

Troy's Sauces (Organic)

	C	F	Cb
Ginger Sauce, 1 Tbsp	5	0	1
Peanut Sauce, 1 Tbsp	30	2	1

Timpone's: *Per ½ Cup*

	C	F	Cb
Spaghetti Sauce: Classic	50	2.5	8
Family Recipe	80	3	7
Mom's	70	3.5	8

Tomaso's: *Per ½ Cup*

	C	F	Cb
Basil & Fresh Garlic; Spicy Eggplant	60	3	7
Black Olive Fresh Basil	40	2	5
Extra Garlic	55	2	8
Fresh Mushroom & Artichoke	50	2	7
Sugo Rosa	105	7.5	8

Tree of Life: *Per ½ Cup*

	C	F	Cb
Pasta Sauce Plus, all varieties	45	0	9
Organic, average all varieties	35	0	8

Walnut Acres: *Per ½ Cup (125g)*

	C	F	Cb
Organic Pasta Sauce, average	50	1	9

Wild Oats: *Per 2 Tbsp (1 oz)*

	C	F	Cb
Wasabi; Seafood Marinade & Grilled	30	3	4
Korean Sesame Marinade & Grilled	30	0	8

Quick Guide

Mayonnaise	C	F	Cb
Regular			
Average All Brands, 1 Tbsp	100	11	0
Bestfoods, Kraft, 1 Tbsp	100	11	0
½ cup, 4 oz	800	88	0
Light/Reduced Fat			
Kraft, 1 Tbsp	50	5	1
Best Foods, 1 Tbsp	45	4	2
½ cup, 4 oz	360	32	4
Hain, Eggless, Tbsp	60	6	2
Hain, Safflower Oil, Tbsp	50	5	2
Hellman's, 1 Tbsp	50	5	1
Wild Oats Canola Oil, 1 Tbsp	100	12	0
Fat Free			
Kraft, 1 Tbsp	10	0	3
½ cup, 4 oz	80	0	16
Smart Beat, 1 Tbsp	10	0	3
Sugar Free: Dukes Mayo, 1 Tbsp	10	12	0

Mayonnaise Style Dressing	C	F	Cb
BAMA Dressing, 1 Tbsp, ½ oz	50	4	3
Gourmayo (French's), 1 Tbsp, ½ oz	50	5	1
Miracle Whip Salad Dressing:			
Regular, 1 Tbsp, ½ oz	40	3.5	2
Light, 1 Tbsp, ½ oz	25	1.5	3
Free, 1 Tbsp, ½ oz	15	0	3
Nayonaise (Nasoya)			
(Tofu Base/Dairy Free/Eggless)			
Regular, 1 Tbsp, ½ oz	35	3	1
Fat-Free, 1 Tbsp, ½ oz	10	0	2

"Take two of these and call me in the morning"

Salad Dressings

Salad Dressings
Average All Brands
Per 2 Tbsp (Approx 1 fl.oz)

	C	F	Cb
Balsamic Vinaigrette: Reg., 1 oz	90	8	4
Light, 2 Tbsp, 1 oz	45	4	2
Fat Free, 2 Tbsp, 1 oz	5	0	1
Blue Cheese: Regular, 2 Tbsp, 1 oz	150	16	2
Regular, ¼ cup, 2 oz	300	32	4
Light, 2 Tbsp, 1 oz	80	8	1
Caesar: Regular, 2 Tbsp, 1 oz	140	14	2
Regular, ¼ cup, 2 oz	280	28	4
Light, 2 Tbsp, 1 oz	50	5	0.5
Coleslaw: Regular, 2 Tbsp, 1 oz	150	12	8
Regular, ¼ cup, 2 oz	300	24	16
Light, 2 Tbsp, 1 oz	90	7	7
French/Italian: Regular, 1 oz	120	11	5
Regular, ¼ cup, 2 oz	240	22	10
Light, 2 Tbsp, 1 oz	70	7	2
Fat/Oil-Free, 2 Tbsp, 1 oz	20	0	4
Ranch: Regular, 2 Tbsp, 1 oz	180	18	3
Regular, ¼ cup, 2 oz	360	36	6
Light, 2 Tbsp, 1 oz	90	8	3
Fat-Free, 2 Tbsp, 1 oz	50	0	2
Thousand Island: Regular, 1 oz	130	12	5
Regular, ¼ cup, 2 oz	260	24	10
Light, 2 Tbsp, 1 oz	50	4	3
Fat-Free, 2 Tbsp, 1 oz	35	0	3

*Enjoy a healthy salad
but don't drown it
in high-fat salad dressings.
Use 'light' dressing to halve
the fat and calories.*

Per 2 Tbsp (Approx 1 fl.oz)

Annie's Naturals	C	F	Cb
Cowgirl Ranch, 2 Tbsp	120	11	3
French; Goddess, avg.	90	9	3
Organic: Buttermilk	70	7	1
No-Fat Yogurt	20	0	3
Red Wine & Olive Oil	160	17	1
Thousand Island	90	7	5
Tuscany Italian	80	7	5
Vinaigrette:			
Balsamic; Cilantro & Lime, 2 T.	100	10	2
Low-Fat: Honey Mustard	45	2	6
Gingerly	40	2	4
Raspberry	35	1.5	5
Roasted Red Pepper	70	6	3
Shiitake & Sesame	120	13	1

Bernstein's			
Creamy Caesar, 2 Tbsp	120	13	1
Fat-Free Cheese & Garlic Italian	10	0	2
Italian	110	12	1
Olive Oil Vinaigrette	90	9	3
Restaurant Recipe Italian	130	13	1
Other varieties, avg., 2 Tbsp	110	11	2
Light Fantastic: Cheese Fantastico	25	1.5	3
Roasted Garlic Balsamic	45	3.5	3

Best Foods			
Dijonnaise, 1 tsp	5	0	1
Dippin' Sauce: Rockin' Ranch	110	12	1
Honey Mustard Madness, 2 Tbsp	90	6	8
Mayonnaise: Just 2 Good! 2 Tbsp	50	4	4
Light, average., all varieties	100	10	2
Real Mayonnaise, average	95	10	0
w. Lime Juice, 2 Tbsp	180	20	0

Bob's Famous			
Ranch Country, 2 Tbsp	150	15	1
Roquefort; Thousand Isl; Blue Chse	140	14	1
Tartar Sauce	170	16	2

Brianna's			
Blue Cheese; Zesty French	130	13	4
Blush Vintage	100	6	12
French Vinaigrette, 2 Tbsp	150	17	0
Honey Mustard; Poppy Seed	130	12	6
Lemon Tarragon	35	8	8
Rich Santa Fe Blend	15	0	3

Salad Dressings (Cont)

Per 2 Tbsp (Approx 1 fl.oz)

	C	F	Cb
Carb Options: Italian	70	8	0
Ranch	155	17	0
Whipped, 30g	90	10	0
Cardini's			
Caesar, 2 Tbsp	160	17	1
Fat-Free Caesar	40	0	9
Light Caesar	80	7	5
Extra Virgin Olive Oil Ital.; Zesty Garl.	120	13	1
Honey Mustard	140	13	5
Kalamata Olive w. Romano Cheese	120	13	2
Lemon Herb	120	13	1
Parmesan Ranch	150	15	2
Poppyseed w. Shallots	160	14	8
Vintage White Wine	110	12	1
El Torito: Cilantro Pepita Caesar	140	14	2
Emeril's: *Per 2 Tbsp*			
House Herb Viniagrette	140	14	2
Kicked Up Gaaalic	150	15	3
Girards: *Per 2 Tbsp*			
Blue Cheese Vinaigrette	100	10	3
Caesar	150	16	1
Lite	80	7	2
Champagne	150	16	2
Lite Champagne	60	5	2
Greek Feta Vinaigrette	110	11	1
Honey Dijon Peppercorn	120	13	7
Olde Venice Italian	120	13	2
Oriental Chicken Salad	120	11	6
Original French	120	13	0
Raspberry	90	10	9
Shiitake Chardonnay	100	9	4
Spinach Salad	80	2	14
Fat-Free: Balsamic/Red Wine, avg.	25	0	6
Caesar	40	0	9
Raspberry	50	0	13

Hidden Valley: *Per 2 Tbsp*	C	F	Cb
Light Ranch: B.L.T.	90	7	5
Light Ranch	80	7	3
w. Sundried Tomato	140	14	2
Regular Ranch: BBQ Ranch	120	12	3
B.L.T. Ranch; Coleslaw	150	15	5
Caesar w. Garlic	120	11	4
French w. Honey & Bacon	150	12	10
Old Fashioned Buttermilk	130	14	2
Original Ranch	140	14	1
Spicy	140	14	2
White Cheddar	130	13	1
w. Bacon	140	14	1
Fat-Free: Original Ranch	30	0	6
Honey & Bacon French	50	0	11
Original Ranch w. Bacon	40	0	5
Ken's Steak House Dressings: *Per 2 Tbsp*			
3 Cheese Italian	110	10	4
Balsamic & Basil Vinaigrette	110	12	1
Chunky Blue Cheese	140	15	1
Country French	130	11	9
Creamy Caesar	170	19	0
Peppercorn Ranch	180	19	2
Ranch	180	20	1
Italian w. Aged Romano	110	12	1
Thousand Island	130	13	4
Lite: Chunky Blue Cheese	80	7	4
Caesar/Olive Oil Vinaigrette	70	6	3
Creamy Parmesan	90	8	3
Ranch	100	9	4
Knott's Berry Farm: *Per 2 Tbsp (1 oz)*			
Honey Dijon, 2 Tbsp	130	13	4
Honey Poppyseed	120	9	10
Oriental Chicken Salad	130	11	5

MINIMAL EXERCISES FOR LAZY SLIMMERS

1. After finishing a set meal, place both hands on edge of table and P-U-S-H back hard!

2. Shake your head vigorously from side to side, every time you are offered a second helping of rich food.

Salad Dressings (Cont)

Salad Dressings (Cont)

Per 2 Tbsp (Approx 1 fl.oz)

	C	F	Cb
Kraft			
Regular Dressings: *Per 2 Tbsp*			
Honey Dijon	115	10	6
Classic Caesar	110	11	0.5
Coleslaw	150	12	8
Creamy Italian	105	11	3
Creamy French	155	15	5
Horseradish Sauce, 1 tsp	20	1.5	1
Roka Brand Blue Cheese	130	13	2
Thousand Island, avg.	125	10	5
Kraft Free (Fat-Free): Italian	15	0	4
Caesar Italian	25	0	4
Other varieties, avg.	45	0	11
Carb Well: Classic Caesar, 2 Tbsp	110	11	0
Italian	70	8	0
Ranch	110	11	0
Roka Blue Cheese	120	13	0
Light: Buttermilk Ranch	60	6	0
Italian, 2 Tbsp	20	1.5	0
Light Done Right!: Catalina	30	1	5.5
Italian; Ranch	75	7	3
Other varieties, avg.	70	6	3
Special Collection: Caesar Italian	100	10	2
Balsamic Vinaigrette	90	8	4
Sweet Honey Catalina; Poppyseed	130	11	8
Other varieties, avg.	55	4	4
Seven Seas, all varieties	90	9	2
Kroger			
Cream Cucumber	155	16	3
Creamy French, 2 Tbsp	130	12	6
Honey French	145	12	9
Poppy Seed	160	14	8
Real Mayonnaise	100	11	0
Zesty Italian	95	9	3
Lite: Zesty Italian	35	2	4
3 Cheese Ranch	80	8	2
Ranch	65	6	3
Fat-Free, avg., 2 Tbsp	30	0	8
Litehouse: Caesar	140	14	1
Chunky Bleu Cheese	150	16	1
Coleslaw	90	7	7
Jalapeno Ranch	120	12	1
Lite Bleu Cheese	70	6	2
Other varieties, avg.	120	13	3
Maple Grove: *Per 2 Tbsp (1 fl.oz)*			
Balsamic Vinaigrette	50	3	6
Regular: Honey Mustard	120	9	9
Parmesan & Pepper	115	11	4
Sweet & Sour	110	7	13

	C	F	Cb
Maple Grove (Cont)			
Fat Free: Balsamic Vinaigrette	5	0	1
Caesar Vinaigrette; Greek	10	0	3
Dijon; Poppyseed	40	0	10
Other varieties, avg.	30	0	8
Low Carb: Dijon	80	8	1
Balsamic; Raspberry Vinaigrette	5	0	1
Lite: Caesar; Pesto Parmesan	65	5	5
Honey Mustard	80	5	9
Romano	40	3.5	1
Marie's: *Per 2 Tbsp*			
1000 Island	190	20	2
Blue Cheese	170	18	0
Caesar	150	13	8
Poppy Seed	190	20	2
Ranch (8 fl.oz ctn), 2 Tbsp	160	16	4
(15.5 fl.oz ctn), 2 Tbsp	170	19	1
Light: Blue Cheese	70	7	2
Ranch	70	7	2
Nasoya: *Per 2 Tbsp*			
Vegi-Dressing (Tofu Base/Dairy Free):			
Thousand Island	60	4	6
Other flavors	60	5	3
Nayonaise: Regular, 2 Tbsp, 1 oz	70	6	2
Fat-Free, 2 Tbsp, 1 oz	20	0	4
Newman's Own: *Per 2 Tbsp*			
Balsamic Vinaigrette, 2 Tbsp	90	9	3
Caesar; Olive Oil & Vinegar	150	16	1
Creamy Caesar	170	18	1
Family Recipe Italian	120	13	1
Parmesan & Roasted Garlic	110	11	2
Parmesan Italiano	140	14	2
Ranch	180	18	2
Sesame Ginger, Low-Fat	35	1.5	5
Two Thousand Island	140	14	4
Lighten Up: Light Italian	60	6	1
Light Raspberry & Walnut	70	5	7
Light Balsamic Vinaigrette	45	4	2
San-J: Tamari Peanut	60	2	9
Tamari Sesame	45	2	5
Tamari Vinaigrette	45	3	4
Fat-Free: Tamari Mustard	25	0	5
S & W: *Per 2 Tbsp (1 oz)*			
Light: Italian	35	0	8
Red/White Wine; Raspberry Blush	40	0	10
Seeds of Change: *Per 2 Tbsp (1 oz)*			
Balsamic/Greek Feta Vinaigrette	60	5	4
Italian Herb Vinaigrette	50	4	4

Salad Dressings (Cont)

	C	F	Cb
Spike Splashes!			
Original, 2 Tbsp	100	11	1
Salt-Free	100	10	2
Fat-Free	10	0	2
Spectrum: *Per 2 Tbsp (Approx 1 fl.oz)*			
Fat Free: Creamy Dill/Garlic	20	0	4
Sweet On. & Garlic; Tstd Sesame	10	0	3
Low-fat: Honey Dijon	35	2	4
Zesty Italian	30	2	1
Organic: Greek Goddess, 2T.	110	11	2
Balsamic Vinaigrette	85	8	3
Provencal Garlic Lovers	55	5	2
Rocky Mountain Ranch	135	14	1
Steel's (Sugar-Free)			
Honey Mustard, 2 Tbsp	180	14	0
Sweet Ginger Lime, 2 Tbsp	140	14	2
Subway Select: *Per 2 Tbsp (1 oz)*			
Premium Collection: Caesar	170	16	1
Lite Blue Cheese; Lite Ranch	80	7	1
1000 Island	130	13	4
Jalapeno Ranch	100	10	1
The Spice Hunter: *Per 2 Tbsp (Mix Prepared)*			
Caesar Salad, 2 Tbsp	150	13	1
Chinese Salad; Garlic & Herb	140	13	2
T. Marzetti's: *Per 2 Tbsp (1 oz)*			
Regular: Balsam./Wild Berry Vinaig.	100	9	4
Buttermilk	180	19	1
Creamy Caesar	150	17	0
Caesar Lite	70	6	2
Italian	100	10	3
Original Slaw	170	16	6
Ranch	160	17	2
Red Wine Vinegar & Oil	130	14	2
Roasted Garlic	150	15	2
Roasted Garlic Vinaigrette	130	10	8
Sesame Oriental	110	9	8
Sour Cream Blue Cheese	170	16	0
Sun Dried Tomato Vinaigrette	130	11	6
Vinaigrette Blue Cheese	120	11	4
Light: Buttermilk Ranch	80	8	2
Chunky Blue Cheese	90	5	5
Original Slaw	100	7	10
Toby's: *Per 2 Tbsp (1 oz)*			
All varieties, average	120	12	1.5

	C	F	Cb
Walden Farms			
Fat-Free, Calorie Free Range, 2 Tbsp	0	0	0
Weight Watchers			
Salad Celebrations Dressings			
Fat Free: Caesar (Single), 0.75 oz	5	0	1
Caesar, 2 Tbsp	10	0	3
Creamy Italian (8 oz), 2 Tbsp	30	0	7
French Style, 2 Tbsp	40	0	9
Honey Dijon, 2 Tbsp	45	0	11
Italian (8 oz), 2 Tbsp	10	0	3
Ranch Style, 2 Tbsp	35	0	7
Ranch (Single), 0.75 oz	25	0	6
Wild Oats: *Per 2 Tbsp (1 oz)*			
Balsamic Vinaigrette; Thousand Isle	80	7	5
Caesar Style	120	12	1
Creamy Peppercorn	100	10	1
Honey Toasted Sesame Ginger	100	10	3
Ranch	120	11	3
Thousand Isle	90	7	5
Wishbone: *Per 2 Tbsp (1 oz)*			
Regular: 5 Cheese Italian	120	10	6
Chunky Blue Cheese	170	17	2
Classic Caesar	110	10	2
Creamy Caesar	180	18	1
French: Deluxe French	120	11	5
Sweet 'N Spicy	140	12	6
Italian: Regular	80	8	3
House Italian	110	10	3
Robusto Italian	90	8	4
Ranch: Original	160	17	2
w. Garlic/Spring Onion	150	15	2
Red Wine; Balsamic Vinaigrette	60	5	3
Russian, regular	110	6	15
Thousand Island	130	12	7
Fat-Free: Chunky Blue Cheese	35	0	7
Italian	15	0	2
Ranch	40	0	9
Dressing & Marinades: Asian	45	2	6
Balsamic Olive Oil & Herbs	40	2.5	4
Lemon Garlic & Herb	50	2.5	4
Tangy Honey Mustard	70	4	10
Ranch Up!	140	15	2
Just 2 Good!: Blue Cheese	45	2	6
Classic/Creamy Caesar; Ranch	40	2	5
Country Italian; Italian	30	2	5
Parmesan Peppercorn Ranch	45	2	6
Thousand Island	60	2	9

Breakfast Cereals

Quick Guide

Cooked Cereals

	C	F	Cb
Buckwheat Groats, roasted:			
Dry, ½ cup, 3 oz	280	2	60
Cooked, 1 cup, 7 oz	180	1	39
Bulgar: Dry, ½ cup, 2½ oz	240	1	53
Cooked, 1 cup, 6½ oz	150	0.5	34
Corn/Hominy Grits:			
Dry, ¼ cup, 1.4 oz	145	0.5	33
3 Tbsp, 1 oz	110	0.5	25
Cooked, ¾ cup, 6½ oz	110	0.5	25
Instant, 1 pkt, 0.8 oz	80	0.5	18
w. Imitation Bacon Bits, 1 oz	100	0.5	22
Cream of Rice, ckd, ¾ c, 6 oz	90	0	20
Cream of Wheat:			
Regular, ckd, ¾ cup, 6 oz	180	0.5	37
Quick, ckd, ¾ cup, 6 oz	95	0.5	20
Instant, ckd, ¾ cup, 6 oz	110	0.5	23
Farina: Cooked, ¾ cup, 6 oz	85	0	18
Millet, dry, ¼ cup, 1 oz	100	0	20
Oat Bran: Raw, ⅓ cup, 1 oz	75	2	21
Cooked, ½ cup	40	1	11
Oatmeal: Dry, ⅓ cup, 1 oz	110	0	19
Regular, ckd, ¾ cup, 6 oz	110	2	19
1 cup, 8 oz	145	3	25
Instant: Regular, avg., 1 oz	100	2	18
Flavored, average	150	2	32
Wheat Hearts, 1 oz dry, ¾ c. ckd	110	1	21

Brans, Wheatgerm, Add-Ons

	C	F	Cb
Bran: Wheat, unprocessed,			
1 Tbsp, 3g	10	0	3
Rice Bran, raw, 1 Tbsp, 5g	16	1	2.5
¼ cup, 1 oz	90	6	14
Oat Bran, 1 Tbsp, 5g	15	0.5	3
⅓ cup, 1 oz	75	2	15
Wheat Germ, 1 Tbsp, ¼ oz	25	1	3.5
¼ cup, 1 oz	105	3	15
Fruit: Dried, average, 1 oz	80	0	21
Banana, ½ medium	50	0	23
Prunes in Syrup, 5, 3 oz	90	0	24
Honey, 1 Tbsp, ¾ oz	65	0	17
Lecithin Granules, 1 Tbsp, 10g	50	5	1
Nuts, Almonds, 6 (¼ oz)	40	4	5
Bee Pollen Granules, 1 T., 8g	25	1	2
Psyllium Husks, 1 Tbsp, 5g	10	0	1

Hot/Cooked Cereals ~ Brands

Per Serving	C	F	Cb
Albers Grits, ¼ cup, 1.4 oz	140	0.5	31
Bobs Red Mil-10 Grain, ¼ c., 40g	180	2.5	35
CarbSense: MiniCarb Instant	170	6	17
Instant Cereal: Country Spice, ½ C.	170	7	15
Roasted Hazelnut, ½ cup	190	9	15
Country Choice Oats, ½ cup, 40g	150	3	27
Dr McDougall's			
Oatmeal: 4 Grains, 2.2 oz	220	2	44
Barley, all varieties, 2.5 oz	270	3	51
Wheat, 2.4 oz	220	2.5	44
Erewhon: Barley Plus, ¼ c., 1.7 oz	170	1	37
Brown Rice Crm, ¼ cup, 1.6 oz	170	1	36
Instant Oatmeal, 1.2 oz pkg	140	2	26
Oat Bran, ⅓ cup, 1.8 oz	170	2.5	31
Health Valley: Hot Cups,			
Apple; 10 Grain, 1 cup	220	2.5	42
Maple; Banana, 1 cup	240	2.5	46
McCann's Instant Irish Oatmeal			
Apple & Cinnamon, 1.23 oz	130	1.5	27
Maple & Brown Sugar, 1.5 oz	160	2	32
Original, 1 oz pkg	100	1.5	18
Steel Cut Oats, ¼ cup, 1.4 oz	150	2	26
Mothers Oat Bran, ½ cup, 1.4 oz	150	3	25
Nabisco: Cream of Rice, ¼ c., 46g	170	0	38
Cream of Wheat: Orig., 3T., 1 oz	120	0	25
Maple Brown Sugar, 1.2 oz pkg	120	0	27
Malto Meal: Orig., 3T., 1.2 oz	120	0.5	26
Maple Brown Sugar, ¼ cup	170	0	37
Natures Path: Apple Cinn.1.7 oz	190	2	38
Average other varieties	200	4	35
Quaker: Oatbran, ½ cup, 1.4 oz	150	3	25
Brown Sugar Bliss, 1 cup, 1.7 oz	190	2.5	39
Honey Nut Heaven, 1 cup, 1.7 oz	190	3.5	38
Multigrain, ½ cup	130	1.5	29
Old Fashioned Oats, ½ cup, 1.4 oz	150	3	27
Stone-Buhr Rice, ¼ cup, 1.4 oz	65	0	14
Sun Country Quick Oats, ½ c.,1.4 oz	130	1	30
Grits: Reg. all types, 1 pkg	130	0.5	31
Instant, all types, 1 pkg, 1 oz	100	1	22
Instant Oatmeal: *Per Package*			
Oatmeal Regular, 1 oz	100	2	19
Bakery Favorites, avg. all types	160	2	33
Breakfast Blast, avg. all flavors	155	2.5	32
Fruit and Cream, avg. all flavors	140	2.5	26
Low Sugar, avg. all flavors	115	2	23
Nutrition for Workers, avg. all flav.	165	3	33
Oatmeal Express, avg. all flavors	205	3	42
Supreme, avg. all flavors	160	3	32
Silver Palate Oatmeal, ⅓ c., 40g	160	2.5	28
Uncle Sam Oatmeal, 1.2 oz	145	3	24

Quick Guide

Cold Cereals
Average All Brands

	C	F	Cb
Bran Flakes, ¾ cup, 1 oz	90	0.5	21
Corn Flakes, 1 cup, 1 oz	110	0.5	24
Granola, ¼ cup, 1 oz	130	4	21
Oat Bran Cereal, ⅓ cup, 1 oz	110	1	22
Puffed Rice, ½ oz	55	0	12
Puffed Wheat, ½ oz	55	0	12
Raisin Bran, ½ cup, 1 oz	85	0.5	20
Rice Crisps, 1 cup, 1 oz	110	1	25
Shredded Wheat, 1 bisc., ¾ oz	80	0.5	18
Sugar-frosted Flakes, ¾ c, 1 oz	110	0.5	26
Wheat Flakes, 1 cup, 1 oz	105	0.5	23

Breakfast Bars: *See Page 137*

Ready-To-Eat Cereal

	C	F	Cb
Arrowhead Mills			
Amaranth, 1 c., 1.2 oz	140	2	26
Bran Flakes, 1 cup, 1 oz	110	1	22
Corn Flakes, 1 cup, 1.2 oz	120	0	27
Kamut Flakes, 1 cup, 1 oz	120	1	25
Maple Buckwheat Flake, 1 c., 1.5 oz	170	1	35
Multi Grain Flakes, 1 cup, 1.5 oz	170	2	33
Nature O's, 1 cup, 1.1 oz	130	2	25
Oat Bran Flakes, 1 cup, 1.2 oz	140	2.5	24
Perfect Harvest, 1 cup, 1.2 oz	140	2	25
Puffed Corn/Rice, avg., 1 c., 0.6 oz	60	1	12
Puffed Kamut, 1 cup, 0.5 oz	60	0	11
Puffed Millet/Wheat, 1 cup, 0.6 oz	60	0.5	12
Rice Flakes, 1 cup, 1.7 oz	180	1	40
Shredded Wheat, 1 cup, 1.7 oz	190	1	38
Spelt Flakes, 1 cup, 1.1 oz	120	1	24
Atkins			
Morning Start: Blueberry, ⅔ cup	100	2	10
Banana Nut Harvest, ⅔ c., 1 oz	115	2.5	11
Crunchy Almond Crisp, ⅔ cup	105	1.5	8
Back to Nature			
Flax and Fiber Crunch, 1 cup, 2.1 oz	200	3	41
Granola, ½ cup, 1.6 oz	170	3	34
Hi Fiber Multibran, ½ cup, 1 oz	70	0.5	22
Hi Protein Crunch, ½ cup, 1.6 oz	150	1	27
Muesli, ¾ cup, 2.3 oz	230	4	48

	C	F	Cb
Barbara's Bakery			
Alpen Original, ⅔ cup, 1.9 oz	200	3	41
Breakfast O's, 1 ¼ cup	130	1.5	22
Brown Rice Crisps; Corn Flakes, 1 c.	110	0.5	25
Crispy Wheats/Soy Essence, ¾ cup	115	0.5	25
Fruity Punch; Puffins, ¾ cup, 1 oz	120	0.5	26
Grain Shop, ⅔ cup	120	1	24
Honey Crunch 'n Oats, ¾ cup, 1oz	115	1	24
Shredded Oats, 1¼ cups, 2 oz	230	2.5	46
Shred. Spoonfuls; Toasted O's, ¾ cup	125	1.5	24
Shredded Wheat, 2 bisc., 1.4 oz	140	1	31
Wild Puffs Caramel, ¾ cup, 1.1 oz	110	1	25
Breadshop			
Cranberry Crunch Muesli, 1 cup	200	3	44
Granola: Triple Berry Cr., ⅔ cup	220	7	36
Other varieties, avg., ½ cup	220	7.5	32
Bulk Cereal Nabisco - Malto Meal			
Apple Zings, 1 cup, 1.1 oz	130	1	30
Balance with Berries, 1 cup, 1.1 oz	110	0.5	26
Cocoa Roos/Dyno-Bites, ¾ c., 1 oz	120	1	27
Frosted Flakes, 1 cup, 1.1 oz	120	0	28
Frosted Mini Spooners, 1 c., 1.9 oz	190	1	45
Golden Puffs, ¾ cup, 1 oz	100	0	25
Mateys/Toasty O's, 1 cup, 1 oz	110	1	25
Toasted Cinnamon Twists, ¾ c., 1 oz	130	3.5	24
CarbSense: *Per ½ Cup*			
MiniCarb Granola, Apple Cinnamon	285	15	29
Cascadian Farms			
Honey Nut O's, 1 cup, 1 oz	120	1.5	24
Multi-Grain Squares, ¾ c., 1 oz	110	0.5	25
Oats & Honey Granola, ⅔ c., 2 oz	240	6	42
Wheat Crunch, ¾ cup, 1 oz	115	0.5	25
Purely O's, 1 cup, 1.1oz	110	2	22
Hearty Morning, ¾ cup, 1.9 oz	200	2.5	43
Raisin Bran, 1 cup, 1.9 oz	180	1	43
Dr McDougall's: Muesli, 2.7 oz	260	3	51
Ener-G (Gluten-Free Cereals)			
Crisp Rice Cereal, 1 cup, 1.7 oz	180	2.5	40
Granola & Trail Mix, ½ cup, 1.8 oz	260	16	2
Rice Nuts, ½ cup, 50g	190	1	41
Erewhon			
Apple Stroodles, ¾ cup, 1 oz	110	0.5	25
Aztec, 1 cup, 1 oz	110	0	26
Banana O's, ¾ cup, 1 oz	110	0	26
Corn Flakes, 1¼ cups, 2 oz	210	2.5	45
Crispy Brown Rice, 1 cup, 1 oz	110	0	25
Fruit'n Wheat, ¾ cup, 1.9 oz	170	1.5	39
Kamut Flakes, ⅔ cup, 1.2 oz	110	1	25
Raisin Bran, 1 cup, 1.8 oz	170	1	40
Whole Wheat Flakes, 1 cup, 2 oz	180	1	42

Breakfast Cereals (Cont)

Ready-To-Eat (Cont)

	C	F	Cb
General Mills (Big G)			
Basic 4, 1 cup, 1.9 oz	200	3	42
Boo Berry, 1 cup, 1 oz	120	1	26
Cheerios: Regular, 1 cup, 1 oz	110	2	22
Apple Cinnamon, ¾ c., 1 oz	120	1.5	25
Berry Burst, all types, 1 c., 1 oz	110	1.5	24
Frosted/Team, avg., 1 cup, 1 oz	120	1	25
Honey Nut, 1 cup, 1 oz	120	1.5	23
Multi-Grain, 1 cup, 1 oz	110	1	24
Chex: Corn, 1 cup, 1 oz	105	0.5	25
Frosted Mini Chex, ¾ cup, 1 oz	110	0.5	26
Honey Nut, ¾ cup, 1 oz	120	1	26
Morning Mix, 1 pouch, 1.15 oz	135	3.5	24
Multi-Bran, 1 cup, 2 oz	190	1.5	46
Rice, 1¼ cup, 1 oz	120	0.5	26
Wheat, 1 cup, 1.7 oz	180	1	40
Cinnamon Tst Crunch, ¾ c., 1 oz	130	3.5	24
Cocoa Puffs, 1 cup, 1 oz	120	1.5	26
Cookie Crisp; Count Choc, 1 c., 1 oz	120	1	26
Fiber One, ½ cup, 1 oz	60	1	11
Fiber One Honey clusters, 1¼ cup	170	1	47
French Toast Crunch, ¾ c., 1 oz	120	1.5	26
Golden Grahams, ¾ cup, 1 oz	120	1	26
Honey Nut Clusters, 1 cup, 2 oz	210	2.5	46
Kix: 1⅓ cup, 1 oz	120	1	25
Berry Berry, ¾ cup, 1 oz	120	1.5	26
Lucky Charms, avg., 1 cup, 1 oz	120	1	25
Oatmeal Crisp: Almond, 1 c., 2 oz	220	4.5	42
Apple Cinamon, 1 cup, 2 oz	210	2	45
Peanut Butter Toast Crunch, ¾ cup	130	3.5	23
Raisin Bran, 1⅓ cup, 2 oz	170	1	42
Raisin Nut Bran, 1¼, 2 oz	200	2.5	44
Reese's Puffs, ¾ cup, 1 oz	130	3.5	23
Total: Brown Sugar & Oats, ¾ cup	110	1	23
Corn Flakes, 1⅓ cup, 1 oz	110	0.5	24
Protein, ¾ cup, 1 oz	120	3.5	11
Raisin Bran, 1 cup, 2 oz	170	1	42
Whole Grain, ¾ cup, 1 oz	120	1.5	26
Trix, avg., 1 cup, 1 oz	120	1	27
Wheaties: 1 cup, 1 oz	110	1	24
Hansen's Natural: Per ½ Cup (2 oz)			
Orange & Chocolate Cereal	230	9	35
Strawberry & Yogurt Cereal	230	9	30
Toasted Nut Crunch Cereal	230	6	39
Tropical Cluster Cereal	210	5	36

	C	F	Cb
Health Valley			
Amaranth; Blue Corn Flakes, ¾ c.	110	0	24
Corn Crunch-Ems!, 1 cup, 1 oz	125	0	27
Empower, 1 cup, 2 oz	220	3	42
Fiber 7 Flakes, ¾ cup	110	0	24
Granola, ⅔ cup	200	1	43
Golden Flax, ¾ cup	205	3	38
Healthy Fiber Flakes, ¾ cup	105	0	23
Heart Wise, 1 cup, 2 oz	215	3	36
Just Flakes, avg., ¾ cup	110	2	19
Oat Bran Flakes, avg., ¾ cup	115	0	24
Oat Bran O's, ¾ cup	105	0	23
Raisin Bran Flakes, 1¼ cup	210	1	47
Raisin Cinnamon Granola, ⅔ cup	200	1	43
Raisin Soy Flakes, 1 cup, 2 oz	205	1	39
Real Oat Bran Alm. Crunch, ½ cup	185	3	34
Rice Crunch-Ems!, 1 cup, 1 oz	120	0	26
Slender, 1 cup, 2 oz	195	1.5	35
Soy Flakes, 1¼ cup, 2 oz	205	1.5	35
Soy O's, 1 cup, 1.7 oz	190	2	31
Crunches & Flakes: Honey, ¾ cup	135	0	31
Other varieties, ¾ cup	210	3	41
Heartland Natural Cereal			
Granola Cereal: Original, ½ cup	300	11	41
Low-fat Raisin, ½ cup	205	3	4
Kashi: Breakfast Pilaf, ½ c., ckd	170	3	30
Cinna-Raisin Crunch, 1 c., 1.76 oz	170	1.5	41
GoLEAN Crunch!, 1 cup, 1.8 oz	205	3	36
Good Friends, 1 cup, 1.8 oz	170	2	43
Heart to Heart, ¾ cup, 1.2 oz	110	1.5	25
Honey Puffed Kashi, 1 cup, 1.2 oz	120	1	25
Kashi GoLEAN, 1 cup, 1.8 oz	180	1	30
Medley, ¾ cup, 1.1 oz	100	1	26
Organic Promise: Cranberry, 1 oz	110	1	26
Autumn Wheat, 1 cup, 1.9 oz	190	1	45
Strawberry Fields, 1 cup, 1.1 oz	120	0	28
Seven in the Morning, ½ cup, 2 oz	210	1.5	47
Puffed Kashi, 1 cup, 0.9 oz	70	0.5	13
Kellogg's			
All-Bran: Bran Buds, ⅓ cup, 1.1 oz	70	1	24
Extra Fiber, 0.9 oz	50	1	20
Original, ½ cup, 1.1 oz	80	1	23
Apple Jacks, 1 cup, 1.2 oz	130	0.5	30
Berry Bones, Scooby-Doo, 1 cup	130	1	28
Cinnamon Krunchers, ¾ cup, 1 oz	130	3.5	23
Complete Oat Bran Flakes, ¾ cup	110	1	23
Complete Wheat Bran Flakes, ¾ cup	90	0.5	23
Corn Flakes: Regular, 1 cup, 1 oz	100	0	24
w. Real Bananas, ¾ cup, 1 oz	110	1	22
Honey Crunch, ¾ cup, 1 oz	110	0.5	26
Corn Pops, 1 cup, 1 oz	120	0	28
Cracklin' Oat Bran, ¾ cup, 1.8 oz	200	7	35

Kellogg's (Cont)	C	F	Cb
Crispix: Regular, 1 cup, 1 oz	110	0.5	25
Cinnamon Crunch, ¾ cup, 1.1 oz	120	1	26
Corn/Rice on One Side, 1 c., 1 oz	110	0	25
Crunchy Blends: Just Right, ¾ cup	200	2	43
Low-Fat Granola w. Raisins, ⅔ cup	200	3	48
Low-Fat Granola, no Raisins, ½ c.	190	3	39
Mueslix, ⅔ cup, 2 oz	200	3	40
Froot Loops: Regular, 1 cup, 1.1 oz	120	1	28
Marshmallow, 1 cup, 1.1 oz	120	1	25
Frosted Bran, ¾ cup, 1 oz	100	0.5	26
Frosted Flakes, Regular, ¾ cup, 1 oz	120	0	28
Fruit Harvest: Banana Berry, ¾ cup	120	1	25
Other varieties, average	110	0	26
Honey Smacks, ¾ cup, 1 oz	100	0.5	24
Lilo & Stitch, 1 cup, 1 oz	110	1	25
Mini Swirlz Cinnamon Bun, 1 cup	120	2	25
Mini-Wheats: Frosted (24)	190	1	44
Frosted Big Bite (5)	180	1	41
Frosted Bite Size (24), 2.1 oz	200	1	48
Frosted Vanilla Creme (24), 1.8 oz	180	1	43
Raisin, ¾ cup, 1.9 oz	180	1	42
Strawberry, ¾ cup, 1.8 oz	170	1	40
Mud & Bugs Chocolate, 1 cup	110	1	25
Nutri-Grain Wheat, ¾ cup, 1 oz	100	1	24
Nutri-Grain Bars: *See Page 137*			
Product 19, 1 cup, 1 oz	100	0	25
Raisin Bran: Regular, 1 c., 2.1 oz	190	1.5	45
Crunch, 1 cup, 1.9 oz	190	1	45
Rice Krispies: Regular, 1¼ cup	125	0	29
Cocoa, ¾ cup, 1.1 oz	120	1	27
Frosted, ¾ cup, 1.1 oz	110	0	27
Treats, ¾ cup, 1.1 oz	120	1.5	26
Smart Start: Antioxidants, 1 cup	185	0.5	43
Healthy Heart, 1 ¼ cup, 2.1 oz	230	2	49
Soy Protein, 1 cup, 2 oz	200	1.5	40
Special K: Regular, 1 cup, 1.1 oz	110	0	22
Fat-Free 10 Vitamin & Min., 1 cup	110	0	25
Fruit & Yogurt, ¾ cup, 1.1 oz	120	1	25
Low Carb Lifestyle, ¾ cup, 1 oz	100	3	14
Red Berries; Rice, 1 cup, 1.1 oz	110	0	25
Vanilla Almond, ¾ cup	110	1.5	25
Smorz, 1 cup, 1 oz	120	2	25
Sponge Bob Squarepants, 1 cup	120	1	26
The Incredibles, 1 cup, 1 oz	120	1	25
Tiger Power, Whole Grain, 1 cup	110	0.5	21
Pop Tarts: Sponge Bob Sq. Pants	195	5	36
French Toast, 1 pastry	220	8	34
Fruit/Frosted, avg. all flavors	200	5	37
Low-Fat, all flavors	190	3	39
Pastry Swirls, avg., 2.2 oz	260	11	37
Snak Stix, 1 pastry, 1.8 oz	200	5	36
Yogurt Blasts, 1 pastry	210	6	37

Mother's	C	F	Cb
Cinnamon Oat Crunch	245	3	48
Cocoa Bumpers, cup	130	0.5	29
Groovy Grahams; Round-Ups, ¾ cup	115	0.5	25
Peanut Butter Bumpers, cup	140	2.5	26
Toasted Oat Bran, ¾ cup	125	1.5	24
Nature's Path			
Corn Flakes, all types, ¾ cup, 1 oz	110	0	25
Eight Grain, ⅔ cup, 1 oz	100	1	23
Flax Plus, ¾ cup, 1 oz	100	1.5	22
Heritage, all types, ¾ cup, 1 oz	115	1	23
Heritage Muesli w. Raspberry, 1 oz	125	3	22
Honeyed Raisin Bran, ¾ cup, 1 oz	110	0.5	23
Multigrain Oatbran, ⅔ cup, 1 oz	100	1	24
Pumpkin Flax Plus, ½ cup, 1 oz	140	6	19
Toaster Pastries (1), 52g	210	4.5	40
Granola: Ginger Zing; Hemp, 1 oz	145	6	20
Avg. other varieties	125	3	22
Optimum: Power Breakfast, 1 cup	190	2.5	40
Slim, 1 cup, 1.9 oz	180	2.5	38
Zen, ¾ cup, 1.9 oz	200	2.5	43
New England Natural Bakers			
Fat Free: Muesli, ½ cup	170	0	39
Granola: Almond Raisin Crisp, ½ c.	255	9	36
Apple Sunrise, ⅓ cup	195	6	30
Berry Good, ⅔ cup	255	6	44
Grateful Date, ½ cup	245	8	37
Honey Crunch; Pecan, ½ cup	295	13	37
Low-fat Granola, ½ cup	205	2.5	41
Marple Almond Date, ½ cup	285	11	39
Peachy Keen, ½ cup	215	7	33
Low-fat Granola, ½ cup	205	2.5	41
Save The Forest: Chocolate Mix	175	10	18
Fruit & Nut Mix	140	6	19
Nut Granola, ½ cup	275	12	35
Granola: Absolutely Nuts, ⅔ cup	225	9	30
Raspberry Razzmatazz, ½ c.	255	9	37
New Morning			
Cocoa Crispy Rice, ¾ cup, 1 oz	120	0.5	26
Cocomotion, ¾ cup, 1 oz	100	0.5	22
Kamutios, 1 cup, 1 oz	120	1	25
Ultimate Oat Bran, ¾ cup, 1 oz	110	2	22
Oatios: Honey Almond, 1 cup, 1 oz	120	1	17
Original, 1 cup, 1 oz	120	1.5	24
Nutritious Living			
Hi-Lo, all types, ½ cup, 1 oz	90	1.5	11
40-30-30 Honey Almd, ¾ c.,1.4 oz	150	5	17

Breakfast Cereals (Cont)

Post	C	F	Cb
100% Bran, ⅓ cup, 1 oz	115	1	22
Alpha Bits, cup, 1 oz	135	1.5	27
w. Marshmallows, cup, 1 oz	120	1	26
Bran Flakes, ¾ cup, 1 oz	115	0.5	24
Carb Well: Cinnamon Crunch, 1 oz	120	2	14
Golden Crunch, 1 oz	110	1	14
Cocoa Pebbles, ⅞ cup, 1 oz	120	1.5	26
Fruit & Bran, 1 cup, 2 oz	210	3	42
Fruity Pebbles, 1.25 cup, 1 oz	110	1	24
Golden Crisp, ½ cup, 1 oz	110	0	25
Grape-Nuts, ½ cup, 2 oz	225	1	47
Grape-Nuts Flakes, ½ cup, 1 oz	115	1	24
Grape-Nuts O's, 1 oz	120	0	28
Honey Bunches of Oats, ¾ c., 1 oz	120	1.5	25
Honey-Comb Strawb. Blasted, 1 cup	120	1	26
Hulk w. Marshmallow Bits, 1 cup	110	0	27
Oreo O's w. M'mallow Bits, ¾ c., 1 oz	110	2	24
Raisin Bran, ⅔ cup, 2 oz	210	1	46
Selects: Banana Nut Crunch, ½ c.	250	6	44
Blueberry Morning, 1 cup, 2 oz	240	3.5	48
Cranberry Almond Crunch, 2 oz	215	3	43
Maple Pecan Crunch, ¾ cup, 2 oz	225	6	39
Great Grains: Crunchy Pecan, ⅔ c.	225	6	38
Raisins Dates Pecans, ⅔ c.	215	4.5	39
Shredded Wheat: Frosted, 1.8 oz	180	1	43
Honey Nut, cup, 1.8 oz	200	1.5	43
Original, 1 cup, 1.6 oz	160	1	36
Shredded Wheat & Bran, 2 oz	200	1.5	48
Toasties Corn Flakes, 1 cup, 1 oz	105	0	24
Waffle Crisp, 1 cup, 1 oz	130	2.5	25

Quaker
Ready to Eat Cereal

	C	F	Cb
Oat Bran, 1¼ cup	210	3	41
100% Natural Granola: ½ cup	220	9	31
Low-fat, ⅔ cup	210	3	44
w. Raisins, ½ cup	230	9	34
Captain Crunch: Regular, ¾ c., 1 oz	110	2	23
Choco-Donuts, ¾ cup, 0.9 oz	100	1	23
Crunch Berries, ¾ cup, 1 oz	110	2	23
Peanut Butter Crunch, 1 oz	110	3	21
Crunchy Corn Bran, 1 cup, 1 oz	90	1	23
Honey Graham Oh's, ¾ cup	110	2	23
Life, all types, ¾ cup	120	1.5	26
Puffed Rice, 1 cup, ½ oz	50	0	12
Puffed Wheat, 1¼ cups, ½ oz	50	0	11
Shredded Wheat, 3 biscuits	220	1.5	50
Unprocessed Bran, ⅓ cup	30	0	11
Bagged Cereal: Cocoa Blasts, 1 cup	130	1	29
Apple Zaps; Fruitany O's, 1 cup	120	1	27
Frosted Flakers, ¾ cup	120	0	28
Frosted/Honey Nut Oats, 1 cup	110	1	24

Quaker (Cont)	C	F	Cb
Bagged Cereal: (Cont)			
Frosted Oats/ Sweet Crunch, 1 c.	110	1.5	23
Rice Crisps, 1 cup	110	0	26
Fruitangy Oh's, 1 cup	120	1	27
Honey Crisp Corn Flakes, ¾ cup	110	0	27
Honey Dipps, 1¼ cup	130	1.5	28

Instant Oatmeal: See Page 94

Bars: See Page 140

Sweet Home Farm	C	F	Cb
Honey Nut Granola, ½ cup, 1.9 oz	200	7	34
Low-Fat Granola, ½ cup, 1.9 oz	180	3	38
Maple Pecan Crisp, 1 cup, 1.9 oz	220	7	36

Trader Joe's	C	F	Cb
10 & 10 Cereal, ¾ cup, 1.7 oz	170	3	31
Banana Nut Clusters, 1 cup 1.9 oz	220	6	38
Blueberry Medley, ¾ cup, 1.7 oz	200	5	36
Corn Puffs Sweetened, 1 cup	120	0	28
Cornflakes, 1 cup, 1.1 oz	110	0	26
Cranberry Almd Clusters, 1 c., 2 oz	220	5	40
Crunch: Cherry Almond, 1 c., 2 oz	210	5	39
Van. Almd/Maple Pecan, 1 c., 2 oz	220	6	38
Essentials, 1 cup, 2 oz	170	3	37
Flakes n'Fruit, 1 cup, 1.1 oz	120	0.5	33
Frosted Flakes, ¾ cup, 1 oz	110	0	27
Golden Flax Cereal, ¾ cup, 1.7 oz	190	3	38
High Fiber Cereal, ⅔ cup, 1.1 oz	90	1	25
Honey Nut O's, ¾ cup, 1 oz	120	1.5	24
Joe's O's, 1 cup	110	2	22
More & Less Apple Cinn.., ⅔ cup	100	1.5	12
Morning Lite, 1 cup, 1.4 oz	140	2	31
Muesli Cereal Blend, ¾ cup, 2 oz	200	1.5	42
Oat Bran Flakes, avg., 1 cup	200	1.5	45
Raisin Bran, 1 cup, 1.9 oz	170	1	44
Shred. Wheats, Bite Size, 1 c., 1.7 oz	170	1	41
Soy Granola, 1 cup, 1.9 oz	220	3	39
Touch of Honey, ⅔ cup, 1 oz	120	1.5	25
Triple Berry O's, ¾ cup, 1 oz	110	1	25
Toasted Oatmeal Flakes, ¾ c., 1.1 oz	110	1	23
Very Berry Clusters, 1 cup, 1.9 oz	200	4.5	36

Uncle Sam	C	F	Cb
Cereal w. Real Mixed Berries, 55g	230	4.5	39
w. Flaxseed, 1 cup, 55g	190	5	38

| Weetabix: 2 biscuits, 1.23 oz | 120 | 1 | 28 |

Weight Watchers	C	F	Cb
Honey Almond Crisp, ¾ cup, 1½ oz	150	2.5	31
Cinnamon Cluster Crunch, ¾ cup	150	1.5	31
Banana Almond Medley, ¾ cup	170	3	31
Puffed Vanilla Wheat, 1 cup, 1.1 oz	100	2	20
Flakes'n Fiber, ¾ cup, 1.1 oz	100	2	18

Grains & Flours	C	F	Cb

Per ½ Cup (8 level Tbsp)

	C	F	Cb
Amaranth, ½ cup, 3½ oz	375	6.5	66
Arrowroot, ½ cup, 2¼ oz	290	0	72
Atkins Bake Mix, low carb, 1 oz	115	2	6
Barley: Regular, ½ cup, 3¼ oz	325	2	67
Pearled, raw, 3½ oz	350	1	78
Flakes, ½ cup, 1½ oz	150	0.5	31
Buckwheat: Regular, ½ c., 3 oz	290	3	60
Groats: Roasted, dry, 3 oz	295	2.5	64
Roasted, cooked, 3½ oz	90	0.5	20
Flour, whole-groat, ½ cup	190	2	40
Bulgur: Dry, ½ cup, 2½ oz	240	1	54
Cooked, ½ cup, 3¼ oz	75	0.5	17
Carob Flour, ½ cup, 1.8 oz	115	0.5	45
Corn Kernels (blue/yellow), 3 oz	75	1	18
Corn Bran, ½ cup, 1.4 oz	90	0.5	34
Corn Flour/Masa, 2 oz, ½ cup	210	2	44
Corn Grits: Dry, ½ cup, 2¾ oz	290	1	62
Cooked, ½ cup, 4¼ oz	75	0.5	16
Corn Germ, toasted, 4 oz	100	1.5	21
Cornmeal: Average All Types			
3 Tbsp, 1 oz	100	0.5	22
½ cup, 2.2 oz	230	1	46
Mixes: same as above	230	1	48
Cornstarch: 1 Tbsp, 8g	30	1	48
½ cup, 2¼ oz	240	1	57
Couscous: Dry, 1 oz (yield 3 oz ckd)	95	0	20
1 cup cooked, 5.5 oz	175	0	36
Farina: Dry, ½ cup, 3 oz	315	0.5	66
Cooked, ½ cup, 4.1 oz	55	0	12
Flax Seeds: Seeds, 2 oz	280	20	20
Ground, 2 Tbsp	60	4.5	4
Flour: *See 'Wheat flour' Next Page*			
Garbanzo (Chick Pea), ½ c., 2 oz	205	3.5	35
Kuzu Root Starch, 1 Tbsp, 10g	35	0	8
Matzo Meal, ½ cup, 2.2 oz	230	0.5	48
Millet: Raw, ½ cup, 3½ oz	375	4	73
Cooked, ½ cup, 4¼ oz	145	1	29
Oat Bran: Raw, ⅓ cup, 1.1 oz	75	2	21
Cooked, ½ cup, 4 oz	45	1	13
Oats, rolled/oatmeal:			
Dry/Groats, ½ cup, 1.5 oz	165	3	28
Cooked, ½ cup, 4.2 oz	75	1	13
Polenta: *See Cornmeal*			
Made Up, ½ cup, 5 oz	220	2	24
Potato Flour, ½ cup, 3.2 oz	355	0.5	72
Psyllium Husks, 1 Tbsp (5g)	35	0	8
Quinoa: Dry ½ cup, 3 oz	320	5	58
Cooked, ½ cup	130	4	17

Grains & Flours (Cont)	C	F	Cb

Per ½ cup (8 level Tbsp)

	C	F	Cb
Rice Bran, ⅓ cup, 1 oz	90	6	14
Rice Flour, ½ cup, 2¾ oz	290	2	63
Rice Polish, ½ cup, 3½ oz	360	0.5	79
Rye Flour: Dark, 1 cup, 4½ oz	415	3.5	88
Medium, 1 cup, 3½ oz	345	2	76
Light, 1 cup, 3½ oz	360	1.5	78
Rye Grain: ½ cup, 3 oz	280	2	59
Flakes, ½ cup, 1½ oz	145	1	30
Semolina, ½ cup, 3 oz	305	1	62
Sorghum, ½ cup, 3.4 oz	330	3	72
Soybean Flakes, ½ cup, 1½ oz	235	10	17
Soy Bean Flour:			
Defatted, 1 cup, 3½ oz	330	1	38
Low-Fat, 1 cup, 3 oz	315	6	32
Full-Fat, 1 cup, 3 oz	370	18	30
Soy Meal, defatted, 1 cup, 4.3 oz	410	3	49
Spelt Flour, ½ cup, 2 oz	195	1	41
Tapioca, pearl: Dry, ½ c., 2.7 oz	275	0	68
3 Tbsp, 1 oz	100	0	25
Teff (Seed) Flour, 2 oz	200	1	40
Tortilla Flour Mix, ½ cup, 2 oz	230	6	38
Triticale: ½ cup, 3.4 oz	325	2	70
Flour, whole-grain, ½ cup	220	1	47
Wheat, average, ½ cup, 3½ oz	335	2	74
Wheat Bran, unproc., 1 oz	60	1	18
Wheat Flakes, ½ cup, 1½ oz	160	1	35
Wheat Germ: ¼ cup, 1 oz	105	3	15
Toasted, ¼ cup, 1 oz	110	3	14
Wheat Flour:			
White, All Purpose/Self-Rising,			
1 level Tbsp, 0.6 oz	60	0	13
½ cup, 2.1 oz	220	0.5	46
1 cup, 4.4 oz	455	1.5	95
Whole Wheat, 1 cup, 4.2 oz	410	2.5	87

Rice

White Rice	C	F	Cb
Raw: Short/Med. Grain, 1 c., 7 oz	720	1	156
Long Grain, 1 cup, 6½ oz	670	1	144
Glutinous, 1 cup, 6½ oz	680	1	150
Cooked Rice (Boiled/Steamed):			
Short/Medium Grain:			
½ cup, 3¼ oz	120	0	27
1 cup (½ Pint), 6½ oz	240	0.5	54
2 cups (1 Pint), 13 oz	480	1	108
Long Grain: ½ cup, 2¾ oz	100	0	22
1 cup, 5½ oz	200	0.5	44
Glutinous/Sticky, ckd, 1 c., 6 oz	170	0.5	36
Parboiled, cooked, ½ cup, 3 oz	90	0	20
Precook./Instant: Dry,½ c., 3½ oz	370	0	80
Cooked, ½ cup, 3 oz	90	0	20
Wild Rice: Raw, 1 cup, 5½ oz	570	13	120
Cooked, 1 cup, 5¾ oz	165	0.5	35

Brown Rice	C	F	Cb
Average of Short or Long Grain			
Raw/Dry: ½ cup, 3½ oz	350	2.5	72
1 cup, 7 oz	700	5	144
Cooked: ½ cup, 3½ oz	110	0.5	23
1 cup, 7 oz	220	1.5	46

Rice Dishes	C	F	Cb
Chinese Fried Rice:			
½ cup, 2½ oz	160	5	21
1 cup, 5 oz (½ Pint)	320	13	42
2 cups, 10 oz (1 Pint)	640	26	84
Mexican Rice: 1 cup	500	12	90
Taco John's, 1 serving (6 oz)	240	8	35
Taco Time, 1 serving (4 oz)	160	2	30
Rice-A-Roni: See Page 74			
Rice Pilaf: Restaurant, 1 cup	270	7.5	43
Bob Evans, 5 oz	165	3	32
Rice w. Raisins/Pinenuts, 1 cup	400	11	70
Risotto, 1 cup	420	18	65
Saffron Rice, 1 cup	370	12	66
Spanish Rice: 1 cup	390	9	72
El Pollo Loco, 4 oz	160	1	33
Taco Cabana, 4 oz	180	5	30
Sticky Thai Rice, plain, 1 cup	170	0.5	36
Sushi Rice, 1 Tbsp	25	0	6
Uncle Ben's: See Page 67			

- Macaroni includes all shapes and sizes; (e.g. spaghetti, fettuccini, shells, tubes, ziti, twists, sheets, cannelloni, manicotti, elbows).
- All regular macaroni products have the same cals/fat/carb. on a weight basis.
- 1 oz Dry = approx. 2½ -3 oz cooked.

Dry Spaghetti/Macaroni

	C	F	Cb
1 oz quantity	105	0.5	21
1lb box/pkg., 16 oz	1680	7	336
Elbows, 1 cup, 3¾ oz	395	2	77
Shells, small, 1 cup, 3¼ oz	340	2	66
Spirals, 1 cup, 3 oz	315	2	61

Cooked Spaghetti/Macaroni

	C	F	Cb
Plain, All Types (no added fat):			
Firm/Al Dente (8-10 mins.), 1 oz	42	0.5	8.5
Medium (11-13 mins.), 1 oz	37	0.5	7.5
Tender (14-20 mins.), 1 oz	32	0.5	7
(Longer cooking increases water absorbed)			
Spaghetti, ½ cup, 2 ½ oz	90	0.5	18
Medium serving, 1 cup, 5 oz	185	1	37
Large (restaurant), 2 c., 10 oz	370	2	74
Elbows/Spirals, 1 cup, 5 oz	185	1	38
Small Shells, 1 cup, 4 oz	150	0.5	31
Protein-fortified: Dry, 1 oz	107	0.5	21
Cooked, 1 cup, 5 oz	230	0.5	44
Spinach/Vegetable: Dry, 1 oz	105	0.5	21
Cooked, 1 cup, 5 oz	180	0.5	37
Whole-wheat: Dry, 1 oz	100	0.5	21
Cooked, 1 cup, 5 oz	175	0.5	37

Fresh Pasta (Refrigerated)

	C	F	Cb
Plain/Spinach/Tomato, average:			
As purchased, 4 oz	325	2.5	64
Cooked, 1 cup, 5 oz	190	1	38
Home-made, without egg:			
Cooked, 1 cup, 5 oz	175	1	35
Buitoni			
Pasta: Angel Hair, 9 oz	230	2.5	43
Fettuccine/Linguini: 9 oz	240	2.5	45
Spinach, 9 oz	260	3	45

Buitoni (Cont):	C	F	Cb
Ravioli: Chicken Parmesan, 9 oz	310	8	45
Four Cheese, 9 oz	330	14	40
Light, 9 oz	230	4	37
Garden Vegetable, 9 oz	250	5	39
Beef Ravioletti, 7 oz	300	7	46
Roast Chicken & Garlic, 9 oz	340	11	47
Tortellini: Cheese & Rst Garlic, 9 oz	270	8	37
Chicken & Prosciutto, 9 oz	330	9	47
Herb Chicken, 9 oz	340	9	52
Mozzarella & Pepperoni, 9 oz	330	10	45
Mushroom & Cheese, 9 oz	270	6	46
Sundried Tomato, 9 oz	310	9	46
Sweet Italian Sausage, 9 oz	330	9	48
Three Cheese, 9 oz	320	7	50
Pasta Sauces: See Page 86			

Noodles

	C	F	Cb
Plain/Egg: Dry, 1 oz	108	1	20
1 cup, 1⅓ oz	145	1.5	28
Cooked, 1 oz	38	0.5	7
½ cup, 2¾ oz	105	1	20
1 cup, 5½ oz	210	2	40
Stir-Fried: 1 cup, 5½ oz	270	9	40
2 cup serving, 11 oz	540	18	80
Yolk Free (Cooked): *Per Cup*			
'No Yolks' *(Foulds)*	210	2	40
Passover Gold *(Manischewitz)*	200	0	42
Chinese: Cellophane/Rice, dry, 1 oz	100	0	25
Chow Mein/hard, dry, 1 oz	150	5	17
Ramen Noodles: See Page 73			
Japanese: Soba, dry, 1 oz	95	0.5	21
cooked, 1 cup, 4 oz	110	1	24
Somen, dry, 1 oz	100	1	22
cooked, 1 cup, 6 oz	225	0.5	49
Japanese Style Pan Fried:			
Maruchan's Yaki-Sobu, 5.6 oz cup	260	3	50
Udon *(Chikara)*, avg., 7.5 oz pkt	250	1	52
Stir Fry *(Yakisoba)*, 3.5 oz serving	220	2	44
Thai Kitchen: See Page 75, 83			

Egg Roll Skins/Won Ton

	C	F	Cb
Egg Roll Skins:			
(Golden Dragon) 1 pce, 1 oz	80	0	18
(Wung Hung) 4 skins, 4 oz	300	0	64
Won Ton Wrappers:			
(Dynasty) 10 wrappers, 2.1 oz	170	1	36
Egg Roll/Spring Roll Wrapper:			
(Dynasty) 3 wrappers, 2.1 oz	170	1	36

Breads

Note: Most breads have similar calories on a weight basis. However, volume may vary.

For example, 1 oz of bread may equal 1 slice regular bread or 2 slices of a lighter bread.

It is best to weigh bread used and calculate on 1 oz bread = 70 calories.

Quick Guide

Bread

Average All Varieties:

	C	F	Cb
Thin slice (¼") 1 oz	70	1	13
Extra thin slice ¾ oz	55	0.5	10
Light thin slice, 0.6 oz	40	0.5	7.5
Toasting slice, 1.2 oz	85	1	16
Thick slice (³⁄₈"), 1.5 oz	105	1.5	20
Large thick (½"), 2 oz	140	2	26
1-lb Loaf, 16 oz	1120	6	208

Toast has same calories as bread used.

1 Toasting Slice:			
w. 2 tsp fat spread	175	10	16
w. 2 tsp "light" spread	120	5	16
w. 1 Tbsp fat spread	185	12	16
w. 1 Tbsp "light" spread	135	7	16

Breads

	C	F	Cb
12-Grain, 1½ slice	120	1.5	23
Batard (8 oz), thick slice, 2 oz	140	0.5	28
Boule, ½" thick, 2 oz slice	130	0	29
Bran style/Dark, 1 oz	70	1	14
Bread w. Soy Isoflavones, 1.2 oz	80	2	11
Buttermilk, average, 1½ slice	120	1.5	24
Caraway Rye, 1 oz slice	70	0	15
Challah, 1 oz slice	85	2	14
Chapati, 2.2 oz	200	7.5	30
Ciabatta, 1 slice, 0.7 oz	50	0.5	11
Corn Bread, average, 1 pce, 3 oz	180	7	30
Cracked Wheat Sourdough, 1½ oz	130	0.5	27
Croissants: *See Page 113, 173*			
Crustless Bread, regular slice ¾ oz	40	0.5	8.5
Crusts Only, regular slice, ¼ oz	30	0	7
Date & Nut, 1 oz slice	90	1	14
'Enriched' Breads, average, 1 oz sl.	75	1	18
Flax & Sunflower Round, 1.2 oz	90	2	18
Foccacia: Plain, 2 oz portion	150	4	23
Cheese & Garlic; Pesto, 2 oz	170	8	21
Tomato & Olive, 2 oz	120	2	20
French Stick/Baguette, 1 oz slice	70	1	15

Breads (Cont)

	C	F	Cb
French Toast, 1 slice, 2¼ oz	160	7	18
Sticks (Aunt Jemima), 1 pce, 1 oz	75	3	12
Garlic Bread/Toast:			
Small slice + 1 tsp spread, ¾ oz	80	5	7
Med. slice + 2 tsp spread, 1½ oz	160	10	14
Thick slice + 3 tsp spread, 1.8 oz	220	14	20
Pepperidge Farm, 1 slice, 1.4 oz	160	10	15
Hemp Bread, 1.2 oz	95	2	12
Italian Bread, 1 oz slice	75	1	15
Light Bread, avg., 0.8 oz slice	40	0.5	8
Lower Carb (higher Protein/fiber), average all brands, 1 oz	60	1	7
Melba Toast, 2 pces	25	0	6
MultiGrain: 1 slice, 1 oz	75	1	14
Nut/Health Nut, 1 oz slice	85	2	15
Oatmeal/Oatbran Bread, 1 oz sl.	70	1	13
Party Breads (Pepp. Farm): Rye, 1 sl.	15	0.5	3
Dijon; Pumpernickel, 1 sl.	18	0.5	3.5
Pita: Average all types,			
Small (4" diam) 1 oz	75	0.5	15
Large (6½" diam) 2 oz	150	1	30
Extra Large (9" diam) 4 oz	300	1	60
Popovers (1), no butter	90	2	14
Poppyseed (Vienna), 0.8 oz sl.	55	1	10
Pumpernickel, 1 oz slice	75	1	15
Cocktail size, 0.4 oz	30	0.5	6
Raisin Bread, 1 oz slice	80	1.5	15
Raisin Walnut, 2 oz slice	160	3.5	29
Roman Meal, 1 oz slice	70	1	14
Country Potato & Oat, 1½ oz	110	1.5	20
Rye: Average, 1 thin slice, 1 oz	75	1	13
1 thick slice, 2 oz	150	2	25
Cocktail size, 0.4 oz	25	0.5	4
Sandwich Bread, 1 oz slice	70	1	13
Sandwich Pockets, Reg., 2 oz	150	1	30
Sourdough, 1½ oz slice	100	1	20
Sourdough French, 1 oz	75	0	14
Spelt, 1.2 oz	90	3	14
Sprouted 7-Grain, 1.5 oz slice	110	1.5	18
Squaw, 1.1 oz slice	85	0.5	13
Tacos/Tortillas: *See Page 104*			
Turkish/Middle Eastern, 1 oz sl.	80	1.5	16
Wheat-Free Breads: Spelt, 1.2 oz	70	0	14
Healthseed Rye, 1.6 oz	90	1	20
Kamut, 1.2 oz	80	0	16
Millet, 1.5 oz	100	1	20

Breads ✦ Bread Rolls ✦ Croutons

Bread Brands

	C	**F**	**Cb**
Controlled Carb Gourmet			
High Fiber, 1 slice, 1 oz	80	2.5	11
Zero Net Carb, 1 slice, 1 oz	60	1	7
Ener-G: Gluten-Free Breads			
Brown Rice Bread, 1 slice, 38g	130	6	18
Light Brown Rice, 1 slice, 19g	70	4	9
Corn Loaf, 1 slice, 19g	40	2.5	8
Light Tapioca, 1 slice, 19g	70	3	10
Ezekiel			
Low Carb: Wheat, 0.8 oz	70	4	4
Savory Herb, 0.8 oz	60	2.5	4
Genesis 1: 29, 0.8 oz	80	2	14
Nature's Path: *Per Slice (2 oz)*			
Manna: Carrot Raisin; Millet Rice	130	0	28
Cinnamon Date	150	0	29
Fruit & Nut	140	1	27
Sun Seed	160	2	29
Whole Rye	150	0	32
Whole Wheat; Multigrain	125	0	26
Oroweat: *Per Slice*			
100% Whole Wheat, 1.3 oz	100	2	19
Carb Counting Multigrain, 1 oz	60	1.5	9
Pepperidge Farm: *Per Slice*			
100% Whole Wheat	85	1	15
Apple Walnut Swirl	80	2	14
Golden Swirl	95	2	15
Hearty 7-Grain	100	2	18
Light Style, average	45	0	9
Raisin w. Cinnamon	85	2	14
Pillsbury			
Popovers: Perfect (1), ¹⁄₁₀ container	95	2	19
Original, w. skim milk, butter & eggwhites (1), ¹⁄₆ container	95	0	18
Original, w. whole milk & whole eggs (1), ¹⁄₆ container	140	5	18
Ralph's: Breakfast Blend, 1 sl., 2 oz	180	3.5	33
Sara Lee: *Per Slice*			
Delightful White, ¾ oz	45	0.5	9
Honey Wheat, 1 oz	70	0.5	14
Multi-Grain, 1.4 oz	100	1	19
Schwan's: *Per Serving*			
Cheese & Herb Biscuits (1), 34g	110	6	11
Chse Stuffed Bread w. Sauce, 56g	155	5	20
Five Chse Garlic French Bread (1), 96g	330	20	26
French Baguette Bread, ¼ loaf, 49g	120	0	25
French Dinner Rolls (1), 51g	130	1.5	24
Frozen Bread Dough, ¹⁄₈ loaf, 56g	140	1.5	27
Southern Style Biscuits (1), 62g	200	10	23
Wonder: Sandwich, 1 slice, 1 oz	70	1	14
Light (Low-Fat), 1 slice, ¾ oz	40	0.5	9

Bread Rolls & Buns

	C	**F**	**Cb**
Brown 'n Serve, average, 1 oz	80	2	15
Carb Monitor *(Pillsbury),* 1.1 oz roll	70	2	11
Ciabatta Roll, 3½ oz	230	4	41
Concha (Mexican Sweet Bread), 3 oz	400	19	50
Dinner Rolls: 1 small, 1 oz	85	2	15
1 medium (3" diam), 1½ oz	130	3	23
English Muffins, avg., 2 oz	140	2	27
Frankfurter/Hot Dog: 1¼ oz	100	2	19
1½ oz size	120	2	23
French: 1 medium, 1.3 oz	110	1	24
1 large, 3 oz	240	2	52
Hamburger: Regular, 1½ oz	120	2	23
Large, 3 oz	240	4	46
Hoagie/Submarine, 4¾ oz	400	8	77
Hot Cross Bun, Medium, 2.3 oz	185	5	31
Kaiser Roll, 2 oz size	170	3	18
Onion Roll, 2 oz size	170	2	24
Parker House Roll, 0.7 oz size	65	1	12
Party Roll, 0.6 oz	55	1	10
Sandwich Roll, 1.6 oz size	120	2	23
Soft Pretzel Bun *(J & J),* 3 oz	235	3	50
Sourdough Roll, 1¼ oz size	100	1	20
Sweet Rolls, 1 oz	100	2	20
w. Icing, average	160	6	20
Wheat Roll: Small, 1 oz	75	0.5	14
Medium, 1½ oz	110	1	20

Breadsticks, Croutons

	C	**F**	**Cb**
Breadsticks: Salt Sticks, plain, 1 oz	110	1	20
Fresh baked (1), 2 oz	180	2.5	34
Boboli, 1.75 oz	130	2	22
Stella D'oro: Sesame (1)	50	2	7
Plain/Onion/Wheat, 1 pce	40	1	7
Keebler/Lance, 2 sticks	30	0.5	6
Croutons: Seasoned, 2 Tbsp, ¼ oz	35	1.5	4
9 small or 6 large, ¼ oz	35	1.5	4
Fat-Free *(Pepp. Farm),* 2 Tbsp	30	0	5

Bread Products

	C	**F**	**Cb**
Bread Crumbs, dry:			
Plain or seasoned, 1 oz	110	1	20
1 rounded Tbsp, 10g	35	0.5	6
1 cup, 3½ oz	390	5	73
Corn Flake Crumbs, 1 oz	110	1	20
Graham Cracker Crumbs, 1 oz	115	1	21
Keebler, 1 cup, 4¼ oz	520	14	84
Bread Dough: Frozen, 1 slice	75	1	14
Refrigerated, French, 1" slice	60	1	13
Wheat/White, 1" slice	80	2	14
Coating Mixes: Average, 1 oz	110	3	20
Featherweight, 1.4 oz pkg	70	0.5	17
Stuffing: Average, dry mix, 1 oz	110	1	10
Made-up, ½ cup, 4 oz	180	9	11

Bagels • Tacos • Rice Cakes

Quick Guide

Bagels

	C	F	Cb
Average All Brands			
Plain/Onion:			
1 mini/bagelette, 1 oz	80	1	15
1 small bagel, 2 oz	160	1.5	30
1 medium bagel, 3 oz	240	2	45
1 large bagel, 4 oz	320	3	60
Bagel Chips (New York Style),			
4 slices, ¾ oz	90	2	17
Pizza Bagel, 6 oz each	380	7	60
Bagel Bites (Ore-Ida), 4 pces	190	7	25
Bagel Crisps (Burns Ricker), 1 oz	150	9	28

Bagel Brands

	C	F	Cb
Amy's Kitchen, average, 3½ oz	235	2	50
Awrey's, 2.7 oz each	190	0.5	42
Controlled Carb Gourmet			
High Fiber Bagel (1), 2 oz	160	5	22
Individual Wrapped (1), 2 oz	80	2	20
Zero Net Carbs (1), 2 oz	120	2	14
Costco Bakery: Plain, 4 oz	300	1	61
Everything, 4 oz	330	3.5	62
Enjoy Life, all types, 3.2 oz	270	6	50
Lenders, all flavors, avg., 3.6 oz	270	2	53
Oroweat: Oatmeal, 3.4 oz	270	4	49
Multi-Grain, 3.4 oz	260	1.5	51
Sara Lee: Mini, average, 1 oz	70	2	15
Toaster Size, all types, 2.2 oz	165	0.5	34
3.5 oz Size (95g): Plain	270	2	50
Other flavors, avg., 3.5 oz	260	2	50
4 oz Size (113g): Heart Healthy	220	1.5	47
Apple Cinnamon	310	1.5	64
Banana Walnut	350	7	61
The Works	330	3.5	62
Other varieties, average	300	1.5	61
Western: All flavors, avg., 3 oz	230	1	47
Bagel Sandwiches: See Page 173			
Fast-Foods: See Page 183			

Bagel Spreads

	C	F	Cb
Cream Cheese:			
Plain: 2 Tbsp, 1 oz	80	8	2
2 oz mini-tub	160	16	4
Reduced Fat: 2 Tbsp, 1 oz	60	5	2
2 oz mini-tub	120	10	4
Flavors: Lox, 1 oz	75	6	1
Raisin Walnut, 1 oz	90	6	8
Strawberry, 1 oz	60	3	7
Sundried Tomato, 1 oz	80	7	2
Vegetable, 1 oz	60	6	1

Rice Cakes

	C	F	Cb
Average All Types/Brands:			
Regular size, 1 cake, 9g	35	0	7.5
Hain, Mini, average, 3g each	12	0.5	2
Lundberg, all types, 15g each	60	0.5	14
Quaker: Large, all flavors, 13g each	50	0	11
Crispy Mini's, average, 15g	70	2	12
Quakes, avg., 31 pces, 1 oz	110	4	19
Westbrae, 1 cake, 7g	25	0	5

Taco Shells & Tortillas

	C	F	Cb
Tacos: Mini Size (1)	25	1.5	2
Regular size, all types (1)	55	3	6
Super Size (1)	90	4	11
Salad Shell, flour (Azteca), 1.4 oz	180	11	19
Tortilla (Soft Taco), each	85	2	15
Corn Tortilla: 6", 1.2 oz each	45	0.5	9
Flour Tortilla: each, 1.75 oz	160	3	28
Low-fat	110	1.5	22
Burritos, 1 tortilla, 2.3 oz	190	5	32
Low-fat	110	1.5	22
Tostada Shells, each	55	3	6
La Tortilla Factory			
Fat Free Flour Tortillas:			
Burrito size, 2.5 oz	120	0.5	34
Soft Taco, 1.8 oz	90	0	24
Low Carb Low-Fat Tortillas:			
Large, 1.26 oz	80	3	19
Original; Flavors, 1.26 oz	50	2	11
Mission Foods			
Tortillas: *Per 6" Tortilla*			
Flour, 1.7 oz	150	4	25
Low Carb Flour, 1.47 oz	110	2.5	18
Low Carb Whole Wheat, 1 oz	80	2	12
White Corn, 1.8 oz	120	2	25
98% Fat-Free Burrito, 10"	160	0.5	33

Rev. Dr Robert Schuller

*"Inch by inch
Life's a cinch"*

*"You'll never win
If you don't begin!"*

Crispbreads

Per Crispbread/Cracker

	C	F	Cb
Ak-Mak: Sesame, 5 crackers, 1 oz	115	0	19
Finn Crisp: Original, rye,1	35	0	7
Other types,1 crispbread	19	0	3
Kavli Norwegian: Thin,1	17	0	3
Thick,1 crispbread	20	0	3
Malsovit Meal Wafers,1	75	4	7
New York Flatbread Crisps, 1	35	0	7
Ry-Krisp: Natural, 1 crispbread	20	0	3
Seasoned,1 crispbread	30	0	5
Sesame,1 crispbread	25	1	3
Ryvita: Dark/Light, 1 piece	26	0	4
WASA: Delikatess (1)	25	0	5.5
Fiber (1); Sesam (1)	30	1	5
Original (1)	35	0.2	7.5
Runda (1)	55	1.5	9
Wheat Dore (1)	50	1	9
Westbrae Rice Wafers (7), 15g	50	0	11

Matzos

Manischewitz

	C	F	Cb
American Matzos, 1 board, 1 oz	115	2	22
Passover Matzos, 1 board, 1.1 oz	130	0	27
Passover Egg Matzos, 1.1 oz	130	2	27
Egg 'n Onion Matzo, 1 oz	112	1	23
Thin Salted Tea Matzos, 0.9 oz	100	0	21
Unsalted; Whole Wheat, 1 oz	110	0	24
Dietetic Matzo Thins, 0.83 oz	90	0	19
Crackers: Miniatures, 1 cracker	9	0	20
Passover Egg Matzo, 1 cracker	11	0	20
Matzo Meal, 1 cup, 4¾ oz	515	2	110
Matzo Farfel, 1 cup, 2.7 oz	180	0.5	60
Grape Matzo, 1 oz each	110	0	25

Quick Guide

Crackers

Average All Brands: Per Cracker

	C	F	Cb
Cheese Crackers: Plain, 1" square	5	0	0.5
Small, octagonal	10	0	1
Round (2" diam.)	15	0	1.5
Sandwich (Peanut Butter)	35	1	4
Graham, 2½" square,1 cracker	30	0.5	5
Melba Toast, plain, 1 piece	20	0	4
Oyster & Soup Crackers, ¼ oz	60	2	10
(40 small oysters/20 lge hexagons)			
Rice Crackers: 1 small	9	0	2
Rice Snax *(Amsnack)*, ½ oz	60	1	12
Saltines, 2 crackers	25	1	4.5
Snack-type, 1 round cracker	15	0	3
Soda, 1 cracker, ½ oz	60	2	10
Water Cracker *(Carr's)*, regular, 1	32	0	7
Small, 1 cracker	14	0	4
Wheat, thin, 1 cracker	9	0	2
Zweiback Toast, 1 piece	30	0	5

Quick Guide

Cookies

Average All Brands: Per Cookie

	C	F	Cb
Biscotti: Small, 0.5 oz	65	2.5	10
Regular, 1 oz	130	5	20
Chocolate Chip Cookies:			
Small/Thin 0.5 oz	55	3	7
Regular, 1 oz	110	6	15
Large, 2.3 oz *(Mrs Fields)*	280	13	38
Jumbo, 4 oz	450	22	64
Oatmeal/Oatmeal Raisin:			
Small/Thin 0.5 oz	50	1.5	8
Regular, 1 oz	95	3.5	15
Large, 2.3 oz *(Mrs Fields)*	280	12	39
Jumbo, 4 oz	380	14	62
Peanut Butter:			
Small/Thin 0.5 oz	60	3	7
Regular, 1 oz	125	6.5	14
Large, 2.3 oz *(Mrs Fields)*	310	16	34
Jumbo, 4 oz	500	25	54
Low-Fat Cookies			
Choc Chip (Low-Fat), 1 oz (1)	100	1	21
Oatmeal Raisin (Fat-Free), 1 oz (1)	90	0	20
Peanut Butter (Low-Fat), 1 oz (1)	105	2	14

Crackers ◆ Cookies (Cont.)

Brands	C	F	Cb
Per Cookie/Cracker (Unless Indicated)			
Archway			
Coconut Macaroon	105	6	12
Apple/Date-filled Oatmeal	100	3	16
Apricot/Strawb.-filled Oatmeal	100	3	16
Frosty Lemon/Orange	110	4	17
Ginger Snaps: Regular/Iced (5)	170	7	26
Reduced Fat (5)	135	4	25
Lemon Snaps (5)	150	7	23
Molasses	115	3	20
Oatmeal: Regular; Raisin	105	4	17
Iced	120	5	18
Peanut Butter; Pecan Icebox	120	6	15
Sugar Cookies (1)	100	3	16
Atkins			
Cookies; Crackers, avg. all	140	9	10
Meringue Cookies, avg. all flav. (1)	5	0	1
Sesame; Whole Wheat, crackers (2)	45	3	4
Austin			
Crackers: *Per Package*			
PB/Cheddar/Peanut Butter Chse	190	10	22
Dolphins & Friends	140	5	20
Cheese w. Cheddar Jack S'wich	200	11	23
Sandwich Crackers: Grilled Chse	200	10	24
PB & J	200	10	24
Toasty Crackers, Peanut Butter	200	10	24
Wheat Crackers, Cheddar	200	10	24
Zoo Animal Crackers 1 pkg (60g)	250	4	50
Baker's: *Per Cookie (3 oz)*			
Peanut Butter	320	10	52
Peanut Butter & Jelly	310	9	55
Vegan Peanut But. Choc. Chunk	320	11	53
Other varieties, average	320	6	58
Barbara's Bakery			
Cookies: Fig Bars, avg. (1)	60	0.5	14
Animal Cookies, Vanilla (8)	120	4.5	18
Crisp Cookies; average (1)	80	4	9
Snackimals, avg. (10)	120	4	19
Crackers: Cheese Bites (22), 1 oz	120	3	20
Organic Go Go Grahams (8), 1 oz	130	4	22
Rite Lite Rounds, avg. (5)	60	2	11
Wheatines, average (4)	55	1	11
Brent & Sam's			
Cookies: Chocolate Chip (2)	130	6	18
Chocolate Chip Pecan (2)	145	8	16
Key Lime White Chocolate (2)	135	6	19
Raspberry Chocolate (2)	125	6	17
White Choc. Macadamia (2)	145	8	17

Carr's	C	F	Cb
Crackers: Table Water (5)	70	1.5	13
Monterey: Hearty Wheat (3)	60	2	9
Savory/Sesame (3)	70	3	9
Entertainer; Whole Wheat (2)	80	3.5	11
Cocktail, Croissant Orig. Gold (22)	140	3	21
Cookies: Bisc. for Tea (2)	140	6	20
Choccines (3)	150	9	16
Ginger Lemon Cremes (2)	140	7	19
Hob Nobs (2)	140	6	19
Imperials: Milk Chocolate (2)	140	7	18
Dark Choc (2)	150	7	19
Milk Choc & Creme	140	7	18
Petites Bijoux (4)	140	5	21
Cookies &			
Cookie Bars: M&M's (1)	170	9	20
Milky Way (1); Snickers (1)	180	11	21
Peanut Butter (1)	150	9	17
Twix (1)	180	10	21
Country Choice			
Ginger Snaps (5)	120	5	19
Sandwich Cremes (2)	130	5	19
Soft Baked: Peanut Butter	100	5	13
Avg. other varieties	100	4	16
Vanilla Wafers (7)	120	5	19
Dove			
Cookies: *Per Serving*			
Beyond Chocolate Chunk (1)	110	6	13
Chocolate Walnut Oasis (1)	110	6	13
Chocolate Walnut Rendezvous (1)	110	6	13
Milk Chocolate Moment (3)	160	9	20
Mint Chocolate Serenade (3)	160	8	19
Toffee Chocolate Tango (3)	160	8	20
Dr Soy: Average (2)	85	2	5
Entenmann's			
Soft Baked Milk/Choc Chip	100	5	13
Estee (Fructose Sweetened)			
Chocolate Chip; Fudge Cookies	40	2	5
Coconut Cookies, Oatmeal Raisin	35	1.5	5
Sandwich Cookies	55	2	6
Vanilla; Lemon	35	1.5	5
Famous Amos			
Choc Chip (4)	140	7	19
Choc Chip & Pecan (4)	150	8	18
Chocolate Creme Sandwich (3)	160	6	25
Oatmeal Choc Chip & Walnut (4)	140	7	18
Oatmeal Raisin (4)	140	6	20
Low-Fat: Gingersnaps (1 pkg)	200	3	41
Lemonsnaps (1 pkg) 1.75 oz	200	2.5	42

Per Cookie/Cracker (Unless Indicated)

Grandma's	C	F	Cb
Peanut Butter Sandwich Creme (5)	210	10	28
Rich 'N Chewy, Choc Chip, pkg.	270	12	39
Vanilla Sandwich Creme (5)	210	10	30
Homestyle Big:			
Fudge Chocolate Chip (1)	190	7	28
Oatmeal Raisin (1)	180	6	30
Peanut Butter (1)	200	10	24
Chocolate Chip (1)	200	9	28
Mini S'wich: Peanut Butter (9)	155	7	21
Vanilla (9)	150	7	22
Cookie Bites: Choc. Chip, 1 pkg	210	9	29

Great American Cookies			
Doozies:			
Chewy Chocolate Supreme	205	8	30
Chewy Pecan Supreme	210	11	25
Chocolate Chip; Snickerdoodle	240	11	32
M&M	240	11	32
Oatmeal; Double Fudge	240	10	34
Peanut Butter M&M	280	15	30
Peanut Butter Supreme	260	14	28
Pecan Supreme	250	13	30
Sugar	195	9	27
White Chunk Macadamia	225	9	32
Big Bites: Peanut Butter Supreme	130	7	14
White Chunk Macadamia	140	8	15
Other varieties, avg.	130	5	19
Big Bite Doozies: Choc Chip	355	17	47
M&M varieties	395	19	53
Sugar varieties, avg.	340	15	48
Colossal: M&M	510	24	68
Cups: Original Cookie Cup	275	13	37
Peanut Butter	255	13	30
Cakes, avg. 1 slice, ⅛ cake	670	30	95
Brownies: Cheesecake Brownie	400	21	48
Cheesecake Chocolate Swirl	485	25	60
Fudge	495	22	67
Fudge Nut	525	27	63

Hain	C	F	Cb
Cookies: Animal (9), 1 oz	125	2.5	23
98% Fat-Free, all types (11)	110	0	23
Crackers: Cheese Bites (22)	120	1.5	23
Cookie Jar Bits (Rice Cakes), (17)	60	0.5	12
Oyster Crackers, Fat-Free (36)	60	0	13
Veg/Rice/Sesame Crackers (11)	140	6	19

Health Valley			
Cookies: Fat Free, avg. all flavors (3)	100	0	24
Cafe Creations, Choc. Chip (1)	100	5	13
Choc./Dble Choc. Chunk (1)	125	7	15
Cookie Cremes, avg. (2)	125	5	19
Oatmeal: Raisin (1)	95	3.5	14
Avg. other varieties (1)	100	4	14
White Chocolate Chunk (1)	135	7	17
Low-Fat, Biscotti/Amaretto (2)	120	3	23
Crackers: Corn Bread (1)	15	0.5	3
Graham: Amaranth; Oat Bran (1)	15	0	3
Original Amaranth/Oat Bran (1)	20	0.5	4
Low-Fat/Whole Wheat, all flavors (1)	10	0	2
Original Rice Bran (1)	18	0.5	3

Hershey's			
Cookies: Hershey's w. Almonds (2)	150	9	16
Almond Joy Cookies (2)	150	9	17
Reese's Cookies (2)	150	8	17
York Cookies (2)	160	9	17

Joseph's Cookies			
Lite Cookies: Almd; Choc Chip (2)	100	5	13
Choc Peach	90	4	12
Nut & Raisin (2)	30	1	7
Oatmeal Raisin (2)	100	2	18
Pecan Double Fudge (2)	90	3	14
Vanilla (2)	25	1	8
Sugarfree Cookies: Oatmeal (4)	115	5	15
Chocolate Walnut (4)	115	6	15
Lemon (4)	100	4	15
Other varieties, avg., (4)	105	5	14
Kalahari Rusks, avg. all types (1)	110	3	18

Success is 1% Inspiration and 99% Perspiration.

Crackers ✦ Cookies (Cont)

Keebler	C	F	Cb
Crackers:			
Club: Orig.; 50% Red. Sodium (4)	70	3	9
33% Reduced Fat (5)	70	2.5	12
Grahams: Regular (8), 1 oz	130	3.5	23
Low-Fat varieties (8), 1 oz	110	1.5	23
Munch'ems, average (38), 1 oz	140	4.5	22
Toasted, Regular varieties (5)	80	3.5	10
Town House: Regular (5)	80	4.5	9
Reduced Fat (6)	60	1.5	11
Wheatables: Reduced Fat (19)	140	4	22
Other varieties, average (19)	140	6	20
Cookies: Chips Deluxe:			
Soft & Chewy (1)	70	3	11
Rainbow (1)	80	4	10
Chocolate Lovers; Coconut (1)	80	4.5	10
Chips Deluxe, avg., 1 pouch	120	5	18
Mini's (4), average	150	10	18
Country Style Oatmeal w. Rais. (2)	130	6	18
Danish Wedding (4)	130	6	18
E.L. Fudge: Original (2)	140	6	19
Butter w. Dble Fudge Creme (2)	180	9	23
Double Stuffed (2)	180	9	23
S'mores Blasted (2), avg.	180	9	24
Fudge Shoppe:			
Deluxe Grahams, regular (3)	140	7	17
Double Fudge 'n Caramel (2)	140	8	20
Fudge Sticks (3), avg.	150	8	19
Fudge Stripes: Regular, avg. (3)	160	8	21
Reduced Fat (3)	130	5	21
Grasshopper (4)	140	7	19
Mini's (4)	150	7	20
Mini Grahams (10)	160	8	22
Iced Animal (6)	140	5	22
Sandies Cookies: Reduced-Fat (1)	80	3.5	11
Cookies (1) avg. all flavors	80	5	9
Mini Pecan (4)	160	10	17
Soft Batch (1)	80	3.5	11
Vienna Fingers: Regular (2)	150	6	21
Reduced Fat (2)	140	4.5	23
Wafers: Vanilla Wafers (8)	150	6	22
Mini Vanilla (18)	150	6	21
Reduced-Fat (8)	130	3.5	25
Vanilla Sugar Free (4)	130	10	19
Keto			
Cookies (1), 1 oz	160	9	6
Ketogenics, avg., 1.76 oz	250	19	26

Kraft	C	F	Cb
White Cheddar Chse Nips (27), 1 oz	150	7	19
Teddy Graham Bearwiches (1)	150	7	21
100 Calorie Pack, 4.4 oz	100	3	15
Kroger			
Cookies: Fudgie Sticks Wafers (3)	125	7	16
Fudgie Stripes Shortbread (3)	160	8	21
Old Style Pecan Shortbread (2)	150	9	15
Crackers: Cheese Bits (31)	135	5	20
Socialites (12)	150	8	17
Lance			
Chocolate Chip, Bite Size (1)	130	6	18
Dunking Sticks, each	180	10	22
Oatmeal Creme (1)	240	10	35
Peanut Butter Creme, 1 pkg.	230	12	26
Toastchee Poppers Pouch	150	8	15
Low Carb Enchantments			
Sugar Free Cookies, avg. (1), 1 oz	150	9	11
Little Debbie			
Apple Flips	150	5	24
Figaroos (1), 1.5 oz	150	3.5	31
Fudge Rounds (1)	150	6	23
German Choc Cookie Rings	140	8	18
Ginger Cookies	90	3	15
Marshmallow Pies, avg. (1)	185	7	28
Marshmallow Supremes (1)	135	5	22
Nutty Bar (2)	310	18	32
Oatmeal Creme Pies (1)	140	2	29
Peanut Butter & Jelly Sandwich	140	5	22
Peanut Clusters (1)	205	11	23
Raisin Creme Pies (1)	140	5	23
Star Crunch Comic Snacks (1)	145	6	22
Crackers: Chse w. P'nut Butter (4)	140	8	16
Toasty w. P'nut Butter (4)	140	7	16
Lu			
Cookies: Marie Lu (3)	160	6	25
Le Fondant Wafers (4)	175	10	19
Le Petit Beurre (4)	150	4	26
Le Petit Ecolier, avg. (2)	130	6	17
Pim's: Chocolatier (3)	155	9	17
Orange; Raspberry (2)	95	3	16
Manischewitz			
Matzo Boards: See Page 105			
Biscotti: Toffee Crunch Macaroons	50	2.5	7
Cappuccino Chip	70	2.5	10
Chocolate Macaroons, each	45	2	8
Matzo Cracker, Miniatures	9	0	2
Whole Wheat Crackers	9	0	2

Per Cookie/Cracker (Unless indicated)

Miss Meringue	C	F	Cb
Meringue Classiques: *Per 4 Pieces*			
Choc./Mint/Triple Choc Chip	100	1.5	20
Other varieties (4)	85	0	20
Meringue Minis: *Per 13 Pieces*			
Orange (13)	110	0	27
Toasted Coconut	120	1.5	26
Other varieties	85	0	20

Mrs Fields Cookies: *See Fast-Foods Section*

Mother's			
ABC Cinnamon Grahams (1)	10	0.5	1.5
ABC Sugar Cookies (1)	10	0.5	2
Butter Cookies (6)	160	8	21
Candy Chip (4)	150	6	23
Checkerboard Wafers	40	2	5
Chocolate Sandwich Creme (3)	170	8	23
Chocolate Chip: Cookies	80	4	11
Cookies (bag) (1)	30	1	5
Chocolate Chip Parade	35	1.5	5
Cocodas Coconut	30	2	4
Cookie Parade: Animal (8)	150	8	19
Cookie (4)	140	7	18
Circus Animal (1)	25	1	3.5
Fudge Circus (6)	140	7	20
Double Fudge	90	4.5	12
English Tea/Taffy Sandwich	90	3.5	13
Flaky Flix Fudge/Vanilla	70	3.5	8
Fudge & Mint (2)	150	8	21
Fudge Gauchos (2)	180	8	26
Hawaiian Chocolate Chip (2)	180	11	20
Iced Chocolate (2)	155	7	22
Iced Lemonade (2)	160	8	22
Peanut Butter Gaucho	95	4	13
Pecan Shortbread (2)	160	9	19
Iced Raisin (2)	170	8	24
Oatmeal Cookies: Regular	55	2.5	9
Chocolate Chip	65	2	11
Oatmeal Raisin Cookies	30	2	4
Oatmeal Walnut Choc. Chip	70	2.5	10
Oatmeal Cremes (2)	180	7	27
Striped Shortbread Cookies	55	2.5	8
Sugar Cookies	70	3	10
Sugar Free Lemon Creme (3)	160	7	23
Sugared Lemon	75	4	10
Vanilla Cremes (2)	180	7	26
Vanilla Wafers (8)	135	5	22

Murray SugarFree Cookies	C	F	Cb
Choc Chip & Pecan (3)	160	9	19
Double Fudge (3)	140	7	23
Fudge-Dipped Wafer: Vanilla (4)	140	10	19
Shortbread (5)	130	7	20
Gingersnaps (7)	130	5	23
Lemon/Choc Cremes (3)	130	7	18
Lemon Wafers (4)	130	10	19
Oatmeal (3)	150	7	21
Peanut Butter (3)	140	9	16
Shortbread (8)	140	6	21
Shortbread Pecan (3)	170	11	19
Vanilla Sugar Wafers (4)	130	10	19

Nabisco			
Crackers:			
Flavor Orig.: Better Cheddars, avg. (1)	5	0.5	1
Cheese Nips, avg. (1)	5	0.2	0.5
Chicken in a Biskit (1)	15	1	1.5
Sociables Crisps (1)	10	0.5	1
Swiss Crisps/Cheese; Thins (1)	10	0.5	1.5
Vegetable Thins (1)	10	0.5	1
Barnum's Animal Cracker (1)	15	0.5	3
Honey Maid Graham, sticks (1)	10	0	2
Wheatsworth, ½ oz	80	3.5	10
Premium: Saltine, avg. (1), 1 oz	15	0.5	2
Fat Free (1)	15	0	2.5
Other varieties (1)	15	0.5	2.5
Unsalted Tops	30	2.5	3
Wheat Thins: Orig., (8) ½ oz	70	3	10
Big Wheat Thins (10)	140	6	20
Ranch (14)	150	7	19
100 Calorie Packs, 4.4 oz	100	3	16
Cookies:			
100 Calorie Packs: Cheese Nips	100	3	15
Chips Ahoy!, 1 pkg	100	3	18
FruitSnacks (Mixed Berry)	100	0	24
Oreo (Thin Crisps), 1 pkg	100	2	20
Biscos Sugar Wafers, 1 oz (8)	140	6	21
Cameo Creme Sandwich	65	2.5	10
Chips Ahoy!: Candy Blasts (1)	80	4	10
Chocolate Chip (1)	80	4	10
Chewy Chocolate (1)	50	2.5	7
Chunky varieties; Cremewiches (1)	80	4	10
Mini Chips Ahoy! (1)	30	1.5	4
Snack Saks, 1 oz (31)	170	8	21
Peanut Butter (1), 0.5 oz	80	4	9
Reduced Fat (1)	45	1.5	8
Soft Baked Chunky (1)	120	5	19
Sticks (9), 1 oz	140	6	21

Crackers ◆ Cookies (Cont)

Per Cookie/Cracker (Unless Indicated)

Nabisco (Cont):	C	F	Cb
Fig Newtons: Reg. (2), 1.1oz	110	2.5	22
Snack Pack, 2 pces, 1 oz	100	2	22
Snackable Dessert, avg. (2)	120	3	25
Fat-Free Fig (1)	100	0	22
Fruit Newtons, avg. (2)	110	2	22
Cobblers, Apple/Peach (1)	70	0	17
Raspberry/Strawb. & Yogurt (1)	130	3	26
Ginger Snaps (1)	30	0.5	6
Grahams	15	0.5	3
Honey Maid: Grahams, all types (2)	30	0.5	6
Low-Fat Cinnamon Grahams (2)	30	0.3	6
Imperio (1)	85	3.5	8
Lorna Doone Shortbread (1)	40	2	5
Mallomars (1)	60	2.5	8.5
Marshmallow Twirls (1)	130	5	21
Morelianas, 1 oz	125	5	19
Nilla Wafers: Original (1)	15	1	3
Reduced-Fat Original	15	0.3	3
Reduced-Fat Chocolate	15	0.2	3
Nutter Butter: Bites, each	15	0.5	2
S'wich Cookie, 1 oz	125	6	18
Real Peanut Butter, 1.9 oz	130	6	19
Oatmeal/Iced Oatmeal (1)	50	2	8
Oreo: Original, 3 cookies	160	7	24
Snack pkg, 2 oz	270	12	40
Reduced-Fat, 3 cookies	150	4.5	26
Choc. Creme; Coffee'n Creme (3)	170	7	24
Double Delight: Mint'n Creme (2)	140	7	20
P'nut Butter & Choc Creme (2)	140	6	20
Double Stuf, 2 cookies	140	7	20
Fudge-Covered, 1 cookie	100	5	13
Handi-Snacks (1), 1 oz	130	5	21
Mini Oreo: 9 pieces, 1 oz	140	6	21
Snack Pack, 1.2 oz (35g)	170	7	25
Uh-Oh!, 3 cookies	170	7	24
100 Calorie Packs (1) 4.8 oz	100	2	20
Pecanz (1)	90	5	9
Pinwheels, Choc./Marshmallow	130	5	21
Social Tea Biscuits (1)	20	0.5	3
Teddy Cheddy Crackers (24), 1.1 oz	130	4	23
Teddy Grahams Snacks, all types (1)	5	0.1	1

Newman's Own	C	F	Cb
Alphabet Cookies, avg. (10)	110	3	22
Champion Chip: Expresso Choc (4)	150	7.5	21
Double Choc Mint Chip (4)	165	8	21
Choc Creme Filled Choc. (2)	130	4.5	20
Chocolate Chip (4)	155	7	21
Chocolate Chocolate Chip (4)	160	8	20
Creme Filled Chocolate (4)	130	4.5	20
Fig Newman's: Fat Free, 2 bars	120	0	28
Low-Fat, 2 bars	140	2	28
Ginger-O's, Creme Filled Ginger (2)	120	4.5	19
Orange Choc Chip (4)	140	7	21
Snack Pack, 46g bar	135	0	32
Tops & Bottoms Wafers (6)	120	3	21
Peak Freans			
Assorted Creme (2)	135	6	19
Fruit Creme (2)	130	5	20
Arrowroot; Ginger Crisp (2)	155	4.5	27
Nice Biscuits (2)	160	6	25
Petit Beurre (2)	130	4	22
Shortcake (2)	140	7	18
Pepperidge Farm			
American Collection: Sante Fe	120	4.5	18
Sausalito, Choc Macadamia (1)	140	8	18
Average other flavors	140	7	16
Chocolate Chunk Big Cookies (1)	140	8	15
Dessert Bliss: Choc. Alm.; Mint Choc. (3)	160	8	22
Distinctive: Bordeaux	35	1.5	7
Brussels (3)	150	7	20
Brussels Mint; Milano (2)	130	7	16
Chantilly Raspberry (2)	120	3	23
Double Choc. Milano	75	4	9
Geneva	55	3	7
Milk Choc. Bordeaux/Milano	60	3	7
Mint/Orange Milano	60	3	7
Homestyle: Choc Chip; Gingerman	45	2.5	6
Lemon Nut Crunch; Shortbread	60	3	7
Mini: Chessmen (9)	145	6	21
Milano (6)	160	8	18
Mint Milano (6)	170	9	20
Nantucket: Choc Chunk Minis (4)	150	8	20
Double Choc Chunk (1)	140	7	18
Soft Baked: Oatmeal Raisin (1), 31g	135	5	21
Other varieties	130	7	16
Goldfish Crackers: Plain (55)	140	6	19
Flavor Blasted (51)	150	8	17
Giant Flavor Blasted, avg. (31)	145	7	19
Graham Snacks: Average (38)	140	5	22
Cookie varieties (4)	20	0	2

Per Cookie/Cracker (Unless Indicated)

	C	F	Cb
Pirouline: 8 rolls, 1 oz	130	3.5	23
Rumbly Grahams			
Cookies: Chocolate Chip (23)	135	4.5	22
Cinnamon: Honey (20)	140	5	22
Ritz			
Original Cracker, ½ oz	80	4	10
Dinosaurs (28), ½ oz	65	2	11
Flavor Assortment, ½ oz	80	4	10
Mini Ritz, Original Bite Size (33)	155	8	19
Ritz Bits Sandwiches: Cheese, 1.5 oz	230	14	23
Graham Cracker S'mores, 1.2 oz	165	7	25
w. Peanut Butter (14)	140	8	18
Peanut Butter Go-Pak, 1 oz	155	8	18
Cheese, 1.5 oz	220	14	23
Ritz Chips, all varieties (33), 1 oz	140	6	20
Snack Mix, Cheddar Baked Snacks	205	9	27
With Peanut Butter, 1.4 oz	195	9	24
With Real Cheese, 1.4 oz	200	11	22
Stay Fresh: Reduced Fat, 0.5 oz	65	2	11
Whole Wheat (5), 0.5 oz	70	2.5	11
Other varieties, avg., ½ oz	85	4	11
Santa Fe Farms			
Fat Free, average, 1 pkg	120	0	26
Snackwell's (Nabisco)			
CarbWell: Grahams (2)	120	7	18
Shortbread (2)	110	6	16
Chocolate Chip: Bite Size (13)	130	4	22
Sugar Free (3)	170	8	23
Cookie Cakes (1)	50	0.5	12
Creme Sandwich (2)	110	3	20
Devil's Food Cake, Fat Free (1)	50	0	12
Golden Devil's Food Cake (1)	55	0.5	11
Sugar Free: Fudge Brownie	90	3.5	17
Oatmeal (1)	95	2.5	17
Shortbread (3)	130	5	22
Sandwiches: Creme Packs 2 Go!	205	5	38
Chocolate (2)	110	3	20
Sugar Free varieties(3)	160	6	24
South Beach Diet (Kraft)			
Cookies: Peanut Butter, 1 pkg	100	5	14
Oatmeal Chocolate Chip, 1 pkg	100	5	16

Stella D'Oro	C	F	Cb
Almond Delight, 1 oz	160	8	18
Almond Toast, 1 oz	115	2.5	21
Anginetti, 1 oz	130	3.5	22
Biscotti, avg., 0.7 oz	100	4.5	13
Breakfast Treats: Mini, 1 oz	125	3.5	21
Choc.; Cinn.; Original, 0.8 oz	90	3	15
Coffee Treats: Angel Wings, 1 oz	170	12	14
Anisette Sponge (2)	90	1	18
Anisette Toast/Mini (3)	125	1	27
Toast, avg. all, 1 oz	100	2	19
Roman Egg Biscuits, 1.1 oz	130	4	21
Egg Jumbo, 1.1 oz	125	1.5	26
Lady Stella, Assorted, 1 oz	125	4.5	20
Margherite: Avg., (2), 1 oz	130	5	20
Mini, 1.1 oz	150	5	24
Swiss Fudge (2), 1.1oz	170	9	22
Sunshine: Grab Bags Crackers (1)	5	0.5	0.5
Heads & Tails, 1.5 oz	210	9	28
Hi-Ho Crackers, avg. (1)	15	0.5	2
Krispy: Original; Whole Wheat (1)	10	0.3	2
Oyster & Soup, 17 crackers	70	1.5	12
Fat-Free (1)	10	0	2.5
Unsalted Tops (1)	15	0.3	2
Party Mix: 1 pkt, 1.7 oz	230	9	32
Reduced Fat, ½ cup, 1 oz	130	3	21
Snack Mix: Original, ½ cup	130	4.5	21
Get Nutty, ½ cup	150	9	16
Big Crunch; Dble Chse, avg.,½ c.	170	4	16

"He misses the way you used to bend over and pat him!"

Crackers ◆ Cookies (Cont) ◆ Refrigerated

Per Cookie/Cracker Unless Indicated

Trader Joe's	C	F	Cb
All Butter Shortbread			
w. Apricot/Raspberry Filling (2)	145	8	17
w. Chocolate Filling (2)	125	7	15
Brownie Bites (3)	150	7	20
Chocolate: Almond Laceys (2)	155	10	13
Chip Dunkers (2)	145	6	21
Coated Choc. Chip Dunkers (2)	190	9	25
Cinnamon Butter Sticks (5)	145	7	18
Crispy Crunchy varieties (12)	145	7	19
Fat Free: Fig Bars (2)	130	0	31
Lemon (4)	100	0	24
Ginger Animal (7)	140	6	19
Lemon Crisp (5)	120	4	19
Low-Fat varieties (15)	120	1.5	19
Meringues: Cappuccino (4)	85	0	20
Chocolate (4)	100	2	20
Fat Free (5)	105	0	25
Mint (5)	100	1.5	20
Milk Choc. Macadamia Laceys (2)	145	10	13
Southern Style Pecan (4)	150	9	15
Swiss Almond Crunch (4)	135	8	14
Teddies, Vanilla (12)	135	5	21
Triple Ginger Snaps (6)	135	5	21
Way More Chocolate Chips (3)	160	11	14

Triscuit			
Original (15), 1 oz	120	5	20
Thin Crisps (15)	135	4.5	21
Baked Whole Wheat: Wafers (7)	145	5	22
Cheddar (6)	135	5	20
Reduced Fat (8)	125	3	21
Deli-Style Rye; Rsted Garlic (8)	145	5	22
Garden Herb, Whole Wheat (6)	135	4.5	20

Wild Oats			
Ginger Snaps (1)	30	1	4
Crunchy Peanut Butter (1)	30	1.5	3
Oatmeal Raisin (1)	25	1	4
Sandwich cremes, avg., (3)	190	7	28
Water Crackers (1)	15	0.5	3

Zesta			
Saltine: Whole Wheat (3)	60	1.5	11
Fat Free, 5 crackers	60	0	13
Original, 5 crackers	60	1.5	11
Red. Sodium; Unsalted Tops (5)	60	1.5	11
Soup & Oyster, 45 crackers	70	3	10

Thaw, Bake & Serve

Cookietree: *Per Cookie*	C	F	Cb
Buttersugar; Cinn. Apple Oatmeal	120	5	17
Choc. varieties; Pecan/Macadam.	130	7	17
Cookie w. M&M's; Dble Fudge	120	6	17
Peanut Butter/Chocolate	130	7	17
Raisin Oatmeal	110	3.5	18

Grands! Biscuits			
Extra Rich	210	12	25
Blueberry; Golden Corn	190	7	28
Butter Tastin'; Buttermilk	190	10	24
Reduced Fat	170	7	27
Flaky; Homestyle; Southern Style	200	10	24
Hungry Jack: Avg. all types (1)	100	4.5	14
Jewel: Biscuits (2)	100	1.5	20

Pillsbury Cookies: *Per 1 oz*			
Cookies: Peanut Butter (1)	125	6	16
Chocolate Chip, Reduced Fat (1)	105	3	19
Double Chocolate Chip Chunk (1)	135	7	17
Oatmeal Chocolate Chip (1)	125	6	17
Ready To Bake: P. Butter Cup (1)	185	9	24
Choc. Chip with Walnuts (1)	125	7	14
Sugar (1)	125	5	19
Refrigerated Dough: Sugar (1)	130	1.5	19
Choc Chip w. Walnuts (1)	130	7	16
Chocolate Chip (1)	140	7	17
Cookies w. M&Ms (1)	130	2	18
Double Choc Chip & Chunk (1)	140	7	17
Peanut Butter (1)	120	6	15

Toll House *(Nestlé)*			
Cookies: Choc Chip Caramel (1)	100	4.5	16
Fudge (1)	110	5	15
Ultimates: Chocolate Chip			
& Chunks w. Pecans (1)	200	11	23
Choc. Chip Lover (1)	200	10	25
Peanut Butter Cup (1)	195	10	24
White Choc. Macadamia Nut (1)	200	11	23
Walnut Chocolate Chip (1)	115	6	14
Refrigerated Dough: Sugar (1)	110	5	18
Chocolate Chip (1)	130	6	20
Chocolate Chunk (1)	150	6	22
Peanut Butter Choc Chip (1)	100	5	13

Cakes, Pastries, Croissants

Ready-to-Eat

	C	F	Cb
Angel Food: Plain, no oil, 2 oz	120	0	25
Plain with oil, 2 oz	160	1.5	25
w. Cream Frosting	230	7	37
Apple Fritters, 3 oz	360	22	38
Apple Pie: *See Pies/Tarts Page 116*			
Baklava, 1½" square, 1½ oz	110	6	13
Banana w. Butter Cream, 3 oz	300	13	40
Black Forest, 3 oz	230	10	34
Brownie, 3.5 oz	420	25	52
Bundt, 3 oz	300	17	35
Carrot Cake: Plain, 3 oz	230	8	41
w. Cream Cheese Frosting	380	21	42
Cheesecake: Small serving, 3 oz	260	18	24
Large serving, 5 oz	430	30	40
w. Low-Fat Cheese/fruit, 3 oz	150	8	30
Cheesecake Factory: See Fast-Foods Section			
Denny's Cheesecake, 1 slice, ⅙	580	38	51
Cherry Cobbler, 5 oz	350	10	62
Chocolate Cake: Plain, 3 oz	220	11	40
w. Chocolate Frosting, 3 oz	320	15	42
& Cream Filling, 3½ oz	360	21	43
Churros, 1 stick, 1½ oz	150	8	18
Cinnamon Crumb Cake, 4 oz	450	23	57
Cinnamon Roll, Large, 6 oz	630	27	87
Coffee Cake, 2½ oz	230	7	38
Concha: Small, 2½ oz	250	8	38
Large (5" diameter), 5½ oz	550	18	84
Cream Cheese Crumb, 4 oz	410	20	52
Cream Puff (custard fill), 4½ oz	300	18	26
Creme Horns, each	190	13	19
Croissants: *See Next Column*			
Cupcake: Plain, 1½ oz	140	6	25
w. Frosting	170	7	30
Danish Pastry: Small, 2 oz	220	10	25
Large, 4 oz	440	20	51
Date Nut Roll, ½" slice	80	2	12
Devil's Food, w. Frosting, 3 oz	460	25	55
Donut Holes, 1¼" balls, 2 oz (5)	220	10	30
Donuts: *See Page 115*			
Eclair, Choc., Cust. fill, 3½ oz	240	14	23
Fried Twinkie (1)	420	34	45
Fig Bars, average, each	150	3	30
Fig Cake, ½ piece	110	2	21
Fruit Cake, Dark/Light, 1½ oz	165	7	26
Fudge Nut Brownie, each	340	13	56
Funnel Cake (1), 9"	390	1	85
Gingerbread: From mix, 3" sq.	200	6	37
Honey Bun, each	330	13	47
Jelly Roll, ¹⁄₁₀ roll	150	2.5	29
Key Lime Pie, 4.5 oz	440	22	54
Kolacky, Apricot/Rasp., ½ oz (1)	60	3.5	8
Lemon Cake, 2½ oz piece	220	9	40

Ready-to-Eat (Cont)

	C	F	Cb
Lemon Poppy Seed Creme, 3 oz	310	15	40
Marble Cake, 1 slice, 4 oz	380	14	60
Mississippi Mud Pie, 4 oz	380	24	37
Mud Cake, 1 piece, 3½ oz	350	16	48
Muffins: *See Next Page*			
Orange Creme (Ring), 3 oz	300	15	40
Pineapple Upside Down, 2½ oz	230	9	37
Peach Melba, 3½ oz	300	8	52
Strawberry Creme, 3 oz	290	14	40
Strudel Bites, ¾ oz	85	4	12
Pecan Twirls, 1 piece	110	5	16
Pecan Pie, 3 oz	330	13	51
Pies & Tarts: *See Page 116*			
Pound Cake, 3 oz	420	27	42
Sponge: Plain, 2½ oz	190	3	36
w. Cream & Strawberry	325	8	38
w. Chocolate Icing	300	12	38
Raisin Bun, 1 bun, 2¼ oz	180	2	37
Strudel, fruit, average, 3 oz	280	8	45
Sweet Roll, average, 1½ oz	155	7	24
Swiss Rolls, each	170	9	23
Tarts: *See Page 116*			
Tiramisu, 5 oz	400	29	30
Toaster Strudel, 2 oz	190	10	26
Turnovers, fruit, average, 3 oz	270	12	36
Zeppole (Italian Donut), 1	65	1	12
Starbucks: *See Page 255*			

Croissants

	C	F	Cb
Average All Brands			
Plain/Butter/Cheese: Mini, 1 oz	115	6	13
Small, 1½ oz	170	9	19
Medium, 2 oz	230	12	26
Large, 2½ oz	270	14	31
Sweet Croissants: *(aprox. 3oz)*			
Almond Filled	330	18	39
Butter with Apricot Glaze	320	17	31
Chocolate Filled	360	19	43
Raspberry & Cream Cheese	260	12	34
Au Bon Pain: *See Page 187*			
Burger King: *Croissan'wich, See Page 194*			
Dunkin' Donuts: Plain Croissant	330	18	37
Pizza; Spanish Cheese	520	35	33
Sara Lee: All Butter, 1½ oz	180	9	19
All Butter Petite, 1 oz	120	6	13
Starbucks: *See Page 255*			
Croissants Sandwiches: *See Page 173*			

Muffins, Sweet Rolls

Quick Guide | C | F | Cb

Muffins: Ready-To-Eat
Average All Types:

	C	F	Cb
Small, 1 oz	80	3	12
Medium, 2 oz	160	6	24
Large, 3 oz	240	9	36
Extra Large, 4 oz	320	12	48
Giant, 6 oz	480	18	60
Super Size, 8 oz	640	24	96
English Muffin, 2 oz	150	2	29

Brands ~ Ready-To-Eat

	C	F	Cb
Awreys: Blueberry, 2.25 oz	210	9	29
Raisin Bran, 2.5 oz muffin	190	7	30
Carl's: Blueberry Muffin	340	14	49
Bran Raisin Muffin	370	14	61
Controlled Carb Gourmet			
Almond Muffins, 3 oz	210	15	28
Grandpa's: Original, 3 oz	280	11	40
99% Fat Free, 5 oz	360	1	74
Hostess: Mini, average, each	55	3	7
Fruit Pie, avg., 4.5 oz	480	21	70
McDonald's: Apple Bran, 4 oz	300	3	61
My Favorite Muffin: Plain, 6 oz	660	30	75
Chocolate Chip, 6 oz	630	33	81
Fat Free, avg., 6 oz	360	0	80
Oroweat: Cinnamon Rais., 2.4 oz	180	1.5	28
Extra Crisp; Sourdough, 2 oz	140	1	28
Health Nut, 2.3 oz	180	3.5	31
Otis Spunkmeyer: *Per Whole Muffin (4 oz)*			
Banana Nut, 4 oz	480	24	60
Cheese Struedel	440	20	60
Wild Blueberry	420	22	48
Our Daily Muffin: Each, 3 oz	150	0	31
Pepperidge Farm: Average	150	3	28
Ralphs: Banana, 4.5 oz muffin	470	21	62
Blueberry, 4.5 oz	410	16	60
Bran & Raisin, 5 oz	380	8	78
Sara Lee: Blueberry	220	11	27
Corn	260	14	30
Starbucks: *See Fast-Foods Section*			
Uncle Wally's: Rich & Moist, 4 oz	390	20	48
All Natural; Gourmet, 2 oz	140	2	28
Fat Free Gourmet, 2 oz	125	0	28
Van de Kamp's: Banana Nut, 4 oz	500	32	48
Almond Poppy Seed, 4 oz	460	25	54
Blueberry, 3.8 oz	420	24	48
Chocolate Chip, 3.8 oz	480	28	53
Zen Bakery			
Bran Muffin (1)	110	2.5	19
Oat Bran Muffins (1)	135	3	23
Fast-Food Restaurants: *See Page 183*			

Muffin Mixes | C | F | Cb

Prepared: Per Muffin

	C	F	Cb
Atkins: Muffins, average	70	1	8
Betty Crocker: Apple Streusel	210	8	33
Blueberry	160	6	25
Choc Chip; Cinn. Streusel	170	8	23
Fat Free, all flavors	120	0	26
Duncan Hines: Blueberry, reg.	120	3	21
Bakery Style: Pecan Crunch	220	11	27
Avg. all other flavors	200	7	32
Oat Bran Blueberry	110	4	17
Oatmeal & Apples/Walnuts	210	9	30
Entenmann's			
Little Bites Muffins*: Per Pouch*			
Fudge Brownies, 2.1 oz	280	15	34
Blueberry, 1 pouch, 1.76 oz	190	9	26
Gold Medal: Apple; Blueberry	250	8	41
Chocolate Chip w. Glaze	330	12	51
Cornbread varieties	140	3.5	25
Variety	105	7	9
Average other flavors	280	8	46
Krusteaz			
Carb Simple, avg., 2 oz	150	5	20
Sweet Rewards: Low-Fat	230	1.5	51

Sweet Rolls & Buns

Note: Weigh for actual weight as can be 10-50% higher than label weight.

	C	F	Cb
Cinnabon: Classic	815	32	117
Caramel Pecanbon, 1 roll	1100	56	141
Minibon, 1 roll	335	13	49
CinnaPretzel	755	6	156
CinnaPoppers (3)	370	21	41
Cinnabon Stix (5)	380	20	41
Entenmann's			
Gourmet Cinn. Rolls, ½ roll, 2 oz	220	8	33
Hostess: Honey Bun, Glazed, 2.7 oz	320	19	34
Actual weight up to 3.9 oz	460	27	49
Iced/Frosted, 3.5 oz	410	24	42
Little Debbie: Pecan Spinwheels, 1 oz	110	4	16
Pillsbury: Cinnamon Roll, 1.5 oz	150	5	23
Reduced Fat, 1.5 oz	140	3.5	24
Svenhard's: Viking Size Cinn. Bun, 4 oz	650	35	79
Actual weight up to 5.6 oz	650	35	79
Label data based on 4.8 oz	560	30	68
Van de Kamp's			
Cinnamon Roll (1) 1.1 oz	140	7	17
Zen Bakery			
Cinnamon Raisin Roll, ½	100	1	21

Donuts

Quick Guide	C	F	Cb
Donuts			
Average All Brands			
Plain, 1¾ oz	210	12	25
Sugared, 1¾ oz	220	11	27
Glazed, 2 oz	250	12	34
Chocolate Iced, 2 oz	260	14	29

Brands	C	F	Cb
Dolly Madison			
Regular, 1¾ oz	270	12	40
Gem varieties, ½ each	65	3	8
Powdered Mini, ½ each	60	3	8
Dunkin' Donuts			
Apple N' Spice Donut	200	8	29
Blueberry Cake Donut	290	16	35
Boston Kreme Donut	240	9	36
Chocolate Frosted Cake Donut	360	20	40
Chocolate Glazed Cake Donut	290	16	33
Cinnamon Cake Donut	330	20	34
Glazed Cake Donut	350	19	41
Jelly Filled Donut	210	8	32
Kreme Filled (Choc./Vanilla)Donut	270	14	38
Old Fashioned Cake Donut	300	19	28
Powdered Cake Donut	330	19	36
Sugar Raised Donut	170	8	22
Entenmann's			
Dark Choc. Frosted, 2 oz	280	19	27
Frosted Devil's Food, 2.3 oz	310	19	34
Glazed Buttermilk, 2¼ oz	270	13	35
Iced Buttermilk, avg., 2.3 oz	285	16	34
Milk Chocolate Frosted, 2.4 oz	310	19	35
Powdered, 1¾ oz	230	14	25
PopEms (bite size): *Per 4 pieces*			
Glazed (4) 2 oz	240	12	31
Glazed Devil's Food (4) 2 oz	240	11	33
Popettes (bite size), 3 pces, 1.8 oz	240	15	24
Hostess			
Cinnamon Sweet Rolls, 2.3 oz	210	7	34
Regular: Plain, 1 oz	140	7	15
Chocolate Frosted, 1½ oz	180	11	19
Powdered, 1½ oz	150	8	19
Old Fashioned Glazed, 1½oz	260	13	33
Blueberry, 1½ oz	210	13	21
Hostess O's, Raspberry, 2 oz	230	10	34
Donettes: Plain, ½ oz	70	4	8
Frosted, 0.5 oz ea	65	4	7
Crumb, 0.7 oz ea	80	3.5	8
Powdered, ½ oz ea	60	3	8

Brands (Cont)	C	F	Cb
Jewel: Cinnamon Spiced, 2 oz	230	15	24
Krispy Kreme			
Chocolate Brownie Deluxe	300	17	33
Chocolate Glazed Cruller	290	15	37
Chocolate Iced Glazed	250	12	33
Chocolate Iced Kreme Filled	345	20	38
Chocolate Iced w. Sprinkles	270	12	38
Cinnamon Twist	225	9	33
Glazed Cruller	240	14	26
Glazed Kreme Filled	345	20	38
Maple Iced Cake	270	13	35
New York Cheesecake	325	19	35
Original Glazed	205	12	22
Powdered Cake	285	14	37
Traditional Cake Doughnut	230	13	25
Doughnut Holes, 4 pieces	210	10	29
Little Debbie			
Donut Sticks, 1.6 oz pkg	210	13	21
3 oz pkg	390	23	39
Mickey			
Egg Fluff (2) 1.65 oz	210	11	25
French Twirl (2) 1.65 oz	240	16	21
Jumbo, avg. all types (1) 1.5 oz	190	11	21
Mini (2) 1 oz	130	8	15
Tastykake			
Plain, 1½ oz	190	10	22
Cinnamon, 1½ oz	180	8	26
Frosted Rich, 2 oz	260	16	28
Glazed, Mini (6) 2½ oz	270	12	38
Powdered Sugar, Mini (6) 2½ oz	280	13	38
Van De Kamp's			
Plain (1) 1.25 oz	180	8	18
Chocolate (1) 1.4 oz	180	10	21
Powdered (1) 1.5 oz	170	9	22
Crumb (1) 1.5 oz	160	7	23
Cinnamon (1) 1.5 oz	190	10	25
Glazed Blueberry Cake (1) 2.5 oz	290	17	32
Glazed Choc. Donut Holes (4)	250	11	37
Zingers			
Devil's/Vanilla Food, 2 cakes	280	8	50

Full Nutritional Data
~ See Author's Website
www.CalorieKing.com

115

Pies & Tarts

Quick Guide

Pies: *Average All Brands (9")*

Apple; Blueberry; Cherry:	C	F	Cb
Small, ⅛ pie, 4½ oz	340	16	46
Medium ⅙ pie, 7½ oz	565	27	76
Large, ¼ pie, 9½ oz	720	34	97
Extra Large, ⅓ pie, 12 oz	905	43	122
Whole Pie (9"), 38 oz	2870	135	390

Other Pies: *Per Small Serving (⅛ of 9" Pie)*

Chocolate Cream Pie	345	22	38
Custard; Coconut Custard	270	14	31
Lemon Chiffon Pie	360	14	50
Lemon Meringue	330	13	52
Pecan Pie	480	25	59
Pumpkin Pie	230	10	30
Strawberry Pie	230	9	37

Brands ~ *Per Serving*

Denny's: Apple Pie, 7 oz	485	24	64
Chocolate Peanut Butter, 6 oz	655	39	64
Entenmann's			
Homestyle Apple, ⅙ pie, 4.3 oz	340	12	56
Hostess: Fruit; Cherry, 4.5 oz pie	480	20	68
Lemon, 4.5 oz pie	500	24	66
Long John Silver's			
Chocolate Cream Pie	310	22	34
Pecan Pie	370	15	23
Pineapple Cream Pie	290	13	39
Marie Callender's			
Per ⅕ Pie: Apple	865	49	92
Blueberry	885	57	76
Boysenberry	860	57	82
Cherry	900	58	87
Banana Cream	630	28	67
Chocolate Cream	535	29	66
Coconut Cream	650	32	64
Per ¼ Pie: Fresh Strawberry	615	28	89
Mince	885	59	97
Lemon Meringue	550	23	76
Pumpkin	615	28	80
Tastykake: Fruit, average	270	11	41
French Apple	330	12	55
Coconut Creme	370	20	42
Lemon Pie	300	13	45
Sara Lee: See Page 118			
Weight Watchers: See Page 118			

Pastry & Pie Crusts

	C	F	Cb
Pie Crust: Baked, 9" diameter shell			
1 Pie Shell, 6½ oz	880	56	72
2-crust Pie, 9", 11¼ oz	1240	82	112
Piecrust Sticks, 8 oz	960	64	90
Choux Pastry, raw, 1 oz	60	4	3
Filo Pastry: 4 sheets, 2½ oz	210	2.5	40
Athens: 5 sheets, 2 oz	180	1.5	37
Mini Dough Shells, 2, 8g	35	2	2
Pepp. Farm, 2 sheets, 1½ oz	120	1	25
Flaky Pastry, 1 sheet, 6 oz	780	72	18
Puff (*Pepp.Farm*), ½ sheet, 4.5 oz	510	33	42
⅛ sheet, 1½ oz	170	11	14
Bake & Fill Shell, 1.7 oz	190	13	16
Pizza Crust, ⅛ whole	90	1	16
Bisquick: Baking Mix,			
Original, ⅓ cup, 1½ oz	160	6	25
Reduced Fat, ⅓ cup, 1½ oz	150	2.5	27
Betty Crocker, 9", ⅛ shell	110	7	9
Boboli, Thin Pizza Crust, ⅕, 2 oz	170	3.5	28
Hershey's Choc Crust, ⅛	110	5	14
Jewel, ⅛ of 9" crust	130	8	13
Keebler Graham Cracker, ⁸⁄₁₀ of 9"	110	5	14
Reduced Fat, ⅛	90	3.5	14
Shortbread Crust, ⅛	110	5	14
Graham Crackers Minis (1)	120	6	15
Mrs Smith's Deep Dish, 9" (⅛)	130	7	14
Nabisco Oreo, ⅙ of 9" crust	130	7	19
Honey Maid Graham, ⅙, 1 oz	150	8	18
Nilla Pie Crust, ⅙, 1 oz	140	7	18
Pet-Ritz, all types, ⅛, ¾ oz	90	5	11
Pillsbury (All Ready), ⅛ pie, 1 oz	120	7	13

Pie Filling (Canned)

Average All Brands

Apple: ½ cup, 4¼ oz	120	0	30
21 oz Can	600	0	145
Apricot, 2 Tbsp	70	0	17
Blackberry, Blueberry, Cherry, 4 oz	120	0	28
Chocolate, Coconut, 4 oz	140	3	33
Lemon, ⅓ cup, 4 oz	130	1.5	28
Mincemeat, 4 oz	190	1	45
Peach, Strawberry, ⅓ cup, 4 oz	100	0	23
Pumpkin, 4 oz	40	0.5	9
Raisin, 4 oz	130	0	30
Raspberry, Black/Red, 4 oz	120	0	30
Strawberry, ⅓ cup, 4 oz	100	0	23

Cakes, & Pastries – Packaged

Cakes & Pastries

	C	F	Cb
Banquet: Cream Pies, avg., 1/3 pie	350	21	39
CarbSense: Per Serving (Prepared)			
Brownie, 1/12 pk	220	17	11
Carrot Cake, 1/9 pkt	280	20	10
Cheesecake Factory: See Fast-Foods Section			
Dolly Madison: Honey Bun, 3.75 oz	440	25	49
Cinnamon Sweet Rolls (1)	210	7	34
Dunkin' Stix, 1 stix	170	9	20
Eli's Frozen Cheesecakes: Per 1/8 Pkg (3 oz)			
Cookies N Creme; Choc. Caramel	320	23	11
Keylime; Original, average	320	22	26
Entenmann's			
All Butter Loaf, 1/6 loaf, 2 oz	210	9	30
Bavarian Cream Danish, 1/8, 2 oz	190	7	30
Cheese Danish Twist, 1/8	220	12	27
Cheese-Filled Crumb Coffee, 2 oz	210	10	26
Chocolate Fudge, 1/6 cake, 3 oz	260	13	39
Coffee Cake: Cheese Topped, 1/9, 2 oz	200	9	26
New York Crumb, 1/8, 2 oz	270	14	31
Golden Loaf (Light) 1/8, 1.7 oz	120	0	28
Gourmet Cinn. Rolls, 1/2 roll	220	8	33
Light Raspberry Twist, 1/8, 1.8 oz	120	0	29
Little Bites: Blueberry, 1 pouch	190	9	26
Chocolate Chip, 1 pouch	210	10	28
Fudge Brownie, 1 pouch	280	15	34
Louisiana Crunch, 1/9, 3 oz	340	15	49
Pecan Danish Ring, 1/8	250	15	25
Raspberry Danish Twist, 1/8	220	11	28
Muffins/Rolls: See Page 114			
Glenny's Slim Carb Cheesecake: Per 1/6 Cake			
Natural New York, 3 oz	210	13	15
Other varieties, 3.5 oz	135	1	23
Grands!: Cinnamon Roll (1)	300	7	54
Hostess: Per Cake Unless Indicated			
Cinnamon Streudel Cake (1)	170	6	28
Chocodiles	230	11	36
Crumb Coffee	170	6	28
Cup Cake, each	180	6	30
Ding Dongs	170	9	23
Hearty Muffin, average	620	33	73
Ho Ho's, each	125	6	17
Honey Bun: Glazed, 2.7 oz	310	15	39
Actual weight up to 3.9 oz	460	27	49
Mini Muffins (3)	230	14	24
Raspberry Zinger (1)	200	8	30
Snoballs	170	5	32

Hostess (Cont)	C	F	Cb
Twinkies, 1 cake, 1.5 oz	145	4.5	27
Vanilla Zinger (1)	210	7	36
Zingers (1)	200	7	33
Jewel Bake Shop			
Choc Mini Cookies, 1 cake	100	12	30
Cinnamon Swirl Bread, 1 oz slice	160	2.5	30
Creme Horns, 1 horn	190	13	19
Elephant Ears, 2.5 oz	340	22	34
Fancy Jelly Roll, 1/6 roll, 2.7 oz	190	2.5	38
French Torpedo Roll, 2.7 oz	170	1	35
Gourmet Cinn. Rolls, 6 oz roll	640	29	88
Key Lime Meringue Pie, 1/6, 5 oz	340	12	55
Krispy Kreme			
Tarts (Packaged): Per Tart			
Apple Pie	400	19	54
Cherry Pie	410	19	56
Coconut Pie	450	21	61
Peach Pie	370	17	51
Little Debbie			
Brownies (1)	290	13	40
Choc Chip Snack Cake (2), 2.4 oz	290	1.5	39
Coffee Cake (2), 2 oz	200	6	35
Creme-filled Strawb. Cupcake (1)	200	10	26
Devil Squares, 2 cakes, 2.2 oz	280	13	39
Frosted Fudge , 1.5 oz cake	200	10	25
Honey Buns, 1.75 oz bun	230	13	24
Marshmallow Pie (1)	180	7	28
Oatmeal Creme Pie (1)	170	7	26
Pecan Spinwheels, 1 roll	100	4	16
Swiss Cake Rolls, 2 cakes	270	12	40
Tiny Cakes (2)	140	15	42
Zebra Cakes, 2 cakes, 2.6 oz	340	16	46
Manischewitz: Cheesecake, 3 oz	230	19	16
Marie Callender's (Frozen)			
Cobbler: Berry, 1/4 pie, 4 oz	280	13	35
Peach, 1/4 pie, 4 oz	270	13	36
Mrs Smith's			
Cream Pies: Oreo, 1/6, 4.3 oz	380	17	54
Choc Chip Delight, 1/6, 4.9 oz	410	18	59
Moose Tracks, 1/6, 4.5 oz	495	29	51
Silk Pies: avg., 1/9 pie	565	40	50
Slices: Apple; Peach, 1 pce	265	13	37
Dutch Apple, 1 piece	240	10	37
Pies: Egg Custard, 1/10 pie	250	12	30
Peach Cobbler, 1/8 pie	230	10	34

Cakes & Pastries (Cont)

Pepperidge Farm	C	F	Cb
Turnovers (Frozen): Apple, 3.2 oz	290	15	36
Raspberry, 3.2 oz	290	15	35
3-Layer Cakes: Coconut, ⅛, 2.5 oz	260	14	33
Golden, ⅛ cake, 2.5 oz	260	13	34
Fruit Squares: Apple/Blueb./Cherry	210	10	27
Rich's: Chocolate Eclairs (Frozen)	190	9	24
Bavarian Creme Eclair	220	12	25

Sara Lee (Frozen)

Bites: *Per Serving*	C	F	Cb
Choc. Dipped Orig. Cheesecake (5)	100	7	8
Choc. Dipped Praline Pecan (5)	90	6	8
Triple Choc. Fudge Brownie (1)	90	4	12
Cheesecake: *Per Slice*			
Chocolate French, ⅕ cake	430	22	52
Choc. Swirl New York Style, ⅙	470	29	45
French Classic, ⅕ cake	410	25	41
French Strawberry, ⅙ cake	320	14	43
New York Style, ⅙ cake	350	21	35
Original Cream Cherry, ¼ cake	350	12	55
Original Cream Classic, ¼ cake	340	18	38
Original Cream Strawberry, ¼ cake	330	12	49
Cakes: *Per Slice*			
Coffee Butter Streusel, ⅙ cake	190	9	25
Coffee Crumb, ⅛ cake	190	8	30
Coffee Deluxe Cinnamon Rolls w. Icing (1)	320	15	41
Coffee Pecan, ⅙ cake	140	13	23
Layer Cakes: *Per ⅛ Whole*			
Layer Coconut, ⅛ cake	260	14	33
Layer Double Chocolate, ⅛ cake	260	13	33
Layer Fudge Golden, ⅛ cake	260	13	34
Layer Vanilla, ⅛ cake	260	14	32
Pound Cakes: *Per ¼ Whole*			
All Butter, 2.6 oz	220	15	34
Free & Light, ¼ cake	200	4	39
Strawberry Swirl, ¼ cake	290	11	44
Pies			
French Silk Pie, 1 slice, 4.8 oz	340	21	34
Tangy Lemon Meringue Pie	220	5	41
Tropical Coconut Cream Pie	330	19	37
Cobbler Anytime Pie: Apple, 4 oz	350	17	47
Blackberry, 4 oz	350	17	48
Peach, 4 oz	340	17	4

Sara Lee (Cont)	C	F	Cb
Oven Fresh Pies (9″, 37 oz Box): *Per Slice (4.6 oz)*			
Apple Pie, ⅛	340	16	46
Cherry Pie, ⅛	320	14	44
Dutch Apple Pie, ⅛	350	15	53
Mince Pie; Blueberry Pie, ⅛	370	15	55
Peach Pie, ⅛	330	13	50
Pumpkin Pie, ⅛	260	11	37
Raspberry Pie, ⅛	360	16	50
Southern Sweet Potato Pie, ⅛	280	10	45
Signature Selection Pies: *Per Slice*			
Caramel Applenut, ⅑	370	18	45
Chocolate Dream Pie, ⅛	440	24	54
Cinnamon French Apple, ⅒	360	15	48
Dulce de Leche Caramel Swirl, ⅑	400	26	37
Fruits of the Forest, ⅑	340	17	41
Golden Peach, ⅒	340	16	46
Gourmet Cherry Deep Dish Pie, ⅑	380	18	50
Key West Lime Pie, ⅛	400	25	41
Lemon Grove Meringue Pie, ⅒	350	16	51
Orchard Apple Deep Dish Pie, ⅒	400	24	43
Southern Pecan Pie, ⅑	520	24	70
Strawberries & Cream Pie, ⅛	400	27	33
Traditional Pumpkin Pie, ⅒	250	9	34
TastyKake: Chocolate Jnr, 3.4 oz	340	12	54
Creme Filled Koffee Kakes, 3 oz	390	19	51
Koffee Kake Junior, 2½ oz	270	10	42
Van de Kamp's			
Angle Food Ring, ⅛ cake	130	0	29
Banana Square Cake, ¼	410	18	60
Bear Claw, 1 pce, 2 oz	250	14	27
Carrot Square Cake, ¼	520	33	54
Cinn. Raisin Danish, 1 pce, 2 oz	245	12	16
Crumb Cake, ⅛ cake, 2.5 oz	330	18	39
Fruit Danish, 1 pce, 2 oz	230	12	28
German Chocolate Cake, ¼	290	16	36
Pies: Apple; Cherry, avg., ⅙ pie	360	23	36
Pumpkin Pie, ⅙ pie	340	14	48
Pecan; Sweet Potato, ⅙ avg.	390	16	58
Weight Watchers: *Per Serving*			
Brownie à la Mode	190	4	33
Carrot Cake, 3.3 oz	220	3.5	34
Chocolate Mousse	180	4	24
Chocolate Eclair	150	4	25
Choc. Chip Cookie Dough Sundae	190	4.5	35
Double Fudge Brownie Parfait	260	5	43
Double Fudge Cake	150	4.5	20
French Style Cheesecake	170	4	28
Key Lime Pie, 3.3 oz	200	6	34
Mississippi Mud Pie	160	5	24
Peanut Butter Pie, 3.3 oz	210	6	37
New York Style Cheesecake	150	5	21

Cakes, Cookies & Dessert Mixes

	C	F	Cb
Made As Directed			
Arrowhead Mills: *Per Serving (Prep'd)*			
Cookie (1), avg. all types	100	4.5	11
Perfect Harvest Muffin, 1/2 pkg	270	12	40
Wheat Free Brownie, 1/20 pkg	160	7.5	21
Aunt Jemin			
Coffee Cake, 1/8 cake, prep.	180	6	27
Banquet			
Dessert Bakes: *Per Serving (Prep'd)*			
Apple Crisp, 1/6 pkg	210	3.5	41
Choc. Cherry Decadence, 1/6 pkg	310	5	62
Chocolate Lava Cake, 1/7 pkg	370	7	73
Cherry Cobbler, 1/6 pkg	250	4	50
Betty Crocker			
Cakes (Super Moist): *Per 1/2 Cake (Prep'd)*			
Butter Recipe Yellow	250	11	36
Chocolate varieties	280	15	34
Cinnamon Swirl	280	11	42
Devil's Food	270	13	35
White	230	10	34
Other flavors, average	270	13	35
Per 1/10 Cake (Prepared): Carrot	320	15	45
Sour Cream	280	12	43*
If using No Cholesterol Recipe, deduct 40 cals and 4g fat.			
Other Cakes: Pound Cake, 1/8	260	8	45
Angel Food Cake, 1/12 mix	140	0	32
Gingerbread Cake, 1/8	210	5	39
Pineapple Upside Down, 1/6	390	13	65
Sunkist Lemon Bar (1)	140	4.5	24
Brownie Mixes: *Per 1/20 Pkg (Prep'd)*			
Chocolate Chunk varieties	180	9	25
Dark Chocolate	170	7	25
Fudge	170	7	24
Original Supreme	160	6	27
Peanut Butter; Walnut	180	9	23
Turtle (Caramel & Pecan)	170	8	23
Cookie Mix: *Per 2 Cookies (Prep'd)*			
Rainbow Chocolate Candy	150	7	22
Other varieties, average	170	9	21
Complete Desserts: *Per 1/6 Pkg*			
Apple Crisp	270	6	53
Hot Fudge Cake	430	13	75
Peach Cobbler	290	7	55
Warm Delights: *Per Bowl*			
Cinnamon Swirl Cake	400	12	70
Fudgy Choc. Chip Cookie	340	11	58
Other varieties, average	365	12	62

	C	F	Cb
Betty Crocker (Cont)			
Muffin Mix: *Per Muffin (6.5 oz)*			
Apple Streusel	200	6	34
Blueberry; Golden Corn	160	6	24
Chocolate Chip	220	10	30
Triple Berry	120	3	22
Twice the Blueberries	160	4	26
Wild Blueberry	190	7	21
Other varieties, average	130	4	21
Snackin' Cake: *Per 1/9 Pkg*			
Banana Walnut	180	6	27
Cinnamon Swirl	210	9	28
Chocolate varieties	200	8	30
Carb Monitor: *Per Serving (Prep'd)*			
Brownie: Choc Chunk, 1/16 pkg	150	9	20
Walnut (1), 1/16 pkg	160	11	20
Cookie, 2 cookies, 1/14 pkg	130	7	18
Muffin (1), 1/12 pkg	160	9	27
Dr Oetker: *Per Serving (Prep'd)*			
Chocolate Chip Cookie Mix, 1/12	170	7.5	24
Muffin Mix, 1/12 pkg, average	170	2	30
Simple Organic Cake Mix, 1/12	255	11	32
Duncan Hines			
Angel Food, 1/12 whole	140	0	30
Brownie Mix (low-fat recipe)			
1/18 pkg, avg. all types	180	9	23
Cookies, all flavors, 1 cookie	65	3	8
Moist Deluxe Cake Mix:			
Average, 1/12 pkg, prepared	290	15	36
Lower Fat Recipe, 1/12 pkg, prep.	200	5	36
Estee: Brownie, 1 pce, 2"x 2"	50	2	12
All cakes, 1/5 cake	200	4	38
Choc. Chip Cookie, 1 cookie	45	2.5	6
Ghirardelli: *Per Serving (Prepared)*			
Brownie, 1/16 pkg	200	10	27
Chocolate Chip Cookie (1)	280	13	38
Dble Choc Muffin (1)	250	10	37
Jell-O No Bake Cheesecakes: *Prep'd As Directed*			
Cherry/Strawberry, 1/9 pkg	290	10	43
Chips-Ahoy!, 1/6 pkg	260	9	46
Chocolate Silk Dessert, 1/6 pkg	180	6	34
Oreo, 1/6 pkg	270	9	48
Peanut Butter Cup, 1/8 pkg	290	15	38
Real, 1/6 pkg	220	5	47
Krusteaz: Cinn. Crumb Cake, 1"	230	7	38
Lemon/Key Lime Bar, 2" bar	160	3.5	29
Muffins: Blueberry (1)	150	4	26
Peach Cobbler (1)	270	6	46
Fat-Free varieties (1)	130	0	30
Carb Simple Muffins			
Banana Nut (1)	180	7	19
Other varieties (1), average	170	5	22

Frostings ◆ Baking Ingredients

Cakes & Dessert Mixes (Cont)

Made As Directed

	C	F	Cb
No Pudge			
Fudge Brownie, 1/12 pkg, prep'd.	120	0	28
Pamela's			
Ultra Chocolate Brownie, 1/16 pkg	170	8	23
Oil Free, 1/16 pkg	110	1.5	24
Pillsbury			
Moist Supreme: *Per 1/2 Cake (Prepared)*			
Angel Food Cake	140	0	31
Devil's Food Cake	270	14	34
French Vanilla; German Choc.	250	11	34
Funfetti	260	11	36
Streusel Coffee, 1/16 cake	260	11	37
Other flavors, average 1/12 cake	250	10	35
Thick 'n Fudgy Deluxe Brownie *(Prepared)*			
Caramel Swirl, 1/12 pkg	200	8	27
Cheesecake Swirl, 1/18 pkg	150	8	19
Choc./Vanilla Frosted, 1/16 pkg	190	9	27
Double Choc, 1/16 pkg	160	7	23
Fudge, 1/20 pkg	170	8	33
Fudge Toffey, 1/20 pkg	170	8	23
Chocolate Chunk, 1/16 pkg	170	8	22
w. Walnuts, 1/12 pkg	200	11	24
Muffins, avg. all types (1)	185	6	30
Robin Hood			
Angel Food Cake, 1/2 cake	115	0	27

Cake Frostings

	C	F	Cb
Betty Crocker			
Rich & Creamy, average, 2 Tbsp	150	8	15
Whipped, all flavors, 3 Tbsp	110	5	20
Easy Flow Icing, 2 Tbsp	150	8	18
Duncan Hines: *Per 2 Tbsp (1.2 oz)*			
Creamy Homestyle, avg all flavors	140	5	22
Pillsbury: *Per 2 Tbsp (approx. 1/2 Tub)*			
Chocolate Cream Cheese	140	6	21
Coconut Pecan	160	10	17
Cream Cheese; Lemon	150	6	23
French Vanilla	160	6	25
Milk/Chocolate; Choc. Fudge	140	6	21
Rainbow Chip	140	5	23
All other flavors, average	150	6	23
Decorators, Choc., 1 Tbsp	70	2	11

Baking Ingredients

	C	F	Cb
Almond Paste:			
(Marzipan), 1 oz	125	7	12
Baking Powder: Regular, 1 tsp	3	0	0.5
Cream of Tartar, 1 tsp	2	0	0.5
Baking Mix *(Bisquick)* :			
Original, 1/3 cup, 1 1/2 oz	160	6	26
Reduced Fat, 1/3 cup, 1 1/2 oz	150	2.5	27
Butter/Margarine, 1/2 cup, 4 oz	820	91	0
Carob Flour, 1/2 cup	90	0.5	26
Chocolate Baking Bars: *Average All Brands*			
Unsweetened, 1 oz	140	14	8
Grated, 1 cup, 4 1/2 oz	680	68	36
Semi-sweet, 1 oz	140	9	16
Bitter-sweet/White Baking 1 oz	160	8	20
Chocolate Baking Chips: *Average All Brands*			
Milk Choc./Semi Sweet 1 oz	160	9	18
1/4 cup, 1 1/2 oz	240	12	30
1 cup, 6 oz	960	48	120
Mini Kisses (Hershey), 1 pce	5	0.5	1
M&M's Minis, Nestle Morsels, 1 oz	140	8	18
Reeses Peanut Butter Chips, 1 oz	160	8	16
Cocoa Powder, Baking: *Nestle,* 1 T.	15	1	3
1/3 cup, 1 oz	80	4	12
Hershey's, 1 Tbsp	20	0.5	3
1/3 cup, 1 oz	115	3.5	21
Coconut, dried: Unsweet., 1 oz	190	18	7
Sweetened/flaked, 1 oz	135	9	12
1/2 cup, 1.3 oz	175	12	18
Toasted *(Baker's),* 1 oz	170	13	17
Coconut Cream/Milk: *See Page 39*			
Cornstarch, 1 Tbsp	30	0	7
Flour, white: 1 Tbsp, 0.6 oz	55	0	12
1 cup, 4.4 oz	450	1	95
Whole Wheat, 1 cup, 4.2 oz	360	2	84
Flavor Extracts: *Average All Brands*			
Imitation, 1 tsp	15	0	3.5
Pure Extract, 1 tsp	20	0	4
Almond, Vanilla, 1 tsp	10	0	3
Fruit Pectin: Swtnd, 1 Tbsp, 1/2 oz	35	0	10
Unsweetened, 1 Tbsp	2	0	0.5
Gelatin, dry, 1/4 oz pkg	30	0	0
Lemon/Orange Peel, 1/4 cup	30	0	4
Rennin, 1 pkg (11g)	12	0	1
Sprinkles, all types, 1 Tbsp, 1/2 oz	45	0	9
Vinegar, avg. all types, 1 oz	4	0	2
Whey, sweet, dry, 1 oz	90	0.5	20
Yeast: Active, dry, 1/4 oz pkg	15	0	2
Bakers, compressed, 1 oz	25	0	3
Brewers; Torula, 1 oz	80	0.5	11
Fleischmann's, 0.6 oz pkg	0	0	0

Puddings, Desserts, Gelatin

Ready-To-Serve

	C	F	Cb
Instant Pudding, Reg., ½ cup	170	4	30
Reduced Calorie: *D-Zerta;* Estee	70	0	12
Jell-O, sugar-free, ½ cup	80	2	11
Royal, sugar-free, ½ cup	100	2	17
Del Monte Pudding Snacks	130	4	24
Fat-Free Vanilla	90	0	20
Dr McDougall's Rice Pudd., 3 oz	310	1.5	69
Hershey's Portable Pud., 2.25 oz	100	3	16
Hunt's Snack Pack: *Per 3.5 oz Cup*			
Puddin' Cakes: Choc Brownie	180	7	27
German Choc Cake	160	3.5	30
Puddin Pie: Lemon Meringue	130	2.5	27
Apple; Choc Mud	170	7	26
Dessert Favorites, avg. all flavors	140	5	22
Jell-O			
Pudding Bites, average 1 pouch	90	1.5	18
Pudding & Pie Filling: *Per ¼ Pkg*			
Cook & Serve, average, prep.	100	0	22
Instant, regular, avg.	100	0	25
Fat & Sugar Free, avg.	30	0	8
Pudding Snacks: Fat-Free, 4 oz	100	0	23
Cheesecake Snack, 4 oz	150	4.5	25
Chocolate; Creme Savers, 4 oz	160	5	28
Smoothie Snacks, 4 oz	100	2.5	20
Jewel: Chef's Kitchen			
Rice Pudding, ½ cup, 4.5 oz	230	8	35
Tapioca Pudding, ½ cup, 4.5 oz	170	8	35
Jolly Rancher: Reg., 3.5 oz cup	100	0	25
Sugar-Free, all flavors, 3.5 oz cup	10	0	2
Kozy Shack: Avg. all types, 4 oz	140	4	25
Lite, 4 oz	110	1	22
Creme Caramel Flan, 1 cup, 4 oz	160	2	28
Kraft Handi Snacks: *Per Cup (3.5 oz)*			
"Doubles", avg. all flavors	125	3.5	22
Chocolate Pudding Fat-Free	85	0	21
Rice Pudding	140	6	19
Tapioca; Vanilla Pudding	115	3.5	20
Kroger: *Per Container*			
Peaches & Cream w. Natural Flav.	180	2.5	36
Whipped Varieties	145	2.5	27
Manischewitz: Choc., ½ cup	110	0.5	26
Passover Gold Noodle, ½ cup	140	2	28
President's Choice			
Key Lime Pie (36 oz) ⅛ pie, 4.5 oz	440	22	54
Mississippi Mud Pie (36 oz) ⅓ 4 oz	380	24	37

Ready-To-Serve (Cont)

	C	F	Cb
Swiss Miss Pudding Snacks			
Swirls, Choc. Pudd. Snacks, 3½ oz	150	5	23
Tapioca: 1 pudding cup, 3½ oz	120	3.5	21
Fat-Free varieties, 3½ oz	90	0	20
Weight Watchers (Frozen)			
Chocolate Mousse, 2¾ oz	190	5	31

Homemade Puddings

	C	F	Cb
Apple Tapioca, ½ cup	150	0	32
Bread Pudding, ½ cup	250	8	40
Blancmange, ½ cup	140	5	19
Chocolate, ½ cup	190	6	30
Corn Pudding, ½ cup	135	4	21
Crème Brûlée, ½ cup	400	35	16
Plum Pudding, 2 oz	170	3	32
Rice with Raisins, ½ cup	200	4	38
Sponge Pudding, 3½ oz	340	16	45
Tapioca Cream, ½ cup	110	4	15
Trifle, ½ cup	180	7	26

Custards

	C	F	Cb
Custard Mix: Jell-O (Americana) Golden Egg			
Dry, ⅙ pkg	80	0	19
Prep. w. 2% milk, ½ cup	140	2.5	19
Jello Flan, w. 2% milk, ½ cup	140	2.5	20
Royal-Flan: Prep. w. 2% milk, ½ c.	130	2.5	18
Homemade Custard			
Baked: Plain, ½ cup, 4½ oz	150	7	16
w. skim milk, artif. sweetened	70	3	4
Boiled, ½ cup	165	7	18

Meringues

	C	F	Cb
Meringue Swirl, ½ cup	50	0	8
Meringue Shell, 1 oz shell	100	0	16
(Add extra calories/fat/carbohydrate for fillings)			

Jell-O • Cups • Parfait

	C	F	Cb
Gelatin Mix: *Jell-O, Royal ~ Made Up*			
Regular, all flavors, ½ cup	80	0	18
Sugar Free/Low Calorie, ½ cup	8	0	0
Creme Gelatin/Parfait: *Per ½ Cup*			
Ida Mae, ½ cup	60	2	10
Winky: Strawberry (109g)	110	1.5	22
Rainbow (130g)	100	0	24
Reser's, Dessert Parfait (110g)	100	2	19
Mrs Crockett's Kitchen, Str. Parfait	160	4	26
Gel Snacks (Jell-O): Regular, 3.5 oz	70	0	17
Sugar Free, 3.2 oz	10	0	1
X-Treme Cups, 2.5 oz	100	0	24
X-Treme Sticks, 2.2 oz	60	0	16

Pancakes & Waffles

Quick Guide

	C	F	Cb
Pancakes			
Plain: Average All Types			
Small (3" diam.), ¾ oz	50	2	6
Medium (4" diam.), 1¼ oz	85	3.5	11
Large (5" diam.), 2½ oz	175	7.5	22
Add Extra for Syrups/Butter			
Pancake Syrup: Regular, 1 Tbsp	50	0	13
¼ cup	210	0	52
Lite, 1 Tbsp	25	0	6
¼ cup	100	0	26
Butter/Margarine: Regular, 1 T.	100	11	0
Whipped, 1 Tbsp	70	7.5	0
Waffles			
Homemade: 7" waffle, 2½ oz	245	13	26
From Mix: 7" waffle, 2½ oz	205	8	28

Frozen Breakfasts

	C	F	Cb
Aunt Jemima			
Pancakes: Mini (13)	240	4	46
Syrup Dunkers, Mini (13)	520	4	114
Waffles: Homestyle (2)	190	5	32
Syrup Dunkers, 8 sticks	370	7	74
French Toast: Cinnamon Sticks (5)	330	11	54
Homestyle; Cinnamon, avg., (2)	230	6	36
Syrup Dunkers, 5 pieces	540	13	101
Eggo *(Kellogg's)*			
French Toast Sticks, avg. (2)	215	6	36
Toaster Swirlz, set of 4, 47g	115	3	20
Farm Rich			
French Toast Sticks, avg. (5)	300	14	40
Pillsbury			
Pancakes: Mini, average, (14)	425	7	88
Chocolate Chip (3)	270	5	51
French Toast Sticks (6)	360	7	69
Dunkables Cinn. Bites/Icing (3)	140	4.5	23
Toaster Strudel, avg. (1)	190	9	26
Krusteaz			
Pancakes: Mini (12)	220	2.5	43
Buttermilk (3)	280	4	52
French Toast: Average, 1 slice	115	2.5	18
Sticks, 4 sticks	230	5	41

Restaurant-Style: *See Fast-Foods Section*
Frozen Egg Breakfasts: *See Page 47*

Pancake Brands

	C	F	Cb
Atkins: All-Purpose, 2 tsp. dry mix	30	0	5
Bake Mix, ¼ cup dry mix	80	0.5	8
Aunt Jemima			
Syrup Dunkers (frozen), 13 mini	520	4	114
Pancake & Waffle Mix:			
Original, ⅓ cup, prepared	250	8	37
Complete, ⅓ cup, prepared	160	2.5	32
Buttermilk Pancake Batter:			
½ cup, 4 x 4" pancakes	270	3.5	51
Betty Crocker Pancake Mixes			
Complete Original/Buttermilk, 3	200	3	39
Bisquick (Shake 'N Pour), 3	200	3	38
CarbSense: ½ cup dry mix	160	2	7
2 pancakes prepared	320	15	9
Hungry Jack Pancakes			
Mixes: *Per ⅓ Cup (Prepared)*			
Buttermilk: Complete, ⅓ cup	150	1.5	31
Original, w. 2% Milk, Oil, Egg	250	8	37
w. Skim Milk, Oil, Egg Whites	180	1	37
Extra Lights: Complete	150	2	30
Microwave (frozen): Pancakes (3)	270	4.5	51
Krusteaz: Carb Simple, prepared,			
3 x 4" pancakes	180	5	23
Northern Pines: 3 x 4" pancakes	380	7	71

Frozen Waffles

	C	F	Cb
Aunt Jemima: Blueberry (1)	95	3	15
Buttermilk (1)	100	2.5	17
Eggo *(Kelloggs):* Banana Bread (1)	95	3	15
Chocolate Chip, 1 waffle	100	3	16
Cinnamon Toast/Homestyle (1)	90	3	15
Nutri-Grain (1)	85	2.5	14
Special K (fat-free), 1	95	0.5	18
Waf-fulls, all types (1) 2 oz	155	5	25
GO-LEAN *(Kashi):* Average (1)	90	1.5	16
Hungry Jack: Blueberry, 1 waffle	105	4	17
Buttermilk; Homestyle (1)	95	3	15
Mini Funfetti (1)	65	2	11
Nature's Path: Average (1)	120	4	18
Lifestream: Gorilla; Koala, avg.	110	3.5	17
Other varieties, avg. (1)	120	4	17
Pillsbury: Waffles, avg. (1)	90	2.5	15
Waffle Sticks (6) & syrup	340	7	64
Van's: Belgian Original (1)	110	2.5	16
97% Fat Free (1)	80	1	15
Mini Homestyle (4)	115	3.5	18
Carb Manager: Butter Pecan (1)	50	3	4
Other varieties (1)	110	5	16

Sugar, Syrup, Jam, Honey

Sugar

	C	F	Cb
White Sugar, granulated:			
1 level teaspoon, 4g	15	0	4
1 heaping teaspoon, 6g	25	0	6.5
1 cube, ½"	24	0	6.5
Single portion, 1 packet	25	0	6.5
1 Tablespoon, 12g	48	0	12
1 ounce, 1 oz	110	0	20
1 cup, 7 oz	770	0	203
1 pound	1760	0	464
Brown Sugar: 1 Tbsp, 13g	50	0	13
1 ounce, 1 oz	109	0	28
1 cup, not packed, 5 oz	540	0	140
1 cup, packed, 7¾ oz	845	0	218
Powdered/Confectioners:			
Sifted, 1 cup, 3½ oz	385	0	98
Unsifted, 1 cup, 4¼ oz	460	0	117
Cinnamon Sugar, 1 tsp	15	0	4
Dextrose, 1 oz	110	0	27
Fructose, 1 tsp	15	0	4
3 Tbsp, 1 oz	110	0	27
Glucose, 1 oz	110	0	27
Glucose Tablets (Dex 4), 1	15	0	4
Palm Sugar, 3 Tbsp, 12g	45	0	11
Piloncillo (Brown Sugar), 3oz Cone	325	0	81
Turbinado Sugar, 1 oz	110	0	27
Unrefined Cane Sugar, 1 oz	110	0	27

Sugar Substitutes

	C	F	Cb
DiabetiSweet, 1 teaspoon	9	0	4
(Carbohydrate as Sugar Alcohol)			
Equal: Tablet/Liquid	0	0	0
Granulated, 1 pkg	4	0	1
Powdered, sachet, 0.04 oz	0	0	0.5
Sugar Lite, 1 tsp	8	0	2
NutraSweet Spoonful, 1 tsp	2	0	0.5
Nutra Taste; Sweet One, 1 pkt	0	0	0
PerfectSweet, 1 tsp	15	0.5	4
Shugr (Swiss Diet), 1 tsp	0	0	0
Sorbitol, 1 tsp	110	0	27
Splenda: Powder, 1 cup	96	0	24
Sachet, sachet	0	0	0.5
Granular, 1 tsp	5	0	1
Sugar Blend, for Baking, ½ cup	385	0	96
Sprinkle Sweet, 1 tsp	2	0	0.5
Stevia, 1 pkt	0	0	0
Sugar Delight, 1 pkt	8	0	2
Sugar Like (Bateman's), 1 tsp	4	0	1
Sugar Twin: 1 pkt	3	0	1
Sugar Substitute, 1 tsp	2	0	1
Sweet 'N Low, 1 pkt	0	0	1
Walgreens Wal-Sweet, 1 pkt	0	0	0
Weight Watchers; Whey Low, 1 tsp	4	0	1

Honey, Jam, Preserves

Average All Brands	C	F	Cb
Honey: 1 tsp, ¼ oz	22	0	5.5
1 Tbsp, ¾ oz	65	0	17
1 ounce, 1 oz	86	0	23
1 cup, 12 oz	1030	0	269
Single Portion, ½ oz pkg	43	0	11
Jams/Jellies/Marmalade/Preserves			
Regular, 1 tsp, ¼ oz	18	0	5
1 Tbsp, ¾ oz	65	0	16
1 ounce	90	0	22
Single Portion, ½ oz pkg	38	0	11
Apple/Fruit Butters, 1 T., 0.6 oz	20	0	6
Fruit Spreads: Regular, 1 tsp	16	0	4
Low Sugar, 1 tsp	8	0	2
Low Cal. (Featherweight), 1 tsp	4	0	1
Jelly: Regular, 1 tsp	18	0	4.5
Imitation, Low Calorie, 1 tsp	4	0	1

Syrups, Molasses

	C	F	Cb
Syrups: Average All Brands			
(Corn/Rice/Maple/Pancake/Sundae/Waffle)			
Includes Aunt Jemima, Cary's, Karo, Hershey's,			
Hungry Jack, Log Cabin, Mrs Butterworth's			
Regular/Dark/Light Color:			
1 Tbsp, ½ fl.oz	55	0	14
¼ cup (4 Tbsp)	220	0	55
Single Portion: 1½ oz pkg	170	0	42
Lite: 1Tbsp	25	0	6
¼ cup (4 Tbsp)	100	0	25
Sugar-Free: Atkins, all types	0	0	0
Cary's, 2 Tbsp, 1 oz	18	0	5
Cozy Cottage, 2 Tbsp, 1 oz	10	0	3
Da Vinci, 2 Tbsp, 1 oz	0	0	1
Honey Cream Syrup, ¼ c., 2 oz	220	0	55
Molasses: Dark/Light: 1 T., ¾ oz	55	0	14
1 cup, 11½ oz	880	0	224
Blackstrap: 1 Tbsp, ¾ oz	47	0	13
1 cup, 11½ oz	750	0	208

Ice Cream Toppings

Average All Types & Brands	C	F	Cb
(Hershey's, Kraft, Smuckers)			
Butterscotch, Caramel, 2 Tbsp	140	1	30
Chocolate: Hot Fudge, 2 Tbsp	140	4	22
Fat Free Chocolate, 2 Tbsp	100	0	23
Pineapple, Strawberry, 2 Tbsp	110	0	28
Smuckers: Guilt-Free/Lite, 2 T.	100	0	24
Magic Shell, 2 Tbsp	210	15	18
Milky Way, 2 Tbsp	130	3.5	24

Candy, Chocolate

Quick Guide

Chocolate
Average All Brands

	C	F	Cb
Milk Chocolate, regular:			
Plain/Nuts/Fruit, average, 1 oz	150	10	13
1½ oz Bar	225	15	23
2 oz Bar	300	20	30
4 oz Block	600	40	60
8 oz Block	1200	80	120
1 Pound, 16 oz	2400	160	240
Dark/White Chocolate, 1 oz	150	10	16
Sugar Free *(Hershey's)* 1 pce, 0.3 oz	225	14	23
Chocolate-coated:			
Almonds, 5-6, 1 oz	160	11	11
Clusters, nut, 2, 1 oz	160	11	15
Coffee Beans, 1.4 oz	180	10	23
Creme/Cordial Centers, 1 oz	120	4	21
Fudge, 1 oz	125	5	18
Macadamias, 2-3 pces, 1 oz	180	13	11
Mints 1 med., 11g	45	1	9
Nougat & Caramel, 1 oz	120	4	21
Peanuts, 12 med., 1 oz	160	11	15
Raisins, 30 med., 1 oz	120	4	21
Cooking Chocolate:			
Sweet/Semi-sweet, 1 oz	160	8	20
Chips, ¼ cup, 2½ oz	210	12	24
Unsweetened, 1 oz	150	15	8
Dipping Choc *(Bakers),* ½ oz, 1T.	80	5	9
Carob: Plain, 1 oz	160	11	9

Brands & Generic

Per Piece/Serving

	C	F	Cb
Abba Zaba, 2 oz bar	250	5	48
Absolutely Almond, 2.5 oz bar	380	23	40
Aero Bar *(Nestlé),* 1.45 oz bar	210	13	26
After Dinner Mints, 1 small	45	1	9
After Eight Mint *(Nestlé),* each	35	1.2	6
Air Head, 2 bars, 1 oz	120	1	30
Allen Wertz: Simply Sugar Free			
Coffee Time (decaf), 4	45	1.5	8
Coffee Toffee, 6	120	3	23
Other types, 4	120	2.5	24
Almond Joy: 1.76 oz bar	230	13	28
King Size, 2 pces, 1.7 oz	425	24	53
Snack, 1, 0.68 oz bar	90	5	11
Bites (8)	90	6	9
Swoops, 1 cup, 1.26 oz	200	12	20
Almond Roca, 3 pces	220	15	19
Sugar Free, 3 pces	205	15	16
Almonds, sugar-coated, 7, 1 oz	130	5	20

Brands & Generic (Cont)

Per Piece/Serving

	C	F	Cb
Almond Clusters *(Trader Joe's),*			
2 pce, 1.2 oz	210	14	5
Altoids *(C & B),* each	3	0	1
Amazin' Fruit, 1 bag, 1.9 oz	180	0	41
Andes: Creme de Menthe; Cherry Jubilee			
Choc covered Patty, (3), 1½ oz	180	3	35
Thins, avg. all flav., (8), 1.4 oz	210	13	22
Anthon Berg: Cognac, each	180	8	25
After Dinner Sweet:			
Marzipan w. Madeira, 1.4 oz	175	7.5	26
Marzipan Brod	120	7	13
Asteroid *(Nestlé),* 1.9 oz	260	10	40
Atomic Fireball, 1 piece	35	0	9
Baby Ruth: King Size, 3.7 oz bar	480	24	66
2.1 oz bar	280	13	34
Fun size, each	100	4.5	17
Snack, 1 bar, ¾ oz	100	5	12
Baci *(Perugino),* each	85	5	8
Bar, 1.58 oz	230	15	27
Bar None, 1.5 oz bar	240	14	23
Barley Sugar, 1 pce, 0.2 oz	25	0	6
Baskin-Robbins, 3 pce, 0.5 oz	60	1	13
Big Hunt, 2 oz	230	3	47
Bit-O-Honey, 1.7 oz	200	3.5	41
Chews, 6 pces, 1.4 oz	170	3	34
Blow Pops, each	50	0	14
Bon Bons (1)	25	0	6
Bonus Bar, 2.1 oz bar	290	16	34
Boston Baked Beans, 30 pces, 1 oz	135	5	20
Brach's: Almond Supremes (11)	215	13	22
Butterscotch Disks (3), 0.6 oz	70	0	16
Caramel Clusters (3), 1.5 oz	225	13	2
Choc Bridge Mix (16), 1.3 oz	185	8	26
Circus Peanuts, each	25	0.6	13
Double Dippers (15)	215	12	23
Golden Butter Toffee (3)	80	2	15
Malted Milk Balls (15), 1.3 oz	190	7	30
Milk Maid Caramel (18)	170	6	28
Orange Slices (2), 1.3 oz	130	0	32
Breath Savers, all types, each	10	0	2
Brite Crackers, 1 bag, 1.5 oz	140	0	32
Breath Savers, all types, each	10	0	2
Brite Crackers, 1 bag, 1.5 oz	140	0	32
Brock: Candy Corn (10) 0.7 oz	75	0	18
Gummy Bears; Sour Balls, each	26	0	6
Lemon Drops, each	20	0	5
Orange Slices, each	35	0	9
Spice Drops, each	12	0	3
Starlight Mints, each	20	0	5
Toffee, each	25	0.8	5

Brands & Generic (Cont)

Per Piece/Serving	C	F	Cb
Bubble Gum: See 'Gum' Page 131			
Buncha Crunch, ½ cup, 1.4 oz	200	10	26
Burnt Peanuts, 40 pces, 40g	190	8	32
Butterfinger: 2.1 oz bar	270	11	41
King Size, 3.7 oz bar	480	18	75
Fun size, each	100	4	15
Mini, each	45	1.5	7.5
Snack (2) 1.3 oz	170	7	27
Crisp Bar: 1.76 oz bar	250	13	33
Minis, 4 pieces	220	11	29
Butterfinger B.B's, 1.7 oz bag	220	9	34
Buttermints, 18 pces, 1½ oz	160	0	40
Butterscotch: 5 pces	120	2.5	28
Buttons (Walgreens), 3, 18g	70	0	16
Chips (Hershey's), 1 oz	160	8	20
Discs (Sathers), 3, 0.6 oz	110	0	24
Candy Apple, medium, 6.5 oz	260	4	54
Candy Cane, medium, 5", ½ oz	50	0	12
Candy Corn, 1 oz	110	0	27
4 oz Pkt: 24 pces, 1½ oz	150	0	37
Candy Jar Mix (Jewel), 3, 17g	70	0	17
Candy Necklaces, 20g each	80	0.5	20
Caramels: each	30	1	6
Chocolate, each	25	0.3	6
Creams, 3 pces, 1¼ oz	130	3	23
2.75 oz pkt, 5 pces, 1½ oz	160	3.5	30
Hershey's Classic Caramels:			
Soft 'n Chewy, 3 pces	80	2.5	13
Choc Creme Filled, 3 pces	80	3	13
Caramel Nips, each	30	1	6
Caramel Popcorn, 1 cup, 1 oz	120	1.5	26
Caramel Truffles (Godiva), 1 pce	110	6.5	11
Caramello (Hershey's), 1.6 oz bar	220	10	28
Snack, 0.66 oz	90	4	12
Cadbury: 1.6 oz bar	210	9	29
Kingsize, 2.7 oz bar	360	16	49
Certs: Breath Mints, 1 pce	6	0	2
Sugar-free, 1 piece	7	0	2
Charleston Chew, 1 bar, 53g	230	7	40
Chews, all types, 1 oz	110	1	25
Chocolate Mints (Hershey's), each	20	0.5	4
Chocolate Parfait Nips, each	30	1	5
Chuckles Jelly: each	35	0	9
Jujubes (Hershey's), each	10	0	3
Chunky Bar (Nestlé), 1.4 oz	210	11	24
Chupa Chups, 1 pce, 0.42 oz	50	0	11
Cinnamon Bears (Walgreens), 5	150	0	38
Cinn. Buttons (Walgreens), 3 pce	70	0	17
Cinnamon Drops (Sathers), 19 pce	150	0	36

Per Piece/Serving	C	F	Cb
CocoaVia Crunch Bars, average	80	2.5	14
Coconut Stacks, 4, 41g	190	6	33
Coffee Go Coffee/Cappuccino, ea.	18	0.4	4
Coffee Rio-Gold, each	15	0.5	1
Collard & Bowser, Eng. Toffee (2)	80	4	12
Conversation Hearts (Necco), 1 lge	16	0	4
Cote d'Or: Bouchee, each	130	8	12
Chokotoff, each	210	9	30
Nougatti	150	8	19
Bar & Nuts, 1.3 oz	220	18	12
Cotton Candy, 1 oz	110	0	28
Cough Drops: See Page 131			
Cracker Jack, 1.25 oz box	150	2.5	29
Creme Savers (Sugar-Free) 1 pce	10	0.5	2.5
Crisped Rice: Almond, 1 bar	130	6	18
Choc Chip, 1 bar	115	4	18
Crispy Rice Snacks (Hershey's), 1 bar	60	2	9
Crows, 12 pieces, 1.5 oz	140	0	35
Crunch: 5 oz bar	725	38	90
King Munch, 2.75 oz bar	400	20	51
1.55 oz bar	230	12	29
Fun size, each	50	2.5	7
Snack (3), 1½ oz	220	11	28
Pieces, ¼ cup, 38g	190	10	25
White Bar, 1.4 oz bar	220	13	23
Carb Select, 1.1 oz	140	11	18
Crunch Berries Treats, 1.6 oz bar	190	4.5	36
Decadence (NuBar) Bar, 1.3 oz	140	2.5	30
Doctor's Carbrite, 12 pces	30	2	4
Dots, 12 dots, 1.5 oz	140	0	35
Double Dip Stick, 1 stick	16	0.5	3
Dove: Promises, 5 pieces, avg	210	13	24
Single, 1 bar, 1.3 oz	200	12	22
Dark/Milk Bar, 6 oz	900	55	103
Drops Candy (Hershey's), 9 pces	100	0	24
Dum Dum Pops (Spangler), 1 pop	25	0	6
Endulge (Atkins): Per Serving			
Candy Bits, avg., 1 oz bag	150	8	16
Caramel Nut Chew Bar, 1.23 oz	175	9	17
Chocolate Almond Bar, 1.1 oz	180	13	14
Chocolate/Crunch Bar, 1.1 oz	130	12	3
Chocolate Peanut Bar, 1.1 oz	135	13	3
Peanut Butter Cups (3), 1.2 oz	195	13	17
Peanut Caramel Cluster, 1.23 oz	170	9	13
Wafer Crisp Bars (2), 1 oz	155	9	15
English Toffee, 1 pce	48	3	5
Eda's Sugar Free, all flav., 5, ½ oz	40	0	15

Brands & Generic (Cont)

Per Piece/Serving

	C	F	Cb
Estee Dietetic Candies:			
Caramels, all flavors, 1 pce	30	1	5
Chocolate, Dark/ Mint, ½ bar	200	14	23
Gummy Bears; Gum Drops, 1 pce	7	0	1.5
Hard Candies: Butterscotch (2)	25	0	6
Peppermint (3)	30	0	7
Lollipops; Mint/Toffee (5)	60	0	15
Lollipop	30	0	8
Milk Chocolate, ½ bar, 4 oz	230	17	17
Peanut Butter Cups, 1 cup	40	3	3
Fructose Sweetened, 1 cup	40	2	3
Peanut Brittle, ⅓ box, 1.5 oz	240	9	28
5th Avenue: 2 oz bar	280	12	37
King Size bar	460	20	64
Snack Size, 0.58 oz	75	3.5	10
Fanny May: Single Wrapped Pieces			
Mint Meltaway Patty, 1.5 oz	250	17	22
Pixie, 1.5 oz	215	12	24
Trinidad, 1.5 oz	205	11	24
Fast Break *(Reese's)*, 2 oz	275	13	35
Ferrero Rocher: each	75	5	6
3 pces, 1.3 oz	220	15	17
Fifty 50 Snack Bars:			
Peanut Butter, 2	200	14	16
Almond Choc., 7 pce, 1½ oz	210	15	20
Crunch Choc., 7 pce, 1.1 oz	160	11	19
Fruit & Nut Choc., 7 pce, 1½ oz	200	14	21
Milk Choc., 3 pce, ½ bar, 43g	210	14	25
Mint Bars, 8 bars, 1 oz	140	9	16
Fluffy Stuff *(Charms)*, 0.6 oz bag	70	0	17
Fondant: Choc-coated, 1.2 oz	130	3	28
Mint, 1 oz	105	0	27
Franklin Crunch 'N Munch:			
all varieties, average, 1.25 oz	170	7	30
Fran's: Gold Bar, 1.75 oz	260	14	34
Gold Bites (Almonds), 1	130	7	17
Frootsies, 12 pces	145	3	29
Fruit Crystals *(Walgreens)*, 3 pces	70	0	17
Fruit Drops, each	6	0	1
Fruit Gems *(Sunkist)*, 3, 1.1 oz	105	0	26
Fruit Leathers, average, 0.5 oz	45	0	12
Fruit Pastilles, 1 roll, 1.4 oz	100	0	26
Fruit Rolls, 1 roll	80	0	20
Fruit Roll-Ups, ½ oz	50	0	12
Fruit Runts *(Walgreens)*, 1T., ¼ pkt	60	0	14
Fruit Shapes *(Fruitfield)*, 1 oz (10)	100	0.5	23
Fruit Waves, 0.5 oz	50	0	12
Fudge: Chocolate/Vanilla, 1 oz	115	3	20
with Nuts, 1 oz	120	4	21
Choco. Marshmallow, 1 oz	120	5	18
w. Nuts, 1 oz	125	5.5	18
Peanut Butter, 1 oz	105	2	21

Per Piece/Serving

	C	F	Cb
Ghirardelli: Milk/Dark Chocolate,			
1.25 oz bar	185	12	20
w. almonds, 1.5 oz bar	220	14	25
Creme filling, 3 pces, 1.5 oz	220	12	26
Godiva: Hearts, each	45	2	4
Almond Butter Dome, 1 pce	80	6	6
Bouchee au Chocolate, 1 pce	220	13	23
Cordial Assortment, each	60	2.5	9
Gold Ballotin, 1 pce	70	3.5	9
Milk/Dark/Ivory Assortment, each	75	4	8
Nut & Caramel, each	75	4	6
Truffle Amaretto, 1 pce	110	6.5	12
Golden Almond Bar, 1 bar	520	34	40
Golden 111 Bar, 1 bar	500	30	52
Go Lightly: Box Candies, 4	60	0	15
Bags: Assorted Taffy, 6	140	3	36
Vanilla Caramels, 5	150	6	31
Super Free Choc Crunch (7) 1½ oz	180	13	23
Goobers Peanuts, 1 pkg, 1.4 oz	210	14	22
Good 'N Fruity: 1 box, 1.8 oz	140	1	35
Snack Size, 1 box, 17g	60	0	15
Good & Plenty *(Hershey's)*: 1.8 oz box	160	0	40
Snack Size, 1 box, 17g	60	0	14
GooGoo Cluster, 1 bar, 1.75 oz	240	11	32
Gubor Surprise (3) 1.5 oz	235	15	22
Gum Drops: 1 small	15	0	3
1 large, 0.4 oz	40	0	7
6 oz pkt: 4 pces, 1.4 oz	130	0	31
Gummi Bears: 8 bears, 1½ oz	140	0	32
Gummi Novelties *(Walgreens)*, 6	150	0	22
Gummi Savers, each	12	0	3
Gummi Sweet Tarts, 1 bug, 1.5 oz	150	0	34
Gummi Watch, 1, 2 oz	105	0	24
Gummi Worms, each	25	0	5
Guylian: Milk Choc., 8 squares, 1 oz	126	9	15
Dark Choc., 8 squares, 1 oz	117	9	14
Halvah *(Joyvah)*: Plain, ½ bar, 2 oz	390	25	18
Choc.coated Sesame, ½ bar, 2 oz	380	23	20
Hard Candy: All flavors, 1 oz	110	0	28
1 regular piece	18	0	5
Heath: Original, 1.4 oz bar	210	12	24
Bites, 1 piece	15	1	1.5
Snack, 0.33 oz	50	3	6

Brands & Generic (Cont)

Per Piece/Serving

	C	F	Cb
Hershey's: Kisses, avg. all var. (1)	25	1.5	3
Bar: 1.55 oz bar	240	14	25
King Size bar, 2.6 oz	410	25	38
w. Almonds, 1.45 oz bar	230	14	20
Cookies 'n' Creme, 1.55oz bar	230	12	26
Bites: Almond Joy (8)	100	6	10
Cookies 'n' Creme (8)	90	5	10
York (9)	90	1.5	19
Milk Choc w. Almond (7)	90	6	8
Cookies 'N Mint: 1.55 oz bar	230	12	27
Snack, 0.6 oz	90	4.5	11
Crunchy Cookie Cups, 1.4 oz	210	12	23
Hugs: Regular (1), 4.5g	25	1.5	3
Regular (9), 40g	220	13	23
w. Almonds (9), 40g	230	13	22
Milk Chocolate: 1.55 oz bar	230	13	25
Eggs, candy coated (4)	90	4	12
Snack, 0.6 oz	90	5	10
Kingsize, 2.6 oz bar	400	23	42
7 oz bar, ⅓ bar	200	12	21
w. Almonds Snack, 0.6 oz	100	6	9
w. Almonds, 1.45 oz bar	235	15	20
Miniatures: 5 pces, 1.5 oz	230	13	25
Kisses, 1 bag	420	24	44
Nuggets: Snack, avg. all bars (1)	50	3	6
P'nut Butter Crispy Rice, (1)	230	13	25
Special Dark Choc., 1.45 oz bar	230	13	25
Sweet Escapes: 1.4 oz bar, avg.	180	7	27
Snack, avg. (1) 0.7 oz	80	3.5	12
Swoops, avg., 1 cup, 1.26 oz	190	11	20
Whoppers, 10 pieces	100	4	16
Candy-Coated Eggs:			
Milk Choc (4), 0.6 oz	90	4	12
w. Almonds (4) 0.6 oz	100	6	9
Sugar Free: Choc. Candy (3)	215	13	24
Dark Chocolate Candy (5)	220	13	24
Chocolate w. Almonds (5)	225	14	23
Peanut Butter Cups Minis (5)	210	12	23
1 gram Sugar Carb: Choc. Bar, 1 oz	130	11	18
w. Soy Crisps, 1 oz	120	10	16
w. Almonds, 1 oz	110	12	16
Honeycomb: Plain, 1 oz	115	0	27
Choc-coated, 1 oz	125	1	28
Hot Tamales: 1 box, 60g, 2.1 oz	220	0	55
Sathers, 19 pces, 1.4 oz	150	0	36
Ice Blue Mints *(Walgreens)*, 3, 17g	70	0	17
Jawbreakers *(Sathers)*, 3, 17g	70	0	17
Jellies, 3 medium, 1 oz	120	0	30

Per Piece/Serving

	C	F	Cb
Jells Raspberry *(Joyva)*, each	70	1	8
Jelly Beans: Small, 22 beans, 1 oz	100	0	24
Regular, 12 beans, 1 oz	100	0	24
1 bean	8	0	2
Sugar Free	135	0	34
Jumbo, 1 bean	20	0	5
Jewel, 13 beans, 1.4 oz	140	0	36
Sathers/Walgreens, (17) 40g	150	0	37
Wonderbeans, 33 beans	100	0	24
Jelly Bellys: each	4	0	1
32 pces, 1.4 oz	150	0	37
Sugar Free Beans/Sours (31), 1.4 oz	80	0	37
Sugar Free Fruit Slices, 8 pces, 1.4 oz	60	0	30
Jelly Rings *(Jewel)*, 3, 1.5 oz	160	0	39
Jolly Rancher: Candy (1)	40	0	9
Fruit Chews (3), 1.4 oz	150	1.5	33
Hard Candy (3), 18g	70	0	17
Jolly Jellies, 7 oz	120	0	30
Lollipops, 1 pce, 0.6 oz	60	0	16
Sugar Free, 4 pces, 0.5 oz	35	0	14
Junior Mints, 1.84 oz box	210	3.5	40
16 pces, 1.4 oz	160	2.5	34
Juicefuls: Red Raspb., (3), 0.6 oz	60	0	13
Assorted Fruits, 1 pce	20	0	5
Jujubes, all types (6), 1.4 oz	5	0	3
Juju Mix *(Sathers)*, 11 pce, 1½ oz	150	0	36
Juju Toys, 6 pce, 1.5 oz	150	0	37
Jujyfruits, 1 box, 0.2 oz	40	0	10
Kit Kat: 1.5 oz bar	235	11	29
2.8 oz bar	400	20	50
Big Kat, 1.94 oz	290	15	35
Bites (7), 1.4 oz	200	10	25
King Size, 3 oz bar	495	25	62
Miniature, 0.35 oz	50	2.5	6.5
Multipack/Snack Bar each	80	4	10
Krackel: 2.6 oz bar	330	18	38
Snack size, 0.6 oz	85	4	12
Kraft: Caramels, (5), 40g	160	3.5	33
Kudos: 1 oz bar, avg. all types	120	5	20
M&M's Milk Choc Minis, 0.8 oz	90	2.5	17
Snickers, 0.8 oz	100	3.5	16
Lance: Popscotch, 1.2 oz pkg	160	6	24
Chocolaty Peanut Bar, 2 oz bar	320	18	30
Peanut Bar, 1.8 oz pkg	260	14	24
Lemon Drops (3) ½ oz	50	0	12
Sugar Free *(Walgreens)*, 5, ½ oz	35	0	14
Lemonhead, 10, ½ oz	60	0	14

Candy, Chocolate (Cont)

Brands & Generic (Cont)

Per Piece/Serving	C	F	Cb
Licorice: Average all types, 1oz	100	0	25
Bites (Switzer), each	10	0	2
Chews (Panda), each	10	0	1
Tid Bits, each	5	0	1
Twists: Black/Red, avg. 1 pce	30	0	7
American Licorice Co.: Laces, 1	35	0	8
Stick, (1) 0.5 oz	45	0	11
Choco Sticks, (4) 1.4 oz	145	0	35
Red Bites, 1.4 oz	140	0	34
Super Red Ropes, 1 rope, 2 oz	200	0	46
Vines, 1 pce	70	0	17
Lifesavers: Large size, 1 candy	15	0	4
Regular, all flavors, 1 candy	10	0	2
1 Roll (14 candies), 1.14 oz	130	0	32
Creme Savers (1)	25	0.5	4
Gummi Savers, 1.5 oz roll	140	0	32
Lollipops Fruit, 1 pce, 0.4 oz	45	0	11
Pepomint, 4 mints	60	0	15
Sugar-Free Delites: Per Candy			
Orchard Fruits; Summer Blend	5	0	2
Butter Toffee; European Collect.	10	0.5	3
Creme Savers (1)	10	0.5	2.5
Lik-m-aid (Nestlé), 1.7 oz	60	0	15
Lindt: Lindor, Balls, average	75	6	5
Amaretto Balls	65	5	5
Milk Chocolate, 1.4 oz pce	210	12	23
Lollipops, each, 0.2 oz	20	0	5
Lollipops C Pops (Glenny's), each	35	0	8
M & M's: Plain, 1.7 oz pkg	235	10	34
Milk Chocolate, 1 pce	5	0.2	0.5
20 pce, 0.6 oz	80	4	10
¼ cup, 1.8 oz	255	10	37
Almond Choc., 1.3 oz pkg	200	11	21
1.5 oz pkg	230	13	25
Crispy, 1.5 oz	205	8	31
Minis, Mega Tube, 1.1 oz tube	150	7	21
Mega: Milk Choc (27), 1.4 oz	200	9	28
Peanut (12), 1.4 oz	210	11	24
Peanut: 1.7 oz pkg	255	13	30
Fun Size, 0.7 oz pkg	110	5	13
Peanut Butter: 1.6 oz pkg	250	14	26
Fun Size, 0.7 oz pkg	110	6	12
Mamba, 9 pce, 1½ oz	160	2	36
Marathon (Snickers) Bar, 1.9 oz	225	7	32
M.Azing, 1 bar, 1.5 oz	220	12	29
Mars Bar: All varieties, 1.76 oz	240	13	31
Fun size, 1 bar	95	5	12
Marshmallow Egg, 1 egg	110	0	26

Per Piece/Serving	C	F	Cb
Marshmallows: Firm/Soft, 1 oz	90	0	23
Regular size, 6 pce, 33g	110	0	26
Mini-Marshmallow, ½ oz, 30g	100	0	24
Choc-coat. Twists (Joyva), each	95	2	10
Fluff, 2 Tbsp, 18 g	60	0	15
Kraft: Mini, ½ cup	80	0	10
Creme, 2 Tbsp	40	0	10
Jet-Puffed, 5 pcs	90	0	23
Funmallows, each	25	0	6
Miniature, ½ cup	100	0	25
Teddy Bear, ½ cup	50	0	12
Marzipan, 1 oz	140	7	16
Mauna Loa: Choc. 2.5 oz bar	420	29	36
Choc. coated Macadamias (9)	230	17	19
Mega Fruit Gummi, each	10	0	2
Mexican Hats (9)	100	0	24
Mentos, each	10	0	2
Mike & Ike: 1 pkg, 2.1 oz	220	0	55
19 pce, 1.4 oz	150	0	36
Milkfulls (Storck), 6 pces, 1.4 oz	170	3	35
Milk Chocolate: See Hershey's			
Milk Choc. Crisp, 1.45 oz bar	205	11	22
Milk Duds (Hershey's), 7 pces	170	6	28
Milk Shake Bar, 1.8 oz bar	220	7	37
Milky Way: Midnight Bar, 1.75 oz	220	8	36
Regular Bar, 2 oz	270	10	41
Fun size, 2 bars, 1.4 oz	180	7	28
King Size, 3.63 oz bar	480	18	72
Miniatures (5) 43g	190	7	30
Pop'ables (13) 39g	200	7	28
Choc. Covered Caramels, 2 oz	200	8	30
Milky Way Lite, 1.57 oz	170	5	34
Miniatures, 1.4 oz pkg (5)	150	4.5	29
Mints: Uncoated, 1 oz	100	0	23
1 small mint (¾" diam.)	7	0	2
1 large mint (1½" diam.)	30	0	7
Mon Cheri (Ferrero), 4 pces, 45g	260	18	20
Mounds: 1.75 oz bar	255	13	31
Snack, 0.68 oz	90	5	11
Mr Goodbar: 1.75 oz bar	280	18	25
King Size, 2.6 oz bar	420	26	38
Snack, 0.6 oz	100	6	9
Miniatures (1)	45	2.5	5
Bites (9), 1.4 oz	230	14	21
Necco Candy Wafers (3) 57g	15	0	4
Nestle Toll House, 2 pces, 2 oz	260	14	34
Neuhaus, average all types	80	5	7
Newman's Own, Pepp. Cups, 1 pkg	170	11	20
P'Nut B. Cups (Milk/Dark), 3, 1 pkg	180	12	17

Brands & Generic (Cont)

Per Piece/Serving	C	F	Cb
Nibs, all types, 1 pouch, 0.5 oz	45	0	10
Nips (Pearson), all flavors, 2, 14g	60	2	10
Nite Bite (Glucose Bar)	100	3.5	15
Nothing But Nuts Butter Toffee			
3 Tbsp, 1 oz	200	15	9
Nougat, 2 pces, 1 oz	115	1	25
Chocolate Covered, 1 oz	120	4	20
Nougat Nut Cream, 3.5 oz	340	31	50
Now & Later (Nabisco), 1 pkg	270	2.5	63
Nutrageous Bar (Reese's), 1.8 oz	275	16	27
Snack, 0.6 oz	90	5	9
Oh Henry! 1.8 oz bar	240	10	32
100 Grand, 1.5 oz bar	190	8	30
Orange (Lindt), 6 block, 40g	190	10	24
Orange Slices: Jewel, 3, 41g	140	0	36
Walgreens, 3, 43g	150	0	36
Pastel Mints (Walgreens), 33 pce	150	0	38
Patteez (Sweet n' Low), ½ ctn, 5	120	2.5	32
PayDay Bar: 1.85 oz bar	260	14	27
King Size, 3.4 oz	480	26	50
Snack, 0.7 oz	100	5.5	10
Peanut Bar, 1.6 oz bar	210	14	20
Peanut Butter Bars, 3 pces, 18g	80	1.5	10
Peanut Butter Cups: See Reese's; Newman's Own			
Peanut Brittle, 1 oz	130	5	20
Sugar Free (Judy's), ¾ cup, 1 oz	75	6	2
Peanut Riesen (5), 41g	190	7	28
Peanuts, choc-covered, each	25	1.5	2
Pearson's Mint Patties, (5), 38g	150	2.5	31
Pecan Roll, ⅓ bar, 40g	200	10	26
Peppermints, 7 small, 0.5 oz	50	0	12
Hershey's, 3 pces	60	0	15
Peppermint Twists (2), 13g	60	0	12
Pez, 1 roll	30	0	6
Planters: Choc. Peanuts (25) 7 oz	220	13	20
Orig. Peanut Bar, 1.6 oz	230	14	22
Pop'ables: Average, 13 pces, 1½ oz	200	8	28
12 oz Package	1600	64	224
Positively Pecan, 2.5 oz bar	390	24	38
Pralines: Small, 0.3 oz	38	2	5
1 large piece, 1.4 oz	180	10	24
Pretzels: Choc-covered,			
3 minisize, 1.15 oz	150	5.5	23
1 regular, 1 oz	130	4.5	20
Pretzel Flipz (Nestlé), 8 pces, 1 oz	130	5	19
Raisinets, 1 pkg, 1.7 oz	210	8	33

Per Piece/Serving	C	F	Cb
Raspberry Cream, each	80	2.5	5
Reception Sticks (4)	70	2	12
Red Hot Dollars, 7 pces	100	0	24
Reese's: Chocolate Bar, 2.8 oz	420	24	43
Candy (Multipack), each	95	5.5	10
Miniatures, each	40	2.5	4
Peanut Butter Bites (7)	90	5	10
Mini, 1 pce	40	2.5	4
Peanut Butter Cups: 1.6 oz pkg	250	14	25
Kingsize, 2.8 oz	420	24	43
Mini, 1 pce, 0.27 oz	45	2.5	4
Peanut Butter Eggs (1), 0.6 oz	90	5	9
Reese's Pieces (25), 1.6 oz	225	10	26
ReeseSticks, Kingsize, (2), 1.5 oz	230	13	23
Snack Size, 1.2 oz (34g)	190	11	19
Swoops, 1 cup, 1.26 oz	180	10	17
Fast Break, 2 oz	120	13	35
1 gram Sugar Carb, 1.1 oz	160	12	17
Rice Krispies Treats (Kellogg's):			
Average all varieties	110	3.5	19
Rice Crunchy Bars, 19g bar	60	0	14
Riesen Choc. Chew, (5) 1.4 oz	180	7	29
Peanut & Milk Choc, (5)	190	7	28
Ritter Sport: Plain Choc, 50g	260	16	26
w. Hazelnuts, ½ pkg, 50g	290	19	24
Rocky Road, 1.8 oz bar	240	11	34
Robin Eggs: Large (2); Mini (10)	70	2	13
Medium, 4 pces	90	2.5	16
Rolo: All types (3), 0.64 oz	90	2.5	12
Mini Bites, 19 pieces, 1.4 oz	190	9	26
Root Beer Barrels (3) 0.5 oz	65	0	16
Ross Chocolate Bar: White, 1.2 oz	130	13	3
Almond; Crunchy, 1.2 oz	140	13	4
Russell Stover Candy: Creams (1)	60	2	9
Almond Delight, 2 oz	290	17	32
Caramel Bar, 46g	230	7	34
Jelly Cups (P/Nut Butter), 2, 34g	140	9	14
Mint Dream	160	8	19
Pecan Roll, 50g	260	18	23
Low Carb: Pecan Delight (2), 1.4 oz	180	13	24
Cups (3), 1.3 oz	170	11	23
Mint Patties, 1.4 oz	190	11	27
Sugar Free Dark Choc., 5 pces	220	15	21
Salt Water Taffy (Sathers), 5, 43g	150	2.5	34
Scooby-Doo! (Fruit Snacks), 10 pces	100	0	24
Seashells (Guylian), 1 shell	65	4	6
See's Candies: Average all Flavors			
Brittles (2), 1.3 oz	220	15	18
Caramels & Chews, 2 pieces	175	10	19
Creams, 2 pieces	180	9	24
Little Pops, 4 pieces	60	2	11
Lollypops (1)	80	2.5	14
Nut Clusters, 3 pieces	225	16	16

Brands & Generic (Cont)

Per Piece/Serving	C	F	Cb
Sesame Crunch, 3 pces	80	4	7
Signature Treasures (Nestlé):			
Choc. Creme, 3 pieces, 1.2 oz	210	13	21
Creamy Caramel, 3 pieces, 1.3 oz	175	9	23
Dark Choc Mint, 4 pieces, 1.5 oz	220	10	30
Peanut Butter, 4 pieces, 1.6 oz	260	17	23
Strawberries & Creme, 3 pces	195	12	21
Simply Lite, ½ ctn, 36 pieces	130	5	18
Simply Sugar Free: See Allen Wertz			
Sixlets (Hershey), 24 pces	90	3.5	14
Skittles: Sour, 1.8 oz bag	200	2	44
Orig./Trop./Wild Berry, 2.17 oz	240	2.5	54
Fun Size, 1 bag, 0.7 oz (20g)	80	1	17
King Size, 4 oz bag	440	4.5	100
Large bag (16 oz), ¼ cup, 1.5 oz	170	2	37
Mint (Pepp./Sprmint), 1.6 oz pkg	180	2	40
Skor Toffee Bar, 1.4 oz	220	13	24
Smarties Candy Rolls, 1 roll	25	0	5
Snackwell's Raisin Dips, 5 oz	160	5	34
Snickers: 2.07 oz bar	280	14	35
3.7 oz bar	510	24	63
Creme Egg, each	170	10	19
Cruncher, 2.54 oz	370	21	41
King Size, ½ bar, 1.2 oz	170	8	21
Marathon Bar, avg., 1.9 oz	225	7	32
Miniatures, each	40	2.5	5
Munch Bar, 1.4 oz bar	230	15	17
Pop'ables, 13 pieces, 1½ oz	190	9	24
Snack (2), 40g	190	10	24
Sno Caps, 2.3 oz pkg	300	13	48
Soft Chews (Maalox), 1 chew	20	0.5	4
Soft 'N Chewy Butter Toffee, ea.	30	0.5	7
Soft Drops (9)	100	0	24
Soft Hot Dollars (11)	90	0	23
Sonic Boom Pops (Walgreens), ea.	60	0	14
Sour Brite Crawlers, 13 pces	140	0	31
Sour Punch: All types, 2 oz	190	1	45
1 straw	20	0	5
Spearmint Leaves: Jewel, 5, 40g	140	0	35
Walgreens, 5, 1½ oz	150	0	38
Spice Drops, 10 pces, 1½ oz	130	0	33
Spree Candies: Original, 8 pces	60	0	14
Chewy Spree, 8 pces	50	0	12
Starburst: Candy Canes, 0.5 oz	70	0	18
Fruit Chews, each	20	0.4	4
2 oz pkg	240	4.5	48
Fruit Twist, each	35	0	8
Fruit Twist, 2 oz pkg	190	1	45

Per Piece/Serving	C	F	Cb
Starburst (Cont)			
Jellybeans, 1.5 oz	150	0	38
Jellybean Egg, 2 oz	200	0	51
Tropical Fruit, 2.07 oz pack	240	4.5	48
Starlight Mints, 3 pces, ½ oz	55	0	14
Suckers (Walgreens), 1 sucker, 11g	45	0	11
Sugar Babies, 1.7 oz pkg	190	2	43
Sugar Coated Peanuts, 1 oz	120	8	10
Sweet 'N Low: Chews, each	14	0	3
Coffee Cremes (1)	70	5	10
Sugar-Free Hard Candy, each	8	0	2
Wafer Bars, avg. (1)	55	3	7
Mint Patteez (1)	25	0.5	7.5
Sweet Escapes: See Hershey's			
Sweet Success Bars, 1 bar	120	4	23
Sweet Tarts (Nestlé), 7 pces, ½ oz	50	0	13
Symphony: 1.5 oz bar	240	15	22
Snack: Chocolate (1), 0.6 oz	90	5	10
w. Almds & Toffee (1), 0.5 oz	80	5	7
Taffy, 1 pce, ½ oz	55	0.5	12
3 Musketeers: 2.13 oz bar	260	8	46
Fun Size, each	70	2	13
Miniatures, each	25	0.5	5
Pop'ables (10), 41g	180	6	31
Tang-a-Roos: 1 roll	25	0	6
Tarts (Walgreens), 4 pce, 15g	60	0	15
Tails (Walgreens), 8 pce, 15g	60	0	15
Tastetations (Hershey's), 3	60	1.5	12
Terry's Choc Orange, (5), 1.5 oz	230	12	27
Tic Tac, all varieties, each	1.5	0	0
Toblerone: 50g (1.76 oz bar)	270	15	32
1 bar, 100g (3.5 oz)	540	30	63
⅓ bar, 33g	180	10	21
Toffees, Regular, 1 oz	150	9	15
Toll House Bars, 2 pieces, 2 oz	130	6	18
Tongue Torchers (Walgreens), 3	70	0	17
Tootsie Pops, Mini (3)	50	0	13
Tootsie Roll, 2.25 oz roll	230	5	26
Trolli Gumm Candy, avg., 5 pces	120	0	29
Truffles: Regular, 1 pce, 0.4 oz	60	4	5
Large (Godiva), 0.75 oz	110	6.5	12
Extra Large (J.Schmidt), 1½ oz	220	13	24
Turtles (Nestlé), avg., each	85	4.5	10
Twists (Sugar Free): Licorice; Strawberry, 6 twists, 40g	140	0	32
Twix: Caramel 2 pce pkg	280	14	37
King Size, 3 oz pkg	405	20	52
Fun Size: 0.5 oz	80	4	10
2 oz pkg, 2 bars	280	14	37
Peanut Butter, 1.8 oz	280	17	28
Snack, 1 cookie, 0.5 oz	80	5	8

Candy ✦ Gum ✦ Cough Drops

Brands & Generic (Cont)

Per Piece/Serving — **C** **F** **Cb**

	C	F	Cb
Twizzlers: Twists, 4 pieces, 1.6 oz	160	1	36
Pull 'n' Peel Cherry (1), 1 oz	100	0	25
Velamints Sugar Free, 2 pce	5	0	1
Werther's: Original, 3 pce, 15g	60	1	13
Chocolates (5), 20g	110	6	13
Sugar-Free, 3 pieces	20	0.5	7
Whatchamacallit Bar, 1.6 oz	230	11	28
Snack (1), 0.57 oz	80	4	10
Whitman's: Pecan Roll, 2 oz roll	300	20	26
Sampler, 3 pces, 1.4 oz	200	11	25
Assorted; Dark Chocolate, 1 pce	65	3	9
Snoopy Treats, 2 pces	190	10	24
Sucratrol Mint Pattie, 1 oz	120	7	17
Whoppers, 9 pce	100	3.5	15
Wonka			
Laffy Taffy: Orig., 5 bars, 1.5 oz	170	2	38
Stretchy & Tangy, 1 bar, ½ oz	60	1	12
Yogurt Candy: Plain, 1 oz	120	6	15
Coated Raisins, 1 oz	120	4	21
York Mints 1.5 oz patty	145	5	34
Snack size, 0.5 oz	50	1	11
Peppermint Patties, 3	150	2.5	30
Peppermint Patties Bites, 15 pces	160	3	33
Sugar Free, Mini (1), ½ oz	35	1	9
Swoops, 1 cup, 1.26 oz	190	11	21
Zachary Old Fash. Creme Drops (3)	170	3	36
Zagnut: 1.75 oz bar	230	10	31
Snack size (1), 0.5 oz	70	3	9
Zero Bar, 1 pce, 0.6 oz	70	2.5	12
Zingos, 3 pce, 2g	5	0	2

Gum ~ *Per Piece*

Per Piece — **C** **F** **Cb**

	C	F	Cb
Bazooka, each	30	0	7
Beechies	6	0	2
Big League Chew	10	0	2
Bubble Gum Balls *(Hershey's)*	10	0	2
Bubble Yum	25	0	6
Sugarless	10	0	3
Candilicious	30	0	2
Carefree (Sugarless/Regular)	5	0	1
Chiclets	5	0	1
Clorets, stick	10	0	2
Dentyne	6	0	1
Estee, bubble/regular	5	0	2
Extra *(Wrigley's),* Sugar-Free (1)	5	0	2
Freshen-Up	13	0	2
Hubba Bubba: Regular	23	0	6
Sugar-free, average	14	0	0.5
Ice Breakers, 1 stick	5	0	2
Sonic Boom Bubble Gum	15	0	3
Sticklets	7	0	2
Super Bubble	15	0	4
Trident: Original; White	5	0	1
Soft Bubble Gum	9	0	1
Wrigley's, all flavors	10	0	2

Carob Candy

Per Piece/Serving — **C** **F** **Cb**

	C	F	Cb
Carob: Plain/Natural, 1 oz	160	11	9
Carob Coated: Raisins, 1 oz	130	8	15
Almonds/Peanuts, 1 oz	150	10	14
Malt Balls, 1 oz	135	8	15
Caramels, 1 oz	110	4	18
Dates, 1 oz	125	5	20
Soybeans	145	9	16
Trail/Party Mix, 1 oz	140	9	15
Carob Chips, unsweetened, 1 oz	140	7	19
Carob Bars: Plain/Nut, 1 oz	160	11	13
Fruit & Nut, 1 oz	155	10	13
Mint/Orange, 1 oz	160	11	14
Carafection: Cashew Coconut Crunch, ½ Bar, (42g) 1.5 oz	250	14	5
Caroby Natural Touch, 3 oz	450	27	36

Cough Drops

— C F Cb

	C	F	Cb
Beech Nut, 1	10	0	2
Diabetic Tussin, 1 drop	0	0	0
Halls Defense Vit. C, 1 drop	15	0	4
Halls Fruit Breezers, 1 drop	15	0	4
Halls Menthol Drops, 1 drop	15	0	4
Sugar Free, 1 drop	5	0	4
Halls Plus, 1 drop	20	0	5
Helps Cough, all flavors, 1	15	0	3
Listerine Lozenge (Amer. Chicle)	10	0	2
Luden's Throat Drops, all flavors, 1	10	0	2
Sugar Free, 1 drop	0	0	0
Pine Bros, 1 cough drop	10	0	2
Ricola: Cough Drops, 1 drop	15	0	3
Sugar-Free Lemon Mint, 2 mints	0	0	1
Rite Aid, Menthol Cough, 1 drop	10	0	3
Robitussin: Regular, 1 drop	15	0	3
Honey Cough, 1 drop	40	0	10
Sugar Free Throat, 1 drop	10	0	3
Sunny Orange Vit. C, 1 drop	10	0	3
Rolaids/Sodium Free, 1	5	0	1
Sathers Peppermint Lozenges, 1	15	0	3
Squibb Cough/Throat Loz.'s, 1	15	0	4
Sucrets *(Beecham)* Lozenges, 1	10	0	2
Wintergreen Loz. *(Walgreens),* 1	15	0	3

Cough Supressant Liquids: *See Page 142*

Popcorn

Home-Popped Popcorn

	C	F	Cb
Popping Corn Kernels:			
2 Tbsp, 1 oz	100	1	22
(makes approx. 3½ cups)			
Air-popped (no oil), plain, 1 oz	100	0	22
1 cup (6g)	30	0	4
Oil-popped, plain, 1 oz	140	8	10
1 cup (11g)	55	3	4
Popcorn Oil, 1 Tbsp	120	14	0

Microwave Popcorn

	C	F	Cb
Average All Brands (Popped)			
Butter: Regular, 1 cup	35	2	4
Light, 1 cup	25	1	4
Act II Popcorn:			
Butter, 1 cup, 0.3 oz	35	2	4
4 cups, popped, 1 oz	140	8	16
Light Butter, 1 cup, 0.2 oz	25	1	4
5 cups, popped, 1 oz	125	4	20
Butter Lovers,1 cup, 0.3 oz	45	3	4
3.5 cups, 1 oz	160	10	14
Butter Lovers (Reduced Fat), 1 c.	30	1.5	4.5
4.5 cups, 1 oz	130	6	20
American Fare (K-Mart):			
Butter, 1 cup, 0.3 oz	35	2.5	4
3.5 cups, 1 oz	130	9	14
Light Butter, 1 cup, 0.3 oz	30	1	4
3.5 cups, 1 oz	100	4	17
Healthy Choice: Butter, 6 cups	100	2.5	22
Natural, 6 cups, 1 oz	100	2	22
Jolly Time: America's Best, 1 cup	20	0	5
Blast O Butter: Regular, 1 cup	45	3	5
Light, 1 cup	30	1.5	4
Healthy Pop, 1 cup	20	0	4
Kettle Mania, 1 cup	60	4	5
Mallow Magic, 1 cup	60	5	5
Newman's Own: Butter, 1 oz	170	11	16
Light Butter Flavor, 1 oz	110	3	20
Orville Redenbacher's: *Popped*			
Movie Theater Butter, 1 cup	40	3	4
4 cups, popped, 1 oz	170	12	16
Light Movie Theater Butter, 1 cup	25	1	4
5 cups, 1 oz	125	5	20
Smart Pop!: Butter, 7½ cups	110	2	30
Mini Bags, 6 cups	100	2	24
Tender White, 3½ cups	180	13	14
Pop Secret Popcorn: *Popped*			
94% Fat Free, 6 cups	125	2	23
Jumbo Pop Butter, all types, 3 ½ cups	170	11	18
Light Butter, 6 cups	135	5	20
Movie Theater Butter, 4 cups	180	12	12
One-Step, 4 cups	160	10	12
Other varieties, avg., 4 cups	160	10	16

Bagged Popcorn

	C	F	Cb
Average All Brands (Ready-to-Eat)			
Regular: Plain, ½ oz pkg	80	5	7
1 oz pkg	160	10	14
4 oz pkg	640	40	56
Box (store/airport), 2 oz	320	20	28
Bag (9″ high x 5″ wide), 3 oz	480	30	42

Brands ~ Bagged Popcorn

	C	F	Cb
Act II Popcorn: Supreme, ¾ cup	130	5	22
Butter Toffee: ¾ cup, 1 oz	110	1	27
w. Peanuts, ¾ cup, 1 oz	120	2.5	22
Boston's: Fat Free, ⅔ cup, 1 oz	100	0	23
Lite, 2 cup, 1 oz	140	6	19
Gourmet Super Prem., 2 c., 1 oz	160	11	13
40% Less Fat, 2¾ cup, 1 oz	140	6	17
Cracker Jack: Original, ½ c., 1 oz	120	2	23
Fat Free varieties, ¾ cup, 1 oz	110	0	26
Crunch 'N Munch: ½ cup, 1 oz	140	5	22
Buttery Toffee, ⅔ cup, 1 oz	150	6	22
Caramel w. P'nuts, ⅔ cup, 1.2 oz	140	3.5	25
Fiddle Faddle: Skippy ¾ c., 1 oz	130	3	23
Honey Nut, ½ cup, 1 oz	130	3.5	24
w. Real Planters Peanuts, ⅔ cup	130	3	24
Jay's: Fat Free Caramel Corn, 1 oz	110	0	24
Korn Krunch: *(Kornfections Treasures):*			
Almond Pecan (Sugar Free), 1 oz	150	8	19
Orville Redenbacher:			
Popcorn Cakes, avg. (8) ½ oz	65	1	12
Pre-Popped: Clusters, ½ cup, 1 oz	135	5	22
Drizzles, avg., ⅔ cup, 1 oz	160	6	24
Savory, avg., 2¾ cups, 1 oz	165	10	16
Pizza Hut Cheese Pizza, 2 oz bag	360	26	26
Poppycock: Pecan Delight, 1 cup	300	14	40
Just Be Nuts!, ¼ cup, 1.3 oz	190	15	13
Wild Oats, all types, 2.5 cup, 1 oz	160	10	15

Movie Theater Popcorn

	C	F	Cb
Small (7 cups): Plain	400	27	30
with Butter	580	47	30
Medium (16 cups): Plain	900	60	70
with Butter	1170	90	70
Large (20 cups): Plain	1150	76	90
with Butter	1500	116	90

Potato Chips, Pretzels, Tortilla Chips

Potato Chips/Crisps

Average All Brands	C	F	Cb
Regular:			
Plain or flavored, 1 chip	9	1	1
17 chips, 1 oz pkg	150	10	15
4 oz quantity	600	40	60
Lay's Stax, avg. all, 1 oz	150	10	15
Pringles: 14 crisps, 1 oz	160	11	15
Large, 5.75 oz can	920	63	86
Snack Stack, 23g tub	140	9	12
100 Calorie Pack, 18g tub	100	6	13
Ruffles, 14 chips, 1 oz	160	10	14
Reduced Fat: *Pringles,* 1 oz	140	7	20
Crunch Tators, 1 oz	140	7	19
Sun Chips; Terra, average, 1 oz	140	7	19
Lowfat/Baked, average, 1 oz	115	1.5	23
Fat Free: *Childer's/Louise's,* 1oz	100	0	22
Pringles, 1 oz	70	0	15
Lay's Wow!, 20 chips, 1 oz	75	0	17
Ruffles Wow!: 17 chips, 1 oz	70	0	17
Cheddar Sour Crm (15) 1 oz	70	0	16
Low Carb: *Atkins* Crunchers, 1 oz	110	3	8
Carb Solutions, 1 oz	135	5	3
Q-Smart (Quaker), 3.03 oz pkg	120	4.5	9
Tastemorr, average, 1 oz	130	5	8

Corn & Tortilla Chips

Average All Brands	C	F	Cb
Corn Chips: Avg. all types, 1 oz	160	10	15
8 oz bag	1280	80	120
Doritos: (12), 1 oz	150	7	20
Nachos; 4-Cheese, 1 oz	140	8	17
3D's Nacho Cheesier (32) 1 oz	130	5	19
Rollitos (17) 1 oz	160	10	16
Fritos (Sabrositas), 1 oz	155	9	17
Pringles, Torengos (13), 1 oz	140	9	15
Tortilla Chips: Average, 1 oz	150	8	22
(1 oz = approx. 12 chips or 13 strips)			
Boston, Baked, 13 chips, 1 oz	110	1.5	23
Doritos: 18 chips, 1 oz	140	6	20
Light, 13 chips, 1 oz	130	5	20
Wow! Nacho Cheesier, 1 oz	90	1	18
Edge (Doritos/Tostitos), 1 oz	140	8	9
CarbSense Soy Chips (15) 1 oz	140	8	12
Frito-Lay, Baked, (15) 1 oz	120	3.5	21
Garden of Eatin', 1 oz	145	7	18
Keebler Suncheros Light, 1 oz	150	8	18
Kettle, average, 1 oz	140	6	18
Munchies Mix, ¾ cup, 1 oz	135	6	18
Padrino Reduced Fat, 1 oz	130	4	22
Torengos, 13 chips, 1 oz	150	9	16
Utz Lowfat Baked, 8 chips, 1 oz	120	1.5	23
Wild Oats, 14 chips, 1 oz	150	7	18

Pretzels

Average All Brands	C	F	Cb
Hard Baked Pretzels: *Per Pretzel*			
1 oz	110	2	22
Sticks, thin, 2¼" (9/oz), each	12	0	3
Twists, thin, ¼" thick, (5/oz), 1	25	0.2	5
Dutch (2¾"x 2⅝") ½ oz, 1	55	1	11
Sourdough *(Shultz),* ¾ oz, each	80	0	17
Fat Free Pretzels:			
Snyders (1), 1 oz	100	0	22
Mini (20), 1 oz	110	0	25
Utz Wheels/Nuggets, 1 oz	100	0	22
Rold Gold: Sticks (48), 1 oz	100	0	23
Sourdough Nuggets (12), 1 oz	100	0	23
Sourdough Hards (1), ¾ oz	80	0	17
Thins (12), 1 oz	110	0	24
Twists (8), 1 oz	110	0	23
Tiny Twists/Sticks (18), 1 oz	100	0	23
Low Fat Pretzels:			
American Fare Mini Twists, 1oz	120	1	23
Frito-Lay, Rold Gold:			
Butter Checkers 20 pcs., 1 oz	110	1.5	22
Braided Twists (8), 1 oz	110	1	23
Choc-coated *(Nestlé),* 1 oz	130	6	20
White Fudge covered *(Nestlé),*			
1 oz, 7 pieces	140	6	19
Yogurt *(Wild Oats)* 8 pcs., 1.4 oz	210	10	27
Soft Pretzels (Twists) average:			
Plain: Regular, 2.5 oz	190	0	41
King Size, 5 oz	390	0	83
Big Cheese, 5 oz	380	7	61
Peanut Butter filled *(Tr. Joe's)* 1 oz	160	7	18
Auntie Anne's: See Fast-Foods Section			
CarbSense, Soy Pretzels (15)	115	3	12
Frito-Lay Pretzels			
Flavor Twists, 23 pces, 1 oz	160	10	16
Braided Twists, 8 sticks, 1 oz	110	1	23
Rold Gold Flavor Rush, ⅓ oz. 1 oz	150	7	20
Snyder's of Hanover Pretzels			
Logs (7), 1 oz	120	1	21
Homestyle (15), 1 oz	120	1	25
Mini (20), 1 oz	110	0	25
Super Pretzel: Soft Pretzels (1)	175	1	36
Softstix (2)	145	3.5	23
Soft Pretzel Bites (5)	140	0.5	29
Pretzelfils: Onion Veggie (2)	150	4	24
Pepperjack; Pizza (2)	140	3.5	22

Snacks — C F Cb

Note: Actual weight of packaged snacks is usually 5-10% more than label Net Wt. For accuracy, weigh snack and allow extra calories for any extra weight.

	C	F	Cb
Bacon Cheese Crackers, 1 oz	140	6	14
Baja Bob's Soy Munchables, 1 oz	120	4	7
Banana Chips, ¼ cup, 1 oz	150	8	20
Beef Jerky, average, 1 oz	70	1	3
Beef Sticks (Frito-Lay's) 0.3 oz	50	4	1
Bugles: Original, 1⅓ cup, 1 oz	160	9	18
Baked Bugles, 1½ cup, 1.1 oz	130	3.5	23
Carb Slim, Low Carb Bites, 1 oz	155	9	14
Cajun Jerky, 1½ oz	150	6	6
Carrot Chips (Hain)	160	9	26
Cheddar Lites (Health Valley) 1 oz	120	3	21
Cheese Crackers, 1 oz	130	6	18
Cheese Filled (Frito-Lay's)	210	11	24
Cheese Curls: 1¼ cup, 1 oz	160	9	19
Reduced Fat (Utz), 1 oz	140	6	21
American Fare, 1¼ cup, 1 oz	140	5	22
Cheese Nips (Nabisco), 38, 1 oz	190	7.5	19
Cheese Puffs: Average, 1 oz	150	10	15
Lowfat, 1 oz	140	5	20
Health Valley, 1½ cup	110	3	21
No Fries, 1 oz	110	0	23
Cheese Straws, 4 pieces	110	7	8
Cheese Twists, 23 twists, 1 oz	150	8	19
Cheetos: Regular all flavors, 1 oz	160	10	15
Light, cheese flavored, 1 oz	140	6	19
Cheez Balls: 45 balls, 1 oz	150	10	15
Reduced Fat, 45 balls, 0.73 oz	100	4.5	13
Cheez Bopps (Boston's), (28) 1 oz	130	6	17
Cheez Curls/Doodles, 1 oz	160	12	15
Cheez Mania (Planters), 35, 1 oz	160	10	15
Cheez It: White Cheddar, 1 pkt (26)	160	7	18
Original (27)	160	8	16
Reduced Fat (29)	135	4.5	20
Chex Mix (General Mills):			
Bold Blend; Peanut, ½ cup	145	6	20
Other varieties, avg., ½ cup	135	4.5	22
Chip's Chips: Snackers, avg., 1 oz	135	7	2
Cheese Thins, avg., 1 oz	135	8	0
Churros (Mex. Pastry) 10", 1.2 oz	140	9	12
Cinna Chips (T.J. Cinn.) 3, 1 oz	110	4	19
Combos (Oven Baked):			
Crackers, 1⅓ cup, 1 oz	140	7	18
1 cup, 3 oz	420	21	54
Pretzels, 1⅓ cup, 1 oz	130	4.5	19
1 cup, 3 oz	390	14	57
Cookies: See Pages 105-112			
Corn Chips: See Page 133			

Snacks (Cont) — C F Cb

	C	F	Cb
Corn Crunchies/Spirals, 1 oz	160	10	15
Corn Crisps (Pringle), 1 oz	140	7	18
Corn Nuts: ⅓ cup, 1 oz	130	4	20
1.7 oz bag	220	7	34
Corn Puffs: Health Valley, 2 c., 1 oz	120	1.5	25
Pirate's Booty, 1 oz	130	5	18
Wotsits (Walker), 21g pkg	110	6.5	11
Dunkaroos, 1 tray, 1 oz	130	4.5	20
Flavor Twists (Fritos), 1 oz	160	10	16
French's Potato Sticks ¾ c., 1 oz	180	12	16
Funyun's: Onion flavor, 1 oz	140	7	18
Mini, 1 oz	270	13	35
Girlfriend's Booty, 1 oz	120	4.5	18
Goldfish (Pepperidge Farm): 1 oz	140	7	18
2 oz pkg	280	14	36
Gold-N-Chees (Lance), 1⅜ oz	180	7	23
Handi Snacks (Kraft), Bearwiches	150	7	21
Honey Mustard Onion Pieces			
(Snyder's) 1 pkg, 2 oz	280	12	38
Hot Peanuts (Lays), 1¾ oz pkg	310	25	10
Jerky (Beef), 1 oz stick	70	1	3
Keebler: Wheatables Snack Mix,			
Toasted Honey, ½ cup, 1 oz	130	5	20
Peanut Butter Crunch, ½ c., 1 oz	160	7	20
Chse & P'nut Butter			
Sandwich Cookies, 1 pkg	250	12	30
Koolstuf, all flavors, 1.3 oz bar	130	3	27
Lance Sandwich: Bonnie, 1 pkg	160	7	23
Capt. Wafers; Choc-O-Mint, pkg	190	10	23
Sour Dough w. Cheddar, 1 pkg	240	15	23
Other varieties, average, 1 pkg	200	10	23
Lunchables: Fudge Brownie	250	9	42
'S'Mores	200	6	35
Munchos, 16 pieces, 1 oz	160	10	16
Nabisco: Chips Ahoy, 1.3 oz	165	8	21
Chips Ahoy! Cookie Barz, 35g	180	10	23
Nutter Butter Bites (10)	150	6	20
Oreo, 1.3 oz	160	7	23
Oreo Cookie Barz, 1 bar	180	10	21
S'Mores	200	6	35
Sportz, Cheese Nips (38), 1 oz	190	7.5	19
Sweet Crisps (18), 1 oz	180	5	15
Nibblers (Snyder's): Regular (13)	130	5	23
Fat Free (16)	110	0	25
Onion Rings (Lance), 1 pkg	120	6	16
Oriental Mix (Rice Snacks), 1 oz	155	7.5	15
Rice Snacks (Wild Oats) ⅔ c. 1 oz	110	0	25
Oyster Crackers (Bradshaw's), 1 oz	140	5	14
Party Mix (Flavor Tree) ¼ c., 1 oz	160	11	14

Snacks (Cont)

Snacks (Cont)

	C	F	Cb
Peanut Butter Nuggets (8), 1 oz	150	8	14
Pirate's Booty w. White Ched., 1 oz	130	5	18
Pita Snax, avg., (34) 1 oz	115	1.5	22
Popcorn: See Page 132			
Pork Skins/Rind: Baken-ets, 1 oz	160	10	0
Gram's Crunchies, avg., 1 oz	150	10	4
Grande, ⅔ cup	80	5	0
Lance, 1 pkg	65	4	1
Potato Chips: See Page 133			
Potato Puffs (Health Valley) 1 oz	110	3	21
Potato Skins (TGI Friday's), 1 oz	150	9	17
Potato Sticks (French's), ¾ c., 1.1oz	180	12	16
Puffs, 1⅔ cups, 1 oz	140	8	17
8 oz pkg	1120	64	136
Quakes: Corn Rings (25)	135	4.5	21
Mini Rice Snacks: Apple Cinn. (8)	65	0	15
BBQ (10); Ranch (10)	75	2.5	12
Caramel Corn (7)	55	0	13
Nacho/Cheddar Cheese (9)	70	2.5	11
Chocolate (7)	65	1	13
Sour Cream & Onion (10)	75	2.5	12
Ranch Puffs (No Fries), 1 oz	110	0	23
Rice Chips, Bar-B-Q/Onion, ½ oz	70	3	9
Santitas (Frito-Lay), 1 oz	140	6	20
Sesame Sticks (Cityfarm), 1 oz	160	11	13
Snack Crackers (No Fries), 1 oz	110	0	24
Soy Crisps, avg. 1 oz	130	2	18
Soy Nuts: Dry Roasted, ¼ cup, 1 oz	140	7	10
Choc-coated, 1 oz	140	8	14
Dr Soy Soy Nuts BBQ, 1 oz	180	8	8
Spicers Wheat Snacks, 1½ oz	150	7.5	18
Sun Chips (Frito-Lay), 1 oz pkg	140	6	19
TastyKake: Koffee Kake Jnr	250	8	40
Chocolate Jnr	320	12	50
Creme Filled Koffee Kakes	360	14	54
Toast/Cheese Crackers, 1 pkg	205	10	23
Tortilla Chips: See Pages 133			
Tostitos: Regular, average, 1 oz	140	8	18
Fat Free, 1 oz	90	0	20
Trail Mix (Nuts/Seeds/Dried Fruit):			
Regular, 3 Tbsp, 1 oz	130	8	13
Tropical, 3 Tbsp, 1 oz	120	5	19
w. Chocolate Chips, 1 oz	140	9	13
Dr Soy Trail Mix, 1 oz	110	4	12
Turkey Jerky Teriyaki (Oberto)	80	0.5	0
Vegetable Snacks/Chips, 1 oz	130	4	24
Veggie Chips, 1 oz	130	5	18
Veggie Stix, 1 oz	140	7	15
Wahoos, 1 oz, 23 pces	140	8	18
Weight Watchers: Chse Curls, ½ oz	70	2.5	18
Apple Chips, ¾ oz pkg	70	0	18
Yogurt Raisins, 1 oz	130	6	20

Fruit Snacks

	C	F	Cb
Betty Crocker: Per Serving			
String Things, 1 pouch, 0.75 oz	80	1	17
Lucky Charms Fruit Shapes,			
1 pouch, 0.9 oz (25g)	80	0	20
Squeezit, average, 1 bottle	100	0	25
CapriSun Juicers, 1 oz	80	0	19
Kellogg's Disney Fruit Snacks (25g)	80	0	20
Fruit Streamers, 1 roll (0.8 oz)	80	0	17
Nabisco: Rugrats; Wacky Faces (1)	80	0	18
Blues Clues; Dora the Explorer (1)	60	0	14
Fruit Rolls, 1 roll, 0.74 oz	80	2	16
100 Calorie Fruit Snacks, 1.1 oz	100	0	24
Sunkist: All flavors, 1 pch, 0.9 oz	80	0	21
Fruit Snack Cups: See Page 146			

Vending Machines

	C	F	Cb
Brownie, frosted	180	9	24
Cheese Balls, 1 oz	150	8	16
Choc Chip Cookies, 4	130	7	19
Choc Milk, 8 fl.oz	225	9	26
Coca-Cola Classic, 12 fl.oz	140	0	35
Diet Coke, 12 fl.oz	1	0	0
Corn Chips, 1 oz	160	10	15
Danish Pastry, 2 oz	220	10	25
Donut, plain, 1¾ oz	210	12	25
Fruit Pie, 4 oz	290	13	46
Granola/Cereal Bars	130	3	26
Hershey's, 1.55 oz bar	240	14	25
Hot Fries, 1 oz	140	10	11
Kellogg's Rice Krispies Treat	120	1.5	26
Lance: Captain's Wafers, 1 pkg	230	12	26
Big Town, 1 pkg	250	11	38
M & M's: Plain, 1.7 oz	240	10	34
Peanuts, 1.7 oz	250	13	30
Milk: Whole, 8 fl.oz	150	8	12
Reduced Fat, 2%, 8 fl.oz	120	5	12
Milky Way, 2 oz	270	10	41
Onion Rings, 1 oz	120	6	16
Orange Juice, 8.75 fl.oz	120	0	28
Peanuts, roasted, 1 oz	165	14	6
Popcorn, plain, 1 oz	160	10	14
Pork Skins, 1 oz	160	10	0
Potato Chips, 1 oz	150	10	15
Reduced Fat, 1 oz	140	7	20
Pretzels, 1 oz	110	2	22
Raisins, ½ oz pkg	40	0	9
Reece's Peanut Butter Cups, 1.8 oz	280	17	28
Snickers, 2.1 oz bar	280	14	35
Tortilla Chips, 1 oz	150	8	22

Note: Actual weight of bars is usually 5-10% more than label Net Wt. Weigh bar and allow extra calories.

Breakfast Bars

	C	F	Cb
Barbara's Bakery: Multigrain, 1.3 oz	120	1.5	25
Puffins Cereal & Milk Bars, avg.	135	2	24
Carborite Cereal Bar, all types (1)	50	2.5	4
General Mills: Milk 'n Cereal Bars			
Cinnamon Toast Crunch, 45g	180	4	33
Peanut Butter Toast Crunch	190	5	33
Other varieties, average	160	4	29
Health Valley Cereal Bars (1)	130	2	27
Kellogg's			
Cereal & Milk Bars, avg., 0.8 oz	105	3	17
Nature's Path: Crispy Rice, avg.	115	3	21
Flax Plus; Hemp Plus, average	170	5	29
Granola: Apricot 'n Nut	180	7	28
Cranberry Soy	170	5	28
New England Natural Bakers			
Save the Forest Bars (1)	125	4.5	19
Nutri-Grain Bars			
Twists Bar	140	3	26
Cereal Yogurt Bars, 1.3 oz	140	3	27
Mini's, 1.5 oz pouch	160	3	32
Muffin Bars	165	4	31
Chewy Bars, average, 1 bar	110	3.5	18
Chewy Bites, avg., 1 pouch	130	6	20
Post, Honey Bunches of Oats Bar	130	3	26
Quaker			
Breakfast Squares, avg., 2.1 oz	220	4	44
Fruit & Oatmeal Bites (3)	140	2.5	27
Breakfast Graham Bar (1), avg	130	3.5	23
Fruit & Oatmeal Bars (1), avg.	130	2.5	27
Granola Bars: *See Page 140*			
Slim-Fast Optima Bkfast Bars	180	6	22
Low Carb Breakfast Bars, avg.	180	6	19
South Beach Diet (Kraft)			
High Protein Cereal Bars (1), 35g	140	5	15
Special K Cereal Bars, avg., 0.8 oz	95	1.5	18

In eating, one third of the stomach should be filled with food, one third with drink, and the rest left empty.
~ Gitten, the Talmud

Other Bars

	C	F	Cb
Per Bar			
AdvantEdge			
Carb Control Crisp Bar	230	7	27
Carb Control Nutrition Bar	200	7	21
Complete Nutrition Bar	210	5	27
All Goode Organics: *Per 1.73 oz Bar*			
Cashew Almond Passion	190	8	24
Chocolate flavors, average	200	8	29
Honey Nut Harvest	160	3.5	32
Nutty Choc Apricot	200	10	26
Alpen: *Per 3.5 oz Bar*			
Cereal Bars: Fruit & Nut	395	9	71
Apple & Blackberry w. Yogurt	420	12	73
Fruit & Nut w. Chocolate	430	15	68
ABB Rivets, 45g pkt	200	7	18
Arbonne Balanced Nutr., 1 bar	190	4.5	24
Atkins: Endulge *(See Page 125)*			
Average all varieties	220	11	22
Avid Source *(Mission Nutrition)*	240	6	22
Balance: Balance Bars, 1.7 oz	200	6	23
Balance Plus Bars, 1.76 oz	200	6	22
Carb Well: Caramel 'n Choc., 1.7 oz	200	8	22
Chocolate Fudge, 1.7 oz	190	6	23
Chocolate Peanut Butter, 1.7 oz	200	8	22
GoMix, 1.5 oz bag	200	7	22
Gold Crunch Bars, avg., 1.7 oz	210	6	23
Gold Bars, avg., 1.7 oz	210	7	22
Outdoor Bars, 1.7 oz	200	6	22
Trail Mix Energy Bar, 1.8 oz	210	7	22
Barbara's Bakery Granola, ¾ oz	80	2	14
Bariatrix Proti-Bar: (15g Protein)			
Caramel Nut, 40g	150	4.5	14
Bear Valley: Meal Pack, 3.75 oz	410	12	56
Big Whey (Next Nutrition), 100g	420	16	38
Bumble Bar, average	210	12	26
Biochem: Strive, avg.	190	9	24
Ultimate Protein Bar, 78g	290	4.5	19
Bio-Tech, Bio-Protein, 81g	300	7	39
Body Smarts: Choc. P'nut Crunch	210	6	34
Yogurt Berry Crunch	200	5	35
Boost, Choc./Strawb. Crunch	190	6	30

Granola, Sports & Diet Bars (Cont)

Note: Actual weight of bars is usually 5-10% more than label Net Wt. Weigh bar and allow extra calories.

Other Bars (Cont)

Per Bar

	C	F	Cb
Boulder Bar Endurance, 2.5 oz	220	4	13
Bumble Bar, 1.6 oz	210	11	26
Carb Options, 1.76 oz bar	200	8	17
Carb Sense Soy Energy			
Blueberry Crisp, 2 oz	235	6	33
Mocha Cappuccino Crisp, 2 oz	255	9	31
Peanut Butter Crisp, 2 oz	250	7	21
Carb Solutions: Sugar Free, 1 oz	170	7	14
Good Mornings, 1 oz bar	150	7	14
Taste Sensations: Per Bar (60g)			
Chocolate Toffee Hazelnut	260	13	15
Other varieties, avg.	250	10	16
Carb Watchers: Lean Body, 2.5 oz	290	9	22
Choc Peanut Butter	280	7	26
Other varieties, average	270	8	20
Carb Wise: Crisp Bars, avg., 50g	200	9	24
Gold Bar, 50g	190	7	18
Choc. Peanut Crunch, 60g	210	10	23
Choc. Raspberry Crunch, 60g	240	9	24
Choc. S'Mores Crunch, 60g	240	9	24
Lemon Yogurt Crunch, 60g	210	9	23
Carbolite: Choc Almond, 1.75 oz	230	17	25
Choc Crisp Bar, 1.75 oz	250	17	27
Milk/Dairy Choc, avg., 1.75 oz	250	19	28
CarboRite Bars, 1.06 oz	120	5	13
CarbRite Diet *(Doctor's)*, 2 oz	200	35	23
Champion Nutrition: SnacBar	180	3	24
Cheetah *(NutraFig)*, 2.25 oz bar	210	2	43
Choice, all types, 1.23 oz bar	140	4.5	19
Clif Bars: Luna Bar, average, 1.5 oz	180	4.5	27
Builders Bars, 2.5 oz	270	8	30
Luna Glow, 1.23 oz	155	7	15
Mojo Bar, average, 1.5 oz	200	8	23
Nutrition Sustained Energy (68g):			
Apricot; Cranb. Apple Cherry	250	3	48
Designer Whey: Zanzibar	320	9	31
Gourmet Bars, avg. all flav., 2.7 oz	260	7	7
Detour, 2.8 oz bar	310	10	25
Dexatrim All in One, 1.76 oz	180	5	21
Dr Phil's Shape Up! Bars, avg.	240	7	29
Dr Soy: Protein Bar, Lemon, 1.76 oz	180	2.5	24
Chocolate/Peanut, 1.76 oz	180	4.5	25
Healthy Snacker, avg., 1.7 oz bar	180	6	23
Low Carb Snacker	170	7	26

Per Bar

	C	F	Cb
EAS Advantage Edge			
Carb Control, average, 2.12 oz	200	5	21
HP Energy Bar, avg., 2.46 oz	260	5	37
Complete Nutrition, 2.12 oz Bar:			
Choc Caramel	240	7	32
Iced Oatmeal Raisin Crisp	220	5	31
EAS Myoplex			
Deluxe Bar, average, 3.2 oz	340	7	44
Lite Bar, average, 1.97 oz	190	4	28
Carb Sense, average, 2.5 oz	250	7	20
EAS Results for Women			
Weight Management Bar, 1.94 oz	190	5	17
Complete Energy Bar, 1.67 oz	200	6	28
ELEV8: Protein & Fruit Trail,			
All Fruit Blend, 66g bar	210	3	32
Cocoa & Coconut, 66g	230	6	32
Ensure Chewy Choc P'nut, 2.12 oz	230	6	35
Extreme Body, 3 oz bar	340	8	24
Extreme Ripped Force, 45g	160	3	33
Fi-Bar Nectar Granola Bars, 1 oz	100	0	22
Chewy & Nutty Bar, 1.2 oz	140	4.5	22
Fit! *(Medifast)*, 1.5 oz bar	160	4	20
Fruitein Energy Bar, 1.3 oz	130	3	18
General Mills Momentum Bars, 1.4 oz	150	3.5	17
GeniSoy: Low Carb Crunch, 1.5 oz	185	6	18
Soy Protein Bars, avg., 2.2 oz	235	4.5	33
Xtreme, avg., 1.5 oz	200	8	23
Xtreme Crunch, avg., 1.5 oz	170	3.5	27
Glenny's: Light 'n Crispy, ½ oz	65	2.5	9
Slim Carb: Double Fudge, 1.3 oz	140	4	19
Other varieties, 1.3 oz	90	4	2
Glucerna Meal Replacement, 2 oz	220	7	32
GNC ProCrunch: Choc Crisp	260	7	34
Peanut Butter Crunch	260	7	34
Cookies n' Cream; S'Mores	250	4	37
Govinda's: Hemp Bar, 1.5 oz	170	9	22
Bliss Bars, average all types	230	15	25
Greens + Bar: Avg., 2 oz	170	6	20
Hempower Bars, 1.6 oz	170	6	22
Hansen's (1.4 oz): Active Nutr., avg.	140	3.5	20
Natural Crunch, avg. all flavors	185	3	37
Natural Functional, avg. all flav.	190	5	25
Health Valley Fruit/Granola Bars	140	0	34
Healthy Recipes *(Novartis)*	150	4	21
Healthy Shape n Slim, 1.7 oz	150	2	28
HeartBar, Orig., Cranberry, 50g	190	3	27

138

Granola, Sports & Diet Bars (Cont)

Per Bar	C	F	Cb
Henry's Top Vine: Roundup, 1.4oz	165	5	26
Honey Peanutty, 1.4 oz	230	17	10
Hershey's Smart Zone, avg, 50g	210	8	21
High Protein: Peanut Butter, 4 oz	420	16	45
Other varieties, average	335	8	36
HMR Benefit Bar, 1.1 oz	160	5	22
Iron-Tek, Vanilla Fudge, 2.73 oz	290	5	21
Jay Bar, average, 2 oz	230	10	27
Jenny Craig: Choc/Yogurt, 1.97 oz	220	5	33
Oatmeal Raisin, 1.97 oz	210	3	35
Milk Choc; Lemon Meringue	210	5	32
Joyride (Next Nutrition)	340	12	27
Joyva Sesame Crunch, 1.1 oz	190	15	15
Kashi Golean: Bars, avg., 2.7 oz	290	5	35
Crunchy!, avg., 1.76 oz bar	160	3	32
Kellogg's: Krave, Bars, 1.7 oz avg.	200	7	29
Keto Bar: Chocolate types, 65g	270	8	24
Average other flavors	250	7	24
Mini Bar, 32g, avg. all flavors	130	4	12
Kid Sport Bars, avg, 1.76 oz	200	6	29
Kong (Next Nutrition)	460	11	58
Kudos: Apple Nut Crunch	90	3	15
Chocolate Chip	130	5	20
Peanut Butter	130	6	18
M&M's; Snickers, average	100	4	16
Larabar: Apple/Cherry Pie, 1.6 oz	190	9	22
Banana Cookie Dough, 1.8 oz	255	15	24
Lean Body, 76g	280	6	15
Lindora: Chocolate Chip	140	2	15
Other varieties, average	150	4.5	18
Luna Bars, average, 1.5 oz	180	4.5	27
Marathon (Snickers): Energy, 2 oz	220	7	30
Low Carb, average, 1.7 oz	170	7	19
Protein, average, 2.8 oz	290	8	40
Medifast Fit! 1.5 oz bar	160	4	20
Metabolife, average, 2 oz bar	230	6	36
Met-Rx: "Big 100", avg., 100g	360	5	53
Protein Plus, 3 oz bar	310	8	25
MLO Bio Protein, 2.85 oz	300	7	39
Mojo Bar, average, 45g	190	8	23
MRM Response, 2.1 oz	235	5	20
Muscle Tech: Nitro-Tech, average	290	8	33
Meso-Tech, avg., 3.11 oz	340	8	44
Meso-Tech Lite, avg., 2.12 oz	220	6	16
Myoplex: See EAS			
Nabisco, HoneyMaid Bars, 37g	150	4.5	27
Natrol Prolab, 1.76 oz bar	190	6	12
Naturade, Total Soy, 2.1 oz	250	8	32
Nature Valley: Chewy, average	140	6	24
Crunchy, average	190	7	28
Sweet & Salty, avg., 1.2 oz	165	8	20

Per Bar	C	F	Cb
Nature's Best: Solid Protein, 2.75 oz			
Choc./Peanut Butter; S'Mores	290	7	12
Other varieties, average	290	4	11
Nature's Plus: Energy Bar, 1.45 oz	140	4.5	24
Chi Chinese Herbal, 1.5 oz	140	4	20
Calcium Almond Blitz, 1.5 oz	150	2.5	29
Spiru-tein, all flavors, 1.4 oz	150	4	20
New You: Peanut Butter, 1.65 oz	185	5	25
Choc Chip; Lemon Crisp, 1.65 oz	170	3	26
Next Proteins: Designer Whey, 78g	290	9	23
Detour, 2.8 oz	330	10	25
U-Turn Protein, 2.8 oz	300	8	26
NiteBite (Time-release Glucose Bar)			
Choc. Fudge; P'nut Butter, 25g	100	3.5	15
NuBar Decadence, 1.3 oz	140	2.5	30
Nutiva: Hempseed, 1.4 oz	210	14	11
Flax Chocolate, 1.4 oz	200	12	19
NutriSystem Sweet Success, 2.1 oz	220	3	33
Nutrilite: Protein Bars, average	250	9	22
Meal Replacements, average	230	8	30
Odwalla Energy Bars: Chocolate	240	6	40
Choc. Chip Peanut/Crunch, avg.	250	7	39
Carrot; Cranberry C Monster	220	2.5	47
Super Protein	240	5	31
Opti-Pro Meal	290	5	40
Organic Food Bar: Avg., 2.4 oz	300	12	35
Almond-Flax Bar, 1.4 oz	170	6	21
Perfect Rx Nutrition Bar, 100g	340	3	50
Phil's Bar, 50g	200	6	22
Planters CarbWell			
Peanut Butter Crunch, 35g	160	12	16
Caramel Choc Crunch, 38g	180	13	17
PR Bar Ironman, 49.6g	190	6	22
Power Bar: Harvest Dip'd, avg., 2.3 oz	255	5	45
Harvest; Performance, avg, 2.3 oz	240	4	45
Power Crunch, average, 1.3 oz	190	9	13
Premier: Protein Eight, 2.4 oz	285	8	23
Protein Meal Replacement, 2.5 oz	280	8	20
Complete Nutrition, 48g	190	4.5	28
Odyssey Protein, 80g	310	11	29
Odyssey Slim Advantage, 60g	250	12	23
Pria (Power Bar): Bars, 1 oz	115	3	16
Carb Select, avg., 1.7 oz	195	8	21
Promax: Average, 2.7 oz bar	290	6	40
Rampage Bar, 2.75 oz	310	9	31
Protein Complete, avg., 1.97 oz	220	6	28
Protein Plus: Average, 2.75 oz	290	5	38
Carbselect, average	270	11	32

Granola, Sports & Diet Bars (Cont.)

Other Bars (Cont)

Per Bar

	C	F	Cb
Prozone Nutrition Bar, 50g	195	6	18
Pure Protein High Protein, 1.76 oz	190	6	17
Pure Fit, average, 2 oz bar	235	6	27
Quaker Chewy Granola Bars			
Chewy (Regular): Avg. all flavors	120	4	20
Peanut Butter/Chocolate	120	3.5	20
Cookies & Milk, average	120	3.5	20
Dipps: Choc Chip	150	6	21
Peanut Butter	150	7	18
Fruit 'N Crunch, average	160	3.5	31
Trail Mix, average	150	5	24
Wholesome Favorites, avg. 1.2oz	110	2	22
Rapunzel: Crisp, 20g	100	7	11
Coco; Rio; Tango, average	230	17	16
Real Protein, 2.75 oz bar	290	5	28
Resource, OptiSource Mini Bar	90	2.5	10
Restart: Peanut Butter, 1.25 oz	130	2.5	18
Strawb. Banana; Chocolate	130	2.5	21
Revival Soy Bars *(Direct):* *Per Bar*			
Choc. Temptation	220	3.5	30
Apple Cinnamon; Marshm. Krunch	220	3	33
Peanut Butter/Choc Pal, avg.	240	6	32
Low Carb, average all flavors	250	9	33
Russell Stover: Pecan Delight, 2 pieces	240	16	22
Pecan Delight Sugar Free, 2 pces	130	9	15
Diabetx : Toffee Square, 1 oz	100	7	14
Pecan Delights, 1 oz	130	9	16
SCAN Diet, 45g	160	2.5	26
Slim-Fast Bars			
Optima: Breakfast Bars, avg.	180	6	22
Meal Bars, average	220	5	35
Snack Bars, average	120	4	20
Muffin Bars: Banana Nut	150	8	18
Blueberry; Choc Chip, avg.	140	5	22
Low Carb Diet: Breakfast Bars, avg.	180	6	19
Meal Bars, average	200	7	21
Snacks, average	120	3	16
Original: Brkfst & Lunch Bars, avg.	140	5	20
Chewy Granola;Layered, avg.	220	5	35
Meal-On-The-Go, average	220	5	36
Skippy Snack Bars, average, 1.2 oz	185	11	18
SlimWhey, average, 1.1 oz	120	3	14
Snackwell's: Cereal Bars	120	0	26
Other varieties	130	3	26
Solo GI, average, 47g	180	6	25

Per Bar

	C	F	Cb
Spiru-tein Energy Bar, 1.4 oz	170	4	22
Steel Bar (ABB), 2 oz	330	6	52
Strive (*Biochem*), avg., 2.1 oz	200	6	25
The Sports Club/LA:			
Caramel Cr./Choc P'nut (16g prot.)	200	5	22
P'nut Butter Fudge (13g prot.)	185	9	13
Think Protein Bar, 2.3 oz	280	9	18
Think Thin! Low Carb Diet, avg. all bars, 2.1 oz	250	10	22
Tiger's Milk: 35g Bar	130	2.5	24
Peanut Butter varieties	150	7	18
Protein Rich	150	5	18
Tiger Sport, 65g	230	2	43
Tri-O-Plex, Peanut Butter, 4.2 oz	360	11	34
Ultimate Lo Carb: Honey Almd	270	10	24
Amaretto Irish Cream	140	6	1
Choc Brownie Nut	165	7	2
Creamy Peanut Butter	270	9	4
Ultimate Lo Carb 2: Choc Peanut	230	6	25
Choc S'Mores; Black Forest, avg.	230	6	25
Other varieties, avg.	250	8	25
Ultimate Protein Bar, 78g	290	4.5	19
Usana: Fiberg Bar, 48g	100	1.5	23
Nutrition Bar: Wild Berry	150	2.5	23
Peanut Butter Crunch	150	4	20
Vyo-Pro *(AST)* Chocolate, 2.2 oz	210	7	17
Whole Foods: Everyday Bars, avg.	190	4.5	18
Choc Fudge/Raspberry	172	4	17
Honey Peanut Yogurt	200	4.5	18
Worldwide Sport Nutrition:			
Pure Protein Bars, 2.75 oz			
Peanut Butter	310	10	24
Honey Nut; Maple Pecan	310	9	26
Other varieties, average	290	7	27
You Are What You Eat, 56g	220	5	39
Zanzibar (Designer Whey)	320	9	31
Zoe Flax & Soy, Choc., 1.8 oz	200	6	33
Zone Perfect, average, 1.76 oz	210	7	24

'*Life is what happens to you when you're making other plans.*'

~ Betty Talmadge

Nuts

Per 1 oz Unless Indicated

	C	F	Cb
Acorns, raw 1 oz	105	7	12
Almonds, Dried/Dry Roasted:			
Whole, 24-28 med., 1 oz	170	15	7
½ cup, 2½ oz	420	37	17
Chopped,½ cup, 2¼ oz	380	34	16
Sliced, ½ cup, 1⅔ oz	280	25	12
Choc. coated (5-6), 1 oz	160	11	14
Oil Rstd *(Blue Diamond)*, 1 oz	175	17	3.5
Honey Roasted, 1 oz	170	13	8
Almond Meal (partially defattened)			
1 cup (not packed), 2¼ oz	260	11	11
Brazil Nuts, 8 medium, 1 oz	185	19	3.5
Cashews, Dry or Oil Roasted:			
14 large/18 med./26 small, 1 oz	165	14	10
½ cup, 2.4 oz	400	33	23
Honey Roasted, 1 oz	160	12	11
Chestnuts, avg. all: Dried, 1 oz	105	1	22
Raw/Fresh, 5-6 nuts, 1 oz	60	0	13
Canned, water chestnuts			
sliced/whole/drained, 1 oz	23	0	5
Coconut: Flesh, 1 oz	100	10	4
Raw: 1 pce. (2"x2"x½"), 1.6 oz	160	15	7
½ medium (4½" diam.)	650	62	30
Dried (Desiccated):			
Unsweetened, 1 oz	187	18	17
Sweetened: Shredded, 1 oz	140	9	13
Grated, ½ cup, 1.3 oz	185	12	18
Cream (canned), ½ cup, 5.2 oz	285	26	12
Milk (canned), ½ cup, 4 oz	225	24	3
Water (center liq.), ½ c., 4¼ oz	23	0	4.5
Filberts or Hazelnuts:			
Shelled, 18-20 nuts	180	18	4.5
Chopped, ¼ cup	180	18	4.5
Ground, ¼ cup	120	12	3
Ginkgo Nuts, can., 14 med., 1 oz	90	4	21
Hickory, 30 small nuts	190	18	5
Macadamia Nuts, shelled:			
Raw, 7 med./14 small, 1 oz	200	21	4
½ cup, 2.3 oz	460	48	10
Oil roasted, 1 oz	205	22	3.5
½ cup, 2.4 oz	490	52	8
Choc. coated, 2-3 pces, 1 oz	180	13	15
Mixed Nuts: 18-22 nuts, 1 oz	175	13	7
Planters: Dry Roasted/Honey	170	15	7
Oil Roasted, all types	180	16	7
Sweet Roasts, 26 pces, 1 oz	160	12	10
Kettle: Choc Lover's Mix, 1 oz	140	7	16

Per 1 oz Unless Indicated

	C	F	Cb
Nut Toppings:			
Chopped, 1 Tbsp, ¼ oz	40	4	1.5
Peanuts:			
Raw/Dried: In shell, 1 oz	117	10	3
Shelled, 1 oz	160	14	4.5
Boiled, ½ cup, 1.1 oz	102	7	7
Roasted, 30 lge./60 sml., 1 oz	165	14	6
1 cup, 5.1 oz	860	76	22
Chopped, 3 Tbsp, 1 oz	165	14	6
Planters: Oil Roasted, 1 oz	170	15	5
Beer Nuts, 1 oz pkg	170	14	7
Choc-coated, 1 oz pkg, 2½ oz	220	15	19
Cocktail, oil roasted, 1 oz	170	14	5
Dry Roasted, 1 oz	160	14	6
Honey Roasted, 1 oz	150	11	10
Honey/Roasted, 1 oz	160	13	7
Spanish Oil Roasted, 1 oz	170	14	5
Sweet 'n Crunchy, 1 oz	140	8	16
Pecans: Kernel halves, 1 oz	190	19	5
(20 Jumbo or 31 large halves)			
1 cup halves, 3.8 oz	685	71	13
Chopped, ½ cup, 2 oz	380	30	10
Oil Roasted, 1 oz	205	20	4.5
Honey Roasted, 1 oz	200	18	5
Pilinuts, dried, ¼ cup, 1 oz	205	23	1
Pinenuts, dried, 1 Tbsp, 10g	50	5	1.5
Pistachios: Unshelled, ½ cup, 2 oz	165	14	7
Shelled, ¼ cup, 45 nuts	165	14	7
Lance, 1⅛ oz package	180	14	8
Planters: Dry Roasted, 1 oz	170	15	6
Fruit 'n Nut Mix, 1 oz	140	9	13
Nut Topping, 1 oz	180	16	6
Tavern Nuts, 1 oz	170	15	6
Trail Mix, 3 Tbsp, 1 oz	140	9	15
Sesame Nut Mix: Planters, 1 oz	160	12	8
Soy Nuts: Dry Roasted, 1 oz	130	6	9
½ cup, 3 oz	390	18	28
Dr Soy: Choc coated, 1 oz pkg	140	7	13
Flavors, average, 1 oz	150	7	8
Walnuts:			
Black: 15-20 halves, 1 oz	175	16	3.5
Chopped, ¼ cup	190	18	4
Ground, ¼ cup	120	12	2.5
English/Persian:			
14 halves, 1 oz	185	18	5
Chopped, ¼ cup	195	19	5

Seeds • Supplements

Seeds

	C	F	Cb
Alfalfa Seeds, sprouted, ½ c., ½ oz	5	0	1
Caraway, Fennel, 1 tsp	10	0.5	1
Cottonseed Kernels, rst., 1 Tbsp	50	4	2
Flax Seeds, 3 Tbsp, 1 oz	150	10	11
Lotus Seeds, dried, ½ c., ½ oz	50	0.5	10
Poppy Seeds, 1 tsp	15	1	1
Pumpkin & Squash Seeds, whole:			
Roasted/Tamari, 1 oz	125	5.5	3
½ cup (32g)	140	6	3.5
Dried, 1 oz	155	13	5
Safflower Kernels, dried, 1 oz	150	11	10
Sesame Seeds: Dried, 1 Tbsp, 9g	50	4.5	2
Roasted/Toasted, 1 oz	160	14	7
Sunflower Kernels/Seed:			
Dry Roasted, 1 Tbsp, 8g	45	4	1.5
¼ cup, 1 oz	160	14	6
Oil Roasted, ¼ cup, 1 oz	180	17	6
Watermelon, dried, ¼ cup, 1 oz	160	14	4.5

Quick Guide

Peanut Butter: *Average All Brands*

1 teaspoon, 6g	35	3	1.5
1 Tbsp, 0.6 oz, (17g)	105	8.5	3.5
2 Tbsp, 1.2 oz, (34g)	210	17	7
1 oz Quantity (28g)	170	14	6
½ cup, 5 oz	850	70	30
Jif: Reduced Fat, 1 Tbsp	100	6	7.5
Creamy; Crunchy; Simply, 1 Tbsp	105	8	3.5
Peanut Butter & Honey, 1 Tbsp	95	7.5	5.5
Peanut Wonder, 1 Tbsp	45	1.5	6
Smucker's: Honey Swtnd., 1 Tbsp	100	8	4
Goober Grape/Strawb., 1 Tbsp	90	5	4
Skippy: Carb Options, 1 Tbsp	100	8.5	1
Reduced Fat, 1 Tbsp	100	6	7.5
Squeez'it, 1 Tbsp, ½ oz	105	8.5	3.5

Other Nut & Seed Butters

	C	F	Cb
Almond Butter, 1 Tbsp, ½ oz	105	8	3
Almond Butter Honey Roasted	90	7	5.5
Beanut Butter, 1 Tbsp, ½ oz	90	5.5	7
Cashew Butter, 1 Tbsp, ½ oz	90	7	4.5
Cashew Peanut Date Butter	95	7	4
Hazelnut Butter, 1 Tbsp	100	10	2.5
Nutella, 1 Tbsp	100	5.5	12
Pecan Butter, 1 Tbsp	110	11	3.5
Pistachio Butter, 1 Tbsp	100	8.5	5
Sesame Butter/Tahini, 1 tsp	30	3	1
1 Tbsp, ½ oz	90	8.5	3
Soy Nut Butter, 1 Tbsp	85	6	2.5
Sunflower Seed Butter, 1 Tbsp	95	8	4

Supplements

	C	F	Cb
Aloe Vera Juice, undiluted, 2 fl.oz	5	0	1
Barlean's Flax Oil, 3 capsules	27	3	0
Cod Liver Oil, 1 Tbsp	120	13	0
Evening Primrose Oil, capsules, 1	5	0.5	0
Fiber Supplements: Tabs, 1	1	0	0
Bios Life 2, 1 packet	10	0	2
Metamucil, 1 packet	5	0	0
Regular, 1 rounded Tbsp	34	0	8
Sugar-Free, 1 Tbsp	6	0	1
Fish Oil Capsules, average, 1	10	1	0
Flax Oil Capsules, 2	10	1	0
Garlic Tablets/Capsules, each	3	0	1
Lecithin Granules, 1 Tbsp, 10g	50	5	1
Protein; Powders, average, 1 oz	100	0.5	0
Tablets, 20 tabs, ½ oz	70	0	0
Seaweed: Dried, 1 oz	85	0.5	22
Soaked, drained, 1 oz	15	0.5	3
Spirulina, 1 tablet	2	0	0.5
Vitamins/Minerals: Tabs/Caps, 1	2	0	0
Vitamin E Capsules, each	5	0.5	0
Viactiv Chews (1)	20	0.5	4
Yeast: Tablets, 2 tabs	4	0	0.5
Flakes, 1 heaping Tbsp, ⅓ oz	30	0.5	4
Powder, 1 heaping Tbsp, ½ oz	50	0.5	6

Cough & Pharmaceutical

	C	F	Cb
Cough/Cold Syrups: *Per Tablespoon*			
Regular: w. sugar, 1 Tbsp	35	0	9
w. alcohol, 1 Tbsp	46	0	9
Sugar-Free *(Diabetic Tussin),* 1 T.	0	0	0
Cough Drops/Lozenges: *See Page 131*			
Antacids: Average, 1 tablet	4	0	1
Liquid, 1 Tbsp	6	0	1
Sudafed Syrup, 1 tsp	14	0	3
Tylenol Liquid: Child, 1 tsp	17	0	4
Extra Strength, 1 tsp	11	0	3

Nut eaters are healthier and live longer say medical researchers.

Nuts are a nutritious source of protein, antioxidants, vitamins, minerals, healthy fats and fiber.

Their fat and fiber content can help to lower blood cholesterol, but watch the quantity if overweight.

Weights As Purchased	C	F	Cb
Acerola, 1 cup, 20 pcs, 3½ oz	30	0	7.5
Apples: whole, average all varieties:			
1 small (4 per lb), 4 oz	55	0	14
1 medium (3 per lb), 5½ oz	70	0	17
1 large (2 per lb), 8 oz	110	0	28
1 extra large, 11 oz	150	0	37
without skin, 1 medium	60	0	15
Candy/Caramel Apple, 1 med.	170	0	42
Nut Coated, 1 medium	230	5	46
Apricots: 1 small (12 per lb)	17	0	4
1 medium (8 per lb), 2 oz	25	0	6
1 large (5-6 per lb), 3 oz	35	0	8
Avocado (w/out seed/skin):			
Average, ½ medium, 3½ oz	160	15	6
1 salad slice, ½ oz	25	2	1
Mashed/Puree, 2 Tbsp, 1 oz	50	4.5	2
¼ cup, 2 oz	90	9	4
Californian, ½ medium, 3 oz	160	14	8
Mashed/Puree, ½ c., 4 oz	210	18	12
Florida, ½ medium, 5½ oz	170	13	14
Mashed/Puree, ½ c., 4 oz	125	10	9
½ cup cubed, 3 oz	105	8	8

Note: Avocados are nutritious and contain no cholesterol. Fat is mainly monounsaturated and benefits blood cholesterol. Excellent substitute for butter or margarine.

	C	F	Cb
Banana: 1 small (6" ~ 4 per lb), 4 oz	90	0	23
1 medium (7" ~ 3 per lb), 5 oz	105	0	27
1 large (8" ~ 2½ per lb), 7 oz	120	0	30
1 extra large (9"), 9 oz	135	0	35
w/out skin, 1 oz	25	0	6
Berries: (Blueberries/Black/Boysenberries)			
½ cup, 2.5 oz	40	0	10
1 pint, 14 oz	225	1	56
Breadfruit, ½ cup, 4 oz	115	0	28
Cactus Pear, 1 fruit, 3½ oz	40	0	9
Cantaloupe: Flesh/no rind, 1 oz	8	0	2
½ small, 20 oz (w. rind/seeds)	125	1	30
½ medium, 28 oz (w. rind/seeds)	175	1.5	42
1 slice, 2.5 oz (w/out rind)	20	0	6
1 cup pieces/balls, 5.5 oz	25	0	13
Carambola (Star Fruit), 1 med	50	0	4
Cassava, ⅓ cup, 2½ oz	120	0	27
Cherimoya (Custard Apple), 4 oz	80	1	18
Cherries: Sweet, 8 fruit, 2 oz	30	0	7
½ lb (30 cherries)	110	0	27
Sour, 8 fruit, 2 oz	30	0	7
½ lb (30 cherries)	110	0	7
Clementine, 1 med., 3 oz	50	0	15

Weights As Purchased	C	F	Cb
Coconut: Fresh,			
1 piece, 2"x2"x ½", 1 oz	100	10	3
Shredded, fresh, ½ cup	140	13	6
Sweetened, dried, ½ cup	235	16	22
Crabapples, ½ cup slices, 2 oz	40	0	9
Cranberries, ½ cup, 2 oz	20	0	5
Currants: Per ½ Cup			
European Black, raw, 2 oz	35	0	8
Red & White, raw, 2 oz	30	0	7
Custard Apple, raw, 4 oz	110	1	27
Dates: See Dried Fruits			
Dragon Pearl Fruit, med., 11.6 oz	100	0.5	23
Durian, flesh, 4 oz	165	6	28
Elderberries, ½ cup, 2½ oz	55	0	13
Feijoas, 1 medium, 2½ oz	35	0	7
Figs: green/black: 1 med., 2 oz	40	0	10
1 large, 3 oz	60	0	15
Fruit Salad, fresh, average,			
½ cup, 3½ oz	60	0	15
1 cup, 7 oz	120	0	30
Gooseberries, raw, ½ c., 2½ oz	30	0	7
Grapefruit: Average all types,			
½ fruit, 10 oz (6 oz flesh)	50	0	12
1 cup sections w. juice, 8 oz	75	0	18
Grapes: Average, 1 cup, 5½ oz	105	0	25
1 small bunch, 4 oz	75	0	18
1 medium bunch, 7 oz	130	0	32
1 large bunch, 16 oz	305	0	75
Granadilla, flesh, 2 oz	95	0	23
Groundcherries, ½ cup, 2½ oz	35	0	9
Guava: 1 fruit, 4 oz	80	0	15
½ cup, 3 oz	55	0	12
Honeydew, 1 wedge, (⅛ of 7" diam.),			
8 oz (with skin)	50	0	12
1 cup cubes/balls, 6 oz	60	0	14
Honey Murcots, 1 only, 5 oz	45	0	11
Jaboticaba, flesh, 4 oz	75	2	15
Jackfruit, flesh, ⅛ average, 4 oz	105	0	25
Jambos (Brazil Cherry), flesh, 4 oz	35	0	8
Java-Plum, 4 plums, ½ oz	25	0	6
Jujube, 3 oz	65	0	16
Kiwifruit: 1 medium, 3 oz	45	0	11
1 large, 4 oz	60	0	15
Kumquats, 5 medium, 3½ oz	60	0	15
Kiwano, ½ medium, 5 oz	35	0	8
Langsat, Duku, 1 medium, 2 oz	25	0	5
Lemon: 1 medium, 4 oz	20	0	5
1 wedge, 1 oz	5	0	1.5
Peel, 1 Tbsp	4	0	1
Limes, 1 medium (2" diam.), 2 oz	20	0	5
Loganberries, froz., ½ cup, 2½ oz	40	0	9

Fresh Fruit (Cont)

Weights As Purchased	C	F	Cb
Longans, 5 fruit, ½ oz	10	0	2.5
Loquats, 4 fruit, 2¼ oz	30	0	7
Lychees, 4 fruit, 2¼ oz	32	0	7
Mamey Apple: 1 whole, 3 lb	430	4	100
¼ fruit (1 cup flesh), 7 oz	100	1	23
Mandarin: 1 small, 3 oz	35	0	9
1 medium, 4 oz	45	0	11
1 large, 6 oz	50	0	12
Mango: flesh, ½ cup sl., 3 oz	55	0	14
1 whole, medium, 11 oz	205	0.5	53
Melon, avg, 1 cup, cubes/balls, 6 oz	60	0	14
Monstera Deliciosa (Taxonia), Edible part, 4 oz	50	0	11
Mulberries, 20 fruit, 1 oz	15	0	3
Nashi Fruit (Asian Pear), 1 med., 7 oz	85	0	21
Nectarines: 1 medium, 4 oz	50	0	12
1 large, 5½ oz	60	0	14
Oheloberries, ½ cup, 2½ oz	20	0	5
Olives (Pickled): Green, 10 lrg, 1½ oz	45	5	0.5
Ripe, Greek Style, 10 med., 1 oz	70	7	2
Ripe (Black) Californian:			
1 small/medium	5	0.5	0.3
1 large/extra large	6	0.5	0.5
1 jumbo	7	0.5	0.5
1 colossal	11	1	0.5
1 super colossal	13	1	1
Oranges: Average all varieties,			
1 small, 5 oz (with skin)	45	0	11
1 medium (3" diam.), 7 oz	60	0	15
1 large, 10 oz	85	0	21
Flesh only, 1 cup, 6 oz	80	0	19
Californian Valencia,			
1 medium (2¾" diam.), 6 oz	60	0	15
Californ. Navels (3" diam.), 7 oz	70	0	17
Sunkist Navel, 14 oz	130	0	30
Florida Orange, 1 medium, 7 oz	70	0	17
Peel, 1 Tbsp	0	0	0
Papaya: ½ cup, cubed, 2½ oz	30	0	7
1 medium, (5"x3" diam.), 16 oz	120	0	28
Green (unripe), ½ cup, 3½ oz	20	0	5
Passionfruit, 1 medium, 1¼ oz	20	0	4.5
PawPaw (see Papaya)			
Peaches: 1 small/donut, 3 oz	30	0	7
1 medium (4 per lb), 4 oz	40	0	10
1 large, 6 oz	60	0	15
1 extra large, 10 oz	90	0	22

Weights As Purchased	C	F	Cb
Pears: Bartlett, 1 small, 4 oz	80	0	20
1 medium, 6.5 oz	95	0	24
1 large, 8 oz	120	0	30
1 cup slices, 6 oz	95	0.5	24
Asian, 1 medium, 7 oz	85	0	21
Bosc, 6.5 oz	95	0	24
D'Anjou, 1 medium, 8 oz	120	0	30
Forelle, 1 medium, 7 oz	90	0	22
Red Pear, 5 oz	85	0	20
Seckel (Wash'ton), 2¼ oz	35	0	9
Pepino, ½ medium, 4 oz	20	0	4
Persimmons: Native, 1 oz	30	0	7
Japan (2½"d. x 2½"h), 7 oz	120	0	30
Seedless (Maui), 1 md., 5 oz	100	0	25
Pineapple (no skin):			
1 thin slice, (½"), 2 oz	28	0	7
1 thick slice, (¾"), 3 oz	40	0	10
1 cup, diced, 5½ oz	75	0	19
1 medium, 1½ lb (peeled)	325	0	82
Wedges (*Del Monte*), 12 oz pkg	168	0	42
Canned: *See Page 146*			
Pitanga, 3 fruit, 1 oz	6	0	1
Plaintains, ½ cup slices, 2½ oz	90	0	22
Plums: Average all types,			
Mini/Damson, (1" diam.), ½ oz	8	0	2
Small (1¾" diam.), 2 oz	30	0	7
Medium (2¼" diam.), 3 oz	45	0	10
Large (2½" diam.), 4 oz	65	0	15
Pluot (plum-apricot), 1 med., 5 oz	80	0	19
Pomegranates, ½ fruit, 5 oz	55	0	13
Pummelo, flesh, ½ cup, 4 oz	35	0	8
Prickly Pears, 1 fruit, 5 oz	50	0	11
Quince, 1 medium, 3½ oz	55	0	14
Rambutan (Rambotang),			
Red/Yellow, 1 medium, 2 oz	15	0	4
Raspberries, ½ cup, 2 oz	30	0	7
Rhubarb, raw, ½ cup, 2 oz	15	0	3
Sapodilla (Chico), 1 md., 7½ oz	140	2	33
Sapotes, ½ medium, 5.5 oz	150	0	37
Satsuma Tangerine, 1 med., 3 oz	50	0	15
Soursop, 1 cup pulp, 8 oz	150	0	38
Strawberries: 1 cup, 5½ oz	45	0	10
6 medium/3 large, 2 oz	15	0	3
1 pint, 14 oz	115	0	28
Chocolate Dipped, 2 medium	45	2.5	6
Sugar Apples, ½ cup pulp, 4 oz	120	0	30
Tamarillo, 1 medium, 3 oz	20	0	3
Tamarind, 1 fruit, ¼ oz	5	0	0

Fresh Fruit (Cont) ◆ Dried Fruit

Weights As Purchased	C	F	Cb
Tangelo: 1 small, 4 oz	30	0	7
1 medium, 5 oz	40	0	9
1 large, 7 oz	55	0	12
Tangerine, 1 medium, (2½" diam.), 4 oz	45	0	11
Tangor, 1 medium, 4 oz	35	0	7
Tomatillos, (3) 3 oz	20	0	5
Tomato: 1 small, 3 oz	15	0	4
1 medium, 5 oz	20	0	5
1 large, 7 oz	30	0.5	7
1 jumbo (salad/steak), 10 oz	50	1	11
Grape, 3 medium	8	0	2
Yellow Tear Drop, 4 medium, 1 oz	8	0	2
Cherry: 1 medium, ¾ oz	5	0	1
1 cup, 5¼ oz	27	0	6
Slices: (Medium Tomato):			
Thin slice, ½ oz	3	0	1
Medium (¼" thick), ¾ oz	4	0	1
Thick (⅜"), 1 oz	5	0	1
Fried Green Tomato, 1 slice (36g)	70	5.5	4.5
Canned Tomatoes/Products: *See Page 85*			
Tree Tomato (Tamarillo), 3 oz	20	0	5
Ugli Fruit, Tangelo type, 5 oz	40	0	8
Watermelon: Flesh only/no rind, 1 oz	9	0	2
1 cup cubes or balls, 5½ oz	45	0	11
Regular Long Shape:			
1 thick (1") slice (¼ circle, 4½" radius)			
9 oz w. rind (5½ oz no rind)	50	0	12
1 thin (½") slice (¼ circle)	25	0	6
1 thick (1") slice (½ circle)			
18 oz w. rind	100	1	24
1 whole melon (15" long, 7½"diam.)			
20 lb w. rind/10lb no rind	1360	7	340
Seedless Round Shape:			
Medium Size (13 lbs, 8¼" diam.)			
Edible Weight (no rind), 4 lbs	550	3	137
Wedge (⅛ whole melon),			
26 oz (with rind)	70	0.5	17
Flesh only (no rind), 8 oz	70	0.5	17
Wax Jambu (Rose Apple), 2 oz	10	0	2

Dried Fruit

	C	F	Cb
Apples, 5 rings, 1 oz	75	0	18
Apricots, 8 halves, 1 oz	65	0	15
Banana Chips, ½ cup, 1½ oz	160	5	18
Banana Flakes, 4 Tbsp, 1 oz	80	0	20
Cranberries, swtn, dr., ⅓ c, 1.4 oz	130	0	33
Currants, ¼ cup, 1¼ oz	100	0	24
Dates: 5 medium dates, 1½ oz	120	0	28
Large Calif., 3 dates, 2 oz	160	0	37
½ cup, chopped, 3 oz	240	0	57
Date Crumbles (*Bob's Redmill*),			
1 oz, ¼ cup	90	0	23
Figs, 3 medium figs, 2 oz	145	0	34
Longans; Lychees, 1 oz	80	0	19
Mango Slices, 4 strips, 1 oz	70	0	15
Mixed Fruit, 1 oz	70	0	16
Papaya Spears, 1 oz	75	0	17
Peaches, 2 halves, 1 oz	60	0	14
Pears, 3 halves, 2 oz	75	0	17
Pineapple, 1 oz	80	0	18
Prunes (dried Plums): w. pits, 1 oz	60	0	14
1 Medium (60/lb)	16	0	4
1 Large (50/lb)	22	0	5
1 Extra Large (40/lb)	27	0	6
Without pits, 4 med., 1 oz	70	0	17
Cooked: w. sugar, ½ c, 5 oz	200	0	47
w/out sugar, ½ c, 4½ oz	125	0	33
Raisins: 2 Tbsp, 1 oz package	90	0	22
½ cup, 2.8 oz	260	0	62
CinnaRaisins, 1.4 oz pkg	135	0.5	32
Sunsweet: Fruitlings, ⅓ c., 1.5 oz	130	0	31
Plums (5) 1.4 oz	100	0	24

Candied Glacé Fruit

	C	F	Cb
Apricot, 1 medium, 1 oz	100	0	25
Cherry, 3 large, ½ oz	50	0	12
Citron/Fruit Peel, 1 oz	90	0	21
Fig, 1 piece, 1 oz	90	0	21
Ginger, 1 oz	95	0	23
Pineapple, 1 slice, 1¼ oz	120	0	30

Fruit Leather/Rolls

	C	F	Cb
Average All Brands, 1 oz	100	0	24
Fruit By The Foot, 1 roll, ¾ oz	80	0	17
Fruit Gushers, 1 pouch, 1 oz	90	1	20
Fruit Roll-Ups, 1 roll, ½ oz	50	0	12
Stretch Is. Leathers, 2 pcs, 1 oz	90	0	21
Sunkist Fruit Roll, 1 roll	75	0	18
Other Fruit Confectionery/Snacks/Bars: *Page 137*			

Eat at least 5 servings of fruit and vegetables every day . . . and Enjoy Better Health!

145

Canned/Bottled Fruit ◆ Fruit Snacks

Canned/Bottled Fruit

Solids & Liquids:	C	F	Cb
Per ½ Cup (Approx. 4 ½ oz)			
Apples, sweetened	70	0	17
Apricots: In water/diet	35	0	9
In juice/lite	60	0	15
In syrup	105	0	27
Black/Blueberries: Heavy syrup	115	0	30
In light syrup	110	0	26
Cherries, pitted, in water	55	0	14
In light syrup	85	0	21
In heavy syrup	110	0	28
In extra heavy syrup	130	0	33
Maraschino, 5, 1 oz	50	0	13
Pie, ⅔ cup, 5 oz	60	0	14
Fruit Salad: In water/diet	35	0	9
In juice/Light	60	0	16
In heavy syrup	95	0	25
Gooseberries, Light syrup	90	0	23
Grapefruit: Juice pack	45	0	15
In light syrup	75	0	20
Lychees, ½ cup, 4.5 oz	105	0	26
Mixed Fruit: In water/diet	40	0	10
In fruit juices/light syrup	60	0	15
In heavy syrup	100	0	25
Peaches (halves/slices): In water/diet	30	0	8
In juice/light	50	0	14
In light syrup	70	0	20
drained, ½ peach	40	0	11
In heavy syrup	100	0	26
Pears: In water/diet	35	0	10
In juice/light	60	0	16
In heavy syrup	100	0	26
Pineapple: All types			
In own juice	70	0	17
In heavy syrup	90	0	22
Slices, drained, 2 slices			
In own juice, drained	30	0	7
In heavy syrup, drained	45	0	11
Plums: In water	50	0	14
In juice	75	0	20
In light syrup, 3 plums	85	0	21
In heavy syrup, ½ cup	160	0	41
Prunes: In heavy syrup	120	0	32
In Liqueur, ½ cup, 125g	280	0	70
In Water, ½ cup	135	0	32
Raspberries, in heavy syrup	120	0	30
Strawberries: In water	25	0	7
In heavy syrup	120	0	31
Tropical Fruit Salad: In light syrup	80	0	18
In heavy syrup	95	0	21

Fruit Snack Cups

	C	F	Cb
Deli/Take-Out: Small, 6 oz	70	0	16
Large, 12 oz	140	0	32
Yogurt & Fruit Cup, 15 oz	380	4.5	75
Del Monte Fruit Cups: *Per 4 oz cup*			
Fruit Cocktail: In water/diet	40	0	11
In juice/light	55	0	15
In light syrup	80	0	21
In heavy syrup	95	0	25
Mandarin Orange cup	70	0	17
Mandarin Oranges: In water	40	0	10
In light syrup	80	0	20
Peach/Pear/Lite	50	0	13
Fruit Rageous cup	90	0	22
Carb Clever: *Per ½ Cup (4.2 oz)*			
Fruit Cocktail	40	0	11
Peaches, chunks/slices	30	0	7
Pears, chunks/slices	40	0	10
Fruit to Go, 4 oz cup	70	0	18
Pop Top Snack Cans:			
Fruit Cocktail, 8½ oz can	190	0	47
Lite Sliced Peaches, 8¼ oz can	115	0	28
Dole Fruit Bowls			
4 oz Bowls: Peaches/Mandarin Or.	70	0	17
Mixed Fruit	80	0	19
Pineapple/Tropical Fruit	65	0	15
Fruit n Gel Bowls 4.3 oz: Reg.	90	0	22
Reduced Sugar	50	0	13
Mott's: Healthy Harvest, 4 oz cup	50	0	13
Blues Clues; Fruitsations, 4 oz c.	90	0	22
Tree Top: Fruit Rocketz, 1 tube	45	0	11
Natural Apple, 1 Pkg., 4 oz	50	0	12
Vons: Mixed Fruit,			
In heavy syrup, 1 cup, 4.5 oz	90	0	22
In lite syrup, 1 cup, 4.5 oz	60	0	13

Apple & Fruit Sauces

	C	F	Cb
Apple Sauce:			
Regular/sweetened, 2 Tbsp, 1.1 oz	23	0	5
4 oz package cup	80	0	20
½ cup, 4.5 oz	90	0	22
Mott's Cinnamon, ½ cup, 4.5 oz	110	0	27
Cranberry Sauce: Whole Berry, 1 T.	15	0	3
¼ cup, 2½ oz	110	0	27
Jellied Cranberry, ¼ cup	110	0	27
Fruit Sauces & Purees:			
Average all fruit types, 2 Tbsp, 1 oz	25	0	6
½ cup, 4 oz	100	0	24

Vegetables	C	F	Cb
Alfalfa Sprouts, ½ cup, ½ oz	12	0	1
Artichokes, Globe/French:			
1 medium, 4½ oz	72	0	14
1 large, 7 oz	110	0	21
Artichoke Heart: Plain, 1 piece	8	0	2
Marinated, 1 piece	15	2	2
Asparagus, raw/froz.: 4 med. spears	12	0	2
Cuts & Tips, ½ cup	17	0	3
Bamboo Shoots, ckd, ½ c, 2 oz	7	0	1
Beans: Green/Snap, ½ c, 2 oz	20	0	4
10 beans (no shell), 2 oz	20	0	4
Dried Beans, average all types: (Kidney, Brown, Haricot, Lima, Mung, Navy, Pinto, Red, White)			
Raw: 2 Tbsp, 1 oz	95	0.5	18
1 cup, 7 oz	665	3	126
Cooked: 1 oz	35	0	7
½ cup, 3 oz	105	0	21
Bean Sprouts, avg., ½ cup, 2 oz	17	0	3
Beets: Raw, 1 beet (2" diam), 3 oz	40	0	8
Cooked, ½ cup, slices, 3 oz	40	0	8.5
1 beet, 2" diam., 1¾ oz	24	0	5
Beet Greens, ckd, ½ c., 2½ oz	20	0	4
Bell Pepper: See Peppers			
Bitter Melon/Gourd, 1 c. pces, 1.6 oz	14	0	2
Black Eyed Peas, ckd, ½ c., 2 oz	100	0.5	18
Bok Choy (Chinese Chard) 3 oz	12	0	2
Breadfruit, ¼ small fruit	100	0	26
Broadbeans (Fava Beans):			
Green (in pod), raw: 4 pods (3½ oz w. shell; 1.2 oz beans)	30	0	6
1 cup beans (no shell), 4½ oz	110	1	22
Mature Seeds: Raw, 1 c., 5.3 oz	512	2	87
Cooked, ½ cup, 3 oz	94	0	17
Broccoli: Raw, chopped,1 cup, 3 oz	35	0	6
3 Florets, 2½ oz	30	0	5
1 Spear (5" long) 1.1oz	13	0	2
1 Whole: Medium size, 14 oz	163	2	26
Large, 21 oz	245	2	40
1 Head (no stalk), 11 oz	128	1	21
1 Stalk, small (5" long), 5 oz	58	0.5	10
BroccoSprouts, 1 cup, 1 oz	16	0	2
Brussel Sprouts: ckd, ½ cup, 3 oz	28	0	6
2 Sprouts, 1½ oz	15	0	3
Butterbeans, cooked, ½ cup, 3 oz	90	0	16
Cabbage, All types/colors, average:			
Raw: 1 Leaf, large, 1.2 oz	8	0	2
Shredded, 1 cup, 2½ oz	17	0	4
½ Large Head (7" diam), 22 oz	150	1	35
Cooked, shredded, ½ cup, 2½ oz	20	0	5
Cactus (Nopal), sliced, 1 cup, 3 oz	14	0	3

Vegetables (Cont)	C	F	Cb
Carrots: Regular thick variety			
1 small, 4 oz	47	0	11
1 medium, 6 oz	70	0	16
1 large, 8 oz	93	0	22
Chopped, 1 cup, 4½ oz	52	0	12
Grated, 1 cup, 4 oz	47	0	11
Slices, 1 cup, 4½ oz	52	0	12
Sticks (4"), 4, 1½ oz	18	0	4
Long thin variety, 1 medium, 2.2 oz	25	0	6
Baby, snack size, 5 medium, 1 oz	10	0	2
Snack Pack, 3 oz	35	0	7
Cauliflower: Raw: 1 cup (pces), 3½ oz	25	0	5
½ medium head, 10 oz	70	0	15
Cooked, 3 florets, 2 oz	12	0	2
Celeriac, ½ cup, raw, 2¾ oz	33	0	7
Celery: 1 large stalk, 11", 2 oz	8	0	2
1 small stalk, 5", 2 oz	2	0	0.5
4 Strips/sticks, ½ oz	2	0	0.5
Chopped, 1 cup, 3½ oz	14	0	3.5
Chard (Swiss), ckd, ½ cup, 3 oz	17	0	3.5
Chayote Squash, raw, 4½ oz	22	0	5
Chick Peas (Garbanzo Beans):			
Dry, 1 cup, 6 oz	620	10	103
Cooked, 1 cup, 6 oz	280	4	47
Chicory, Greens, ½ cup, 3 oz	20	0	4
Chicory/Witloof: See Endive			
Chili Peppers: See Peppers			
Chinese Long Bean, sliced, 1 c., 3.2 oz	45	0	8
Chives, chopped, 1 Tbsp	1	0	0
Choy Sum, 3 oz	13	0	3
Cilantro (Coriander), 1 Cup	10	0	2
Collards, cooked, ½ cup, 3 oz	25	0	5
Corn, yellow/white:			
Raw: Kernels, ½ c., 2¾ oz	80	0.5	19
Ear (5"x 1¾"), raw, 5½ oz	154	1	37
Cooked: Kernels, ½ c., 2¾ oz	77	0.5	18
Cob, cooked, dr: Small, 2¼ oz	60	0.5	14
Large ear, 5½ oz	118	1	28
(Also see Frozen & Canned Corn Page 149-150)			
Courgette: See Zucchini			
Cress, Garden, raw, ½ cup, 1 oz	10	0	2
Cucumber: 1 whole, 11 oz	36	0.5	7
½ cup slices, 2 oz	7	0	1
Mini/Lebanese (1), 3 oz	10	0	3
Daikon Radish, 3 oz	15	0	3
Dandelion Greens, raw, ½ cup, 1 oz	13	0	3
Edamame *(Immature green soybeans):*			
Shelled, 1 cup, 2.6 oz	120	5	11
With shells, 10 pods, 1¼ oz	30	1	3
Eggplant: Raw, ¼ medium, 4 oz	27	0	7
Raw, 1 cup, 1" pieces, 1½ oz	10	0	2.5
1 slice, fried, 1 oz	75	4	10
Endive, Belgian/French: Raw,			
1 med. head (6"), 2½ oz	12	0	2

Vegetables (Cont)

Vegetables (Cont)

	C	F	Cb
Fiddleheads, 3.5 oz	33	0.5	4
Fava Beans: See Broadbeans			
Fennel, 1 cup, sliced, 3 oz	26	0	6
Gai Choy Cabbage, ckd, 1 cup	20	0	5
Gai Lan (Chinese Kale), 3 oz	35	0	7
Garlic, 1 clove	4	0	1
Ginger: ¼ cup slices, 1 oz	22	0	5
Crystallized (sugared), 1 oz	87	0	22
Horseradish, raw, 1 pod, ½ oz	4	0	1
Jerusalem Artichoke, raw, ½ cup	57	0	13
Jicama, raw, sliced, ½ cup, 2¼ oz	24	0	5.5
Kale, 1 cup, chopped	34	0.5	6
Kohlrabi, ½ cup, cooked, 3 oz	25	0	6
Lambsquarters, boiled, 3 oz	27	0.5	4
Leeks, cooked, 1 whole, 4½ oz	40	0	10
Lentils, green/brown: Dry, 1 oz	96	0.5	16
Dry, 1 cup, 6¾ oz	646	2	109
Cooked, 1 cup, 3½ oz	115	0.5	20
Lettuce: 1 c., chop./shred., 1½ oz	7	0	1
Butterhead, 2 leaves, ½ oz	2	0	0.5
Cos/Romaine, ½., shred., 2½ oz	12	0	2
Iceberg: 1 outer leaf, ¾ oz	3	0	1
1 medium head, 15-16 oz	68	0.5	14
Lamb's Lettuce, 2 ½ oz	15	0	1.5
Lima Beans, baby, ckd,½ c., 3 oz	105	0	14
Lotus Root, 10 slices, ckd, 3 oz	56	0	14
Mung Bean Sprouts, ½ cup, 2 oz	17	0	3
Mushrooms: Raw, 1 medium, 0.6 oz	4	0	0.5
Raw, 1 large, sliced, ¾ oz	5	0	1
Raw, ½ cup pieces, 1¼ oz	8	0	1
Cooked, ½ cup pieces, 2½ oz	20	0	4
Mustard Greens, raw, ½ cup, 1 oz	7	0	1
Nopal (Cactus): 1 leaf, 4½ oz	20	0	4
Sliced, 1 cup, 3 oz	15	0	3
Okra, cooked, ½ cup, slices, 2¾ oz	20	0	4
Onions: Raw: 1 small, 2 oz	24	0	6
1 medium, 4 oz	48	0	12
1 large, 8 oz	95	0	23
1 jumbo, 16 oz	190	0.5	46
Chopped, raw, ½ cup, 3 oz	36	0	9
1 Tbsp, 0.3 oz	4	0	1
Slices: 1 cup, 4 oz	47	0	11
1 thin slice, small, 0.3 oz	4	0	1
⅛" slice, medium, ½ oz	6	0	1
¼" slice, large, 1.3 oz	16	0	4
Dehydrated flakes, ¼ c, ½ oz	50	0	12
Rings, breaded/fried, 2 rings	80	5	9
Scallions, 1 medium, 0.5 oz	2	0	0
Spring, ¼ cup, chopped, 1 oz	9	0	2
French's Fried Onions: See Page 72			
Blossom/Blooming: See Fast-Foods (Chili's/Outback)			

	C	F	Cb
Parsley, chopped, ½ cup, 1 oz	10	0	2
Parsnips: 1 medium, 4 oz	85	0	20
Cooked, ½ cup slices, 2¾ oz	55	0	13
Peas: Green, ¼ cup, 1½ oz	35	0	7
Raw, with pods, ½ lb	70	0	13
Snow Peas (8-9 pods), 1 oz	10	0	8
Split, dry, hulled, 1 oz	50	0	10
cooked, 1 cup, 7 oz	235	1	42
Peppers: Sweet, 1 medium, 5 oz	28	0	7
Bell: 1 medium, 5 oz	28	0	7
½ cup, chopped, raw, 1¾ oz	10	0	2
1 ring (3" diam. x ¼" thick)	2	0	0.5
Chile: Green/Red, 1½ oz	18	0	4
Habanero, 1 only, 8g	11	0	2
Pigeon Peas, cooked, ½ cup	94	1	17
Pimientos, 3 medium, 3½ oz	25	0	5
Poi, ½ cup, 4.2 oz	135	0	32
Pumpkin, mashed, ½ cup, 4 oz	25	0	6
Raw, 1" cubes, 1 cup, 4 oz	30	0	7
Pumpkin Flowers, 1 cup, 1.2 oz	5	0	1
Purslane: Cooked, ½ c., 2 oz	10	0	2
Raw, 1" cubes, 1 cup, 4 oz	18	0	4
Potatoes: Raw (with skin)			
1 Baby, Gourmet, 2 oz	45	0	10
1 Small, 3 oz	65	0	15
1 Medium, 5 oz	110	0	25
1 Peeled, 4 oz	90	0	20
1 Large, 8 oz	175	0	40
1 Extra large (Russet), 12 oz	263	0	60
1 Jumbo (Russet), 16 oz	350	0	80
Baked (no fat); large, 10 oz raw:			
Plain, with skin, 7 oz	255	0	58
without skin, 5½ oz	145	0	34
Garlic Potatoes, mashed, 4 oz	136	6	18
w. Skin/Toppings: + 2 tsp fat	270	8	58
+ Sour Cr./Chives, 2 Tbsp	320	6	60
+ Plain Yogurt, 2 Tbsp	260	1	60
+ Grated Cheese, 1 oz	370	9	58
+ Cottage Cheese, 2 oz	315	2	60
Mashed w. milk and fat, ½ c.	113	4	17
Hash Browns: w. Butt. Sce, 2½ oz	125	6	17
Homemade, 1 cup, 2½ oz	188	9	25
Potato Skins: (w. Cheese topping)			
½ whole (8 oz baking), 4 oz	240	13	22
French Fries: Small serve, 2½ oz	220	12	28
Medium serve, 4 oz	350	20	45
Froz., uncooked, 18 fries, 4 oz	178	7	28
Oven-heated, 18 fries, 4 oz	178	7	28
Take-Out, 1 cup, 5 oz	440	25	60
McDonald's: Small, 2.6 oz	230	11	30
Medium, 4 oz	350	16	47

Vegetables (Cont)

	C	F	Cb
Potatoes (Cont)			
Fried, 18 fries, 4 oz	275	15	28
Au Gratin, ½ cup, 4.3 oz	160	9	14
Pancakes, 1 only, 2 oz	207	11	22
Kugel, 5 oz	300	20	26
Puffs, fried, 4 puffs, 1 oz	62	3	9
Scalloped, ½ cup, 4¼ oz	112	5	15
Ore-Ida Frozen Potatoes: See Page 150			
Potato Salad, ½ cup, 4½ oz	180	10	14
Radicchio, 2 leaves, ½ oz	3	0	1
Shredded, 1 cup, 1½ oz	10	0	2
Radish: Avg., 10 only, 1½ oz	7	0	2
Oriental, ½ c. slices, 1½ oz	10	0	2
Rutabagas, ckd., ½ c. cubes, 3 oz	30	0	7
Salsify, ckd, ½ c. slices, 2½ oz	48	0	11
Sauerkraut, ½ cup, 4 oz	22	0	5
Seaweed: Average, dried, 1 oz	50	0	13
Soaked, drained, 1 oz	15	0	4
Nori/Laver, dried, 6 sheets, 1 oz	35	0	5
Shallots, chopped, 1 Tbsp	7	0	1.5
Sorrel, raw, ½ cup, 4 oz	23	0.5	4
Soybeans: Mature, dry, 1 oz	110	5	7
Dry, ½ cup, 3½ oz	385	18	22
Cooked, ½ cup, 3 oz	105	5	6
(Soy Products/Tofu/Tempeh: See Page 77)			
Spinach: Cooked, ½ cup, 3 oz	20	0	3
Creamed, avg., ½ cup, 4½ oz	140	12	8
Raw: 3 leaves/1 cup, 1 oz	7	1.5	1
1 Bunch, 12 oz	80	1	9
Squash: Summer, raw, ½ c., 2¼ oz	10	0	2
Cooked, ½ cup slices, 3 oz	14	0	3.5
Winter, cooked,			
Acorn, ½ cup cubes, 3½ oz	55	0	14
½ medium (10 oz raw wt.)	114	0	30
Butternut, ½ c. cubes, 3½ oz	40	0	10
¼ medium (9 oz raw wt.)	95	0	23
Spaghetti, ½ cup, 2¾ oz	22	0	5
Succotash, ckd, ½ cup, 3⅓ oz	110	1	23
Sweetcorn: See Corn			
Sweet Potatoes: Cooked with Skin (no fat)			
1 medium, 4 oz	103	0	24
No skin, mashed, ½ c., 5½ oz	120	0	28
Swedes, ½ cup, 3 oz	20	0	4.5
Swiss Chard, ckd, chopped, 1 c., 6 oz	35	0	7
Taro, cooked, ½ cup, 2 oz	80	0	20

Vegetables (Cont)

	C	F	Cb
Tomatoes: 1 small, raw, 3 oz	15	0	3
1 medium, raw, 5 oz	26	0	5.5
1 large, raw, 7 oz	36	0	8
Cooked, ½ cup, 4¼ oz	23	0	5
Fried, 1 small, 3 oz	175	13	12
Also See Fruit: Page 145			
Tomatillo, 1 medium, 1.2 oz	10	0	2
Turnips: White, cooked, ½ cup, 3 oz	20	0	4.5
Greens, cooked, ½ cup, 2½ oz	15	0	2
Water Chestnuts: 4 nuts, raw	35	0	8.5
½ cup slices, 2¼ oz, raw	62	0	15
Canned, 1 oz	14	0	3.5
Watercress, 10 sprigs, 1 oz	3	0	1
Yam: Cooked, ½ cup, 2½ oz	80	0	20
Baked, 1 medium (6") 8 oz	260	0	63
1 large (9") 12 oz	396	0	94
Yardlong Bean, 1 pod, ½ oz	7	0	1
Yucca Root, ½ cup, 2.5 oz	60	0	14
Zucchini: 1 medium, 10 oz, raw	45	0.5	10
½ cup slices, cooked, 3 oz	14	0	3

Frozen Vegetables

	C	F	Cb
Birds Eye			
Broccoli/Corn/Red Peppers, ¾ cup	60	1	11
Chopped Spinach, ⅓ cup	30	0	3
Other varieties, average, 1 cup	30	0	6
Baby: Bean & Carrot Blend, 1 cup	35	0	5
Broccoli Florets, 1 cup	30	0	4
Corn, Pea & Bean Blend, ¾ cup	70	0.5	13
Sweet Peas, ⅔ cup	70	0.5	12
White Corn, ⅔ cup	90	1	18
Deluxe Vegetables: *Per Cup*			
Sugar Snap Stir Fry	40	0	7
Broccoli, Cauliflower & Carrots	30	0	5
Broccoli, Carrots & Water Chestnuts	35	0	6
Stir Fry: *Prepared (Includes Pasta)*			
Asparagus, 2 cup	80	0.5	15
Green Bean, 1¾ cup	100	0.5	19
Voila! Meals: *See Page 61*			
Green Giant			
Vegetables: Asparagus Cuts, ½ c.	15	0	2
Corn: Nibblers, ½ ear	70	0.5	14
Extra Sweet Niblets, ⅓ cup	50	0.5	11
S/Western & Rst Peppers, ¾ c.	80	0.5	17
Honey Glazed Carrots, 1 cup	90	3	15
Le Sueur Baby Sweet Peas, ½ cup	60	0	12
Spinach, ½ cup	25	0	3

Vegetables – Frozen, Canned, Bottled

Frozen Vegetables (Cont)   C   F   Cb

Green Giant (Cont)

Veges In Cheese & Cream Sauce: *Prepared*

	C	F	Cb
Alfredo Vegetables, ¾ cup	70	2.5	9
Broccoli, Cauliflower, Carrots, ⅔ cup	60	2.5	8
Cauliflower & Cheese Sce, ½ cup	60	2.5	6
Creamed Spinach, ½ cup	70	2.5	9
Cream Style Corn, ½ cup	110	1	23
Green Bean Casserole, ⅔ cup	110	8	8

Rice & Vegetables: *Prepared*

	C	F	Cb
Cheesy Rice & Brocc., 1 pkt, 10 oz	270	5	50
Rice Medley, 1 pkt, 10 oz	280	4	52
Rice Pilaf, 1 pkt, 10 oz	230	3.5	44
White & Wild Rice, 1 pkt, 10 oz	280	6	51

Ore-Ida (As Purchased):

	C	F	Cb
French Fries: Country, 18 fries, 3 oz	120	4	19
Crispers 20 pces, 3 oz	210	12	23
Crispy Crunchies, 13 fries, 3 oz	160	8	20
Fast Food Fries, 27 fries, 3 oz	180	7	21
Waffle Fries, 8 fries, 3 oz	160	6	22
Golden Crinkles, 12 pces, 3 oz	130	4	17
Golden Fries, 14 pces, 3 oz	120	2.5	20
Oven Chips, 7 pces, 3 oz	160	7	22
Shoestrings, 32 pces, 3 oz	150	6	19
Steak Fries, 7 fries, 3 oz	120	3	17
Zesties, 12 pces, 3 oz	140	5	22
Hash Browns: Toaster, 2 patties	220	12	25
Potatoes O'Brien, ¾ c., 2 oz	60	0	13
Onion Rings: Gourmet, 3 pces, 3 oz	190	9	24
Onion Ringers, 6 pces, 3.2 oz	220	12	25
Sweet Potatoes: 4 oz	80	0	18
Tater Tots: 9 pces, 3 oz	150	7	22
Mini, 19 pces, 3 oz	190	10	19
Onion, 9 pces, 3 oz	160	7	22
Extra Crispy, 12 pces, 3 oz	145	7	19
Twiced Baked: Potatoes, 1, 5 oz	190	7	26

TGI Friday's

	C	F	Cb
Potato Skins, 3 pces, 3½ oz	210	11	20

Wild Oats: Tater Bites, 9 pces, 3 oz

	C	F	Cb
Tater Bites, 9 pces, 3 oz	150	6	21
Shredded Hash Browns, 1 c., 3 oz	70	0	15
French Fries, 14 pces, 3 oz	110	3	17

Eat at least 5 servings of fruit and vegetables every day . . . and Enjoy Better Health!

Canned/Bottled   C   F   Cb

Solids & Liquid

	C	F	Cb
Artichoke Hearts: Plain, 1 oz (1)	10	0	2
Marinated, 1 oz	55	5	2
Asparagus, ½ cup, 4½ oz	20	0	3
Bamboo Shoots, ½ cup, 4½ oz	25	0	4
Bean Salad, ½ cup, 3 oz, no oil	90	0	20
Beans: Green, ½ cup, 4¼ oz	20	0	4
Baked Beans, ½ cup, 4½ oz	120	0.5	26
Butter Beans, ½ cup, 4½ oz	90	0	16
Italian, cut, ½ cup, 4½ oz	30	0	7
Kidney Beans, ½ cup, 4½ oz	105	0.5	19
Lima Beans, ½ cup, 4½ oz	80	0	15
Pinto Beans, ½ cup, 4½ oz	105	1	18
Beets: Sliced/Whole, ½ c., 4½ oz	35	0	8
Crinkle/Pickled (*Del Monte*) ½ c.	80	0	20
Carrots: Sliced, ½ cup	35	0	8
Honey Glazed (*Del Monte*) ½ c.	70	0.5	18
Corn: Kernels, ½ cup, 4½ oz	90	1	18
Drained Solids, ½ cup, 3oz	65	0.5	15
Creamed style, ½ cup, 4½ oz	100	0.5	24
Garbanzo/Chick Peas, 3 oz	100	1	20
Green Chilies: diced, 2 Tbsp, 1 oz	5	0	1
Hearts of Palm (1), 1.2 oz	7	0	1
Mushrooms: ½ cup, 2½ oz	20	0	2
in Butter Sauce, 2 oz	14	1	2
Onions: Pickled, 1 med., ¾ oz	10	0	2
Cocktail, 1 onion	0	0	0
French's Fried Onions: *See Page 72*			
Peas, ½ cup, 3 oz	60	0	10
Peppers: Hot Chili, 1 only, 1 oz	6	0	2
Sweet, undrained, 2½ oz	10	0	3
Jalapeno, w. liq., ½ c. chopped	18	0.5	3
Fried, drain, 2 Tbsp, 1 oz	60	5	3
Salsa, average all types, 2 Tbsp	15	0	3.5
Sauerkraut, undrained, ½ c., 4 oz	25	0	5
Spinach, ½ cup, 3½ oz	25	0	4
Succotash: w. Cr. Style Corn,½ c.	100	1	23
w. whole kernels, undrained	80	1	18
Sweetcorn: *See Corn*			
Sweet Potato: ½ cup, 3½ oz	80	0	20
Candied (*Green Giant*) ¾ cup	240	7	41
Tomatoes, Sundr.: Natural, 5-6 pce	22	0	5
In Oil, drained, 6 pces, ½ oz	60	4	6
Tomato Products: *See Page 85*			
Vegetables, mixed, ½ cup, 4 oz	45	0	8
Yams: in Light Syrup, ½ cup, 4 oz	105	0	25
Candied, ½ cup, 5 oz	170	0	46
Zucchini in Tom. Sce., ½ c., 4 oz	30	0	8

Salads

Take-Out Salads & Vegetables

Avg. All Outlets: Per Serving

	C	F	Cb
Antipasto Salad, 1 cup	140	10	2
Bean Salad, ½ cup	110	4	17
Bulgur Salad, ½ cup	70	2	15
Caesar Salad, Classic, 1 cup	200	14	15
Side Salad, no Dressing	25	0	6
Carrot Raisin: No Dressing, ½ cup	20	0	5
with Dressing, ½ cup	65	5	5
Chef Salad: Regular, no Dressing	620	37	6
w. 2 oz 1000 Island	860	61	8
Chicken Salad Platter, 6 oz	200	8	12
Coleslaw: Traditional, ½ cup	150	8	18
w. Low Cal Dressing	60	1	12
Corn, Mexican, ½ cup	240	12	33
Cucumber: Non-Oil Dressing, ½ c.	60	0	14
w. Oil Dressing, ½ cup	140	12	8
Eggplant Salad, ½ cup	75	5	7
Fettucini w. veges, ½ cup	110	5	15
Garden Salad, no Dressing	35	0	8
Greek Salad, 1 cup	120	10	7
Greek Vegetables, ½ cup	140	12	7
Lettuce, hearts, ¼ head	20	0	4
Lobster Salad Platter, 6 oz	200	8	12
Macaroni Salad, ½ cup, 4 oz	180	13	13
Nicoise, 1 cup	450	32	18
Pasta Salad, ½ cup	160	8	16
Pineapple Coconut Slaw, ½ cup	150	10	14
Potato Salad: Dijon	140	7	17
w. Mayonnaise, ½ cup	170	10	17
Lowfat, ½ cup	110	1.5	21
Rice Salad, ½ cup	150	10	13
Saffron Rice, ½ cup	130	3	24
Spinach Salad, 1 cup	180	13	13
Tomato & Mozzarella, ½ cup	180	14	10
Tabouli, ½ cup	150	6	22
Three Bean Salad, ½ cup	80	5	9
Tortelini w. Basil Pesto, ½ cup	170	10	19
Waldorf w. Mayo, ½ cup	160	12	12

Signature Salads: *Per Serving (6 oz)*
(Supplied to Deli's and Institutions)

	C	F	Cb
Antipasto Salad, 6 oz	510	50	4
Artichoke Salad, marinated	400	41	8
California Medley	120	7	15
Cheese Agnolotti	250	8	23
Chicken Salad	420	33	11
Crabmeat Flavored	450	38	20

Take-Out Salads (Cont)

Signature Salads (Cont)

	C	F	Cb
Egg Salad	300	23	14
Fresh Button Mushroom	190	16	6
Garden Olive	630	67	3
Ham Salad	400	32	14
Prima Pasta Salad	360	30	18
Seafood Pasta Del Mar	170	10	21
Seafood with Crab & Shrimp	420	34	20
Shrimp Salad	360	32	8
Tuna Salad	450	36	14

Fast-Food Restaurants: *See Page 183*

Fresh Salad Packs

Pre-Packaged (Supermarkets)

	C	F	Cb
Dole: Complete Caesar, 3½ oz	170	13	8
Complete Oriental, 3½ oz	120	6	13
Complete Romano, 3½ oz	150	12	9
Complete Spinach Bacon, 3½ oz	170	10	18
Complete Sunflower Ranch, 3½ oz	160	16	5
Special Blends (no added dressing),			
avg. all varieties, 2 cups, 3 oz	15	0	3
Regular Salad Packs (no added dressing):			
Classic Coleslaw, 3 oz	25	0	5
Classic Iceberg, 3 oz	15	0	4
Zesty Italian, 7 oz	110	0	4
Fresh Express: *Per Package*			
Chicken Caesar, 1 pkg, 183g	240	16	13
Chicken Crmy Ranch, 1 pkg, 194g	230	14	15
Chicken Teriyaki, 1 pkg, 193g	250	15	17
Salad Kits: *Per Serving (Prepared)*			
Caesar, 2 cups	160	14	7
Caesar w. Light Dress., 2 cups	100	7	8
Caesar Supreme, 2 cups	150	12	7
Oriental, 2 cups	140	9	13
European, 2½ cups	15	0	3
Ready Pac: Average all types	15	0	2

Salad Toppings

	C	F	Cb
Bacon Bits, average, 1 Tbsp	30	1.5	2
Chow Mein Noodles, dry, ½ cup	120	5	13
Croutons, 2 Tbsp, 10g	35	1	6
Olives, 5 medium	25	2	0
Potato Chips, 1 oz	150	10	15
Sunflower Seeds, 1 Tbsp, 8 g	45	4	1.5
Tortilla Chips, 1 oz	150	8	16

Fruit & Vegetable Juices/Smoothies

Quick Guide

	C	F	Cb
Orange Juice			
Average ~ Fresh or Sweetened:			
½ Cup, 4 fl.oz	55	0	13
Small Glass, 6 fl.oz	82	0	20
Regular Glass, 8 fl.oz	110	0	26
8¾ fl.oz Box	120	0	28
10 fl.oz Bottle	140	0	32
11½ fl.oz Can	160	0	36
16 fl.oz Bottle	220	0	52
20 fl.oz Bottle	275	0	62
64 fl.oz/½ Gallon	875	0	200

Juices ~ Generic

Average All Brands: Per 8 oz Unless Indicated	C	F	Cb
Aloe Vera Juice, unsweet., 2 oz	5	0	1
Apple Juice: 8 fl.oz	120	0	30
10 fl.oz Bottle	150	0	38
16 fl.oz	240	0	60
Carrot Juice: Fresh, 6 fl.oz	60	0	14
Sweetened, 6 fl.oz	75	0	17
Cranberry Juice, Cocktail/Blend	145	0	36
Fruit Blends, average, 8 fl.oz	110	0	27
Fruit Nectars, average, 8 fl.oz	120	0	30
Grape Juice, 8 fl.oz	160	0	40
Grapefruit Juice, 8 fl.oz	115	0	27
Lemon/Lime Juice: 1 Tbsp	3	0	1
1 cup, 8 fl.oz	50	0	15
Concentrate, 1 tsp	0	0	0
Noni Juice: *Tahitian,* 2 Tbsp, 1 fl.oz	5	0	1
Southern Cross Botanicals, 1 fl.oz	6	0	1
Tahiti Traders, 1 fl.oz	20	0	5
Orange Juice, 8 fl.oz	110	0	26
Passion Fruit Juice (Fresh):			
Purple, 1 cup, 8 fl.oz	125	0	34
Yellow, 1 cup, 8 fl.oz	150	0	36
Papaya/Peach Nectar, 8 fl.oz	120	0	31
Pear Nectar, 8 fl.oz	150	0	40
Pineapple Juice, 8 fl.oz	135	0	35
Prune Juice, 8 fl.oz	175	0	45
Strawb./Raspberry Juice, 8 fl.oz	100	0	23
Tangerine Juice, 8 fl.oz	100	0	25
Tomato Juice, 8 fl.oz	40	0	7
Vegetable Juice, 8 fl.oz	50	0	10
Wheat Grass Juice: 1 fl.oz 'Shot'	5	0	1
2 fl.oz 'Shot'	10	0	2

Quick Guide

	C	F	Cb
Fruit Smoothies			
Average All Brands:			
Fruit Only: 8 fl.oz	105	0	25
12 fl.oz	160	0	38
16 fl.oz	210	0	50
24 fl.oz	320	0.5	76
Fruit + Nonfat Milk/Soy:			
12 fl.oz	190	0.5	40
16 fl.oz	250	0.5	53
24 fl.oz	380	1	80
Fruit + Nonfat Frozen Yogurt/Sherbet:			
12 fl.oz	210	0.5	47
16 fl.oz	280	0.5	62
24 fl.oz	420	1	94

Juice Brands

Per 8 fl.oz Unless Indicated	C	F	Cb
100% Fruit Juice Boxes: *Per Box (4.2 fl.oz)*			
White Grape	90	0	22
Average other flavors	60	0	15
Ame			
Sparkling Fruit Juice: *Per 8 fl.oz*			
Ame Dry	60	0	15
Ame Red/Rose	80	0	20
Ame White	90	0	23
Apple & Eve			
Naturally Cranberry	130	0	32
Cranberry/Raspberry Apple	120	0	30
Cranberry Grape	140	0	34
Bright & Early *(Minute Maid)*			
Orange Juice (Chilled/Frozen)	110	0	30
Campbell's			
Tomato Juice: 5.5 fl.oz can	30	0	6
11.5 fl.oz	60	0	13
Capri Sun			
Sport, all flavors, 6.75 fl.oz	60	0	16
Big Pouch: *Per 11.2 oz Pouch*			
Raspberry Lemonade	200	0	50
Average other flavors	170	0	42
Clamato			
Tomato Cocktails, average, 8 fl.oz	60	0	11
Crystal Geyser			
Juice Squeeze: *Per Bottle (12 fl.oz)*			
Blackberry Pomegranate	170	0	43
Orange Lime	160	0	40
Ruby Grapefruit	150	0	36
Average other flavors	140	0	32

Juice Brands (Cont)   C   F   Cb

Per 8 fl.oz Unless Indicated

	C	F	Cb
Dole			
100% Fruit Juice Blends, 8 fl.oz	110	0	27
Donald Duck			
100% Orange Jce (+Calcium), 8 fl.oz	110	0	27
Eden, Organic Apple, 8 fl.oz	80	0	23
Five Alive *(Minute Maid)***:** Frozen Concentrate,			
made up, 8 fl.oz	120	0	30
Florida's Natural			
Cranberry Apple, 8 fl.oz	120	0	30
Orange Juice, 8 fl.oz	120	0	29
Ruby Red Grapefruit Juice, 8 fl.oz	100	0	24
Fruitopia			
All flavors, average, 8 fl.oz	115	0	30
20 fl.oz Bottle	290	0	75
Frulatte Smoothies: *Per Bottle (14 fl.oz)*			
All flavors	195	3	41
Frusia *(Cinnabon)***,** 12 fl.oz	170	0	39
Fuze: *Per 8 fl.oz*			
Energize, 8 fl.oz	100	0	26
Essentials, 8 fl.oz	60	0	15
Refresh, 8 fl.oz	90	0	24
Slenderize, 8 fl.oz	10	0	2
Focus (11% Juice): Mojo Mango	100	0	26
Vitamin Tea	60	0	16
Other varieties, average	90	0	25
Goya Nectar			
Apricot Nectar, 12 fl.oz	130	0	31
Pear Nectar, 12 fl.oz can	240	0	59
Hain: Carrot Juice w. Lutein	80	0.5	16
Veggie Juice w. Lutein, 8 fl.oz	45	0.5	11
Hansen's: Natural Juice Cocktail			
Regular, all flavors, 8 fl.oz	110	0	28
Low Calorie Peach Mango	10	0	4
Apple Varieties, 8 fl.oz	120	0	28
Junior Juice, 4.32 fl.oz box	60	0	15
Juice Slam: *Per Box (6.75 fl.oz)*			
Apple; Paradise Punch	90	0	23
Strawb. Banana; Wildberry	110	0	26
Smoothies: *Per Can (11.5 fl.oz)*			
Fruit Flavors, regular	170	0	43
Lite Cranberry Raspberry	35	0	9

Per 8 fl.oz Unless Indicated   C   F   Cb

	C	F	Cb
Hansen's (Cont)			
Smoothie Blasts: *Per Can*			
Power: Berry Blast	170	0	42
Banana Blast	220	0.5	46
Energy: Island Blast	170	0	40
Colada Blast	190	0	45
Vita Citrus Blast	170	0	43
Energy Smoothies: *See Page 159*			
Hawaiian Punch			
Fruit Juicy: Red, 6 fl.oz	90	0	22
Box, 8.45 fl.oz	120	0	30
Red Light, 6 fl.oz	45	0	11
Hawaii's Own			
Frozen Concentrate: *Per 8 fl.oz (Prep'd)*			
Average all varieties	110	0	28
Hi-C Juice Drinks: Average, 8 fl.oz	120	0	32
6.75 fl.oz box, average	100	0	27
11.5 fl.oz can	180	0	45
Blast, 6 fl.oz pouch	100	0	26
Hood: Apple, 8 fl.oz	120	0	31
Fruit Punch	130	0	32
Orange	120	0	30
Jamba Juice (California): *See Fast-Foods Section*			
Jera's Juice (Boston): *Per 24 fl.oz*			
Berry Blitz	440	2	105
Cape Codder	335	0.5	80
Citrus Burst	320	1.5	75
Mango Passion	290	0	68
Orange Bite; Flu Fighter, avg.	280	1.5	65
Razzle Dazzle	380	1	94
Soy Smoothie (7g protein)	320	3.5	68
Strawberry Smile	345	0.5	84
Triathlete (15g protein)	300	1.5	71
Whey-Out Protein (27g protein)	325	1.5	56
Juicy Juice (Libby's): *Per Box (6.75 fl.oz)*			
Grape	110	0	27
Average other flavors	100	0	24
4.23 fl.oz box, average	60	0	15
Kerns All Nectars			
Canned Juice: *Per Can (11.5 fl.oz)*			
Pear	220	0	54
Pineapple Coconut	280	8	53
Other flavors, average	210	0	52
Kool Aid			
Jammers: Sugar Jammers	10	0	2
Other varieties, 6.75 fl.oz pouch	90	0	24

Fruit & Vegetable Juices (Cont)

Juice Brands (Cont)	C	F	Cb
Per 8 fl.oz Unless Indicated			
Knudsen: *Per 8 fl.oz*			
Fruit Juices: Apple	120	0	30
Cranberry Raspberry	130	0	31
Creamed Papaya	40	0	10
Grapefruit; Just Blueberry	100	0	23
Guava Strawberry	110	0	27
Hibiscus Cooler	90	0	24
Just Concord	160	0	40
Prune	170	0	46
Tomato	60	0	14
Other varieties, average	120	0	30
Sparkling Juice, 8 fl.oz	115	0	30
Nectars: Coconut	140	5	26
Peach	120	0	30
Boysenberry, average	130	0	33
Very Veggie, 8 fl.oz	50	0	11
Simply Nutritious: Mega C	140	0	31
Blackberry Hibiscus Mist	100	0	25
Average other varieties	120	0	30
Krasdale: Cranberry Apple	170	0	42
Cranberry Juice Cocktail	130	0	32
Cranberry Raspberry	150	0	37
L & A: Black Cherry, 8 fl.oz	180	0	45
Grape Juice Plus	160	0	40
Mixed Berry	120	0	30
Prune Juice	180	0	41
Average other varieties	140	0	32

Per 8 fl.oz Unless Indicated	C	F	Cb
Lakewood Organic			
Carrot Pineapple, 6 fl.oz	85	0	19
Coconut, 6 fl.oz	90	1.5	20
Cranberry/Lemonade, 8 fl.oz	90	0	22
Mango, 6 fl.oz	90	0	22
Papaya; Pure Carrot, 6 fl.oz	75	0	18
Pure Cranberry, 6 fl.oz	50	0	12
Pure Pineapple, 6 fl.oz	95	0	23
Pure Prune, 8 fl.oz	165	0	40
Pure Pink Grapefruit, 8 fl.oz	90	0	22
Red Tart Cherry, 6 fl.oz	80	0	19
Super Veggie, 6 fl.oz	40	0	9
Average other varieties, 8 fl.oz	105	0	26
Langers: *Per 8 fl.oz*			
Apple Juice; White Cranberry avg.	120	0	28
Cranberry/100 Varieties, avg	140	0	35
Cranberry Berry	130	0	33
Cranberry Grape; White Grape	150	0	37
Cranberry Raspberry	140	0	36
Diet Apple Juice	60	0	14
Diet Cranberry/Grape	30	0	8
Seasonal Blends: *Per 8 fl.oz*			
Summer	125	0	31
Spring; Autumn; Winter	120	0	30
Frozen Concentrate: *Per 8 fl.oz (Prepared)*			
Cranberry	150	0	36
Other flavors, average	120	0	30
Luzianne: *Per 8 fl.oz (Prepared)*			
Smoothies: Mixed Berry	90	0.5	19
Peach Mango	90	0	19
Strawberry Banana	80	0.5	18
Malibu Beach: *Per 8 fl.oz*			
Teas: Tropical Tea	10	0	3
Beach Peach; Oceanside	10	0	3
Juices: Malibu Mango	10	0	3
Sunset Strawberry; Redondo	10	0	3
Martinellis			
Sparkling Juice: *Per 8 fl.oz*			
Apple-Cranberry	110	0	27
Apple-Grape	120	0	31
Cider	140	0	35
Mauna La'i Hawaiian: 8 fl.oz	140	0	32
Mistic (Mega 24 fl.oz)			
Mega 24 fl.oz: Avg. all flavors, 8 fl.oz	120	0	30
24 fl.oz	360	0	90
Tropicals, all flavors, 8 fl.oz	120	0	31
Lemon Tea, 8 fl.oz	90	0	23
Grape Strawberry, 8 fl.oz	130	0	32
Watermelon Kiwi, 8 fl.oz	110	0	28
Peach Beach, 8 fl.oz	0	0	0
Diet Lemon tea, 8 fl.oz	100	0	24

Juice Brands (Cont)   C   F   Cb

Per 8 fl.oz Unless Indicated

Minute Maid

	C	F	Cb
Orange Juice, Premium, 8 fl.oz	110	0	27
Light Orange Juice	50	0	13
Heart Wise; Kids Plus	110	0	27
Lemonade, all flavors	100	0	28
Premium Blends, avg. all flavors	110	0	27
Simply Orange	105	0	26
Tropical Punches	120	0	31
Juices to Go, avg. all flav., 11.5 fl.oz	160	0	44
Boxed Juices, average, 6.75 fl.oz	90	0	25
Coolers, average, 6.75 fl.oz	100	0	28
Disney, 6.75 fl.oz box	100	0	25
Soft Frozen Lemonade, 12 fl.oz	300	0	77
Frozen Concentrates, 8 fl.oz (Prep'd),			
Average all varieties	105	0	28

Mott's

	C	F	Cb
Apple Juice, 8 fl.oz	120	0	29
Apple Raspb., Fruit Punch, 10 fl.oz	145	0	36
Apple Cranb., Grape Apple, 10 fl.oz	180	0	42
Fruitsations, all flavors, 4 oz	85	0	22
Juice Paks: All flavors, 6.75 fl.oz	100	0	25
Mini Motts, 4.23 oz	60	0	15
Plus Lite Applejuice, 8 fl.oz	60	0	15
Juice Boxes, 6.75 fl.oz	110	0	25

Naked Juice: *Per ½ Bottle (8 fl.oz)*

	C	F	Cb
Antioxidants: Mango Acai	190	3	38
Mighty Mango C	125	0	29
Pomegranate Passion	150	0	38
Very Berry	130	0	30
Immunity: Well Being	140	0	32
Strawberry Banana C; Power-C	120	0	29
Just Juices: Just Carrot	80	0	13
Just Apple	120	0	30
Just Grapefruit	95	0	23
Just O-J	110	0	25
Tangerine Scream	110	0	25
Proteins: Protein Zone	210	3.5	27
Chocolate Karma	190	3	31
Vanilla Chai	170	2.5	27
Very Pro Berry	190	1	30
Quenchers: Just Made Lemonade	110	0	27
Raspberry-ade	90	0	22
Superfoods: Blue Machine	170	1	41
Green Machine	130	0	33
Red Machine	160	3	32

Nantucket Nectars   C   F   Cb

Juice Cocktails: *Per 8 fl.oz*

	C	F	Cb
Carrot Orange Mango	130	0	30
Cranberry	140	0	34
Fruit Punch	130	0	32
Grapeade Guava; Orange Mango	130	0	33
Other varieties, avg.	120	0	30
100% Juice: *Per 8 fl.oz*			
Cranberry Raspberry Grape	150	0	38
Grape Juice	160	0	39
Peach Orange	130	0	31
Pineapple Orange Guava	120	0	31
Premium Orange Juice	120	0	27
Other varieties, avg.	100	0	25
Fruit Juice: Apple Cider	100	0	25
Squeezed Nectar Teas: *Per Bottle (16 fl.oz)*			
Diet Lemon Tea	0	0	2
Original Lemon Tea	90	0	23
NectarFizz, all other varieties, avg.	90	0	23
Nectar Lemonades, avg., 8 fl.oz	130	0	32

Newman's Own

	C	F	Cb
Lemonade (Reg./Pink), 8 fl.oz	110	0	27
Fruit Juice Cocktail: Gorilla Grape	140	0	34
Orange Mango Tango	150	0	37
Razzma Tazz Raspberry	120	0	28

Northland

	C	F	Cb
100% Juice: *Per 8 fl.oz*			
Cranb./Peach/Blackberry; Raspb.	140	0	34
Cranberry Grape	140	0	36

Ocean Spray: *Per 8 fl.oz*

	C	F	Cb
Cranberry Cherry	150	0	39
Cranapple	160	0	41
Fruit Punch; Tangerine	130	0	32
Lite Cranberry varieties, avg.	40	0	10
Grapefruit: 100% Juice	100	0	24
Kiwi Strawb.; Summer Cooler	120	0	31
Lemonade flavors, average	130	0	32
Pink Grapefruit	120	0	30
Ruby Red & Strawberry	120	0	30
Ruby Red & Mango/Tangerine	130	0	31
Ruby Red/ White Cranberry varieties	120	0	31
White Grapefruit	100	0	24
Cranberry: Cranberry Grape	140	0	35
Cranberry Juice Cocktail	130	0	33
Light Style (Low Calorie)	40	0	10
Other Cranberry flavors, avg	150	0	39

Fruit & Vegetable Juices (Cont)

Juice Brands (Cont)   C F Cb

Odwalla

	C	F	Cb
AntioxiDance; Grapefruit, avg	90	0	21
B Berrier; Quencher	120	0	30
Carrot Juice	70	0	15
Carrot, Orange, Apple	110	0	25
Glorious Morning; B Monster	140	0	33
Mo'Beta	150	0	37
Strawberry Lemonade	110	0	28
Super Protein	190	1	35
Wellness Echinacea	150	0	34
Smoothies: Blueberry B Monster	140	0	33
C Monster	160	0	38
Blackberry Fruitshake	150	0	36
Mango Tango	150	1	34
Strawberry Banana	130	0	31
Old Orchard: Apple Juice, 8 fl.oz	120	0	29
Frozen Concentrate: *Per 8 fl.oz (Prep'd)*			
Apple	120	0	29
Other flavors	120	0	30
Orange Julius: Original (Orange, Strawberry),			
16 fl.oz	220	1	54
20 fl.oz	270	1	58
32 fl.oz	440	1	108
Other Drinks: *See Fast-Foods, Page 229*			
PS - Private Selection (Ralphs)			
Lemonade (Premium Juice), 8 fl.oz	110	0	29
Orange Juice, 8 fl.oz	110	0	27
Mango Nectar, 8 fl.oz	140	0	35
Realemon - Realime (Borden)			
Lemon/Lime Juice (from concentrate)			
1 teaspoon	0	0	0
2 Tbsp, 1 fl.oz	6	0	2
Pom Wonderful			
100% Juice: *Per 8 fl.oz*			
Pomegranate	140	0	34
Blueberry; Mango	140	0	34
Cherry	140	0	33
Tangerine	150	0	37
S&W			
Apple Juice, 8 fl.oz	120	0	30
Orange Juice, 6 fl.oz can	90	0	22
Grapefruit Juice, unswt'd, 8 fl.oz	105	0	25
Tomato Juice, 8 fl.oz	30	0	7
Santa Cruz (Organic)			
Apple Juice; Cider & Spice	120	0	30
Concord Grape; White Grape	160	0	40
Orange Mango	130	0	31
Tropical Blend	140	0	33
Average other varieties	100	0	24

Per 8 fl.oz Unless Indicated   C F Cb

Santa Cruz (Cont)

	C	F	Cb
Nectars: Apricot; Cranberry	110	0	27
Average other varieites	120	0	30
Spritzers: *Per 12 fl.oz*			
Cherry	140	0	34
Concord Grape	150	0	36
Raspberry Lemonade	120	0	24
Lemonade; Champagne Style	100	0	26
Other varieties	130	0	33
Juice Boxes: *Per 8 fl.oz*			
Lemon	110	0	28
Orange; Grape, average	100	0	25
Tropical Punch	120	0	31
Simply Juice: *Per Carafe (13 fl.oz)*			
Original; Calcium	185	0	43
Country Stand; Grove Made	110	0	26
Snapple			
Fruit Drink Blends, 8 fl.oz	120	0	29
Grapeade; Orangeade 8 fl.oz	120	0	30
Lemonade, all types	110	0	28
Vitamin Supreme	175	0	44
Diet: Snapple Apple	15	0	4
Kiwi Strawberry	20	0	5
Avg. other flavors	10	0	2
Snap.E Tom			
Tom. & Chile Cocktail, 11.5 oz can	70	0	15
Squeezit			
Average all flavors, 6.75 fl.oz	90	0	23
Stonyfield Farm: *Per Bottle (10 fl.oz)*			
Peach Smoothie	250	3	49
Wildberry; Strawberry Smoothie	250	3	46
Light Smoothies, 10 fl.oz	130	0	41
Sunny Delight			
Florida Citrus, 6 fl.oz	90	0	22
Calcium Rich, 6 fl.oz	150	0	37
Mango Citrus	130	0	31
Smooth (California Style)	130	0	32
Sunny Delight Lite, 6 fl.oz	20	0	5
Tangy Original (Florida Style)	120	0	29
Tropical Fruit Punch, 6 fl.oz	120	0	29
Sunsweet			
Prune Juice/w. Pulp, 8 fl.oz	170	0	43
Tampico: Citrus Punch, 1 cup	110	0	25
Mango/Trop. Frt. Punch, 1 cup	110	0	28
Tang			
Pouches, average all flavors (1)	90	0	24
Mix: *Prepared As Directed*			
Regular (2 Tbsp dry), 6 fl.oz	90	0	23
Light, 8 fl.oz	5	0	0

Juice Brands (Cont)

	C	F	Cb
Per 8 fl.oz Unless Indicated			
Trader Joes: *Per 8 fl.oz*			
Carrot Juice	120	0	30
Ginger Lemonade	110	0	28
Organic Carrots & Greens	80	0	19
Strawberry Lemonade	120	0	25
Strawberry Smoothie	130	1.5	30
Other varieties, average	110	0	25
Trader Darwin's (100%):			
Dairy Free Protein w. Pzazz	150	1	31
Very Green Juice Blend	130	0	33
Avg. other varieties	130	0	31
100% Juice: *Per 8 fl.oz*			
Apple Cranberry Blend	120	0	30
Original Lemonade	120	0	30
Other Apple varieties	120	0	30
All Natural Pasteurized: *Per 8 fl.oz*			
Combat; Lemon Ginger	100	0	25
Cranberry Harvest	130	0	36
Cranberry; White Grape	140	0	36
Garden Patch; Vege -10	50	0	11
Hawaiian Pineapple	110	0	29
Just Pomegranate; Concord Grape	160	0	40
Mango Lemonade	140	0	30
Mango Passion Fruit Blend	130	0	33
Rio Red Grapefruit	140	0	35
Average other varieties	125	0	30
Tree Top: *Per 6.75 fl.oz*			
Apple Juice	100	0	25
Apple Cranberry/Grape	130	0	32
Avg. other varieties	120	0	30
Frozen Concentrate, prep., 8 fl.oz	120	0	29
Tropicana: *Per 8 fl.oz*			
Blends: Berry; P'apple, 8 fl.oz	130	0	32
Essentials: Light 'n Healthy	50	0	13
Healthy Heart/Kids	110	0	26
Immunity Defense; Low Acid	110	0	26
Pure Premium: Orange-Strawb.	130	0	30
Lemonade, 8 fl.oz	190	0	47
Average other varieties	120	0	30
Twister: Average, 8 fl.oz	120	0	30
10 fl.oz bottle	150	0	40
11.5 fl.oz can	160	0	40
Light: Average, 8 fl.oz	35	0	10
10 fl.oz bottle	50	0	11
100% Juice Blends: *Per 8 fl.oz*			
Lemonade & Orangeade	100	0	28
Pineapple Orange	120	0	30
Average other flavors	140	0	33

	C	F	Cb
Per 8 fl.oz Unless Indicated			
V8® Juices & Drinks			
V8 100% Vegetable Juice, 5.5 fl.oz	35	0	7
1 Can, 12 fl.oz	70	0	15
V-8 Splash, all flavors, 8 fl.oz	80	0	19
V-8 Splash Smoothies, 8 fl.oz	90	0	20
Diet V-8 Splash, all flavors, 8 fl.oz	10	0	3
Veryfine			
Grape Juice (100%)	150	0	39
Grapefruit Juice (100%)	90	0	20
Pink	120	0	30
Papaya Punch (100%)	120	0	30
Walnut Acres: *Per 8 fl.oz*			
Organic: Apple	115	0	29
Apricot; Raspberry	130	0	32
Blueb.; Cherry; Concorde Grape	120	0	29
Cranberry	110	0	26
Incredible Vegetable	55	0	12
Peach; Pineapple	120	0	31
Welch's: *Per 8 fl.oz*			
100% Grape Juice	170	0	42
100% Red Grape Juice	170	0	44
100% White Grape Juice	160	0	39
Mountain Berry; Guava Pineapple	140	0	35
Orange Juice	120	0	30
Tomato Juice, 8 fl.oz	50	0	10
White Light Grape Juice	170	0	42
Concentrate: *Per 8 fl.oz Made Up*			
Apple	120	0	29
Grape	160	0	41
Fruit Fantastic	130	0	32
Wild Berry	140	0	36
Fruit Juice Cocktails: *Per 8 fl.oz*			
Grape; Strawberry Breeze	130	0	33
Country Pear; Wild Raspberry	145	0	35
Frozen Concentrates: *Per 8 fl.oz (Prep'd)*			
Grape	150	0	38
100% Grape	165	0	41
Strawberry Breeze	130	0	33
Orange Pineapple Apple	140	0	36
Sparkling Juice	160	0	40
Wild Oats			
Down to Earth, average, 8 fl.oz	140	0	34
Beautiful Juices, average, 8 fl.oz	120	0	27

Nutrition/Energy Shakes & Drinks

Nutritional Shakes/Drinks

Per 8 fl.oz Unless Indicated

	C	F	Cb
180 High Energy, 8.2 fl.oz	120	0	33
180 Sport, 8 fl.oz	15	0	3
ABB: Performance,			
Power Drink, 22 fl.oz	310	0	43
Blue Thunder, 22 fl.oz	300	0	43
Carbo Force, 21 fl.oz	320	0	105
Mass Recovery	380	0	60
Pure Pro Shake, Choc., 12 fl.oz	175	1	6
Weight Gain: Pure Pro, 22 fl.oz	180	0	2
Extreme XXL, 24 fl.oz	1090	0.5	215
AdvantEdge: *Per Container*			
Essential Energy Drink	190	7	21
Carb Control Ready-to-Drink	110	0	2
Complete Nutrition Ready-to-Drink	180	3	29
Airforce: All types, 250ml	0	0	0
AllSport, all flavors, 8 fl.oz	60	0	16
AMP Energy Drink, 8.4 fl.oz can	120	0	32
Amway: Positrim Drink Mix, 1 pkt	270	4	27
Trim Advantage, 11.2 oz	140	3	14
Low-Fat Drink Mix, 8 oz	170	2	28
XS Power Protein Shake, 11 oz	220	6	4
Arizona: Caution Energy, 8.3 oz	130	0	34
Caution Energy Low Carb, 8.3 oz	10	0	1
Atkins: Shake Mix, avg., 2 scoops	130	4	10
Shake Pwdr, avg. all flav., 1 scp	85	4	1
Advantage Shakes, 11 oz can	170	9	4
Balanced: Diet, avg., 11 fl.oz	180	2	35
Choc., Strawb./ Van., 11 fl.oz	230	3	35
Kids Chocolate, 8 fl.oz can	160	3	30
Bariatrix Shakes, 1 serving	100	2	6
Proti-Max Meal, 67g	250	3.5	21
Bawls Guarana, 10 fl.oz	120	0	32
Guaranexx Sugar Free, 10 fl.oz	0	0	0
Big Bang/Energy, 12 fl.oz	180	0	44
Bliss Energy Drink, 8.4 fl.oz	25	0	5
Blue Ox Energy: Citrus, 8.4 fl.oz	120	0	29
Black Cherry; Orange Rush, 8.4 fl.oz	110	0	26
Blue Sky Blue Energy, 8.3 fl.oz	110	0	27
Body Design Shakes: 2 scoops	250	3.5	37
Lite, average, 2 scoops	170	4	16
Body Fuel (w. NutraSweet), 8 fl.oz	4	0	1
Bong Water: Chronic Tonic 12 fl.oz	145	0	36
Green Dreams/Purple Haze, 12 fl.oz	165	0	42
Boost: Nutritional Energy, 8 fl.oz	240	4	41
Boost High Protein, 8 fl.oz can	240	6	33
Boost Plus, 8 fl.oz can	360	14	45
Boost w. Fiber, 8 fl.oz can	240	4	42
Breeze Juice Drink, 8 fl.oz	160	0	31
Carb Solutions Shakes, 2 scoops	120	2.5	3
Carbolite At Last! Shake, 11 oz can	150	3	8

Per 8 fl.oz Unless Indicated

	C	F	Cb
Carboplex (Unipro) mix, ½ cup, 2 oz	210	0	52
Carnation Instant Breakfast			
Powder: 1 envelope, 1.3 oz	215	0.5	39
Carb Conscious, 1 envel., 21g	150	0.5	24
Ready-To-Drink, avg, 11 fl.oz	215	5	39
CeraSport: Liquid, 11 fl.oz	70	0	17
20g package (makes 16 fl.oz)	80	0	19
Champion Lyte: Sports Drink	0	0	0
Champion Nutrition			
Heavywt Gainer 900, 4 sc., 5.4 oz	630	10	101
Ultramet: Regular, 1 pkt, 2.7 oz	280	2	24
Ultramet Lyte, 1 pkt, 2 oz	190	1	17
Ultramet Low Carb, 1 pkt, 2 oz	230	6.5	4
Choice dm: 11 fl.oz	125	25	11
Sugar-Free Shake, 12 fl.oz can	100	2.5	7
Citrucel Fiber Shake, 1 pkg	50	2	6
Crunk!!! Energy Drink, 8.2 fl.oz	120	0	29
Curves Protein Drink (mix):			
Chocolate; Vanilla, 2 scoops	100	1.5	8
made with skim milk, 8 fl.oz	190	2	23
Cytomax: 8 fl.oz	65	0	13
Powdered Mix, 1 scoop	120	1	18
Defcon3 Energy, 10 oz	40	0	10
Designer Whey Protein 1 scoop	90	1	28
Diabetitrim, Vanilla, 1 pkt	90	1	4
Dr Phil's Shape Up!: Shake, 325ml	215	3	21
Mix + Drink, 40g pkt. prep.	150	2.5	14
e10 Energy Drink, 8.4 fl.oz	5	0	0
Elements: Avg., all varieties	125	0	31
Diet Air/Ice, 8 fl.oz	10	0	2
Endura (Unipro), 2 scoops, 1.3 oz	120	0	29
Perfect Protein Shake, 8.3 fl.oz	110	0	28
Energy 69, 8.4 fl.oz	110	0	28
Ensure: High Protein, 8 oz bottle	230	6	31
Enlive! 8.1 fl.oz	300	0	65
Ensure Fiber, 8 fl.oz can	250	6	42
Ensure Plus, 8 fl.oz bottle	360	11	50
Ensure Regular, 8 fl.oz can	250	6	40
Glucerna, 8 fl.oz	235	13	23
Powder, made up, ½ cup	250	9	34
Enterex Diabetic (w/fiber), 8 fl.oz			
Carbohydrates as Maltodextrin	237	9	27
Fruit20 (Veryfine), 8/16/20 fl.oz	0	0	0
Full Throttle (Coca-Cola), 16 fl.oz	200	0	56
Sugar Free	0	0	0
Go Fast Sports: Reg., 11.9 fl.oz	190	0	28
Go Fast Light, 11.9 fl.oz	30	0	1
G-Up, 8.4 fl.oz	220	0.5	55
Gatorade: Energy Drink, 12 fl.oz	310	0	78
Lemonade/Raspb. Lem, 8 fl.oz	50	0	14
ThirstQuencher, 8 fl.oz	50	0	14
Nutrition Shake, 325ml can	370	6	62

Nutritional Shakes/Drinks (Cont)

Per 8 fl.oz Unless Indicated	**C**	**F**	**Cb**
Genisoy: Ultra XT, 1 scoop, 1.4 oz	130	0	18
XT Protein Powder, 1 scoop, 1 oz	100	0	0
Glaceau: Vitamin Water, 20 fl.oz	110	0	28
Smart Water	0	0	0
Glucerna Wt Loss Shakes, 11 oz	290	11	39
GNC Pro Performance: Total, 1 can	180	2	30
Distance, 3 scoops	370	1.5	76
MRP Advanced Sports, 1 pkt	280	3.5	22
Protein 95, 1 scp + 8 fl.oz milk	220	2	16
HMR: 70 Plus, 1 package	110	0.5	13
500	100	10	16
Hansen's: *Per Can (8.3 fl.oz)*			
Energy Original	140	0	36
Power	220	0.5	46
Slim Down	0	0	0
D-Stress; B-Well; Stamina	110	0	31
Diet Red Energy	10	0	3
Smoothies: *See Page 153*			
Hollywood Celebrity Diet, ½ cup	100	0	25
Hydra Fuel *(Tury Labs)*	65	0	16
Impulse Energy Drink, 8.3 oz	110	0	28
invigor8, all types, 8 oz	110	0	27
Isopure Perfect, 1 pkg (88g)	100	0	25
Jarrow: Whey Protein, 1 scoop	90	1	1
Muscle Optimal, 1½ scoops	155	2.5	10
Jones, avg., 1 can/8 fl.oz	120	0	30
Kashi GoLEAN Shakes: Vanilla	220	2.5	36
Chocolate, 325ml can	240	3	38
Powdered, avg., 2 scoops	220	1	32
Keto Nutritional Shake, 8 fl.oz	160	8	2
Knudsen: ReCharge, all flavors	70	0	18
Simply Nutritious, ½ bot., 16 fl.oz	120	0	30
Kombucha: Vit. Enriched, 8 fl.oz	30	0	7
Wonder Drink, 8.5 fl.oz	65	0	16
Lipovitan EB3, 8.2 fl.oz	110	0	29
Lost Energy Drink, 8.3 fl.oz can	100	0	26
Met-Rx: Original, 1 pkt	240	3	18
Lite, 1 pkt	175	1.5	15
Protein Plus, 11 fl.oz	110	1	5
Ultra, 1 pkt	265	2.5	24
Ultra Pure Protein, 11 fl.oz can	170	1	2
RTD 40, 15 fl.oz can	240	3	13
Metabolol: Endurance, 2 scp, 52g	200	5	24
Metabolol II, 2 scoops, 66g	260	3	40
Met Max, mix, 2 scoops	230	2	11

Per 8 fl.oz Unless Indicated	**C**	**F**	**Cb**
Monster Energy: Assult, 12 fl.oz	100	0	27
Low Carb, 12 fl.oz	10	0	3
MRM: Low Carb Protein, 1 scoop	120	2.5	4
Whey Protein Isolate, 1 scoop	115	1.5	1
Whey Pumped, 1 scoop	100	1	5
Myoplex: Original Shake, 17 fl.oz	310	7	20
Carb Sense Shake, 11 fl.oz	140	3.5	5
Powder, 1 pkt, 2.7 oz	270	3	23
Lite Powder, 1 pkt, 2 oz	180	2	17
Naturade: Power Shake, 1 scoop	105	1	10
Protein Booster, avg. ⅓ c. dry	110	1	3
Pure Soy, 2 Scoops (1.3 oz), dry	150	1	21
Ribo-tein, avg., 1 oz scoop	105	1	10
Total Soy: Plus, 1 scoop, 1.3 oz	140	1.5	14
Calcium Shake, Choc., 1.2 oz	120	2.5	15
Menopause Relief, 1.1 oz	120	1.5	16
Ready to Drink: 10 fl oz	205	3	31
Other flavors, avg., 1.4 oz	150	1.5	24
Nature's Best: Isopure	300	0	25
Zero Carb, 2 scoops, 2.1 oz	200	0	0
Low Carb, 2 scoops, 2.3 oz	220	0	10
Perfect Whey, 1 scoop, 0.7 oz	90	1.5	1
Nitro Speed, all flavors, 18 fl.oz	110	0	7
Noni: Tahitian/Pacific, 2 Tbsp	5	0	1
Noni Juice, 1 fl.oz	5	0	1
Liquid Hawaiian/Tahiti, 1 Tbsp	30	0	8
Nutrament *(Mead Johnson),* 12 fl.oz	360	10	52
NuVim, 1 cup, 8 fl.oz	70	0	12
Ny-Tro Pro 40, average	260	1	23
Optifast 800: Powder, 1 serving	160	3	20
Ready-To-Drink, Chocolate	160	3	20
Optimum Pro Complex, 2 scoops	245	2	4
Pedialyte *(Abbott)*	25	0	6
Pimp Juice Energy, 250ml	140	0	33
Piranha Energy *(EAS),* 8.4 oz	140	0	35
Pitbull Energy Drink, 1 can	115	0	29
Power Dream *(Imagine Foods):*			
Java Jolt, 11 fl.oz	240	4.5	42
Mango Passion, 11 fl.oz	320	4.5	65
X-Treme Choc, 11 fl.oz	260	5	48
Vanilla Blast, 11 fl.oz	240	5	39
Powerade: Regular, 12 fl.oz	90	0	25
20 fl.oz bottle	150	0	43
Light, 8 fl.oz	25	0	7
20 fl.oz bottle	65	0	18
Rev-up, all flavors, 20 fl.oz	70	0	17
PowerBar: Recovery, 1 scoop	90	0	20
Endurance, 1 scoop, 0.7 oz	70	0	17
Power Gel, Chocolate, 1.5 oz	110	0	28
Pria, 11 fl.oz	170	5	21

Nutrition/Energy Shakes & Drinks (Cont)

Nutritional Shakes/Drinks (Cont)

Per 8 fl.oz Unless Indicated

	C	F	Cb
ProBalance, 8.45 fl.oz	800	41	156
Pro-Cal 100 (R-Kane), 1 pkt	105	2	7
Red Bull Energy Drink, 8.3 fl.oz	113	0	28
Sugar-Free, 1 can	10	0	3
Red Devil Energy Drink, 12 fl.oz	120	0	31
Red Tiger Energy Drink, 8.2 fl.oz	115	0	28
Resource (Novartis): Plus, 8 fl.oz	360	11	52
Bene Protein, 1 scoop	25	0	0
Health Shake, 4 fl.oz	200	4	35
Shake, 6 fl.oz	270	6	45
Standard 8 fl.oz pak	250	6	40
Diabetic, 8 fl.oz pak	250	11	23
Revenge Pro (Champ. Nutr.), 1 oz	100	0	20
Pro-Score 100, 2 scoops	160	2	1.5
Revival Soy Mix: Plain Soy, 1 pkg	120	2	6
Chocolate Day Dream, 1 pkg	240	3	36
Other varieties, avg., 1 pkg	225	2	33
Rhino's Energy Drink, 250ml can	125	0	31
Ripit Energy Fuel-Power, 8 fl.oz	130	0	32
Rite Aid: Nutritional Suppl., 8 oz	250	6	40
Rite Aid Plus, 8 oz	360	11	50
Rockstar: Energy Drink, 8 fl.oz	110	0	29
Diet Energy Drink, 8 fl.oz	10	0	2
Sav-on Nut'l: 8 fl.oz can	360	13	47
Light, 8 fl.oz can	200	3	33
Scan Diet (Soy-base), 1 scoop	160	3	21
Shark Energy Drink, 1 can	140	0	35
Slim-Fast			
Original: *Per 10.8 fl.oz Can*			
Ready To Drink Shake	220	3	40
Lower Carb Diet Shake	180	9	14
Optima: *Per Serving*			
Shake, 10.4 fl.oz can	180	5	24
Smoothie, 10.4 fl.oz can	190	5	22
Powder Shake Mix: 1 scp, ⅓ cup	100	4	17
w. 8 fl.oz fat-free milk	190	4	29
Snapple: Low Carb, 11.3 fl.oz	90	0	16
Adrenaline, 8.3 oz	140	0	37
Meal Replacement, 11.3 fl.oz	210	0	43
SoBe: Power, avg., 8 fl.oz	120	0	32
Fountain, 8 fl.oz	110	0	30
Ice, 8 fl.oz	110	0	31
Synergy, 11.5 oz	120	0	32
Special Recipes, 8 fl.ox	115	0	31
Juice Elixers, 8 fl.oz	100	0	26
Lean, all flavors, 8 fl.oz	5	0	1
Lizard, avg. all types, 8 fl.oz	120	0	31
No Fear, 8 fl.oz	130	0	36

Per 8 fl.oz Unless Indicated

	C	F	Cb
Solaray Soytein (Protein Energy Meal),			
Natural, 1 heaping scoop, 24g	70	0.5	5
Flav., avg., 1 heaping scoop, 32g	110	1	12
Sport Pharma Biomax, 2 scoops	250	3.5	6
Spiru-Tein Powder, 1 scp, avg., 35g	120	0.5	15
Sunny D Intense Sport, 11.3 oz	60	0	16
Sweet Success (Nestlé):			
Healthy Shake, 10 oz can	200	2.5	32
Fruit Flavors, 10 fl.oz	200	0.5	39
Powder, 2 scoops, 32g (1.1 oz)	100	1	25
Synergy: Mystic Mango, 16 fl.oz	100	0	24
Other flavors, 16 fl.oz	70	0	16
The Sports Club/LA, PTS Protein Powder,			
Choc/Mocha/Van., 2 scoops, 1 oz	112	3	5
Total Balance: 9.5 oz can	230	7	25
Drink Mix, avg., 2 scoops	180	6	21
Twin Lab: Ultra Fuel, 16 fl.oz	400	0	100
RxFuel, 1 pkt	250	0	62
Energy Fuel, 250ml can	0	0	0
Vege Fuel	130	1.5	0
Usana: Nutrimeal, 2 scoops, 43g	150	3.5	20
Fiergy Drink, 2 scoops	120	1.5	31
SoyaMax, 2 scoops	110	1	1
Vital Cal Shake, 7.5 fl.oz can	290	9	43
Walgreens Nutritional Drinks			
Nutritional Drink, 8 oz can	250	6	40
Plus, 8 oz can	350	11	50
Slim for Less, 8 oz can	225	3	40
Weider (Powders)			
Creatine ATP, ½ cup, 1.7 oz	210	0	37
Mass 1000, 1⅓ cups	740	4	146
Ultra Whey Pro, ⅓ cup, 1 oz	110	1	4
Dynamic:			
Muscle Builder, 2 scps, ½ c., 45g	150	1.5	21
Weight Gainer, 4 scps, ⅔ c.,85g	450	3	93
Worldwide: Carbo Rush, 20 fl.oz	285	0	60
Fat Shredder, 20 fl.oz bottle	15	0	4
Pure Protein, 22 fl.oz bottle	170	0	0
Rapid Recovery, 20 fl.oz	280	0	25
Thermo 525, 20 fl.oz bottle	5	0	1
XS Energy Citrus/Energy, 8.4 fl.oz	8	0	0
Zone Perfect: Shake Mix, 2 scps	225	7	23
Protein Powder, 1 scoop	30	0	0
Nutritional Drinks, avg., 8 fl.oz	250	8	27

Quick Guide

Cola Soda Drinks

Average All Brands
Includes *Coca-Cola* and *Pepsi*

	C	F	Cb
8 fl.oz Cup	100	0	25
12 fl.oz Can	150	0	37
16 fl.oz Bottle	200	0	50
20 fl.oz Bottle	250	0	63
24 fl.oz (Pepsi)	300	0	75
1-Liter Bottle (34 fl.oz)	400	0	100
2-Liter Bottle (68 fl.oz)	800	0	200

Other Soda Drinks *(Average All Brands)*

	C	F	Cb
Club Soda, 12 fl.oz	0	0	0
Club Soda Cream, 12 fl.oz	170	0	42
Diet Soft Drinks, avg., 12 fl.oz	0	0	0
Ginger Ale, 12 fl.oz	120	0	30
Lemon Lime, 12 fl.oz	220	0	55
Orange, 12 fl.oz	180	0	45
Root Beer, 12 fl.oz	165	0	41
Tonic Water, 12 fl.oz	135	0	34
Mineral Water: Plain, 12 fl.oz	0	0	0
Sweetened/flavored, 12 fl.oz	150	0	37
w. Fruit Juice, 12 fl.oz	120	0	30
Seltzers: Plain/Diet, 12 fl.oz	0	0	0
Sweetened/flavored, 12 fl.oz	150	0	37
w. Fruit Juice, 12 fl.oz	120	0	30
Soft Frozen Lemonade, 12 fl.oz	300	0	78

Fountain, Movie Theater & Take-Out

Average All Flavors

	C	F	Cb
Small Cup, 12 fl.oz: No Ice	160	0	40
With ⅓ Ice	120	0	30
Regular, 16 fl.oz: No Ice	210	0	53
With ⅓ Ice	160	0	40
Medium, 22 fl.oz: No Ice	290	0	73
With ⅓ Ice	220	0	55
Large, 32 fl.oz: No Ice	420	0	105
With ⅓ Ice	320	0	80

(Note: ⅓ Cup of Ice = ¼ Cup Liquid)

Soda Brands

Per 12 fl.oz Unless Indicated

	C	F	Cb
A&W: Cream Soda	165	0	41
Diet Cream Soda/Root Beer	1	0	0
Root Beer	180	0	45
Albertson's: Cola	160	0	43
Lemon Lime	140	0	38
Other flavors, average	170	0	47

Soda Brands (Cont)

Per 12 fl.oz Unless Indicated

	C	F	Cb
Barq's: Root Beer	165	0	41
Floatz, 12 fl.oz	190	0	48
Barrelhead, Rootbeer	165	0	41
Big Red, 12 fl.oz	150	0	38
Blue Sky: Cola; Orange Cream	160	0	44
Cherry; Raspberry; Root Beer	180	0	45
Grape; Lemon Lime; Dr Becker	140	0	36
Organic, all flavors	170	0	43
Other varieties, average	150	0	39
Bubble Up, 12 fl.oz	160	0	42
Cactus Cooler, 12 fl.oz	150	0	40
Canada Dry: Club Soda	0	0	0
Ginger Ale, all flavors	135	0	37
Tonic Water/Twist Lime	150	0	37
Diet, 12 fl.oz	0	0	0
Clearly Canadian, avg., 11 fl.oz	90	0	33
Coca-Cola: Classic/Caffeine Free	140	0	39
Diet Coke, all flavors	0	0	0
Cherry Coke/Vanilla Coke	150	0	40
Coca-Cola Zero	0	0	0
Cragmont: Cola	165	0	41
Cherry	180	0	45
Diet, all flavors	0	0	0
Crush, all flavors	210	0	52
Crystal Light, all flavors	8	0	2
Diet Coke, all flavors	0	0	0
Diet Rite, all flavors	1	0	0
Dr Diablo, Cola	140	0	35
Dr Nehi, 12 fl.oz	150	0	40
Dr Pepper: Reg./Red Fusion	150	0	40
Cherry Vanilla	140	0	39
Diet, all flavors	0	0	0
Fanta: Orange; Grape	180	0	45
Strawberry; Pineapple	180	0	48
Fresca, 12 fl.oz	4	0	1
Fruitopia: *See Page 153*			
GuS, average all flavors	100	0	25
Hansen's: Diet Soda	0	0	0
Natural Orange Mango, 8 fl.oz	170	0	46
Other flavors, average	150	0	44
Hawaiian Punch, all flavors	180	0	45
Health Valley			
Ginger Ale; Sarsp. Root Beer	150	0	41
Rootbeer Old Fashioned	120	0	30
Hires: Cream; Root Beer	180	0	45
IBC: Root Beer	110	0	29
Cream Soda; Black Cherry	180	0	48
Diet Root Beer	0	0	0

Soft Drinks (Cont)

Per 12 fl.oz Unless Indicated

	C	F	Cb
Icee: Coca-Cola, 12 fl.oz	105	0	27
Barg's; Minute Maid, 12 fl.oz	195	0	48
Smoothee Lemonade, 12 fl.oz	255	0	64
Jolt Cola, 12 fl.oz	150	0	41
Knudsen, Spritzers, average	170	0	43
Lucozade, 7 fl.oz	136	0	34
Mello Yello: Regular	180	0	45
Diet, 12 fl.oz	5	0	0
Minute Maid: Lemonade	160	0	40
Fruit Punch; Grape; Strawberry	180	0	45
Lemonade	160	0	40
Valencia Orange; Mixed Berry	180	0	50
Other regular flavors	165	0	41
Light Valencia Orange	10	0	2
Soft Frozen Lemonade, 12 fl.oz	300	0	78
Mistic: Punch, 16 fl.oz	230	0	57
'N Juice, average	155	0	38
Sparkling, average, 11.1 fl.oz	115	0	28
Mountain Dew: Live Wire; Code Red	170	0	45
Diet flavors	0	0	0
Moxie: Original Elixir	150	0	37
Mr Pibb, Regular	150	0	37
Mug Root Beer	160	0	43
Natural Brew: Vanilla, Cream	170	0	43
Ginseng Cola, Ginger Ale	170	0	43
Orange; Grapefruit, avg.	155	0	39
Nehi (Royal Crown): Cream	180	0	45
Ginger Ale, Quinine Water	135	0	45
Other flavors, average	195	0	45
Orangina: 10 fl.oz bottle	120	0	45
Rouge, 8 fl.oz	90	0	22
Pepsi: Regular/Blue/Caffeine Free	165	0	41
Diet Pepsi	0	0	0
One, 12 fl.oz	1	0	0.5
Twist	160	0	40
Wild Cherry; Vanilla	165	0	43
Perrier, Regular or flavors	0	0	0
Qibla-Gold, 330ml can	185	0	46
Ramblin' Root Beer, 12 fl.oz	180	0	45
RC Cola: Regular; Cherry	160	0	40
Diet Cola	1	0	0
Reed's: Spiced Apple Brew	160	0	41
Ginger Brew, avg. all varieties	145	0	38
7-UP: Regular	140	0	38
Cherry, Gold	155	0	38
Caffeinated	170	0	46
Diet varieties, 12 fl.oz	0	0	0
7-UP Plus, 12 fl.oz	12	0	3
Santa Cruz, Sparkling, all types	150	0	37
Schweppes: Bitter Lemon/Sour	165	0	41
Seltzer	0	0	0
Tonic Water; Ginger Ale	120	0	30

Per 12 fl.oz Unless Indicated

	C	F	Cb
Shasta: Black Cherry	170	0	46
Cherry Cola; Doc Shasta	160	0	40
Club Soda; Diet, all flavors	0	0	0
Cola, regular	170	0	46
Caffeine Free	160	0	40
Cream Soda	190	0	47
Fruit Punch, Pineapple	200	0	50
French Vanilla Cola	180	0	45
Ginger Ale	130	0	33
Orange	200	0	49
Root Beer	170	0	42
Sierra Mist, Lemon Lime	150	0	39
Slice: Lemon Lime	150	0	38
Diet Lemon Lime	0	0	0
Orange	190	0	50
Diet Orange	0	0	0
Sprite: Regular	150	0	37
Diet, 12 fl.oz	4	0	1
Tropical Remix	140	0	38
Squirt: Citrus Burst	150	0	40
Diet Citrus Burst	0	0	0
Ruby Red Soda	170	0	46
Star Ruby: Dry Valencia Orange	100	0	26
Other flavors	95	0	24
Sunkist: Average all flavors	210	0	52
Diet Citrus	0	0	0
Diet Orange	7	0	1.5
Surge, Citrus	170	0	46
TAB, 12 fl.oz	0	0	0
Think!: Root Beer, 8.4 fl.oz	118	0	27
Sparkling Citrus, 8.4 fl.oz	130	0	31
Cola, 8.4 fl.oz	112	0	29
Upper 10 (RC): Regular	150	0	37
Diet, 12 fl.oz	4	0	1
Vernor's: Ginger Ale	150	0	37
Diet, 10 fl.oz	0	0	0
Welch's Sparkling, average	180	0	45
Wild Oats: Down to Earth	150	0	37
Wink, 12 fl.oz	195	0	48

Powdered Soft Drink Mix

Per 8 fl.oz (Prep'd)

	C	F	Cb
Country Time: Lemonade	60	0	16
Other flavors, avg.	85	0	22
Crystal Light, 8 fl.oz	5	0	1
Flavoraid: 1/8 pkg	2	0	0.5
Sugar-Free, 8 fl.oz	5	0	1
Kool-Aid: All flavors	70	0	17
Unsweetened, 6 fl.oz	2	0	0.5
Tang, 8 fl.oz	100	0	24

Instant Coffee

	C	F	Cb
Powder/Granules: Regular or Decaffeinated,			
1 level tsp	2	0	0.5
1 rounded tsp	4	0	1
Ground, 1 Tbsp	5	0	1
Brewed/Percolated, 1 cup, 8 fl.oz	5	0	1
Coffee With Milk/Cream/Creamers:			
Per Cup Coffee (8 fl.oz):			
w. Whole Milk: Dash, 1 Tbsp	10	0.5	1
2 Tbsp, 1 fl.oz	20	1	1.5
w. 2% Milk, 2 Tbsp	15	0.5	1.5
w. 1% Milk, 2 Tbsp	12	0.3	1.5
w. Fat Free Milk, 2 Tbsp	10	0	1.5
w. Half & Half, 2 Tbsp	45	4	1
w. Cream (light coffee), 2 Tbsp	65	6	1
w. *Coffee Mate:* Liquid, reg., 1T.	40	2	5
Liquid Fat Free, 1 Tbsp	15	0	2
Powder, 1 heaping tsp	20	1	2
Sugar ~ Add Extra: 1 heaping tsp	25	0	6
Single portion, 1 package	25	0	6

Flavored Coffee Mixes

	C	F	Cb
Chicory: Instant Coffee, 1 tsp	6	0	1
Coffee Essence, 1 tsp	16	0	4
Caffé D'Vita: Mixes, ½ oz	65	2.5	9
Chai Mixes, ½ oz	125	3.5	21
Sugar Free Mixes, ½ oz	35	2	3
General Foods: Average, ½ oz	60	3	10
Sugar-free, average, 1 tsp	30	1.5	3
Cappuccino Coolers, ½ oz	60	0	15
Maxwell House: Mocha, 1 envelope	100	2.5	17
Mocha, sugar-free, 1 envelope	60	3	7
Van., Irish Cream, 1 envelope	90	1	20
Nescafé: Frothé, all flavors, average	90	1.5	19
Ice Java, 2 Tbsp	80	0	19

Coffee Substitute Mixes

Roasted Cereal Beverages: (No Caffeine)

	C	F	Cb
Cafix Instant Beverage, 1 tsp	6	0	1
Kaffree Roma *(Natural Touch)* , 1 tsp	6	0	1
Postum, Instant Hot Beverage, 1 tsp	12	0	3
Revival Soy "Coffee", 1 Tbsp	5	0	1
Teeccino Caffe, 1 tsp	10	0	2

Vending Machine

	C	F	Cb
Cappuccino, 1 cup, 8 fl.oz	70	4	6

Coffee Shops/Restaurants

Per 8 fl.oz Cup (Unless Indicated)

	C	F	Cb
Coffee (Regular/Percolated/Filtered)	5	0	1
Americano Drip Coffee, 1 cup	5	0	1
Cafe Au Lait: 1 cup, 8 fl.oz	65	2.5	6
Nonfat Milk, 1 cup	45	0	7
Caffe Latté:			
8 fl.oz cup: w. Whole Milk	100	5	8
w. 2% Milk	80	2.5	8
w. Nonfat Milk	60	0	8
12 fl.oz: w. Whole Milk	180	10	14
w. Nonfat Milk	110	0.5	15
16 fl.oz: w. Whole Milk	200	10	16
w. Nonfat Milk	120	0	16
Cafe Mocha (Mochaccino): 1 cup	120	3	15
12 fl.oz	180	4.5	15
16 fl.oz	240	6	15
Cappuccino:			
8 fl.oz cup: w. Whole Milk	70	4	6
w. 2% Milk	60	2	6
w. Nonfat Milk	40	0	6
12 fl.oz: w. Whole Milk	110	6	9
w. 2% Milk	80	3	9
w. Nonfat Milk	60	0	9
16 fl.oz: w. Whole Milk	140	7	12
w. Nonfat Milk	80	0	12
Mocha (with cream):			
8 fl.oz: w. Whole Milk	180	12	16
w. Nonfat Milk	150	8	16
Tall, 12 fl.oz: Whole Milk	290	18	25
w. Nonfat Milk	230	11	26
Iced Mocha (no cream):			
Tall, 12 fl.oz: w. Whole Milk	190	9	24
w. Nonfat Milk	140	2	24
Espresso: Regular	4	0	1
Doppio (Double)	8	0	2
Espresso Con Panna,			
(w. dollop whipped cream)	30	3	1
Espresso Macchiato, regular	15	0.5	2
Frappuccino: Tall, 12 fl.oz.	200	3	39
Grande, 16 fl.oz	270	4	52
Frappuccino Mocha:			
Large/Tall, 12 fl.oz	230	3	44
Grande, 16 fl.oz	310	4.5	59
Iced Latte: *Similar to Caffe Latte*			
Intellicino: 12 fl.oz	150	7	15
Lowfat (2% Milk)	120	3.5	5
Starbucks: *See Fast-Foods Section*			

Hot Chocolate ♦ Caffeine Counter

Irish & Liqueur Coffees

	C	F	Cb
Irish Coffee (no sugar)	175	10	0
Liqueur Coffee, avg. all types	200	10	16

Cocoa & Hot Chocolate

	C	F	Cb
Cocoa (8 fl.oz cup): w. Whole Milk	210	14	19
w. Nonfat Milk	80	8	2
Tall (12 fl.oz): w. Whole Milk	300	20	26
w. Nonfat Milk	120	11	5
Hot Chocolate:			
8 fl.oz cup: w. Whole Milk	200	10	25
w. Nonfat Milk	140	2	25
Tall (12 fl.oz): w. Whole Milk	300	15	38
w. Nonfat Milk	210	3	38
Cinnabon, Mocholatta Chill, 16 oz	410	18	54

Coffee Extras

	C	F	Cb
Chocolate (Cocoa) Topping, ½ tsp	10	0	2
Flavored Syrups: Regular, 2 Tbsp	80	0	20
Sugar-free, 2 Tbsp	0	0	0
Half & Half Cream, 2 Tbsp	40	3	1
Light Whipped Cream, 2 Tbsp	30	2	2
Marshmallows, miniature, 2	20	0	5
Hershey's Chocolate Syrup, 2 Tbsp	100	0	24

Bottled Coffee (Chilled)

Ready-To-Drink: *Per Bottle*

	C	F	Cb
AdvantEdge Coffee House, 11 fl.oz	110	3	3
Arizona Mocha Latte 10½ fl.oz	130	2	24
Blue Luna: Cafe Latte 12½ fl.oz	195	3	36
Lite Cafe Mocha, 12½ fl.oz	114	3	15
Jakada (Folgers) Coffee Latte:			
French Roast, 10½ fl.oz	170	3.5	31
Mocha, Vanilla, 10½ fl.oz	180	3.5	33
Jaradelic (Planet Java), 9½ fl.oz	180	3	34
Kahlúa Cappuccino Shake 15½ fl.oz	195	4	36
Main St Cafe:			
French Vanilla Ice Latte, 12 fl.oz	190	4	31
Meadow Gold Mocha Latte	450	16	61
Nescafe: Caffe Latte	140	3.5	23
Mocha	140	3	26
Royal Mills: *Per Can*			
Hawaiian Kona; Iced, 10.8 oz	125	2	27
Iced Cappuccino, 10.8 oz	165	3	32
Island Mocha, 10.8 oz	220	3.5	42
Kona Blend, 11.5 oz	90	1.5	18
Starbucks: *Per 9.5 fl.oz Bottle*			
Frappuccino: Caramel	200	4	37
Coffee	190	3.5	35
Hazelnut; Mocha	200	3.5	37
DoubleShot, 6.5 fl.oz can	140	6	18

Caffeine Counter

Moderate caffeine intake is not harmful to healthy adults. However, frequent large amounts (over 350mg/day) may cause dependency ('caffeinism') and adversely affect health. To be safe, limit caffeine to 200mg/day. Avoid if pregnant; breast feeding; a child under 8; or have heart arrhythmias.

	Caffeine (mg)
Coffee: Instant, Weak, 1 level teaspoon	45
Medium, 1 rounded teaspoon	70
Strong, 1 heaping teaspoon	100
Decaffeinated, 1 round teaspoon	2
Bags (Folgers), 1 bag (6-8 fl.oz)	115
Ground, 1 Tbsp, 6g	60
Bottled (Ready-to-Drink), 9.5 fl.oz	70
Coffee Shop: Brewed, 8 fl.oz	110 - 150
Cappuccino: 1 cup, 8 fl.oz	80
Tall, 12 fl.oz	120
Large, 16 fl.oz	160
Decappuccino (decaffeinated)	5
Espresso: Regular/Solo	80
Double (Doppio) Espresso	160
Iced Coffee, 12 fl.oz	80
Latte, 12 fl.oz	80
Mocha, 8 fl.oz	90
Hot Chocolate, 8 fl.oz	10
Tea (Black/Green): Weak, 1 cup	20
Medium Strength, 1 cup	40
Strong, 1 cup	70
Herbal Tea	0
Iced Tea, Tall Glass/Can, 12 fl.oz	25
Soda Drinks: *Per 12 fl.oz Can*	
Coca-Cola (Classic/Van./Cherry); *Pepsi* (Reg./Diet)	35
Diet Coke; TAB; RC Cola (Regular)	45
Dr. Pepper (Reg./Diet)	40
Sunkist Orange Soda; *Mr PiBB*	40
Jolt Cola; *SunDrop*	65 - 70
Pepsi One; Mtn Dew; Mellow Yellow; Surge	55
Energy Drinks (w. caffeine): Avg., 8 fl.oz	80
Full Throttle, 16 fl.oz can	150
Red Bull (Regular/Sugar Free), 8.3 fl.oz	80
Tilt (Anheuser-Busch), alcoholic, 16 fl.oz	70
B-to-the-E, alcoholic, 10 fl.oz	60
Chocolate Bars: Milk Chocolate, 2 oz	12
Dark Chocolate, 2 oz	30
Cocoa/Hot Choc. Mix, 1 oz pkt	5
Chocolate Milk, 1 cup, 8 fl.oz	5
Choc Chip Cookies, 1 medium, 1 oz	3
Chocolate Syrup, 2 Tbsp, 1.4 oz	7

Extensive Caffeine Counter ~ www.CalorieKing.com

Quick Guide

Teas

	C	F	Cb
Regular: Bag, Loose or Instant			
Brewed, 1 cup, 8 fl.oz	1	0	0
(Add extra for sugar/milk)			
Herbal: Average all varieties, 1 cup	1	0	0
Bigelow: Apple Orchard, 1 cup	5	0	1
Other Varieties	2	0	0.5
Celestial Seasonings:			
Bengal Spice; Spearmint	5	0	0.5
Lemon Zinger	4	0	1
Roastaroma	10	0	2
Other varieties	2	0	0.5
Bubble Tea, average, 12 fl.oz	240	0	55
Chai Tea *(Starbucks):* See Fast-Foods Section			
Tazo Tea *(Starbucks):* See Fast-Foods Section			

Iced Tea

	C	F	Cb
Average All Brands			
Pre-Sweetened: 8 fl.oz	100	0	25
12 fl.oz	150	0	38
16 fl.oz	200	0	50
Unsweetened: 8 fl.oz	2	0	0

Iced Tea Mixes

Per Serving (1 Cup, Made-Up)

	C	F	Cb
4C Instant	90	0	22
Bigelow Nice Over Ice	1	0	0.5
Carb Options, 1 cup	0	0	0
Celestial Seasonings Iced Delight	4	0	1
Crystal Light Sugar Free	3	0	0
Kool-Aid Fruit T's	70	0	17
Lipton: Instant	0	0	0
Instant Lemon/Raspberry	3	0	1
Lemon	55	0	14
Peach/Raspb, Sugar Free	5	0	1
Nestea: 100% Instant	2	0	0
Decaffeinated	6	0	1
Ice Teasers, all flavors	6	0	1
Peach, Raspberry	90	0	22

> ❝ *A woman is like a teabag. You never know her strength until she's in hot water.* ❞
>
> ~ Eleanor Roosevelt

Bottled & Canned Teas

Per 8 fl.oz Unless Indicated

	C	F	Cb
Arizona: Sweet Tea	90	0	23
Green Tea(s)/Asian Plum; Herb	70	0	18
Diet Green/Lemon	0	0	0
Ginseng Tea	60	0	15
Peach/Raspberry	100	0	25
No Carb, all flavors	5	0	2
Brisk: Raspberry, 1 can	95	0	24
Diet	5	0	1
Lemon: 8 fl.oz can	90	0	23
24 fl.oz Bottle	80	0	22
Hansen's: Natural Iced Tea, 8 fl.oz	70	0	21
Low Calorie Blueberry/Raspberry	10	0	3
Honest Tea: Green Dragon, 16 fl.oz	60	0	18
Lori's Lemon Tea	0	0	0
Knudsen Coolers, all flavors	90	0	23
Lipton (16 fl.oz Bottle): *Per 8 fl.oz*			
No Lemon	70	0	18
Lemon	90	0	21
Peach; Raspberry	110	0	26
Mistic Tropical Cooler, 8 fl.oz	45	0	12
Nantucket: Blueberry Tea, 8 fl.oz	80	0	20
Original Lemon Tea; Half & Half	90	0	23
Diet Lemon Tea	10	0	2
Nestea Iced Tea: Diet Lemon	3	0	0.5
Cool from Nestea, 1 can, 8 fl.oz	80	0	20
Diet Cool from Nestea	2	0	0.5
Lemon/Peach/Raspberry	90	0	22
Sweetened Ice Tea	90	0	23
Oregon Chai: Herbal Bliss, ½ cup	70	0	18
Nirvana/Kashmir Green, ½ cup	80	0	20
Royal Mistic: Regular, 12 fl.oz	145	0	36
Diet, 12 fl.oz	8	0	2
Schweppes, 8 fl.oz	90	0	22
Shasta, 8 fl.oz	80	0	20
Snapple: Reg., sweetened, avg.	105	0	26
Diet/Unsweetened	0	0	0
SoBe: Green/Lemon Tea, 8 fl.oz	90	0	23
20 fl.oz bottle	225	0	57
Ssips *(Johanna Farms),* 8.45 fl.oz	100	0	25
Tazo: Iced Teas, 8 fl.oz	70	0	17
Juiced Teas, 8 fl.oz	85	0	21
Organic Iced Teas, 8 fl.oz	35	0	9
Tropicana: Lemonfruit	100	0	25
Diet Lemon Fruit	15	0	4
Peach/Rasp./Tangerine, 8 fl.oz	120	0	28
11.5 fl.oz can	160	0	40
Twister: Apple Berry, 8 fl.oz	100	0	28
Turkey Hill: Regular	90	0	22
Raspberry Cooler	110	0	28

Alcohol Guide

♦ **Health Hazards: Excessive alcohol intake** contributes to obesity, high blood pressure, stroke, heart and liver disease, some cancers, and even impotence. **Concentration and short-term memory** are reduced as well as sporting performance.

Other alcohol hazards include stomach upsets, menstrual problems, anxiety, headaches, insomnia, work absenteeism, risky behaviors, and social problems.

Excess alcohol contributes to obesity and high blood pressure

♦ **Alcohol contributes to obesity** through its high calories and by lessening the body's ability to burn fat. Fat storage is promoted, particularly in the belly - a health danger zone. Alcohol can also stimulate the appetite.

♦ **Alcohol is potentially more harmful while dieting.** Blood sugar levels may drop with resultant tiredness and further impairment of concentration, reflexes and driving skills - and maybe even the dieter's resolve!

SAFE ALCOHOL LIMITS

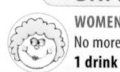 **WOMEN:** No more than **1 drink** per day.

 MEN: No more than **2 drinks** per day.

(At least 2 days a week should be alcohol-free.)

1 DRINK CONTAINS 14 GRAMS ALCOHOL →
- 12 fl.oz Regular Beer (5% Alc.)
- OR 14 fl.oz Light Beer (4.2% Alc.)
- OR 5 fl.oz Wine (12% Alc.)
- OR 1½ fl.oz Spirits (80 Proof)

Note: You cannot save daily drinks for one occasion.

Binge drinking is particularly harmful ~ 4 drinks 'in a row' for males or 3 drinks for females.

For some people, **safe drinking** will mean no alcohol drinks at all. (Even one drink may impair driving skills, particularly if tired; and 3-4 drinks daily has been linked to brain shrinkage in some social drinkers).

♦ **It is advisable not to drink at all if you are:**
- pregnant or trying to conceive
- taking medication or have liver or heart disease (unless approved by your doctor or pharmacist)
- planning to drive, use machinery or play sport
- studying or needing to concentrate
- a child or adolescent

Note: Women and adolescents are more prone to alcohol's ill-effects due to their lower body weight, smaller livers and lesser capacity to metabolize alcohol.

♦ **Ten Hints to Avoid Harmful Drinking:** See Page 172

HOW TO CALCULATE ALCOHOL CONTENT

Percent alcohol on label refers to alcohol volume (ml alcohol/100ml).

100ml = 3½ fl. oz

To convert to grams (weight) of alcohol, multiply the percent volume by 0.8 - since 1 ml of alcohol weighs only 0.8 grams.

EXAMPLE
12 fl.oz Can Beer (5% alcohol)

5% alc.volume = 5% of 12 fl.oz
= 0.6 fl.oz
= 18ml alcohol
(1 fl.oz = 30ml)

Weight (18ml x 0.8) = 14.4g alc.

GOVERNMENT WARNINGS!

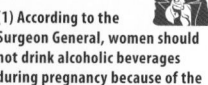

(1) According to the Surgeon General, women should not drink alcoholic beverages during pregnancy because of the risk of birth defects.

(2) Consumption of alcoholic beverages impairs your ability to drive a car or operate machinery, and may cause health problems.

Quick Guide   Alc ~ Alcohol (Grams)   Cb ~ Carbohydrate

Beer

Beer Contains Zero Fat

	C	Alc	Cb
Regular Beer (5% Alc. Vol.)			
7 fl.oz Glass	80	8.5	4
12 fl.oz Bottle/Can/Glass	140	14	10
16 fl.oz Bottle/Can	185	19	13
22 fl.oz Bottle	260	25	20
24 fl.oz Can	280	28	20
32 fl.oz Bottle	370	35	28
40 fl.oz Bottle	470	46	35
50 fl.oz Football	590	57	50
Light Beer (4.2% Alc. Vol.)			
7 fl.oz Glass	65	7	4
12 fl.oz Bottle/Can/Glass	110	12	7
16 fl.oz Bottle/Can	145	16	9
22 fl.oz Bottle	200	22	13
24 fl.oz Can	220	24	14

Non-Alcoholic/Near Beer
(Less than 0.5% alcohol by volume)

	C	Alc	Cb
Average All Brands, 12 fl.oz	80	1	7

Beer Brands

Per 12 fl.oz Serving   Alc ~ Alcohol (Grams)

Percentage alcohol listed below is by volume - not by weight.

	C	Alc	Cb
Amber Ice (5.3% alcohol)	130	15	6
Amstel Light (3.5%)	100	10	5
Anheuser World Select (5%)	165	15	15
Anchor Steam (4.6%)	155	13	16
Arrogant Bastard Ale (7.2%)	190	20	12
Artic Ice (5.3%)	150	15	8
Artic Ice Light (3.9%)	100	11	6
Asahi Super Dry (5.2%)	150	15	11
Aspen Edge Low Carb (4.1%)	95	12	3
Augsburger Bock (4.9%)	170	14	17
Bass (5.51%)	140	16	13
Beck's (5%)	145	14	10
Beck's Light (3.8%)	105	11	6
Big Sky (4.8%)	150	14	12
Big Sky Light (4.5%)	105	13	5
Black Label (5.6%)	155	15	11
Blackhook Porter (4.9%)	160	14	14
Blatz (4.6%)	145	13	13
Blatz LA (2.3%)	75	7	6
Blatz Light (3.9%)	110	11	8
Blonde (4.3%)	140	12	10
Blue Moon: Belgian (5.4%)	170	15	14
Pumpkin Ale (5.8%)	185	16	18
Bud Dry (5%)	130	14	8

Brands (Cont)   Alc ~ Alcohol (Grams)

Beer Contains Zero Fat

	C	Alc	Cb
Bud Light (4.2%)	110	12	7
Bud Ice (5.5%)	150	15	9
Bud Ice Light (4.2%)	110	12	7
Budweiser (5%)	145	14	11
Budweiser Select (4.3%)	100	12	3
Busch (4.6%)	135	13	10
Busch Ice (5.9%)	170	16	13
Busch Light (4.2%)	110	12	7
Carling (4.4%)	140	13	10
Carlsberg (5%)	135	13	10
Carta Blanca (4.0%)	125	11	11
Castlemaine XXXX (4.7%)	140	14	9
Colt 45 Malt (5.6%)	160	15	11
Coors Original (5%)	140	14	11
Coors Extra Gold (5%)	145	14	11
Coors Light (4.2%)	105	12	5
Coors Winter Fest (5.6%)	190	16	17
Corona Extra (4.6%)	150	13	13
Corona Light (4.1%)	105	12	5
Dos Equis Lager (5%)	130	14	9
Drop Top Amber Ale (4.8%)	165	9	15
Fosters Lager (4.9%)	135	14	9
George Killian's: Irish Brown (5.2%)	185	15	15
Irish Red (5%)	160	14	13
Goebel (4.1%)	130	11	12
Goebel Light (3.9%)	110	11	8
Grolsch Premium (5%)	140	14	10
Guinness Draught (4.2%)	125	12	10
Guinness Extra Stout (5.8%)	175	17	14
Hamm's (4.7%)	145	13	12
Special Light (4.1%)	110	14	7
Harp (4.5%)	150	12	13
Heineken (5%)	150	14	12
Heineken Special Dark (5.2%)	175	15	16
Heineken Premium Light (3.5%)	100	10	7
Hop Jack Pale Ale (5%)	185	14	14
Hurricane (5.8%)	160	16	10
Icehouse (5.0%)	135	14	8
Icehouse (5.5%)	150	15	9
Jacob Best Ice (5.8%)	160	16	11
Keystone: Premium (4.4%)	110	12	5
Ice (5.9%)	145	16	7
Light (4.2%)	100	12	5
Killarney's Red Larger (5%)	200	14	23
Killain's Irish Red (4.9%)	165	14	14
King Cobra (5.9%)	170	16	12
Kirin Lager (4.9%)	145	14	11
Kirin Light (3.2%)	95	9	7
Labatt's Blue (5%)	145	14	9

Beers ♦ Ales (with Alcohol Counts)

Brands (Cont)

Beer Contains Zero Fat
Per 12 fl.oz Serving

Alc ~ Alcohol (Grams)
Cb ~ Carbohydrate

	C	Alc	Cb
Leinenkugel's: Original (4.6%)	150	13	14
Light (4.1%)	105	11	6
Lone Star: Regular (4.7%)	140	13	12
Light (3.9%)	110	11	8
Lowenbrau Dark/Special (4.9%)	160	14	15
Magic Hat #9 (4.8%)	140	14	12
Magnum Malt Liquor (5.6%)	155	16	10
Meister Brau (4.5%)	130	13	12
Memphis Brown (4.6%)	120	13	6
Michelob: Regular (5%)	155	14	13
Light (4.3%)	135	12	12
Amber Bock (5.2%)	165	15	15
Golden Draft (4.7%)	150	13	14
Golden Draft Light (4.1%)	110	11	7
Honey Larger (4.9%)	175	14	18
Michelob ULTRA (4.1%)	95	12	3
Mickey's Malt Liquor (5.6%)	160	16	11
MGD (5%)	145	14	13
MGD Light (4.5%)	110	13	7
Miller High Life (5%)	145	14	13
Miller High Life Light (4.5%)	110	14	6
Miller Lite (4.5%)	100	13	4
Milwaukee's Best (4.5%)	130	13	12
Milwaukee's Best Ice (5.9%)	145	16	6
Milwaukee's Best Light (4.5%)	100	13	4
Minnesota's Best (4.9%)	140	14	10
Molson Canadian (5%)	150	14	12
Molson Ice (5.6%)	160	16	14
Molson Special Dry (5%)	145	14	10
Moosehead (5%)	125	14	14
Natural Light (4.2%)	95	12	3
Negra Modela (5%)	155	14	14
Newcastle Brown Ale (4.5%)	140	12	13
Northstone Amber Ale (4.9%)	150	14	8
Olde English "800" (5.9%)	160	16	11
Old Milwaukee (4.6%)	145	13	13
Light (3.9%)	110	11	8
Ice (5.9%)	180	16	15
Old Style (4.7%)	140	13	12
Old Style Light (4.2%)	115	12	7
Olympia Gold Light (2.2%)	70	6	6
Pabst (4.3%)	145	13	12
Pabst Blue Ribbon (4.7%)	145	14	12

	C	Alc	Cb
Pabst Light (3.9%)	110	11	8
Pabst Extra Light (2.2%)	70	6	6
Pearl Light (2.2%)	70	6	6
Pete's Wicked Ale (5.3%)	175	15	17
Piels (4.3%)	125	12	9
Pilsner Urquell (4.4%)	155	13	16
Red Dog (5%)	150	14	14
Red Hook ESB (5.7%)	180	17	16
Red Hook India Pale Ale (4.7%)	180	13	19
Red Stripe Jamaican Ale (5.0%)	155	14	14
Red Wolf (5.4%)	150	15	10
Rolling Rock (4.5%)	120	13	7
Sam Adams Light (4%)	130	11	10
Samuel Adams (4.6%)	170	13	17
Samuel Adams Lager (4.7%)	180	13	19
Sapporo Draft (3.9%)	135	11	14
Schaefer (4.6%)	145	13	12
Schaefer Light (3.9%)	110	11	8
Schlitz (4.6%)	145	13	12
Schlitz Light (3.9%)	110	11	8
Schmidt's (4.6%)	145	13	13
Schmidt's Light (3.9%)	110	11	8
Sheaf Stout, 5.7%	180	16	17
Sierra Nevada: Pale Ale (5.6%)	200	16	12
Big Foot (9.6%)	295	28	25
Porter (5.6%)	200	16	16
Wheat Beer (4.4%)	150	12	12
Silver Thunder (5.9%)	165	17	11
Skyy Sport (5%)	160	14	15
Sol Cerveza Especial (4%)	125	11	11
Southpaw Light (5%)	125	14	7
St Pauli Girl (5%)	135	14	9
Stella Artois, 5%, 330ml	135	14	9
Stroh's (4.6%)	145	13	12
Stroh's Light (4.0%)	130	12	10
Tecate (4.7%)	155	13	16
Tequiza (4.5%)	130	13	9
The Governator (5.2%)	150	15	11
Warsteiner Verum/Dunkel (5%)	155	14	13
Weinhard's: Pale Ale (4/6%)	150	13	13
Hefeweizen (4.9%)	155	14	12
Wheat Hook (4.8%)	150	14	12
Widmer: Hefeweizen (4.7%)	155	13	16
Zeigenbock Amber (4.4%)	145	12	13

Home-Brewed Beer: Similar to regular beers, according to alcohol content.

Cider ✦ Wine (with Alcohol Counts)

Alc ~ Alcohol (Grams) **Cb** ~ Carbohydrate

Non-Alcoholic Brews

	C	Alc	Cb
Less Than 0.5% Alcohol			
Average All Brands (Busch NA, Coors NA, Kaliber, Kingsbury, O'Douls, Old Milwaukee NA, Pabst NA, Stroh's NA, Sharp's, Haake Beck, Texas Select)			
12 fl.oz Can/Bottle	70	1	14
O'Doul's Amber, 12 fl.oz	90	1	18

Cider

	C	Alc	Cb
Alcoholic Cider: Average, 6% alcohol,			
Dry, 12 fl.oz	130	17	12
Sweet, 12 fl.oz	170	17	15
Hardcore Crisp Hard Cider (6%)	190	17	19
Hornsby's: Draft Cider (6%)	170	17	16
Hard Apple Cider (5.5%)	200	16	27
Woodchuck (5%) Amber, 12 fl.oz	200	15	21
Dark & Dry, 12 fl.oz	180	15	17
Granny Smith, 12 fl.oz	165	15	11
Wyder's: Raspb. (4%), 11.5 fl.oz	140	11	15
Peach (5%) 11.5 fl.oz	150	13	16
Pear (5%), 11.5 fl.oz	130	13	14
22 fl.oz bottle	250	25	28

Quick Guide

Table Wines

	C	Alc	Cb
Average All Varieties (11.5% Alcohol)			
Wine Contains Zero Fat			
4 fl.oz 1 small wine glass			
OR ½ large wine glass	90	11	3
6 fl.oz (¾ large wine glass)	135	16	4
8 fl.oz (1 large wine glass)	180	22	6
½ Carafe/Bottle, 375ml	290	34	10
1 Bottle, 750ml	580	68	20

Table Wines

	C	Alc	Cb
Red: Claret/Burgundy/Chianti, 4 fl.oz	80	11	2
Sparkling Reds, 4 fl.oz	90	11	3
Rose: Medium, 4 fl.oz	80	11	2
White: *Per 4 fl.oz*			
Dry (Chablis/Hock/Riesling)	75	11	1
Zinfandel Sweet			
(Moselle/Sauterne), 4 fl.oz	85	11	2
Sparkling, 4 fl.oz	95	11	4

Table Wines (Cont)

	C	Alc	Cb
Champagne: *Per 4 fl.oz Serving*			
Average 1 glass, 4 fl.oz	85	11	2
w. Orange Jce (3:1 orange)	75	8	4
w. Orange Jce (1:1 orange)	65	5	7
Cold Duck, 4 fl. oz	108	11	8
Mulled Wine (Gluhwein), 4 fl.oz	180	14	20
Non-Alcoholic Wine, avg., 4 fl.oz	50	0	12
Reduced Alcohol Wine (6%):			
Average all types, 4 fl.oz	50	0	12
Sake: Rice Wine (16% alc.), 4 oz	125	15	5

Flavored Wine

	C	Alc	Cb
Average All Brands (6% alcohol)			
(Examples: Arbor Mist, Wild Vines, Boones)			
1 small wine glass, 4 fl.oz	80	6	11
1 large wine glass, 8 fl.oz	160	11	21
1 bottle, 750 ml (25.4 fl.oz)	510	36	67

Dessert Wines

	C	Alc	Cb
Madeira (18% alc), 2 oz	85	9	5
Marsala (18%), 2 oz	110	9	11
Port, Muscatel, (18%), 2 oz	85	9	5
Sherry (18%), 2 oz			
Dry, 1 Sherry glass	65	9	0.5
Sweet/Cream, average	85	9	5
Vermouth: Dry (18%), 2 oz	65	9	0.5
Sweet (15%), 2 oz	85	7	8

Cooking Wine

	C	Alc	Cb
Average All Brands			
Red/White: 2 Tbsp, 1 oz	20	3	1
1 cup, 8 fl.oz	160	22	12
Marsala, 2 Tbsp, 1 oz	35	4	2
Sherry, 2 Tbsp, 1 oz	40	4	2

Cooking with Wine:
For alcohol to evaporate, sufficient heat and cooking time (at least 30 minutes) is required.

Red and white table wines would then contain negligible residual calories.

Sweetened wines (marsala/sherry) would contain 10 calories per 1 fl.oz.

Flambé Desserts: Only surface alcohol is burnt off, so negligible reduction in alcohol or calories.

Liquors ◆ Coolers ◆ Cocktails

Spirits/Liquors

Includes Bourbon, Brandy, Gin, Rum, Scotch, Tequila, Vodka, Whiskey.

Note: All spirits with same proof (alcohol) have similar calories and zero fat.

Average All Brands	**C**	**Alc**	**Cb**
80 Proof (40% Alcohol by Volume):			
1 fl.oz	65	9.5	0
1½ fl.oz (1 shot)	100	14	0
3 fl.oz (Double shot)	200	29	0
½ Bottle, 350 ml	810	120	0
1 Bottle, 700 ml	1620	240	0
86 Proof (43% Alcohol):			
1 fl.oz	70	10	0
1½ fl.oz (1 shot)	105	15	0
1 Bottle, 700 ml	1750	250	0
100 Proof (50% Alcohol):			
1½ fl.oz (1 shot)	120	18	0
1 Bottle, 700 ml	2050	300	0

Flavored Spirits ~ Average All Brands			
Includes Malibu Rum; Captain Morgan			
70 Proof (35% Alcohol)			
1½ fl.oz (1 shot)	105	13	3
3 fl.oz (Double shot)	210	26	1

Hard Lemon(ade) & Sodas

	C	**Alc**	**Cb**
Doc's Hard Lemon (5%), 12 fl.oz	170	14	17
Henry's Hard L'ade (5%), 12 fl.oz	285	14	46
Hooch Hard (5.2%), 330ml	215	14	32
Hooch Ice (5.7%), 330ml	230	15	32
Mike's Hard Lem. (5.2%): 11.2 fl.oz	80	10	2
16 fl.oz bottle	345	19	54
Mike's Light Lem. (4%), 11.2 fl.oz	120	10	12
Mike's Hard Iced Tea (5%), 11.2 fl.oz	195	13	27
Rick's Spiked (5.2%), 12 fl.oz	250	14	39
Twisted Tea: Half & Half (5%) 12 fl.oz	250	14	37
Hard Iced/Raspberry (5%) 12 fl.oz	220	14	30
Two Dogs (4.2%), 355ml	205	12	30

Enjoy a beer but watch the portion size. Those footballs hold 50 fl.oz!

Coolers & Premix Cocktails

Ready-To-Drink
Zero Fat Unless Indicated

	C	**Alc**	**Cb**
Arbor Mist: Blenders,			
all flavors (12.5%), 4 fl.oz	100	11	14
Bacardi: Silver (5%), 12 fl.oz	230	14	33
Silver O³ (5%), 12 fl.oz	230	14	33
Silver Raz (5%), 12 fl.oz	230	14	33
Silver Limon (5%)	230	14	33
Silver Low Carb: Black Cherry (4%)	100	12	3
Apple (4%)	95	11	4.5
Ready to Pour (1.75 liter bottle)			
Bahama Mama (10%), 4 fl.oz	130	13	16
Hurricane (12.5%), 4 fl.oz	144	12	16
Rum Island Ice Tea (12.5%), 4 fl.oz	150	12	16
Bartles & Jaymes			
Malt Based Coolers (3.9% alc): *Per 12 fl.oz*			
Black Cherry; Classic Original	200	11	30
Exotic Berry, Juicy Peach	210	11	33
Fuzzy Navel; Hard Lemonade	230	11	38
Margarita, Pina Colada	270	11	48
Raspberry Daiquiri	220	11	38
Strawb. Cosmopolitan/Daiquiri	230	11	35
Raspb. Lemonade, Lusc. Blackb.	230	11	38
B-to-the-E *(Anheuser-Busch)*, 10 fl.oz	150	12	17
Cruzan Island Cocktails (5% alc): *Per 12 fl.oz*			
Jumbie Brew	230	14	32
Mojito	300	14	50
Wazi Koki	285	14	46
Jack Daniels Country Cocktails (5.9%)			
average all flavors, 6.8 fl.oz	170	10	25
Jack Daniels Hard Cola (5%) 12 oz	234	14	34
Jose Cuervo Authentic Margarita (5.9% alc)			
Margarita/ Lime.Strawb. 200ml	180	10	27
Sauza Diablo (5%), 12 fl.oz	260	14	40
Seagram's Coolers (5%)			
Smooth Red/Citrus 12 fl.oz	240	14	35
Skyy Blue (5%), 12 fl.oz	280	14	45
Stolichnaya Citr. (5%), 12 fl.oz	240	14	36
Smirnoff Ice (5%), 330ml	220	13	33
Black Ice (5.5%), 12 fl.oz	240	19	36
TGI Friday's: *Per 3 fl.oz*			
On The Rocks: Margarita (7.5%)	90	6	14
Long Island Ice Tea (15%)	130	11	14
Mudslide (10%)	200	8	18
Blenders (12.5% alc) *Per 3 fl.oz:*			
Mudslide (12.5%)	120	8.5	15
Orange Dream (12.5%)	120	8.5	15
Strawberry Shortcake (12.5%)	115	8.5	12
Tilt *(Anheuser-Busch)* 6.6% alc., 16 fl.oz	390	24	56

Coolers ♦ Cocktails (with Alcohol Counts)

Coolers & Premix Cocktails (Cont)

Ready-To-Drink

The Club *Premix Cocktails (8 oz Can):*
Per 4 oz Serving (½ can)

	C	Alc	Cb
Long Island Ice Tea; Manhattan	220	16	30
Margar.; Screwdriver; Vodka Martini	210	7	40
Mudslide (9g fat)	270	12	41
Pina Colada; Or. Craze; Whisk. Sour	260	10	40
Zima (5.9%), 12 fl.oz	235	15	20

Shooters

Alc ~ Alcohol (Grams)

	C	Alc	Cb
Alabama Slammer	110	14	2
Amaretto Sours	120	6	19
Cranium Meltdown	75	7	2
Duck Fart	85	7	5
Kamakazie	150	20	2
Kool-Aid	160	15	14
Liquid Cocaine	130	13	10
Mud Slide	160	13	17
Fuzzy Navel	120	13	7
Pineapple Bomber	130	11	13
Turbo	110	14	3

Cocktail Mixers

Non Alcoholic ~ No Alcohol Added

Bacardi: *Frozen Concentrate*
(Made Up from 2 fl.oz concentrate)

	C	Alc	Cb
Margarita, 8 fl.oz	90	0	25
Pina Colada, 8 fl.oz	170	0	35
Strawberry, 8 fl.oz	120	0	35
Baja Bob's (Sugar Free), Cocktail/Martini Mix, 4 fl.oz	10	0	2
Daily's Pina Colada, 3 fl.oz	160	0	37
J.Cuervo Margarita, 4 fl.oz	100	0	24
Malibu Beach, all flavors, 8 fl.oz	10	0	3
Mr & Mrs T: Mai Tai, 4.5 fl.oz	140	0	33
Bloody Mary, 8 fl.oz	40	0	9
Margarita, 4 fl.oz	100	0	26
Pina Colada, 4.5 fl.oz	180	0	43
Strawberry Daiquiri, 4 fl.oz	200	0	50
Sweet 'n' Sour, 4 fl.oz	90	0	23
Sauza Margarita, 3 fl.oz	70	0	18
Skyy Cosmo, 4 fl.oz	140	0	36
TGI Fridays: Hurricane, 2.3 fl.oz	60	0	15
Long Island Ice Tea, 3.3 fl.oz	55	0	14
Mudslide, 2.3 fl.oz	120	0	24

Cocktails

Alc ~ Alcohol (Grams)

Made to Standard Recipes
Main Reference: The New American
Bartender's Guide

Zero Fat Unless Indicated

	C	Alc	Cb
Bloody Mary	95	10	16
Blue Lady	230	15	16
Blushin' Russian (9g fat)	365	14	47
Bourbon & Soda	130	19	0
Brandy Alexander (10g fat)	300	20	17
Cerebral Hemorrhage (5g fat)	290	17	32
Chupa Naranjas (w. 1½ oz Tequila)	150	16	8
Collins (with 2 oz Gin)	180	20	11
Cosmopolitan	215	24	12
Daiquiri, average all types	140	19	4
Frozen Daiquiri: no fruit	155	19	6
with fruit (and less Rum)	140	14	10
Gin & Tonic	220	19	22
Grasshopper	280	13	30
Green Fantasy	210	23	11
Harvey Wallbanger (2 oz Vodka)	200	19	17
Highball (1½ oz Whiskey)	110	14	3
Irish Coffee (contains 5g fat)	175	14	6
Kahlua Mudslide: w.milk (3.5g fat)	150	11	10
w. cream (12.5g fat)	230	11	0
L.A. Sunrise	280	26	21
Lady Killer	165	13	20
Leprechaun's Libation	285	31	17
London Rock	165	18	10
Long Island Iced Tea (w. 8 oz Cola)	290	22	31
with Diet Cola	190	22	6
Mai Tai (with 2 oz Rum)	220	21	16
Manhattan	130	17	3
Margarita	150	18	4
Martini	135	20	0
Mind Eraser	160	17	10
Mint Julep	210	29	4
Mojito (with 2 oz Rum)	160	19	6
Pina Colada (contains 12g fat)	325	19	12
Rainbow Room	265	30	14
Screwdriver	160	14	14
Sex On The Beach	240	20	26
Singapore Sling	210	25	9
Spritzer (with 3 oz Wine)	60	8	2
Tequila Sunrise	200	14	25
Tom Collins	210	24	12
Tom & Jerry	170	9	8
Whiskey Sour	150	19	5
White Russian	250	20	16

171

Liqueurs (with Alcohol Counts)

Liqueurs/Cordials

	C	Alc	Cb
Per 1 fl.oz			
Advocaat (36 Proof; 2g fat)	85	4	9
Alizé: Cognac	70	11	2
Gold/Red Passion	105	4.5	11
Amaretto (56 Proof)	110	6	17
Baileys Irish Cream (34 Proof; 5g fat)	95	4	5
Lite (30 Proof; 2g fat)	75	4	7
Benedictine (80 Proof)	90	10	5
Chambord (33 Proof)	105	5	11
Chartreuse (80 Proof)	100	10	7
Cherry Brandy (48 Proof)	80	6	9
Coffee Liqueur (53 Proof)	90	6	11
Cointreau (80 Proof)	100	10	7
Creme de Cacao (54 Proof)	100	6	15
Creme de Menthe (60 Proof)	120	7	14
Curacao (70 Proof)	95	8	6
Drambuie (80 Proof)	105	10	6
Frangelico (48 Proof)	80	6	9
Galliano (80 Proof)	100	10	8
Grand Marnier (80 Proof)	100	10	7
Kahlua (53 Proof)	90	6	11
Kirsch (68 Proof)	80	8	6
Midori (42 Proof), average all types	80	5	11
Ouzo (80 Proof)	90	10	5
Pernod (80 Proof)	75	10	2
Sambuca (84 Proof)	100	10	7
Schnapps (80 Proof)	100	10	4
Southern Comfort (78 Proof)	75	9	3
Starbucks Coffee Liqueur (40 Proof)	80	4	13
Tia Maria (64 Proof)	90	8	9
Triple Sec (60 Proof)	80	7	4

Liqueur Coffee & Hot Drinks

Per Standard Drink			
Liqueur Coffee, avg. all types	200	10	10
Egg Nog	270	10	25
Hot Toddy, w. 2 oz liquor	200	19	17
Irish Coffee, w. 2 Tbsp whip. crm	80	7	4
Mulled Wine (Glühwein), 5 oz	175	14	6

Flavorings/Syrups

Non-Alcoholic (Fat Free)			
Angostura Bitters, ¼ tsp	3	0	0
Ginger Ale, 8 fl.oz	80	0	22
Grenadine/Cassis, 2 Tbsp, 1 oz	70	0	17
Lime/Lemon Juice, 2 Tbsp, 1 oz	10	0	2
Maraschino Cherry, 1 small	8	0	2
Pure Lemon Extract, 1 oz	125	0	17
Sugar Syrup, 2 Tbsp, 1 oz	70	0	17
Sour Mix, 2 Tbsp, 1 oz	10	0	2
Tonic Water, 8 fl.oz	90	0	22

Ten Hints to Avoid Harmful Drinking

1. **Add up the alcohol** you typically drink each day and on social occasions. How does this compare with 'low risk' amounts?

2. **Compare the alcohol** content of different drinks and select the lowest. Request half ounces of alcohol in cocktails and mixed drinks. Dilute them and keep topping off with non-alcoholic drinks.

3. **Go easy on 'Light' beers.** At 4% alcohol, on average, they are still high in alcohol compared to regular beer (5% alcohol).

4. **Try low alcohol** or non-alcohol alternatives such as fruit juices and mineral water. Take your own to parties.

5. **Before drinking alcohol,** quench your thirst with water and non-alcoholic drinks - particularly after vigorous exercise or sport.

6. **Slow the rate of drinking.** Chugging or drinking fast is the major cause of illness and death from alcohol poisoning.

7. **Avoid drinking in 'rounds'.**

8. **Have a non-alcoholic 'spacer'** between drinks (e.g. mineral water, orange juice).

9. **Don't drink on an empty stomach.** Food slows the rate of alcohol absorption.

10. **Keep track of the number of drinks** and know when to stop. Stick to a set limit.

Note: • Alcohol can be very dangerous when taken with prescription or street drugs or when you are very tired.

Extra Info: www.CalorieKing.com

"The doctor told him to cut down to just one glass a day."

Deli, Sandwiches, Wraps

Cafeteria-Style Foods

	C	F	Cb
Apple & Cinnamon, 1.23 oz	130	1.5	26
Beef Stroganoff, 5 oz	195	13	7
Beef Stroganoff w. 4 oz noodles	350	14	36
Chicken Lasagna, 1 piece	300	11	32
Chicken Chop Suey w. 4 oz rice	245	4	37
Deep Dish Burrito, 7 oz	265	13	20
Grnd Beef Casserole, 2 scoop, 6 oz	245	13	17
Italian Meat Sce for Spagh., 5 oz	150	9	9
w. 5 oz Spaghetti	350	10	49
Lasagna, 1 piece	275	11	25
Meatloaf, 3 oz	205	13	4
Ranch Beans, 2 scoops, 6 oz	350	11	45
Red Beans & Rice, 7 oz	280	9	37
Scalloped Potato/Ham, 2 scp, 6 oz	160	6	20
Stuffed Shells in Sauce (1)	105	3	17
Swedish Meatballs (3)	205	12	9
Sweet & Sour Pork/Rice, 9 oz	240	3	40
Swiss Steak w/Mushr. Gravy, 6 oz	280	11	4
Tator Tot Casserole, 2 scoops, 6 oz	260	15	20
Tenderloin Mtrs/Mushr. Gravy, 5 oz	210	13	3
w. 5 oz noodles	395	15	38
Tuna Noodle Casserole, 2 scp, 6 oz	180	6	17
Turkey Tetrazini, 2 scoops, 6 oz	195	7	17
Vegetable Lasagna, 1 piece	250	13	21

Croissants

	C	F	Cb
Unfilled: Medium 1½ oz	180	10	21
Filled: w. Ham (2 oz), Salad	280	14	24
w. Ham (2 oz), Cheese (2 oz)	470	30	20
w. Chick (2 oz) Cheese (2 oz)	470	30	20
w. Turkey/Ham/Chse (2 oz ea.)	580	36	20
Au Bon Pain: Ham & Cheese	340	10	46
Spinach & Cheese	250	9	32

7-Eleven: Page 246

Bagels

	C	F	Cb
Plain: Large, 4 oz (no filling)	320	2	65
with 2 oz Cream Cheese	500	27	54
with 2 oz Lox (Smoked Salmon)	400	4	65

Also see Bagels Section: Page 104
Fast-Foods Restaurants: Page 183
Au Bon Pain: Page 187
Bruegger's: Page 193
Einstein Bros Bagels: Page 207

Sandwiches

No Spreads Unless Indicated
(Includes 2 Slices Bread ~ 3 oz)

	C	F	Cb
BLT (5 strips Bacon, 2 Tbsp Mayo)	600	40	46
Breaded Chicken & Salad	540	28	46
Chicken (5 oz) Salad w. Mayo.	580	30	49
Chopped Liver, Egg, Mayo.	630	25	44
Corned Beef (5 oz) w. Mustard	560	28	44
Cream Cheese w. Olives (5 large)	340	14	46
Egg Salad w. Mayonnaise	570	29	49
Egg Salad Club w. Bacon, Mayo.	780	53	49
Grilled Cheese (3 oz)	540	30	44
Ham (4 oz); Cheese (4 oz), Mayo.	910	56	44
Lobster Salad (4 oz) w. Mayo.	530	27	45
Overstuffed Tuna Salad (7 oz)	870	39	75
Philadelphia Cheese Steak S'wich	550	23	42
Reuben (6 oz Beef/Pastrami, 2 oz Cheese, 2 Tbsp Dressing)	920	60	28
Roast Beef (4 oz) w. Mustard	460	12	45
Roast Pork (4 oz) w. Apple Sauce	500	16	55
Shrimp Salad Club w. Bacon, Mayo.	800	57	48
Sloppy Joe w. Sauce (7 oz)	600	30	45
Steak Sandwich (5 oz cooked)	680	32	41
Triple Cheese (4 oz) Melt	720	45	46
Tuna (5 oz) Salad w. Mayo.	610	23	49
Turkey Breast (5 oz) w. Mayo.	460	18	44
Turkey Breast (5 oz) w. Mustard	360	7	44
Turkey Club w. Bacon, Mayo.	830	38	31
Vegetarian w. Avocado, Cheese	820	49	72

7-Eleven: Page 246
Schlotzsky's: Page 247
Subway: Page 258

Wraps & Roll-Ups

	C	F	Cb
Average All Types (Meat/Chicken/Fish/Veges)			
Small size, approx. 9 oz	500	25	48
Regular, approx. 15 oz	830	40	80
Large, approx. 22 oz	1400	70	134

Fast-Foods Restaurants: Page 183
Au Bon Pain: Page 187
Sonic Drive-In: Page 252
Subway: Page 258
The Wrap: Page 263
WAWA: Page 267

173

Fair & Carnival Foods

Fair & Carnival Foods

	C	F	Cb
Mexican			
Burritos w. Bean/Beef, 17 oz	1100	41	104
Carne Asada, 14.5 oz	820	44	58
Fish Tacos, 1 taco, 5 oz	270	13	31
Nachos w. Cheese, 9" plate	860	59	70
Taco Chicken, 3.3 oz	210	12	16
Tamale (1), 3.5 oz	180	8	21
Taquitos, 5 oz	370	17	43
Greek			
Baklava, 2" square	245	13	32
Falafel, 11.6 oz	660	27	85
Greek Salad, 14 oz	520	48	17
Gyros, 7.5", 12 oz	680	40	55
Spanakopita, 8 oz	200	7.5	23
Italian			
Garlic Bread, ½ loaf, 10 oz	1135	40	147
Pizza Bread Pepperoni, ½ loaf, 12 oz	1115	32	151
Pizza on a Stick, 1 piece	535	28	55
Personal Pizza, 7": Cheese (1)	670	24	80
Pepperoni (1)	795	35	80
Ham & Pineapple (1)	800	31	87
Low Carb			
Beef Patty, wrapped in lettuce, 4 oz	480	33	0
Sandwiches: *Per 7½" Roll*			
Ham, 11 oz	645	39	47
Hot Pastrami, 9 oz	760	17	62
Roast Beef, 11 oz	620	36	46
Philadelphia Cheese Steak, 13 oz	680	36	49
Tuna, 12 oz	830	60	46
Turkey, 11 oz	665	24	65
Veggie, 11 oz	490	23	49
Oriental: Fried Egg Roll, 6 oz	400	19	44
Rice Bowl: Beef, 6" Bowl	880	13	136
Chicken, 6" Bowl	870	15	135
Hamburgers			
⅓ Pound Burger, 7.5 oz	670	41	26
Burger w. Cheese, 6 oz	550	36	25
Hot Dogs/Franks: *With Bun*			
Hot Dog: Regular, (1)	215	14	28
with Chili, 6 oz	450	32	32
with Chili & Cheese, 7.3 oz	500	36	31
⅓ Pound Hot Dog	550	41	31
Foot Long Hot Dog	470	26	41
Corn Dog: Regular, 4 oz	250	14	23
Jumbo, 6 oz	375	21	36
Jumbo Franks w. Bun:			
Bratwurst; Sausage; Kielbasa, avg.	800	60	28

Fair & Carnival Foods (Cont)

	C	F	Cb
Barbeque Items *(Weights with Bone)* **:**			
Beef Stew over Rice, 2 cups	440	14	61
Chicken, 15 oz	740	24	34
Chili, 1 cup	280	11	24
Corn on the Cob, 8" (1), 16 oz	200	1	42
Pork Ribs, 18 oz	1360	68	21
Smoked Turkey Legs (1), 19 oz	1135	54	0
Potatoes & Fries			
Australian Battered Potato, 12 oz	1290	66	155
Baked Potato, 14 oz	435	0.5	100
Fries: French, 7 oz	560	24	70
Cheese Fries, 10 oz	645	38	62
Chili Fries, 10 oz	700	36	83
Chili/Cheese Fries, 13 oz	745	45	57
Curly Fries, 7 oz	620	30	78
Tasti Chips, 40 chips, 6.5 oz	780	33	117
Sweet Potato, 14 oz	405	0.5	97
Ranch Dip, 3 oz	165	14	9
Finger Foods			
Artichoke: Steamed, 6 pieces	65	0	16
Fried, 9 pieces	250	14	24
Chicken Nuggets (6)	340	17	26
Chicken Strips (4), 4.5 oz	445	21	33
Finger Steaks (2), 4 oz	400	20	26
Mushrooms, Fried, 10-12 pieces	395	26	34
Onion Rings, 3 rings	310	13	40
Onion Flower	1320	72	140
Shrimp, Fried, 10-12 pieces, 5 oz	555	30	36
Sweet Potato Strips, Fried, 4 pces	750	30	106
Zucchini, Fried, 4 slices	620	40	42
Salads/Sides			
Baked Beans, 4 oz	140	2	38
Cole Slaw, 5 oz	350	21	37
Pickle, whole (6")	30	0	8
Potato Salad, 5 oz	290	15	35
Popcorn: Plain, small, 3 oz	450	24	48
Large, 6 oz	900	48	96
Kettle Corn: Small, 5 oz	600	15	110
Large, 10 oz	1200	30	220
Cakes, Donuts, Cookies			
Funnel Cake: Plain	760	44	80
Toppings: Cinn. & Sugar, 2 tsp	30	0	8.5
Apple Cinnamon, 2 oz	85	3	36
Strawberries & Cream, 2 oz	70	0	16
Cinnamon Roll, large	730	24	114
Churros, 1½ oz	150	8	18
Donuts, Jumbo Twist, 7.5 oz	905	49	109

Restaurant & International Foods

Fair & Carnival Foods (Cont)

Cakes, Donuts, Cookies (Cont)

	C	F	Cb
Fried Snickers, 5 oz	445	29	42
Fried Oreos, 3 cookies	300	10	33
Fried Twinkie, 1	420	34	45
Cotton Candy, 5½ oz bag	625	0	156
Red Rope Licorice, (24"), 2 oz	200	0	46
Cream Puff, 4.3 oz	500	43	22
Puff-on-a-Stick (4), 8.6 oz	995	86	44
Strawberry Crepe, 4.3 oz	280	14	36
Chocolate Dipped Straw, 1 pce	125	7	15
Fudge, 1.5 oz	200	11	25
Twinkie Dog (Sundae)	500	14	89
Key Lime Pie Bar, 6 oz	635	40	59
Cheesecake on a Stick, 6 oz	655	47	56
Cobbler, 5 oz	350	10	62
Soft Pretzel, 4.5 oz	340	2	70
Candied Apple, 7 oz	330	0.5	80

Ice Cream & Frozen Treats

	C	F	Cb
Dippin' Dots Ice Cream: Small, 4 oz	150	7	17
Medium, 8 oz	305	14	35
Large, 16 oz	600	28	70
Sno-Cone (includes 6 oz syrup)	540	0	132
Frozen Yogurt in sugar cone, 14 oz	475	2	94
Ice Cream: Small, sugar cone, 10 oz	775	42	83
Large, sugar cone, 14 oz	935	54	96
Sherbet, 8 oz	270	4	59
Frozen Banana, choc cover, 5 oz	240	4	53

Drinks

	C	F	Cb
Lemonade, 18 fl.oz	210	0	52
Orange Julius, 20 fl.oz	490	10	96
Strawberry Julius, 20 fl.oz	430	0	98
Icee, 16 fl.oz	235	0	59
Malt, 16 fl.oz	690	33	85
Slushies, 16 fl.oz	260	0	65
Soft Frozen Lemonade, 12 fl.oz	300	0	78
Smoothies: Berry Flavors, 16 fl.oz	350	1	80

Stadium Foods

	C	F	Cb
Sandwiches			
Bacon Burger, 8.3 oz	470	25	34
Cheeseburger, 8.3 oz	450	23	33
Chicken Sandwich: w. Cheese, 8.3 oz	510	29	40
no Cheese, 7.7 oz	460	25	40
w. Bacon, 8.3 oz	530	31	41
Hamburger (1), 7.8 oz	400	19	33
Polish Sausage Sandwich (1), 7 oz	565	33	46
Fries: French Fries, 6.4 oz	470	34	39
Hot Dogs			
Chili Dog (1), 7.7 oz	520	29	45
Hot Dog (1), 6.4 oz	465	21	50
Jumbo Dog (1), 6 oz	440	25	38
Kraut Dog w. Sauerkraut (1), 7.8 oz	490	27	41
Nachos: 40 chips w. 4 oz cheese	1100	59	132
Individual Pan Pizza (6"): *Per 10 oz Pizza*			
BBQ Chicken	630	24	71
Cheese	630	27	71
Pepperoni	660	30	70
Snacks			
Brownie (1), 2.5" x 4.5"	360	18	44
Cheese Sauce, 1.25 oz	100	8	4
Cheetos, 2.75 oz pkg	440	28	42
Chocolate Chip Cookie (1), 2.3 oz	280	12	40
Churros, 8", 3 oz	325	15	42
Doritos Nacho, 2.75 oz pkg	390	20	48
King Size Candy:			
Butterfinger (1), 3.75 oz	485	18	75
Nestle Crunch (1), 2.75 oz	390	21	85
Lays Chips, 2.75 oz pkg	440	28	42
Peanuts in shell, 8 oz	930	80	24
Popcorn: Small (5 cup size)	575	35	56
Large (15 cup size)	950	58	93
Red Vines, 5.5 oz box	560	0	136
Soft Pretzel (1), 8 oz	710	5	147
Beverages: Orange Juice, 12 fl.oz	180	0	2
Beer: Heineken, 16 fl.oz	200	0	16
Light Miller, 16 fl.oz	165	0	10
Miller Draft, 16 fl.oz	205	0	18
Jack Daniels Punch, 12 fl.oz	235	0	34
Wine, White, 9 fl.oz	190	0	6
Lemonade: 32 fl.oz	260	0	63
Strawberry, 32 fl.oz	275	0	71
Sno Cone, 18 oz (incl. 6 oz syrup)	540	0	132
Starbuck's Frappaccino, 12 fl.oz	195	2.5	39

Restaurant & International Foods

Chinese & Asian Dishes

Appetizers

	C	F	Cb
Crab Cake, 63g	105	5	0.5
Curried Meat Triangles, 1 pce	150	5	12
Dumplings: Pork, steamed, 1	40	3	4
Pork, fried, 1 dumpling	75	7	4
Vegetable, steamed, 1	25	0.5	4
Egg Rolls, mini, 3 rolls	100	3	11
Rice Paper Roll, 1	80	2	10
Spring Roll: Small, 1½ oz	100	7	10
Medium, 3 oz	200	12	20
Large, 5 oz	350	15	33
Wonton, 1 only	55	3	4
Soup: Clear, 1 bowl	30	1	4
with Noodles	100	3	12
Chicken & Corn	150	8	8
Rice: Plain, 1 cup (½ Pint), 6½ oz	240	0.5	54
2 cups (1 Pint), 13 oz	480	1	108
Fried: 1 cup, 5 oz	320	13	42
Large dish, 16 oz	1010	40	134
Noodles: Chinese Egg, ckd, 1 cup	200	3	42

Entrees & Mains: Per Whole Dish

	C	F	Cb
Beef Satay, 17 oz	760	50	15
Beef in Black Bean Sce, 17 oz	530	33	17
Beef with Broccoli, 16 oz	650	30	31
Chicken & Almonds, 18 oz	685	50	18
Chicken (sliced) & Broccoli	280	12	13
Chop Suey: Chicken, 20 oz	560	37	7
Pork, 20 oz	680	50	12
Chow Mein, Beef/Chicken, 24 oz	940	60	50
Crab Puff/Rangoon, 1 dumpling	80	4.5	7.5
Crispy Fried Chicken, 8 oz	485	33	12
Egg Drop Soup: w. Noodles, 1 cup	120	3	15
w/out Noodles, 1 cup	70	3	3
Egg Foo Yung w. Sauce, 1 cup	225	12	11
Lemon Chicken, 10 oz	580	32	25
Lo Mein (stir-fried)	620	29	61
Moo Shu Chicken, 2 wrapped crepes	430	16	43
Omelet, Chicken/Shrimp, 16 oz	990	82	10
Steamed Whole Fish, ½ Red Snapper	500	11	1
Sweet & Sour: Fish, 20 oz	1160	58	106
Pork, 18 oz	950	50	92
Vegetable Combination, w. oil, 6 oz	250	17	19
Vegetables, Steamed (no oil), 6 oz	120	1	25
Bubble Tea, average, 12 fl oz	240	0	55
Fortune Cookie: each	25	0.5	5

Cajun & Creole

	C	F	Cb
Alligator, 4 oz cooked	160	2	0
Baked Herb Chicken, 1 serving	850	53	2
Bouillabaisse	400	15	10
Cajun Fried Turkey, 1 serving	630	25	0
Cocktail Sauce, 2 Tbsp	30	0	6
Couche-couche, ½ cup	80	0	17
Crawfish Bisque, 1 serving	500	10	10
Crawfish, cooked, 2 oz	45	0.5	0
Creole Jambalaya, 1 serving	550	30	15
Frog's Legs, steamed (2)	45	0	0
Guinea Fowl, flesh, 4 oz, ckd	160	4	0
Hogshead Cheese, ¼ cup	80	5.5	0
Jambalaya, Shrimp & Crabmeat	520	14	12
Red Beans & Rice, 1 serving	400	17	52
Roasted Quail, w. Bacon on Toast	550	25	15
Remoulade Sauce, 2 Tbsp, 1 OZ	110	11	2
Shrimp Creole, 1 serving	450	20	10
Stuffed Smothered Steak, w. 1 cup Rice	890	50	50
Turtle, cooked, 3 oz	120	3	0

Cuban

	C	F	Cb
Bl. Beans w. Rice (Moros con Cristianos)	510	22	76
Blk.-eyed Pea Fritters (Bollitos de Carita)	80	5	6
Casserole Corn Tamale	445	20	55
Chkn w. Yellow Rice (Arroz con Pollo)	925	49	87
Cuban Bread (Pan Cubano)	80	1.5	10
Donuts in Syrup (Bunuelos)	170	5	10
with Melado	100	5	10
Grilled Plantains	145	0	40
Gypsy's Arm Cake (Brazo Gitano)	260	18	42
Roast Pork S'wich (Pan con Lechon)	640	30	62
Seasoned Beef w. Olives & Raisins (Picadillo)	435	36	10
Shredded Beef (Ropa Vieja)	550	35	10
Taro Root Mash (Pure de Malanga)	315	3	69
Yuca with Citrus Garlic Dressing (Yuca con Mojo)	190	9	25

French Foods

	C	F	Cb
Blanquette d'Agneau (Lamb Stew)	800	30	17
Brioche, 1 cake	280	14	34
Bouillabaisse (Fish Stew)	400	15	10
Coq au Vin (Chicken in Wine)	800	30	16
Coquilles St. Jacques, fried, 6 lge.	300	14	2
Crème Brulée, 1 serving	460	40	21

Restaurant & International Foods

French Foods (Cont)

	C	F	Cb
Creme Caramel (Caramel Custard)	260	10	38
Crepe Suzette, 1x6" crepe w. sauce	220	10	13
Duck a l'Orange	780	35	47
Escargots (Snails), garlic butter (6)	200	10	4
French Stick Bread, 3 slices, 2.2 oz	150	1	35
Frogs Legs, fried, 4 med. pairs	400	20	10
Lamb Noisettes, fried, 2 chops	500	40	1
Mousse au Chocolat	380	15	33
Potage Creme Crecy (Carrot Soup)	360	18	14
Salade Nicoise (Tuna/Oliv./Veg.)	450	13	14
Veal Cordon Bleu (Veal/Ham/Ch)	650	25	18
Vichyssoise (Pot./Leek Soup), 1 c.	200	9	15

Baguette & French Stick: *Page 102, 103*
Croissants: *Pages 113, 173*

German

	C	F	Cb
Bavarian Bread Dumpling, 3 small	330	10	28
Beef Goulash with Veges	520	20	46
Black Forest Cake, 1 slice	380	16	30
Bratwurst, grilled, 1 medium, 6 oz	450	37	2
Chicken: Fried, Viennese-style	530	20	28
Livers w. Apple/On., 6 oz	460	28	10
Herring, Pickled: Rollmops, 4 oz	260	16	3
with Sour Cream, 4 oz	310	20	3
Hot Sausage Curry	300	7	6
Kugelhupf Cake, 1 lge slice, 4 oz	400	23	40
Sauerbraten Pork (Pot Roast)	650	35	15
Torte: Linzer (Alm./Raspb. Jam)	430	18	58
Sacher (Choc./Apricot Jam)	260	12	23
Weiner Schnitzel, 1 medium	750	35	38

Greek

	C	F	Cb
Baklava Pastry: Small	240	13	32
Large, 3¾ oz	400	21	45
Calamari, deep fried, 1 cup	300	13	17
Chicken Kebob Plate	345	13	8
Galactobureko, 1 only			
(Filo, Custard, Pastry in Syrup)	360	15	48
Greek Chicken Salad	400	18	9
Gyros, 4 oz	380	33	6
Hummus & Pita, 4 oz	260	12	30
Kataifi, (Filo, Nut, Pastry in Syrup)	350	11	56
Moussaka, 1 serve, 8 oz	350	22	22
Soup: Argolemono (Egg Lemon Soup			
with Chicken & Rice)	85	6	5
Souvlakia (Lamb), each, 2 oz	120	6	1

Greek (Cont)

	C	F	Cb
Stuffed Tomatoes, 2 only	250	12	17
Taramosalata, 1 Tbsp, ½ oz	40	3	2
Tyropita (Filo/Egg/Cheese Pastry)	350	26	31
Tzatziki (Cucumber/Yog. Dip), 1 T.	20	1	1
Vine Leaves, stuffed, 3 rolls, 6 oz	200	5	13

See Daphne's: *See Fast-Foods Section*

Hawaiian

	C	F	Cb
Ahi Tuna, grilled (6 oz fillet), no fat	220	2	0
Chicken Long Rice, 1 cup, 7 oz	240	14	12
Gyoza, 1 only	55	2	6
Haupia (Coconut Pudd.), 1 pce (4"x 2½")	120	6	17
Hawaiian Sweet Bread, ½" sl., 2 oz	180	4.5	29
Kalua Chicken, 4 oz	280	16	0
Pork, 4 oz	350	24	0
Kim Chee (pickled cabbage), ½ c., 4 oz	20	0	5
Kulolo (Taro Pudding), 1 slice	125	5	19
Lau Lau: Chicken (1) 7 oz	280	21	3
Pork (1) 7 oz	320	26	5
Loco Moco (rice/burger/egg/gravy)	650	27	63
Lomi Salmon, ¼ cup, 4 oz	20	1	2
Malasadas (Donut), 2 oz	240	13	26
Manapua (Char Siu Pork Bun), 2.3 oz	180	8	25
Poi (mashed ckd taro), 1 c., 8½ oz	270	0.5	65
Poke, avg all types, 3 oz	90	1	0
Portuguese Sausage, 2 oz	180	15	2
Potato Salad, ½ cup, 5 oz	170	10	17
Shave Ice *(Matsumoto)*, all flavors:			
w. Icecream, 1 large	300	4	64
w. Beans, 1 large	290	0	72
Spam Musubi: w. Regular Spam	265	11	34
(4 oz rice+1.3 oz Spam/7-Eleven Hawaii)			
Homemade: w. Lite Spam (50% less fat)	220	5	34
Taro Pancake Mix, ⅓ cup (makes 2)	140	2	26
Plate Lunches:			
Chicken Katsu (9 oz) w.2 scp Rice	1110	48	108
+ Macaroni Salad, ¾ cup	1360	68	123
or Tossed Salad + Fr. Dress. (2 T.)	1240	61	111
Hamburger (5 oz) w. 2 scoops Rice	710	24	81
Gravy + Macaroni Salad	1135	49	112
MahiMahi (7 oz) w. 2 scoops Rice	650	12	90
+ Macaroni Salad + Tartar Sce	1150	58	109
or Macaroni Salad, no Tartar Sce	935	34	108
or Tossed Salad + Fr. Dress. (3 T.)	815	27	96
or Tossed Salad, no dressing	670	12	93
Teri Beef (5 oz) w. 2 scoops Rice	790	23	94
+ Macaroni Salad, ¾ cup	1095	47	113
or Tossed Salad, no dressing	800	23	93

Restaurant & International Foods

Indian & Pakistani   C   F   Cb

Per Serving
(Meat dishes allow 4 oz meat/serving)

	C	F	Cb
Aloo Samosa, each	155	12	12
Alu Gosht Kari (Meat/Pot. Curry)	600	40	23
Chicken Korma	500	35	6
Chicken Pilaf (Murgh Biriyani)	700	53	50
Chicken Tikka	260	16	2
Chicken Vindaloo	400	20	8
Chapati/Roti, 7" diam. piece	60	0.5	11
Dal (Lentil Puree): 1 cup, no oil	230	1	37
1 Tbsp Tadka (oil topping)	120	13	0
Dhakla (Lentil Dish), 1" sq., 1 oz	105	5	13
Dhansak, ½ cup	105	3.5	11
Gosht Kari (Meat Curry/Tom./Pot.)	460	25	17
Lamb Pilaf	520	35	40
Lassi (Sweet or Mango), 1 cup, 8 oz	160	4	24
Masala Gosht (Beef/Tom./Gravy)	400	25	18
Mulligatawney Soup, average	300	15	8
Murgh Tikka, 1 cup	300	4	7
Naan Bread, ¼ (8" x 2"), 1 oz	75	2	11
Pappadum, 1 large/2 small	50	3	5
Pesrattu (Lentil Crepe), 9", 2.6 oz	130	5	15
Pork Vindaloo Curry	620	47	3
Rajmah (Kidney Bean Curry), 1 cup	225	5	35
Rogan Josh (Lamb/Yogurt Sce)	500	30	3
Shahi Korma (Braised Lamb)	430	28	3
Tandoori Chicken: Breast	260	13	5
Leg/Thigh portion	300	17	6

Italian Dishes   C   F   Cb

	C	F	Cb
Baked Ziti: Small	370	27	32
Regular	575	42	49
Breadstick (1), 2 oz	120	2.5	25
Broccoli Fettucine Alfredo, reg.	815	23	125
Bruschetta, 2 slices	380	17	53
Calzones, average, all types	840	34	101
Cannelloni, 1 tube, 6 oz	280	15	18
Cheese Breadstick (1), 2.4 oz	180	8	20
Cheese Ravioli w. Sauce	495	17	65
Chicken Alfredo	775	29	82
Chicken Parmigiana, 11 oz	520	22	16
Fettucine Alfredo: Small	525	15	80
Regular	775	22	119
Meat Lasagne, 16 oz	700	36	60
Meat Ravioli	725	22	102
Minestrone Soup, 1 bowl	110	2	18
Shrimp & Scallop Fettucine	595	16	81
Spaghetti w. Marinara: Small	410	6	74
Regular	600	8	111
Spaghetti w. Meatballs: Small	710	31	80
Regular	1010	42	119
Spaghetti w. Meat Sauce: Small	425	8	74
Regular	625	11	111
Vegetable Primavera	610	8	116
Pizza: *Per Slice (⅛ Medium)*			
Cheese: Thin Crust	290	8	21
Thick Crust	375	13	29
Pepperoni: Thin Crust	215	10	21
Thick Crust	290	15	29
Deep Dish Pizza: Pepperoni,			
Medium (11"), 1 slice, (⅛)	445	15	57
Personal (6"), whole	380	10	58
Desserts: Lemon Ice	180	0	45
Gelato: Vanilla (Milk Base), ½ cup	200	15	18
Choc. Hazelnut (Milk), ½ cup	370	29	26
Water Base, ½ cup	100	0	25
Tiramisu, 1 piece, 5 oz	400	29	30

For more listings see Fast-Foods Section.

Sal Monella Restaurant

"I wonder why business is so bad these days?"

For Extra Menu Items
+ Full Nutritional Data
~ See Author's Website
www.CalorieKing.com

Japanese

	C	F	Cb
Sushi Rice: cooked, 1 Tbsp	25	0	5
1 cup, 5¼ oz	380	3	82
Sushi (Maki) Rolls: *Per Piece*			
Average all types (California Rolls; Crm Cheese w. Crab; Eel; Salmon; Shrimp; Tuna; Yellowtail; Vegetable)			
Small (1⅛" diam. x 1⅛" high), 0.8 oz	22	0.5	0.5
Med. (1¾" diam. x 1¾" high), 1.6 oz	44	1	1
Large (2¼" diam. x ⅞" high), 2 oz	55	1.5	1.5
Sushi Packs: *Per Pack*			
Average all types: 6 large pces	335	7.5	7.5
9 medium pieces	405	9	9
12 small pieces	325	12	6
Futomaki (thick roll), 6 pieces	315	1.5	7
Hand Roll (Cone), 2, 6 oz	225	5	5
Inari (rice filled soybean pocket), 4 pce	260	5	46
Sushi-Nigiri (fish on rice):			
average all types, 1 piece	70	0.5	12
Sushi Plate: Assorted, 6 pieces	420	3	36
Combination (Sushi & Sushi Rolls)			
2 Sushi + 6 sm. & 3 med. rolls	400	7	72
Sashimi (Sliced Raw Seafood/Beef)			
Ika (Squid), 4 oz	105	2	0
Hamachi (Yellowtail), 4 oz	165	6	0
Naguro (Yellowfin Tuna), 4 oz	120	1	0
Niku (Beef), 5 oz	200	10	0
Saba (Mackerel), 4 oz	160	7	0
Suzuki (Sea Bass), 4 oz	110	0.5	0
Tako (Octopus), 4 oz	95	1	0
Dipping Sauces: Average, 2 Tbsp	30	0	7
Ginger Vinegar Dressing, 2 Tbsp	20	0	5
Edamame (young green soybeans):			
Steamed/Salad (no pods), 4 oz	60	3	5
Boiled beans (no pods), 4 oz	160	7	12
Katsu-don Pork w. Rice	1100	39	141
Miso Soup w. Tofu pces, 1 cup	85	3	11
Seaweed Salad, 1.5 oz	20	2	0
Sukiyaki (Beef/Tofu/Veg.), 8 oz	400	24	32
Tempura (Batter-fried Shrimp & Veges)			
3 large shrimp & veges	320	18	25
1 shrimp only	60	4	3
Teppan Yaki (Steak, Seafood & Veges)			
10 oz serving	470	30	15
Teriyaki: Beef, 4 oz serving	350	25	4
Chicken, 4 oz serving	260	9	7
Salmon, 6 oz serving	270	8	3
Sake Wine (16% alc.), 3 fl.oz	115	0	7
Yakatori, 1 skewer, 2½ oz	140	5	1

Kosher/Deli Foods

	C	F	Cb
Bagel/Bialy, 1 small, 2 oz	160	2	32
Beiglach (Cheese Knish)	350	17	35
Blintzes: Average, 1 only	120	1	25
w. Sour Crm. & Preserves	370	10	30
Borscht: (no cream), 1 cup	85	3	14
Diet/Reduced Cal., 1 cup	30	1	7
Cabbage Roll (meat/rice), 5 oz	170	6	21
Chicken Broth: 1 cup	80	8	0
with vegetables	100	8	5
with noodles	150	9	16
Lowfat, plain, 1 cup	25	1	0
Cholent, 1 med serve, 1 cup	350	16	48
Chopped Liver: 1 serve, 3 oz	110	6	5
with Egg Salad, ¼ cup	100	7	3
Farfel, dry, ½ cup	90	0.5	21
Hallah (Yeast Bread), 1 sl., 1 oz	85	2	14
Gefilte Fish Balls: Reg., medium, 2 oz	55	2	4
with jelled broth	80	2	6
Cocktail size, 1 oz	30	1	2
Sweet, medium, 2 oz	65	2	4
with jelled broth	95	2	6
Herring: Smoked, 2 oz	120	8	0
in Sour Cream, 2 oz	150	10	0
Kasha, cooked, ½ cup	100	0.5	20
Kipfel (Vanilla/Almd. Cookie), 1 pce	60	2	7
Knaidlach ~ See Matzo Balls			
Knish: Kasha/Potato, 1 only	130	4	22
Cheese, 1 only	350	17	35
Kreplach, beef, 1 piece	40	1	6
Kugel, potato/noodle, 1 serve	300	20	25
Latkes (Potato Pancake), 2 oz	200	11	22
3 Latkes w. Sour Cr./Apple Sce	750	25	95
Lochsen: Plain, 1 cup	130	2	26
Pudding, 1 cup	380	13	48
Lox (Smoked Salmon), 2 oz	65	2	0
Mandelbrot (Almond Bread),			
1 slice, ¼" thick	45	2	5
Matzo *(See Page 105)*, 1 oz board	110	0.5	21
Matzo Balls: 2 small, or 1 large, 2"	90	3	12
Extra large ball, 3"	180	6	24
Matzo Ball Soup:			
Cup w. 2 small or 1 large ball	150	5	27
Bowl w. Chicken & Noodles	325	13	34
Jerry's Deli, large bowl	560	17	56
New York Cheesecake, 4 oz	350	24	26
Pierogi, potato/cheese, 1 pce	90	4	11
Reuben S'wich w. ½ lb corned beef	920	60	28
Schmaltz (Rend'd chick. fat), 1 T.	90	10	0

Restaurant & International Foods

Korean Food

	C	F	Cb
Bibimbab (Vege & Beef on Rice), 1 cup	565	15	89
Bulgogi (Barbeque Beef), 3.5 oz	325	12	15
Galbi (Short Ribs), 16 oz	975	61	16
Gujeolpan (Pancake w. Meat & Vegetables), cup w. 1 pancake	340	11	39
Japchae (Noodle w. Vege & Meat), 1¼ cup	365	19	34
Sides:			
Kimchee (Cabbage Relish), ½ cup	30	0	6
Namool (Assorted Veges) 1 cup	125	6.5	9
Soups: *Per Serving*			
Muguk (Radish & Chive Soup), 6 oz	105	7	6
Samgyetang (Ginseng Chicken Soup)			
no Chicken Skin, 1 cup	520	11	60
w. Chicken Skin, 1 cup	725	35	60
Yuk Gae Jang (Spicy Beef Soup), 1¼ cup	180	13	5

Lebanese/Middle East

	C	F	Cb
Baba Ghannouj, 2 Tbsp, 1 oz (Eggplant/Sesame Dip)	70	6	2
Baklava, 1 pastry, 1¾ oz (Pastry, Nuts, Syrup)	245	18	18
Cabbage Rolls, 1 roll, 3 oz (Cabbage Leaf, Meat, Rice)	100	3	12
Cous Cous, 1 serve (Semolina, Milk, Fruit, Nuts)	400	21	43
Felafel (Chick Pea Fritter):			
Fried, 1 medium, 1 oz	60	4	4
Hummus, ¼ cup, 2.2 oz	105	3	5
Fried Kibbi, 1 piece, 3 oz (Wheat, Meat, Pinenuts)	180	8	15
Kafta, 1 skewer, 1½ oz (Ground Lamb Saus. on Skewer)	85	5	2
Kibbeh Naye, 1 cup, 9 oz (Raw Lamb, Bulgur & Spices)	450	18	28
Lebanese Omelet, 1 serving, 4 oz (Egg, Spinach, Pinenuts, Onion)	200	12	13
Pilaf, 1 cup (Rice, Onion, Rais., Apr. Spice)	400	11	60
Shawourma, 1 serve, 4 oz (Spit Roast Beef)	280	15	2
Shish Kabob, 1 stick, 2½ oz	130	7	2
Spinach Pie, 1 piece, 3½ oz	290	21	20
Sweet Almond Sanbusak, 1 pce (Pastry, Almonds, Spices)	200	15	11
Tabouli, 1 serve, 4 oz	170	14	7
Tahini Sauce, avg., 1 Tbsp	90	8	3

Mexican

	C	F	Cb
Black Bean Soup, 1 bowl	200	3	34
Bueso Fresco, ¼ cup	80	4.5	8
Burritos *(Taco Bell):* Bean	370	10	55
Supreme® Beef	440	18	50
Chili, plain, ¼ cup	90	6	8
Chili con Carne: w. Beans, 1 cup	310	17	15
w/out Beans, 1 cup	370	28	10
Chimichangas, Beef, 5 oz	400	19	43
Chorizo Sausage, 2 oz	265	23	0
Churros, 1½ oz	150	8	18
Corn Chips, ½ cup, 1 oz	160	10	17
Costillas Ribs, 6 oz	675	52	0
Enchilada, average	330	10	49
Fajitas, Chicken (Soft)	200	7	20
Guacamole, 2 Tbsp, 1 oz	120	12	2
Horchata: *Don Jose,* 1 cup, 8 fl. oz	140	4	25
Cacique, 1 pint bottle, 16 fl. oz	320	7	62
Margarita, w. 1½ oz Tequila	160	0	6
Menudo, ½ cup	55	1.5	10
Nachos: *Del Taco,* Regular	395	24	40
Macho Nachos	1145	63	113
Taco Bell: BellGrande®	760	43	80
Supreme®	470	26	42
Nachos: with cheese, peppers,			
1 portion (6-8 nachos), 7 oz	600	33	60
with cheese, beans, ground beef, peppers,			
1 portion (6-8 nachos), 9 oz	570	31	56
Nopal Cactus Salad, 1 serving	130	9	11
Papas Fritas (Fried Potatoes) (1), 4 oz	325	18	40
Piloncillo (Brown Sugar): 1 Tbsp, 13g	50	0	13
Cone, small, 3", 3 oz	325	0	81
Quesadilla, Cheese *(Taco Bell)*	490	28	39
Refried Beans, ¾ cup, 6 oz	160	3	26
Rice Pudding (Arroz con Leche), 4 oz	140	3	24
Sopes (Gorditas), 2 oz	120	0	27
Taco *(Taco Bell):* Regular, Crispy	170	10	13
Ranchero Chicken	270	15	21
Taco Supreme®	220	14	14
Double Decker® Taco	340	14	39
Taco Salad w. Salsa	840	52	85
Taco Sauce, average, ¼ cup	15	0	3
Taco Shell, regular	50	2	8
Tamales, w. Beef/Chicken, avg, 4.5 oz	250	11	27
Taquitos, Beef & Cheese, 4.5 oz	330	15	36
Tostada *(Taco Bell)*	250	10	29
Tortilla, Corn, 6" diam.	70	1	14
Tortilla Chips, 1 oz	150	8	19

Extra Listings of Mexican Dishes:
- **Fast-Foods Section** *(Taco Bell, Del Taco)*
- **Canned Bean/Chili Products:** See Pages 71-76

Mexican (Cont)

	C	F	Cb
Breads: Bolillos, 1 roll, 3½ oz	240	4	42
Telera, 2 oz	150	1.5	19
Mexican Cornbread, 4" square	210	11	19
French Baguette, 2 oz	140	1.5	26
Cakes, Cookies, Pastries			
Banderilla (Pastry Puff), 1 shell	140	10	8
Bigotes, 7"	570	22	44
Calvos, 2½ oz	320	18	38
Capirotada (Bread Pudding), 10 oz	810	38	107
Cinnamon Cookies, 2	125	8	13
Cocadas, 1 oz	120	6	15
Cortadillo, 1 cookie, 1.9 oz	300	11	48
Concha (All Colors):			
Small (3" diam), 2½ oz	250	8	38
Medium (4" diam), 3½ oz	350	11	53
Large (5" diam), 5½ oz	550	18	84
Cream Puff with Custard, 4¼ oz	255	14	25
Cuerno, 2 oz	200	4.5	34
Cuerno Fine, 2¾ oz	330	17	40
Donus (Donuts), 4", 3½ oz	440	21	58
Elotes, 3½ oz	450	24	51
Empanadas (Average all types):			
Small, 2 oz	230	10	28
Regular, 3 oz	300	14	42
Fiesta Cookie, 2¼ oz	280	8	47
Galletas Mixtas (1), 1 oz	100	2.5	16
Guayaba, 3¼ oz	360	14	53
Jelly Rolls, 3¼ oz	240	4	46
Mantecadites (Almond Shortbread), 4½ oz	670	42	64
Mini Pound Cake, 3 oz	260	12	33
Mini Cupcakes, 1¾ oz	180	8	25
Muffins/Nino Enbuelto, large, 6 oz	465	11	48
Novcias, 2¾ oz	290	9	46
Nuez, 3¼ oz	380	17	52
Ojo De Buey, 4 oz	360	15	55
Orejas Ears, 3 oz	310	15	38
Pan Dulce (Mexican Sweet Bread), 1 bun	330	10	45
Panquecitos, 2½ oz	260	11	36
Piedras, 4 oz	470	15	76
Polvorones, 3 oz	370	18	48
Puerquitos, 5 oz	600	24	88
Rebanadas, 3½ oz	390	18	51
Roles De Canela (Cin. Roll), 4½ oz	490	15	81
Roscas, 2¾ oz	360	18	44
Semitas, 3 oz	300	10	46
Sopapillas (flaky pastry puffs), 1 pce	100	7	10
w. Honey & Cream	200	14	18
Strawberry Crème Roll (⅙), 2½ oz	240	5	45

Extra Food Listings ~ See CalorieKing.com

Polish

	C	F	Cb
Cabbage Rolls w. Sour Cr., 2 sm.	220	10	30
Chicken Casserole w. Mush., 1 cup	520	27	5
Kielbasa (Sausages, Onions, fried),			
2 large	350	28	2
Meatballs in Sour Cream,			
3 x 1½" balls	300	16	11
Pierogi, Fruit/Veg, 3" ball	80	2	15
Pork Goulash (Pork/Veg. Stew)	550	21	38
Pot Roast with Vegetables	630	21	28

Soul Foods

	C	F	Cb
Breakfast Sausage, fried, 2 patties	250	17	0
Brunswick Stew, 1 cup, 8.5 oz	320	14	19
Cornbread, home-made, 3 oz	200	7.5	30
Fatback, raw, ¼ oz	60	6.5	0
Ham Hock	90	6.5	2
Hog Maw	45	2.5	0
Hominy, cooked, ¾ cup	110	0.5	25
Hush Puppies, 5 pieces	260	12	35
Kale, cooked, ½ cup	20	0.5	4
Opossum	65	3	0
Oxtail	70	3.5	0
Pig Ear, ¼ ear	50	3	0
Pig Foot, ½ foot	70	5	0
Pig Tail, ⅓ tail	115	10	0
Poke Salad, cooked, ½ cup	16	0.5	3
Pork Brains	40	2.5	0
Pork Chitterlings, simmered, 3 oz	260	25	0
Pork Cracklings, ½ oz	80	6	0
Pork Neck Bones	65	4	0
Pork Skin, 1 cup	70	4.5	0
Pork Tongue, ⅓ tongue	75	5.5	0
Sousemeat	60	4.5	0
Succotash, ½ cup	80	1	17
Sweet Potato Pie, ⅛ of 9" pie	250	12	34
Tripe, 2 oz	55	2	0
Vienna Sausage, 2 small	90	8	1
small	45	4	0.5

Brooklyn

Restaurant & International Foods

Spanish

	C	F	Cb
Arroz Abanda (Fish with Rice)	340	8	31
Arroz Con Pollo (Rice/Chick. Sal)	500	23	50
Clams Marinara, 8 clams	330	16	22
Cochifrito (Lamb w. Lemon/Garlic)	650	25	5
Cochinillo Asado, 2 sl. (Rst Suckling Pig)	300	15	3
Cocido Madrileno			
(Madrid-Style Boiled Dinner)	450	27	18
Flan de Leche (Caramel Custard)	325	9	52
Fritadera de Ternera (Sauteed Veal)	450	27	2
Gazpacho, 1 bowl	60	0	15
Paella a la Valenciana			
(Chicken & Shellfish Rice)	900	42	70
Pollo a la Espanola (Chicken)	475	30	4
Ternera al Jerez (Veal w. Sherry)	660	29	6
Zarzuela (Fish & Shellfish Medley)	530	27	40

Thai Foods

	C	F	Cb
Appetizers: Satay Pork, 1 oz	100	4	2
Spring Roll, 1¼ oz	110	6	13
Soups: Tom Yam (Hot & Sour):			
Spicy Shrimp/Seafood, 1 cup	100	4	6
1 bowl	160	7	10
Vegetarian, 1 cup	50	0	11
Curries: Chicken w. Ginger, 1 cup	390	34	4
Thick Red Curry w. Beef, 1 cup	600	50	7
Thai Chicken Curry, 1 cup	340	23	4
Massaman Curry, 1 cup	680	57	8
Green Curry w. Pork, 1 cup	480	44	5
Pad Thai, Large serving, 18 oz	990	38	125
Fish: Steamed w. Spicy Thai Sce	450	8	46
Crispy Fried, 5 oz	290	15	9
Spicy Chicken (w. veges), stir-fry	450	22	14
Spicy Garlic Tofu w. veges, stir-fry	340	18	18
Sticky Thai Rice: Plain 1 cup, 6 oz	170	0.5	36
w. Coconut & Sesame Seeds, 1 cup	880	28	120
Stir-fried Rice Noodles, 1 c., 5½ oz	270	9	40
Stir-fried Vegetables, 1 cup	100	3	18
Salads: Green Papaya Salad	160	0	40
Spicy Prawn, 9 shrimp	170	3	15
Thai Chicken, 1 serving	330	19	17
Thai Beef Salad, 1 serving	260	9	15
Thai Noodle, 1 serving	410	13	45
Satay Chicken & Peanut Sauce:			
1 satay stick	390	24	20
Sauces: Peanut Satay, ½ cup, 4 oz	160	10	13

Vietnamese

	C	F	Cb
Banh Cuon (Steam Rice w. Pork), 1 roll	105	7	8
Bo Nuong (Beef Satay), 2 sticks	265	9	4
Bo Xao Dau Phong			
(Ginger Beef w.Onion, Fish Sce.)	750	30	10
Ca Chien Gung (Whole Snapper/Ging.)	600	16	6
Canh Chay (Veg./Tofu Soup)	80	3	13
Cari (Curry) Chicken, 1 cup	475	29	16
Cari (Curry) Chicken, w. Rice Noodle,			
cup curry & cup cooked noodles	660	29	60
Cari (Curry) Chicken, w. Steam Rice,			
cup curry & cup rice	650	29	55
Cuu Xao Lan (Curried Lamb,			
Veges in Coconut)	900	40	80
Ga Chien (Crisp Chick + Plum Sce)	900	40	105
Ga Nuong (Chicken Satay + Sce)	240	10	4
Ga Xao Rau (Marinated Chicken			
Braised w. Veg.)	800	26	100
Gio Lua (Lean Pork Pie), ⅙ of pie	245	12	0
Goi Cuon (Cold Spring Rolls), each	60	1	7
Rau Cai Xao Chay (Stir Fried Vege.)	400	15	65
Thit Bo Vien (Beef Balls), 6 balls	225	14	2
Thit Heo Goi Baup Cai, each			
(Spicy Cabbage Rolls w. Pork)	200	7	11
Vietnamese (Cont)			
Soup: *Per Bowl (1½ Cup)*			
Bun Bo Hue (Hot & Spicy Soup			
no Pork Feet	340	9	35
w. Pork Feet	830	45	35
Chicken & Rice Noodle Soup	400	3	55
Pho Bo (Beef Noodle Soup)	410	7	59
Pho Ga (Chicken Noodle Soup)	460	6	58
Pho Tai (Rare Beef & Noodle Soup	440	7	73
Salad: *Per ½ Cup*			
Goi Du Du (Green Papaya Salad)	155	3	29
Sauce: Nuoc Cham (Hot Sauce)	5	0	1

Gourmet & Miscellaneous

	C	F	Cb
Ants Eggs/Larvae, 1 Tbsp	20	0	0
Ants, Choc. coated, 3 Tbsp	140	7	2
Bee Maggots, canned, 3 Tbsp	65	2	0
Caviar, black/red, 1 Tbsp	40	3	0
Caterpillars, canned, 2 oz	60	1	0
Frogs Legs, fried, 1 pair (large)	125	7	0
Haggis, boiled, 4 oz	350	24	22
Locusts, roasted, 1 oz	35	1	0
Silkworms, raw, 1 oz	60	2	0
Snails in garlic butter, 6 large	200	10	4
Snake, roasted, 4 oz	160	6	0

Fast-Food Chains & *Restaurants*

Fast - Foods & *Restaurants*

A&W®

Sandwiches & Burgers	**C**	**F**	**Cb**
Cheeseburger	470	24	40
Cheeseburger Deluxe	510	28	41
Cheeseburger Deluxe Bacon	570	33	41
Cheeseburger Deluxe Double	720	42	46
Cheeseburger Deluxe Double Bacon	800	48	47
Crispy Chicken Sandwich	550	23	55
Grilled Chicken Sandwich	400	13	35
Hamburger	430	22	37
Hamburger Deluxe	460	26	37
Chicken			
Chicken Strips, 3 pces	510	30	33
Hot Dogs: Plain, 3.2 oz	280	17	22
Cheese Dog, 4.4 oz	320	20	25
Coney (Chili), 4.4 oz	310	18	24
Coney (Chili) Chse Dog, 5.4 oz	350	21	27
Fries & Sides: Per Serving			
Fries: French, Regular, 4 oz	310	13	45
French, Large, 5.5 oz	425	18	61
Cheese Fries, 6 oz	390	18	50
Chili Fries, 6 oz	370	15	49
Chili Cheese Fries, 7 oz	410	17	52
Dipping Sauces: Barbeque, 1 oz	40	0	10
Honey Mustard	105	6	12
Sweet and Sour	50	0	12
Poutine, small, 6 oz	420	24	38
Onion Rings, 4 oz	350	20	45
Salads: Coleslaw, Individual	90	6	9
Potato Salad, Individual	160	8	22
Macaroni Salad, Individual	175	9	22
Desserts			
Hot Caramel Sundae	340	9	57
Hot Fudge Sundae	350	11	54
Other Sundaes, avg.	310	8	52
Polar Swirl™: M&M; Oreo, small	840	29	125
Reese's, small	775	36	113
Soft Ice Cream Cone, regular, avg.	250	7	41
Milkshakes & Floats: Per 16 fl.oz			
Chocolate Milkshake	695	29	100
Strawberry Milkshake	665	29	90
Vanilla Milkshake	720	31	97
A&W Root Beer Float	340	5	71
Drinks: Per 20 fl.oz			
A&W Root Beer	300	0	80
Diet A&W Root Beer; Diet Coke	0	0	0
Coca-Cola	300	0	74
Sprite	300	0	72

Applebee's®

	C	**F**	**Cb**
Appetizer: Onion au Gratin Soup	150	8	12
Tortilla Chicken Melt	480	13	50
Veggie Patch Pizza (10") ⅙ pizza	150	9	12
Entree Meals: Includes Sides/Sauces			
Crispy Buttermilk Shrimp	845	34	83
Crispy Orange Skillet w. Noodles	1710	69	209
Fiesta Lime Chkn w. Tortilla Strips	1285	47	136
Grilled Steak Caesar Salad: w. Toast	1295	82	60
no Toast	1190	75	44
Grilled Tilapia, w. Rice Pilaf & Mango	320	6	30
Madeira Steak Tips w toast	910	38	82
Oriental Chicken Salad Roll-Up	710	25	72
Riblets w. sauce + fries	2025	130	106
Sizzling Chicken Skillet	360	4	43
Southwest Philly Roll-Up: w. Salsa	1605	121	60
w. Sour Cream	2230	160	122
Tango Chicken Sandwich	370	9	40
Teriyaki Steak & Shrimp Skewers	370	7	33
Salad			
Grilled Shrimp Skewer	210	2	22
Mesquite Chicken Sandwich	250	4	42
Sides			
Flour Tortilla (12")	305	7	52
Desserts: Per Serving			
Blue Ribbon Brownie			
w. 2 scoops Ice Cream	735	30	105
Chocolate Raspberry Layer	230	3	46
Cheesecake, Berry Lemon	230	7	34
Sizzling Apple Pie w. Ice Cream	1085	56	146
Triple Chocolate Meltdown Cake	725	31	107

For Complete Nutritional Data ~ see CalorieKing.com

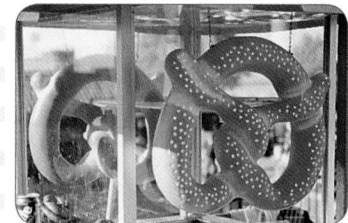

Arby's®

Breakfast: Per Serving	C	F	Cb
Bacon 'n Egg Croissant	410	26	31
Bacon Biscuit	300	17	27
Biscuit: Plain	230	12	26
w. Butter	330	23	26
w. Scrambled Egg	320	18	28
w. Swiss Cheese	270	15	26
Ham 'n Cheese Croissant	350	19	30
Ham Biscuit	270	13	27
Sausage 'n Egg Croissant	510	36	31
Sausage Biscuit	390	27	26
Sourdough Bacon, Egg 'n Swiss	500	29	33
Sourdough Egg 'n Cheese	330	16	31
Sourdough Ham, Egg 'n Swiss	450	23	33
Sandwiches			
Arby-Q	375	11	51
Beef 'n Cheddar	440	21	44
Big Montana	590	29	41
Chicken Bacon 'n Swiss	550	27	49
Chicken Breast Fillet	500	25	48
French Dip 'n Swiss	535	21	51
Giant Roast Beef	450	19	41
Junior Roast Beef	280	9	34
Philly Beef Supreme	715	37	59
Regular Roast Beef	320	13	34
Roast Chicken Club	470	25	39
Super Roast Beef	440	19	48
Market Fresh Sandwiches			
Chicken Salad	770	38	78
Roast Beef & Swiss	780	39	74
Roast Ham & Swiss	700	31	74
Roast Turkey & Swiss	720	27	74
Roast Turkey Ranch & Bacon	830	38	75
Ultimate BLT	780	46	75
Market Fresh Wraps			
Chicken Caesar	680	38	52
Roast Turkey Ranch & Bacon	710	39	48
Southwest Chicken	590	30	45
Ultimate BLT Wrap	650	47	48
Market Fresh Salads: Per Serving			
Asian Sesame:			
w. Almonds, Noodles & Dressing	485	25	40
no Almonds, Noodles or Dressing	140	1	15
Chicken Club Salad: No Dressing	530	33	32
w. Buttermilk Ranch Dressing	860	67	36
Garden Side Salad, no dressing	40	0	8

Arby's® cont..

Market Fresh Salads: (Cont)	C	F	Cb
Martha's Vineyard Salad:			
w. Raspb. Vinaigrette & Almond	500	27	41
no Vinaigrette or Almonds	250	8	23
Santa Fe: w. Dress. & Tortilla Strips	880	62	54
no Dressing or Tortilla Strips	520	29	40
Sauces & Condiments: Per Serving			
Mayonnaise, 0.5 oz	100	11	0
Dipping Sauce: BBQ, 1 oz	40	0	10
Honey Mustard, 1 oz	130	12	5
Dressing: Asian Sesame, 1.9 fl.oz	190	14	15
Buttermilk Ranch, 2 oz	290	30	3
Fat Free Italian, 2 oz	30	0	7
Light Balsamic Vinaigrette, 2 oz	105	6	13
Light Buttermilk Ranch, 2 oz	105	6	12
Raspberry Vinaigrette, 1.9 fl.oz	170	12	16
Santa Fe Ranch, 1.9 fl.oz	270	28	3
Sauce: Arby's, 0.5 oz	15	0	4
Bronco Berry, 2 oz	120	0	30
Cheddar Cheese, 1.5 oz	60	4.5	4
Horsey, 0.5 oz	60	5	3
Marinara, 1.5 oz	30	1.5	4
Red Ranch, 0.5 oz	70	6	5
Tangy Southwest, 2 oz	330	35	5
Sides: Per Serving			
Baked Potato: Plain	200	0	46
w. Broccoli 'n Cheddar	475	23	56
w. Butter & Sour Cream	425	23	48
Deluxe, 10.4 oz	580	34	50
Chicken Fingers: 4 Pack	640	38	42
Combo w. Curly Fries	1050	60	89
Snack w. Curly Fries	600	34	53
Fries: Curly, small, 3.7 oz	340	18	39
Homestyle, small, 4 oz	300	13	44
Potato Cakes (2)	250	15	26
Sidekickers: Jalapeno Bites (5)	310	19	29
Mozzarella Sticks (4)	430	23	38
Onion Petals, 4 oz	330	19	35
Shakes: Chocolate, reg., 13.2 fl.oz	510	13	83
Other flavors, regular, 13.2 fl.oz	500	13	81
Desserts: Per Serving			
Apple Turnover w. Icing	380	12	64
Cherry Turnover w. Icing	380	12	64
Gourmet Chocolate Cookie	200	10	26

For Complete Nutritional Data ~ see CalorieKing.com

Arthur Treachers®

Meals: Per Serving

	C	F	Cb
Fish N Chips	1540	101	132
Fish Sandwich,	480	23	40
Seafood Sampler	3380	270	226
Shrimp N Chips	2050	123	225

Sides

	C	F	Cb
Cole Slaw, 5 oz, 141.5g	215	8.5	34
Hush Puppy (2)	275	10	42

Atlanta Bread Company®

Bagels: Per Bagel

	C	F	Cb
Apple Spice	360	2.5	73
Asiago Cheese	380	10	65
Cinnamon Crisp	330	2.5	68
Everything	320	3.5	60
Low-Carb Cranberry Walnut	110	3.5	16
Poppy Seed	320	5	57
Sesame	360	9	57
Other varieties, average	270	1.5	54

Sandwiches: No Cheese or Dressing

	C	F	Cb
ABC Special on French Roll	420	4.5	61
Peanut Butter & Jelly	600	14	99
Roasted Turkey Breast	430	7	61
Tangy Roast Beef	390	4	56
Tuna, 4 oz	360	32	4
Veggie on Nine Grain	340	5	63
Focaccia: Hot Pastrami	460	10	59
Bella Basil on Tom. & Rosemary	660	35	58
California Avocado on Tom. On.	690	40	71
Chicken Salad, 4 oz	280	21	2
Grilled Chse on French Bread	390	11	57
Honey Maple Ham	410	5	63
Paninis: Chicken Pesto	740	30	78
Cordon Bleu	595	15	76
Cuban Pork Loin	745	30	82
Italian Vegetarian	625	21	81
Turkey Club	750	27	83

Salads: Caesar

	C	F	Cb
Caesar	190	10	11
Chicken Salad on Lettuce	280	21	2
Chopstix Chicken	280	13	24
Extra Croutons, 0.5 oz	50	2	6
Fruit, 10 oz	130	0	34
Greek	200	13	13
House	50	0	11
Tuna Salad on Lettuce	360	32	4
Add Grilled Chicken, 2.5 oz	70	1.5	2

Atlanta Bread ® cont...

Soups: Per Serving (10 oz)

	C	F	Cb
Black Bean & Ham	250	9	40
Chicken Tortilla	190	9	20
Chunky Baked Potato	290	16	30
Classic Chicken Noodle	140	2.5	21
Cream of Broccoli	200	11	19
Creamy Tomato	130	9	10
French Onion w. Toppings	200	10	16
Garden Vegetable	100	1.5	19
Homestyle Chicken 'n Dumpling	290	18	25
New England Clam Chowder	280	16	24
Pasta Fagioli	170	6	24
Spicy Chicken Gumbo	120	2.5	16
Wisconsin Cheese	240	14	21

Breads: Per Thick Slice (2 oz)

	C	F	Cb
ABC Roll, 1 roll	260	1	54
Asiago	160	2	29
Asiago Strip	160	2	28
Challah	160	2.5	29
Cinnamon Raisin Loaf	150	2	30
Cracked Wheat	160	2	30
Muffin Tops: Banana Nut	420	26	39
Blueberry	250	12	31
Chocolate Chip	400	19	52
Mocha	410	20	53
Pumpkin	350	13	54

For Complete Nutritional Data ~ see CalorieKing.com

Au Bon Pain®

Bagels: Per Bagel	C	F	Cb
Asiago Cheese	380	8	59
Cinnamon Raisin	330	1	71
Dutch Apple	470	3.5	99
French Toast	420	7	76
Plain	300	1	61
Spreads: Plain Cream Chse, 2 oz	120	11	4
Smoked Salmon	110	9	3
Sundried Tomato; Veggie, 2 oz	140	12	3

Breakfast Sandwiches: Per Sandwich			
Egg on a Bagel	400	4	63
w. Bacon	480	12	63
w. Bacon & Cheese	560	18	63
w. Cheese	480	11	63

Sandwiches			
Asian Chicken Salad	430	16	50
Chicken & Mozzarella Foccacia	740	24	73
Chicken Tarragon w. Field Onions	800	42	71
Fresh Mozzarella, Tomato w. Pesto	820	43	67
Grilled Chicken w. Blue Cheese	670	29	64
Roasted Trukey Cranberry	555	12	80
Spicy Tuna on Multigrain	690	33	72
Tuna w. Cheddar & Peppers	555	18	62
Turkey w. Guacamole & Swiss	760	28	77
Wraps: Chicken Caesar	590	24	63
Fields & Feta	550	16	90
Mediterranean Wrap	570	22	80
Southwestern Tuna	540	25	68

Brownies: Blonde w. nuts	570	36	57
Choc Chip	480	25	61

Soups: Per Serving (8 oz)			
Broccoli Cheddar	230	16	13
Chicken Noodle	90	2	11
Corn Chowder	240	13	25
Garden Vegetable	40	1	7
Split Pea w. Ham	140	1	23
Vegetarian Chili	170	1	30

Breads: Average, 1.75 oz slice	130	1	27
Bread Bowl (1)	640	3	127
Foccacia (1)	310	3.5	58
Four Grain Bread, 1 slice	315	3	58
Rosemary Garlic Breadstick	200	5	33
Bread Rolls: Hearth (1)	240	2	44
Braided Pain Roll (1)	430	14	62

Au Bon Pain® cont...

Yogurt & Fruit Cups: Per Serving	C	F	Cb
Yogurt & Fruit, average, 15 oz	380	4.5	75
Fruit Cup: Small, 6 oz	70	0	16
Large, 12 oz	140	0	32

Salads: Per Serving (Container)			
Caesar Salad	240	11	23
Chef's Salad	255	14	8
Garden Salad	50	1	10
Gorgonzola & Walnut	340	28	10
Mediterranean Chicken	290	16	14
Thai Chicken	140	2.5	14
Tuna Garden	305	24	25
Turkey Medallion Cobb	370	18	27
Tuna Nicoise	300	15	19

Cookies: Per Cookie			
Chocolate Chip	260	11	41
English Toffee	240	14	26
Oatmeal Raisin	250	9	42
Shortbread	340	22	35

Cakes & Bars: Apple Strudel	410	18	56
Cinnamon Roll	390	12	67
Cherry Strudel	390	19	49
Pecan Brownie	510	31	56
Croissants: Ham & Cheese	340	10	46
Spinach & Cheese	250	9	32
Filled: Plain	250	6	44
Almond	510	25	63
Apple	230	3	47
Chocolate	380	15	61
Raspberry	340	11	55
Sweet Cheese	350	14	52

Muffins: Blueberry	510	19	76
Cranberry Walnut	560	26	69
Chocolate	590	20	83
Corn Chunk	440	18	64
Raisin Bran	530	13	100
Low-Fat: Chocolate Cake	320	2	74
Triple Berry	290	2	61

Drinks			
Mocha Blast, 16 fl.oz	360	11	54
Frozen Mocha Blast, 16 fl.oz	320	13	57
Cappuccino, 16 fl.oz	120	4.5	12
Iced Tea, 22 fl.oz	120	0	30

For Complete Nutritional Data ~ see CalorieKing.com

Fast - Foods & *Restaurants*

Auntie Anne's®

Pretzels: With Butter	C	F	Cb
Almond	400	8	72
Cinnamon Sugar	450	9	83
Garlic	350	4.5	68
Glazin' Raisin®	510	4	107
Jalapeno	310	4.5	59
Original	370	4	72
Parmesan Herb	440	13	72
Sesame	410	12	64
Sour Cream & Onion	340	5	66
Stix, 4 sticks	245	3	48
Whole Wheat	370	4.5	72

Pretzels: Without Butter	C	F	Cb
Almond Pretzel; Whole Wheat	340	1.5	72
Cinnamon Sugar	350	2	74
Garlic Pretzel; Sour Crm & Onion	320	1	66
Glazin' Raisin®	470	0.5	104
Jalapeno	270	1	58
Original	340	1	72
Parmesan Herb	390	5	74
Sesame	350	6	63
Stix, 4 sticks	225	1	48

Dipping Sauces	C	F	Cb
Caramel Dip, 1.5 oz	135	3	27
Cheese Sce; Hot Salsa Chse, avg.	100	8	4
Chocolate Flavored Dip, 1¼ oz	130	4	24
Light Cream Cheese, 1¼ oz	70	6	1
Marinara Sauce, 1¼ oz	10	0	4
Strawberry Cream Cheese, 1¼ oz	110	10	4
Sweet Mustard, 1¼ oz	60	1.5	8

Beverages: Per Serving	C	F	Cb
Auntie Anne's Lemonade, 22 fl.oz	180	0	43
Dutch Ice (20 fl.oz): Kiwi-Banana	270	0	63
Blue Raspberry	230	0	55
Lemonade	450	0	110
Mocha	570	15	105
Orange Crème	400	0	92
Pina Colada; Strawberry	535	0	125
Wild Cherry	300	0	69
Dutch Smoothie: Per 20 fl.oz			
Blue Raspberry	400	14	65
Kiwi-Banana	430	14	68
Lemonade	540	14	95
Mocha	590	23	90
Orange Crème	500	14	83
Pina Colada	470	14	79
Strawberry; Wild Cherry	450	14	74

Backyard Burgers®

Burgers	C	F	Cb
Back Yard Burger ⅓ lb.	470	29	38
Cheeseburger ⅓ lb	520	34	38
Bacon Cheddar	620	42	38
Barbecue Bacon	630	39	47
Black Jack	580	39	36
Chili Cheese	560	36	41
Garden Veggie Sandwich	240	6	47
Jr Burger	310	17	38
Hawaiian	550	33	44
Miz Grazi	530	34	39
Mushroom Swiss	540	36	37
Low-Carb Burger	350	27	3

Chicken Sandwiches	C	F	Cb
Bacon Swiss	390	20	37
Barbecue	280	8	44
Blackened	290	11	39
Buffalo Ranch	540	30	51
Hawaiian Chicken	280	8	45
Honey Mustard	320	11	46
Lemon Butter Chicken	260	9	37
Savory Chicken	230	6	36
Specialities: BLT	270	16	36
Chicken Tenderloins, 3 piece	400	28	22
Chili Dog	340	20	29
Chili Cheese Dog	400	25	29
Hot Dog	310	18	27

Baked Potatoes	C	F	Cb
Chili & Cheddar, 9 oz	330	11	48
Ranch, 7.7 oz	410	22	45
Salsa, 7.7 oz	250	5	47
Traditional/Plain, 6 oz	190	0	43

Fries	C	F	Cb
Chili Cheese Fries, 6.7 oz	350	22	28
Seasoned Fries, regular, 3 oz	260	16	26
Waffle Fries, regular, 3 oz	240	16	23

Salads (No Dressing)	C	F	Cb
Blackened Chicken	160	4	11
Charbroiled Chicken	140	3	11
Garden Fresh	25	0	5

Cobblers: Apple, 6 oz	430	20	61
Blackberry; Peach, 6 oz	420	20	60
Cherry, 6 oz	460	20	68

Shakes: Per 12 fl.oz	C	F	Cb
Chocolate; Strawberry	560	26	79
Vanilla	540	26	71

For Complete Nutritional Data ~ see CalorieKing.com

Restaurants & Fast - Foods

Baja Fresh®

	C	F	Cb
Burritos: *Includes Cheese*			
Baja Burrito: w. Charbroiled Chicken	800	34	70
w. Charbroiled Steak	890	42	70
Bare Burrito: w. Charbroiled Chkn	650	7	99
Vegetarian	590	10	102
Bean & Cheese Burrito: w. Chicken	980	33	99
w. Charbroiled Steak	1070	41	99
Vegetarian	850	31	99
Burrito Dos Manos: w. Chicken	780	25	97
w. Charbroiled Steak	820	29	95
Burrito Mexicano: w. Chicken	810	13	119
w. Charbroiled Steak	900	20	119
Burrito Ultimo: w. Charbroiled Chkn	890	35	87
w. Charbroiled Steak	990	42	87
Grilled Vegetarian	810	32	96
Fajita Burrito w. Chicken	910	37	88
w. Steak	1000	44	88
Enchilado Style:			
(add to any Dos Manos)	640	40	44
Fajitas			
Charbroiled Chkn w. Corn Tortillas	1100	28	146
Charbroiled Steak w. Corn Tortillas	1240	39	146
Nachos: w. Charbroiled Steak	2100	113	166
w. Cheese/Chicken, average	1880	103	166
Quesadilla: w. Chicken & Chips	1350	75	90
w. Charbroiled Steak & Chip	1440	83	90
w. Cheese & Chips	1220	73	90
Vegetarian w. Chips	1270	74	102
Tacos			
Baja Fish Taco w. Breaded Fish	270	13	31
Baja Mahi Mahi Taco w. Fish	260	10	32
Baja Style Taco w. Charbroiled Chkn	180	4	25
w. Charbroiled Steak	210	6	25
w. Wild Gulf Shrimp	190	5	26
Salads			
Baja Ensalada: *No Dressing*			
w. Charbroiled Chicken	310	7	18
w. Charbroiled Fish	360	14	27
w. Charbroiled Steak	450	18	18
Chile Lime Chicken	640	16	75
Chipotle Glaze Charbroiled Chicken	600	22	56
Ensalada w. Charbroiled Mahi Mah	360	14	27
Taquitos: w. Chicken & Beans	770	37	69
w. Charbroiled Chicken & Rice	730	37	67
w. Charbroiled Steak & Beans	800	39	69
w. Charbroiled Steak & Rice	760	40	67

For Complete Nutritional Data ~ see CalorieKing.com

Baskin Robbins®

	C	F	Cb
Hard Scooped Ice Cream			
Classic: Per Regular Scoop			
Chocolate	260	14	33
Chocolate Chip	270	16	28
Chocolate Chip Cookie Dough	290	15	36
Chocolate Fudge	270	15	35
French Vanilla	280	18	26
German Choc Cake	300	16	36
Gold Medal Ribbon	260	13	34
Jamoca	240	13	26
Jamoca Almond Fudge	270	15	31
Mint Choc Chip	270	16	28
Old Fashion Butter Pecan	280	18	24
Oreo Cookies 'N Cream	280	15	32
Peanut Butter 'N Chocolate	320	20	31
Pink Bubblegum	270	14	34
Pistachio Almond	290	19	25
Pralines 'N Cream	270	14	34
Quarterback Crunch	290	17	32
Reeses Peanut Butter	300	18	31
Rocky Road	290	15	36
Vanilla	260	16	14
Very Berry Strawberry	220	11	28
World Class Chocolate	270	15	33
Chocolate Roll Cake: Per Slice (4.1 oz)			
Average all flavors	290	14	36
Low-Fat Ice Cream: Espresso 'N Crm	180	4	32
No Sugar Added Ice Cream, avg.	160	4	27
Ices, Sherbets, Sorbets: Regular Scoop			
Ices, Daiquiri; Margarita	135	0	34
Sherbets, average all flavors	160	2	34
Sorbets, average all flavors	115	0	29
Low-Fat Yogurt (Hard): Regular Scoop			
Average all flavors	200	4	38
Non-Fat Yogurt (Soft Serve): Per ½ Cup			
Vanilla, 4 oz	220	0	46
Other flavors, 3 oz	180	0	34
Shakes, Smoothies, Blasts: Regular (16 fl.oz)			
Shakes: Chocolate Ice Cream	675	26	98
Vanilla Ice Cream	690	33	85
Smoothies: Average all flavors	365	1	82
Blasts: Cappuccino w/whip cream	325	14	44
Cones: Sugar Cone	60	3	7
Cake Cone	25	0.5	4
Waffle Cone: Large	120	1.5	14
Fresh Baked	145	2	3

For Complete Nutritional Data ~ see CalorieKing.com

Ben & Jerry's®   C F Cb

Ice Cream & Frozen Yogurt ~ See Page 32
Novelty Bars ~ See Page 36

Big Apple Bagels®

	C	F	Cb
Bagels: All types, avg., 5 oz	380	2	72
½ bagel, 2.5 oz	190	1	36
My Favorite Muffin® Bagels: Per Bagel (4 oz)			
Honey Grain	310	3	61
Other varieties, average	310	1	66
My Favorite Muffin® Muffins: Per Jumbo			
Blueberry	510	24	66
Blueberry, Fat Free	330	0	78
Chocolate Chip	630	33	81
Chocolate, Fat Free	360	0	84
Cream Cheese: Per 2 Tbsp (1 oz)			
Plain	100	10	2
Honey Cinnamon; Very Berry, avg.	130	12	3
Lite varieties, average	65	5	2
Soups: Per Cup (8 fl. oz)			
Boston Clam/Potato Chowder	210	13	20
Chicken Noodle; Beef Pot Roast	110	4	12
Garden Vegetable	110	1	22
Minestrone	150	3	26
Split Pea w. Ham; Hearty Vege	95	2	16

For Complete Nutritional Data ~ see CalorieKing.com

Big Boy®

Sandwiches			
Big Boy	600	26	35
Brawny Lad™	420	21	30
Buddie Boy	760	34	80
Fish Sandwich	690	48	41
Small Hamburger	445	30	30
Super Big Boy™	830	66	34
Swiss Miss	635	44	28
Tuna Salad Sandwich	545	40	30
Sides & Salad			
French Fries	360	19	45
Chili	315	18	19
Onion Rings	580	41	45
Tartare Sauce, 2 oz	370	40	1
Trio Salad	620	46	18

Blimpie®   C F Cb

Cold Deli Subs: Per 6" Sub on White (w. Cheese)			
Blimpie Best	440	15	51
Club	410	11	50
Ham & Swiss Cheese	410	12	51
Roast Beef	450	13	49
Seafood, no Cheese	350	8	58
Tuna	490	23	51
Turkey	420	11	49
Paninis: Cuban	460	12	50
Grilled Chicken Caesar	560	26	50
Turkey Italiano	390	10	44
Wraps: Chicken Caesar	650	35	56
Zesty Italian	680	33	74
Hot Deli Subs: Per 6" Sub on White			
Grilled Chicken	370	9	50
Meatball w. Cheese	570	27	55
Mexi Max	430	9	65
Steak & Onion Melt w. Cheese	440	16	49
VegiMax	390	7	60
Salads: Chef Salad	210	9	9
Grilled Chicken	350	27	9
Seafood Salad	120	4.5	15
Tuna	260	19	8
Dressings & Sauces: Caesar	210	22	2
Blimpie, 1.5 oz	180	12	24
Soups: Per Serving (⅛ Cup)			
Chicken w. White & Wild Rice	230	12	21
Garden Vegetable	80	0.5	14
Homestyle Chicken Noodle	120	2.5	18
Vegetable Beef	80	5	13
Desserts			
Cookies: Oatmeal Raisin	190	8	27
Sugar	330	17	24
Other varieties, average	200	10	26

For Complete Nutritional Data ~ see CalorieKing.com

Bob Evans®

Breakfast

	C	F	Cb
Combinations: Country Biscuit	845	49	71
Fruit & Yogurt Plate	440	2	96
Home Fries	190	7	28
Lite Sausage Breakfast	500	20	48
Pot Roast Hash Breakfast	740	46	37
Sirloin Steak	415	29	3
Farm Fresh Eggs: Eggs Benedict	420	20	35
Harboiled (1)	65	4	1
Over Easy (1)	90	7	1
Scrambled (1)	160	11	1
Scrambled Egg Beaters (1)	190	12	2
Hotcake: Blueberry (1)	190	5	32
Buttermilk (1)	170	5	28
Omelettes: Cheese	470	40	3
Farmer's Market	620	50	11
Ham & Cheese	495	39	2
Southwestern Chicken	660	51	5
Summer Crepes Combos: Raspb. (2)	435	21	55
Strawberry Banana (2)	425	21	52

Dinners: Per Serving

	C	F	Cb
Beef & Pork: Meat Loaf	620	44	14
Country Fried Steak w. Gravy	535	37	31
no Gravy	480	33	26
Chicken & Turkey:			
Chicken Dinner, Fried (1)	295	15	9
Chicken Dinner, Grilled (1)	215	9	0
Chicken Pot Pie	755	49	46
Chicken-n-Noodles	405	22	32
Turkey Lurkey (Kids) (1)	45	0	1
Seafood: Salmon Dinner	365	23	12
Fried Shrimp Dinner	340	20	8
Kid's Menu: Mac & Cheese	330	12	45
Hot Diggety Dog w. Bun, plain	365	26	23
Mini Cheeseburgers (1)	240	14	20
Pizza Pizzazz	505	23	57
Plenty-O-Pancakes	505	17	79
Quesadilla, Chicken	545	31	39
Spaghetti & Meatballs	525	21	57

Lunch Savors: Per Serving

	C	F	Cb
Chicken & Broccoli Alfredo Pasta	535	21	49
Quesadilla, Chicken	625	36	50
Salads: Cobb w. Grilled Chicken	580	39	9
Country Spinach	555	38	11
Frisco: w. Fried Chicken	500	31	26
w. Grilled Chicken	470	31	9
Wildfire Chkn: w. Fried Chicken	660	29	74
w. Grilled Chicken	630	29	57

Bob Evans® cont...

Lunch Savers (Cont)

	C	F	Cb
Stir-Fry: Grilled Chicken	505	18	55
Grilled Shrimp	465	13	60
Vegetable	285	4	55
Farm Fresh Salad: Chicken Salad	815	46	71
Cobb w. Grilled Chicken	765	50	15
Country Spinach w. Grilled Chicken	630	40	13

Sandwiches & Burgers

	C	F	Cb
Burgers: Bacon Cheeseburger	985	75	31
Cheeseburger	690	46	31
Hamburger	600	38	30
Sandwiches: Big BLT	415	29	29
Bob's BLT & E	795	57	48
Fried Chicken Club	880	59	40
Grilled Chicken Club	820	54	32
Grilled Chicken	435	17	30
Pot Roast	665	31	62
Turkey Bacon Melt	825	47	56
Sides: Onion Rings, 6 oz	460	27	49
Baked Potato Seasoned, Loaded	480	18	57
Baked Potato Seasoned, Plain	250	0	54
Cheddar Broccoli Florets	175	9	14
Coleslaw, 4 oz	195	13	18
Corn, Buttered Sweet, 4.5 oz	165	9	18
Garden Side Salad, 5.3 oz	165	4	26
Home Fries, 5 oz	190	7	28
Mashed Potatoes, 5 oz	120	6	15
Mushrooms, Grilled, 7.9 oz	165	12	10
Rice Pilaf, 5 oz	165	3	32
Specialty Breads: Banana Nut	195	7	30
Cinnamon Swirl Roll, Frosted	555	24	76
Dinner Roll (1)	200	5	34
English Muffin (1)	140	1	28
Garlic Bread, 2 oz	220	16	16
Sourdough, 1.7 oz	130	1	25
Texas Toast, 8 oz	65	1	12

Beverages

	C	F	Cb
Iced Tea: Regular	5	0	1
Blackberry	90	0	23
Raspberry; Strawberry	80	0	20

Desserts, Pies, Sundaes

	C	F	Cb
Apple Dumpling Pie, 1 slice	690	30	100
A La Mode	840	37	119
Banana Cream Pie, 8.6 oz	455	25	52
Cheesecake, Oreo, 6.2 oz	620	38	61
Coconut Cream Pie, 1 slice	465	23	57
Hershey's Hot Fudge Cake, 7.3 oz	605	25	94
Lemon Meringue Pie, 7 oz	535	18	89
Pumpkin Pie, 1 slice	545	27	69
Sundae: Fudge	510	19	78
Reese's	785	35	104

For Complete Nutritional Data ~ see CalorieKing.com

Bojangles®

Cajun & Southern Style Chicken	C	F	Cb
Breast, average	280	17	12
Leg, average	265	16	11
Thigh, average	310	23	11
Wing, average	355	25	11
Sandwiches			
Cajun Filet: w/out Mayo	350	11	41
w. Mayonnaise	450	22	41
Grilled Filet: w/out mayo	235	5	25
w. Mayonnaise	335	16	25
Snacks: Buffalo Bites	175	5	5
Chicken Supremes	335	16	26
Biscuit Sandwiches: Bacon	290	17	26
Bacon, Egg & Cheese	550	42	27
Biscuit (plain)	245	12	29
Cajun Filet	455	21	46
Country Ham	270	15	26
Egg	400	30	26
Sausage	350	23	26
Smoked Sausage	380	26	27
Steak	650	49	37
Fixins': Botato Rounds	235	11	31
Cajun Pintos	110	0	18
Corn on the Cob	140	2	34
Dirty Rice	165	6	24
Green Beans	25	0	5
Macaroni & Cheese	200	14	12
Marinated Cole Slaw	135	3	26
Potatoes, no Gravy	80	1	16
Seasoned Fries	345	19	39
Sweet Biscuits: Bo Berry	220	10	29
Cinnamon	320	18	37

For Complete Nutritional Data ~ see CalorieKing.com

Be sure to balance 'eating out' with adequate fruit and veges.

Boston Market®

Entrees: Per Serving	C	F	Cb
Crispy-Baked Cntry Chkn w. Gravy	440	23	33
Double-Sauced Angus: Meatloaf	510	34	22
Meatloaf & Beef Gravy	580	39	27
Half Sweet Garlic Rotisserie Chicken			
w. skin, ½ whole chicken	590	33	4
Hand-Carved: Honey Glazed Ham	210	8	10
Rotisserie Turkey	170	1	3
Pastry Top Chicken Pot Pie	750	46	57
¼ Chicken: White meat w. skin /wing	280	12	2
no skin or wing	170	4	2
¼ Chicken: Dark meat w. skin	320	21	2
no skin	190	10	1
Hot Side Dishes			
Butternut Squash	150	6	25
Creamed Spinach, ¾ cup	260	20	11
Mashed Potatoes (¾ cup), w. Gravy	230	9	32
Hot Cinnamon Apples, ¾ cup	250	4.5	56
Macaroni & Cheese, ¾ cup	280	11	33
Steamed Vegetable Medley	30	0	6
Sweet Corn	180	4	30
Salads			
Caesar Side Salad	300	26	13
Rotisserie Chicken Caesar Salad	640	44	19
Southwest Chicken Salad	750	49	40
Sandwiches & Burgers			
Chicken Carver w. Cheese & Sauce	670	33	68
Meatloaf Carver w. Cheese	1070	55	102
Turkey Carver w. Cheese & Sauce	690	29	68
Soups: Per Serving			
Hearty Chicken Noodle Soup, 6.7 oz	100	4.5	8
Tortilla Soup w. toppings, 6.5 oz	170	8	18
no toppings, 5.5 oz	80	4.5	7
Desserts: Apple Pie	550	31	66
Caramel Pecan Brownie	900	47	114
Chocolate Brownie	580	23	88
Chocolate Cake	650	32	86
Chocolate Mania	290	16	37
Cornbread	120	3.5	21
Family Size: Apple Pie	350	14	54
Caramel Pecan Brownie	160	8	22
Chocolate Brownie	160	8	22
Molten Fudge Cake	300	19	34
Nestle Toll House Cookie, average	390	19	51
Strawberry Bliss	170	11	16

For Complete Nutritional Data ~ see CalorieKing.com

Restaurants & Fast - Foods

Boston Pizza®

	C	F	Cb
Starters: Cactus Cut Potatoes/Dip	780	41	91
Boston's BBQ Wings	690	42	24
Boston's Pizza Bread, no dip	510	13	83
Soup: Baked Onion	160	4	24
Salads: Caesar, regular size	240	18	15
Greek, regular size	600	57	18
Sirloin Steak w. dressing	640	48	17
Entrees: See CalorieKing.com			
Sandwiches: Boston Brute & Fries	1010	30	144
Boston Cheesesteak & Fries	1640	65	213
Chicken Santa Fe Stromboli & Caesar	720	22	106
New York Steak & Tossed Greens	510	33	12
Pizzas (Medium): Per 2 Slices			
BBQ Chicken	380	12	50
Boston Royal	440	12	54
Californian	320	4	62
Hawaiian	420	10	56
Meatlovers	520	20	58
Spicey	560	24	56
Ultimate Pepperoni	460	20	48
Vegetarian	360	8	54
Other Sizes: See CalorieKing.com			
Pastas (Full Order): Lasagna	670	22	83
Chicken & Mushroom Fettucini	1200	57	134
Spaghetti with Bolognese	780	13	138
Desserts: Chocolate Explosion	880	51	105
New York Cheesecake	620	33	80
For Complete Nutritional Data ~ see CalorieKing.com			

Braum's®

	C	F	Cb
Cinnamon Rolls, with Icing	340	11	56
Frozen Custard, avg. all flavors	185	8	25
Frozen Yogurt: Per Cup (8 fl.oz)			
Vanilla, Peach, Strawb./Banana	260	7	50
Other flavors, average	320	12	50
Ice Cream: Per Cup (8 fl.oz)			
Light: Average all varieties	300	10	52
Premium: Peanut Buttercup	*440*	*28*	*46*
Other flavors, average	380	20	45
Sherbet: Avg. all varieties, 1 cup	140	3	36
Pies (Baked): Average, 1 slice	400	20	50
For Complete Nutritional Data ~ see CalorieKing.com			

Buck's Pizza®

	C	F	Cb
Buck's Deluxe: Med. (12"), 1 sl, ⅙	265	13	28
Large (14"), 1 slice, ⅛	270	13	29
X-Large (16"), 1 slice, ¹⁄₁₂	240	11	38
Small (9"), Whole Pizza	900	44	96
Personal (6"), Whole Pizza	400	17	69

Bruegger's Bagels®

	C	F	Cb
Bagels			
Plain/Salt/Sesame/Garlic	350	2.5	68
Blueberry/Cranb. Or./Cinn. Raisin	340	2	68
Chocolate Chip	310	4.5	69
Everything/Onion/Sundried Tom.	320	2	65
Cream Cheese: Average, 2 oz	180	15	8
Light varieties, average, 2 oz	115	8	6
Hummus, 2 oz	120	7	8
Breakfast Sandwiches: Per Sandwich			
Egg & Cheese	480	15	66
Egg & Cheese & Bacon	560	22	66
Egg & Cheese & Ham	530	17	66
Egg & Cheese & Sausage	695	33	66
Sandwiches			
Bagel: Chicken Fajita	500	12	74
Smoked Salmon	455	10	74
Garden Veggie	390	2.5	80
Herby Turkey	530	14	73
Santa Fe Turkey	480	10	71
Deli: Chicken Breast	440	6	62
Chicken Salad w. mayo	460	12	67
Ham w. mustard	445	4.5	77
Turkey w. Mayonnaise	480	14	65
For Complete Nutritional Data ~ see CalorieKing.com			

Burgerville®

	C	F	Cb
Hamburger	300	15	29
Cheeseburger	350	19	29
Double Beef Cheeseburger	430	25	29
Half Pound Colossal	730	45	31
Colossal	520	30	30
Tillamook Cheeseburger	630	40	32
Pepper Bacon Cheeseburger	680	45	28
Gardenburger	460	19	53
Spicy Black Bean Gardenburger	550	32	45
Turkey Burger	540	29	33
Turkey Club Sandwich	540	32	38
Deluxe Crispy Chicken	610	30	56
Crispy Chicken	450	18	55
Grilled Chicken	350	3	45
Halibut Fillet Sandwich	480	27	42
Halibut Fish, 3 pieces	330	16	25
Chicken Strips, 5 pieces	550	30	36
Protein Platter	530	40	6
French Fries: Regular, 5 oz	390	22	44
Large, 6½ oz	510	29	57
For Complete Nutritional Data ~ see CalorieKing.com			

193

Fast - Foods & *Restaurants*

Burger King®

Breakfast	C	F	Cb
Croissan'wich: Egg & Cheese	300	17	26
Bacon/Ham, Egg & Cheese	340	20	26
Sausage & Cheese	410	29	24
Sausage, Egg & Cheese	500	36	26
French Toast Sticks, 5 sticks	390	20	46
Western Omelet Sandwich	330	17	28
Breakfast Syrup	85	0	21
Hash Brown Rounds: Large	395	25	39
Small	230	15	23
Biscuit, Plain	260	13	31
Biscuit & Gravy, 7 oz	420	23	45
Jam, Grape/Strawberry, 1 pkg	30	0	7
Cini-Minis with Vanilla Icing	540	26	71

Burgers & Sandwiches			
Baguettes (Chicken), all types	390	4	57
Bacon Cheeseburger	390	20	31
Bacon Double Cheeseburger	570	34	32
BK Veggie Burger (with mayo)	420	16	46
without mayonnaise	340	8	46
Cheeseburger	350	17	31
Double Cheeseburger	530	31	32
Hamburger	310	13	30
Double Hamburger	440	23	30
The Angus Bacon & Cheese	710	33	64
Low-Carb (no bun)	455	32	4.5
The Angus Steak Burger	570	22	62
Low-Carb (no bun)	260	18	2

Original Whoppers®			
Original Whopper	700	42	52
without mayonnaise	540	24	52
Low-Carb (no bun)	280	20	3
Original Double Whopper	970	61	52
with Cheese, Mayo	1060	69	52
without mayonnaise	810	44	52
Low-Carb (no bun)	540	40	3
Original Whopper JR	390	22	31
without mayonnaise	310	13	31
Low-Carb (no bun)	140	10	1
Tacos (1)	170	8	16

Chicken & Fish			
BK Big Fish Sandwich w. tartar sce	630	30	69
Chicken Whopper	570	25	48
without mayonnaise	410	7	48
Low-Carb (no bun)	160	3.5	3
Original Chicken Sandwich	560	28	52
without mayonnaise	460	17	52
Spicy TenderCrisp Chicken S'wich	720	37	71
without mayonnaise	570	21	70
TenderCrisp Chicken S'wich	780	45	70

Burger King® cont..

	C	F	Cb
Chicken Fries: No Dipping Sauce			
6 pieces	260	15	18
Chicken Tenders: No Dipping Sauce			
5 pieces	210	11	13
Dipping Sauces (1 oz): Buffalo Sce	90	8	2
Honey Flavored	90	0	23
Honey Mustard	90	6	9
Ranch; Zesty Onion Ring	140	15	1
Sweet & Sour; Barbecue	40	0	10
French Fries: Small, 2.6 oz	230	11	29
Medium, 4 oz	365	18	46
Large, 5.6 oz	495	24	63
King Size, 6.8 oz	605	29	76
Onion Rings: Medium, 3.2 oz	320	16	40
Large, 4.8 oz	485	24	60
King Size, 5.6 oz	560	28	68
Sides: Chili, 7.6 oz	190	8	17
Crackers, 0.2 oz	20	0.5	4
Salads (Without Dressing)			
Fire-Grilled: Chkn Caesar, no toast	190	7	9
Chicken Garden, no toast	210	7	12
Shrimp Caesar, no toast	180	10	9
Shrimp Garden	200	10	13
Tender Crisp: Garden Salad, no dr.	410	22	28
Caesar Salad	390	22	25
Side Garden Salad	20	0	4
Garlic Parmesan Toast, ½ oz	70	2.5	9
Salad Dressings: Gdn Ranch, 2 oz	120	10	7
Creamy Garlic Caesar, 2 oz	130	11	7
Fat-Free Honey Mustard, 1.5 oz	70	0	18
Vinaigrette (Sweet Onion/Tom.), 2 oz	110	8	9
Desserts: Dutch Apple Pie	300	13	45
Chocolate Chip Cookies (2)	330	15	47
Hershey's Sundae Pie	300	18	31
Drinks & Shakes: Coffee, Medium	5	0	1.5
Coca-Cola/Sprite/Dr Pepper (with ¼ Ice):			
Kids	110	0	30
Small	140	0	39
Medium	200	0	53
Large	290	0	79
King	390	0	104
Icee (Coke/Minute Maid): Small	110	0	31
Medium, 20 fl.oz	140	0	40
Low-Fat Milk (1%), 10 fl.oz	100	2.5	1
Milk Shakes (Choc./Strawb.): Small	420	13	69
Medium	590	18	97
Large	860	26	142
Orange Juice, 10 fl.oz	140	0	33

For Complete Nutritional Data ~ see CalorieKing.com

194

Restaurants & Fast - Foods

Captain D's Seafood®

	C	F	Cb
Platters: Per Platter			
Broiled Chicken/Fish, average	1015	8	194
Broiled Fish & Chicken	1005	7	194
Broiled Shrimp	1030	8	195
Lunches: Per Lunch Platter			
Broiled Chicken	490	9	63
Broiled Fish/Shrimp	425	7	63
Broiled Fish & Chicken	460	8	63
Stuffed Crab	155	6	16
Carb Counters: Fish Dinner	350	17	19
Chicken Dinner	320	15	19
Low-Cal Fare: w. Rice & Vegetables			
Baked Chicken Dinner	350	3.5	49
Baked Fish Dinner	390	5	49
Baked Salmon Dinner	470	8	58
Shrimp Scampi Dinner	370	5	50
Sandwiches: Broiled Chicken	445	18	29
Broiled Fish	520	18	51
Desserts: Carrot Cake	430	22	49
Cheesecake	425	31	30
Chocolate Cake	300	10	49
Pecan Pie	455	20	64

For Complete Nutritional Data ~ see CalorieKing.com

Caribou Coffee®

Beverages Based on 2% Milk Unless Indicated

	C	F	Cb
Drinks: Per Cup (16 fl.oz)			
Alaskan Fruit Smoothies: Creampop	470	22	66
Passion Green Tea	200	0	48
Strawberry Banana	260	0	65
Wildberry	230	0	57
Coffee Coolers: Caramel	535	18	87
Chocolate	305	5.5	61
Espresso; Coffee, avg.	230	4	47
Mint Oreo	620	26	85
Vanilla	320	7	63
Espresso: Breve	415	34	14
Campfire Mocha	600	18	97
Cappuccino	180	7	18
Espresso	10	0	2
Latte	200	8	20
Macchiato	15	0.5	2
Mocha	480	19	63
White Chocolate Mocha	540	25	69
Skinny Bou Latte: Low Cal	120	0.5	17
Low Carb	1140	122	10
Wild: Caramel Highrise	420	17	55
Hot Apple Blast	435	10	84
Lite White Berry	480	8	94
Mint Condition	580	19	89

Carl's Jr.®

	C	F	Cb
Burgers/Sandwiches			
Bacon Swiss Crispy Chicken	740	28	91
Catch Fish Sandwich	550	27	58
Famous Star Hamburger	585	32	50
Charbroiled: BBQ Chicken S'wich	365	4	47
Chicken Club Sandwich	545	23	43
Santa Fe Chicken Sandwich	610	32	43
Dble Sourdough Bacon Chseburger	920	59	45
Dble Western Bacon Chseburger	915	50	65
Hamburger	290	9	38
Low Carb Chicken Club S'wich	380	21	10
Ranch Crispy Chicken Sandwich	660	31	70
Sourdough Bacon Cheeseburger	550	29	41
Spicy Chicken Sandwich	480	26	48
Super Star Hamburger	790	46	51
The Six Dollar Burger	1000	62	72
Chili Burger	700	35	57
Low-Carb Burger	490	37	6
Spicy BBQ	1030	61	77
Western Bacon Burger	1045	61	79
Western Bacon Cheeseburger	660	30	64
Western Bacon Crispy Chkn S'wich	755	38	72
Potatoes: Plain, no marg.	280	0	63
Bacon & Cheese	635	29	71
Broccoli & Cheese	520	21	71
Sour Cream & Chives	420	14	65
Breakfast: Breakfast Burger	825	46	65
Breakfast Burrito	550	32	37
Loaded Breakfast Burrito	810	49	53
Breakfast Bowl, Low Carb	910	73	5
Breakfast Quesadilla	380	18	38
French Toast Dip (6), no Syrup	450	20	59
Sourdough Sandwich, no meat	410	19	39
Scrambled Eggs & Bacon	745	42	69
Bakery/Desserts: Chocolate Cake	300	12	48
Chocolate Chip Cookie (1)	350	18	46
Strawberry Swirl Chsecake, 3.5 oz	295	17	30
Side Orders: Chicken Stars, 9 pces	405	25	22
Chicken Breast Strips (5)	640	35	45
CrissCut Fries, 5 oz	410	24	43
French Fries, small, 3.2 oz	295	14	37
Hash Brown Nuggets, 4 oz	330	21	32
Onion Rings, 4.5 oz	440	22	53
Salads: No Dressing			
Charbroiled Chicken Salad-to-Go	265	7	17
Garden Salad-to-Go	60	3	5
Buffalo Ranch Chicken Salad	390	16	42

Carvel®

Sundaes: Per Small	C	F	Cb
Thinny-Thin: Fudge No-Fat	380	0	84
Strawberry No-Fat	290	0	63
Classic Regular: Caramel	590	27	73
Bittersweet Fudge; Hot Fudge	600	31	69
Bordeaux Fudge	550	26	69
Strawberry	500	26	58
Metropolitan Coladas: Per Serving (16 fl.oz)			
Pina Colada	400	17	61
Other varieties	370	10	68
Novelties: Per Small			
Flying Sauces 98% Fat-Free,	190	1.5	40
Parfait; Miniature Sundae No-Fat	190	0	42
Parfait; No Sugar Added	200	2.5	42
Old Fashioned Sundae No-Fat	300	0	66
No Sugar Added	360	4.5	76
Uptown Smoothies: Per Serving (16 fl.oz)			
Broadway Banana	310	0.5	49
Grand Central Cooler	290	0.5	73
Other varieties, average	310	0.5	79
Thinny-Thin: Berry Times Square	300	0	73
Grand Central Cooler	250	0	63
Other varieties, average	270	0	68
Creammaccino: Classic, 16 fl.oz	410	24	36
Caramel Cream, 16 fl.oz	590	26	74
Mocha Fudge, 16 fl.oz	610	35	61

Checkers®

~ Same Menu & Data as Rally's Hamburgers®
See Page 240 ~

Cheesecake Factory®

10" Cheesecake: Per Slice			
P. B. Cup Fudge Ripple	930	59	93
Banana Cream	860	63	70
Brownie Sundae	970	63	96
Choc Chip Cookie Dough	1910	72	102
Dulce de Leche	1010	74	83
Kahlua Cocoa Coffee	840	55	80
Keylime Cheesecake	710	49	64
Original Cheesecake	630	45	53
Vanilla Bean Cheesecake	870	64	69
White Choc. Raspberry Truffle	900	62	80

Charley's Grilled Subs®

Subs: Regular w. Cheese & Dressing	C	F	Cb
BBQ Cheddar	790	43	68
Bacon 3 Cheese Steak	935	63	53
Buffalo Chicken, no cheese/dress.	590	23	57
Chicken Bacon Club	610	26	53
Chicken Cordon Bleu	590	21	57
Chicken Philadelphia, no chse/dress.	600	25	55
Chicken Teriyaki, no chse/dress.	505	14	56
Grilled Veggie Delight, no chse/dress.	440	17	59
New York Deli	680	36	55
Philly Ham & Swiss	605	30	55
Philly Steak Deluxe	830	53	55
Philly Steak	830	53	54
Steak Italiano	875	57	54
Turkey Breast, no cheese/dress.	560	20	57
Ultimate Turkey Club	675	34	52
Fresh Salads: Garden w. dressing	280	22	13
Fries (Per Regular): Original	270	8.5	42
Cheddar & Bacon	435	19	54
Cheddar Ranch & Bacon	780	56	57
Ranch & Bacon	710	50	52
Beverages: Natural Lemonade, reg.	170	0	40

Chevys Fresh Mex®

Burritos	C	F	Cb
Veggie w. Tortilla, Marinated Veges, San Antonio Veges, Pico de Gallo & Ranchero Sauce	430	19	49
Catch of the Day			
Fresh Fish, San Antonio Veges, Salsa & Tomalito	430	16	16
Fajitas			
Chicken w. San Antonio Veges & Tomalito	285	6	13
Shrimp w. San Antonio Veges & Tomalito	285	7	13
Veggie w. Marinated Veges, San Antonio Veges & Tomalito	345	28	16
Salad: With Salsa Vinaigrette Dressing			
Chicken, Grilled	535	18	53
Mixed Green	360	16	42
Sides: Black Beans	60	0	11
Guacamole, 2 oz	105	10	3
Mexican Rice	210	3	39
Salsa for Chips, 5 oz	40	0	8
Sour Cream	120	12	2
Tortilla: Corn	80	1	17
El Machino	165	4	27

For Complete Nutritional Data ~ see CalorieKing.com

196

Restaurants & Fast - Foods

Chick-Fil-A®

Chick-Fil-A Sandwiches	C	F	Cb
Chicken Sandwich	410	16	38
Chargrilled Chicken Sandwich	275	3.5	33
Chicken Salad Sandwich	350	15	32
Cool Wraps®: Chicken Caesar	460	10	52
Chargrilled/Spicy Chicken, avg.	395	7	54
Breakfast: Plain Biscuit, 2.8 oz	265	11	38
Biscuit and Gravy	330	15	44
Biscuit: w. Bacon, Egg & Cheese	470	26	39
w. Sausage	490	29	45
Hashbrowns, 3 oz	260	17	25
Chick-n-Minis, 3 count	270	11	28
Chicken Biscuit	420	19	44
Platter: Chicken	630	32	51
Bacon	550	30	44
Breakfast Burrito: Chicken	420	19	39
Sausage	460	24	40
Chicken, Egg & Cheese Bagel	460	18	47
Salads: Chick-n-Strips® Salad	390	18	22
Chargrilled Chicken Garden	180	6	9
Southwest Chargrilled Chicken	240	8	17
Salad Dressing: Per Packet (1.25 oz)			
Caesar Dressing	160	17	1
Raspberry Vinaigrette	80	2	15
Bleu Cheese; Buttermilk	150	16	1
Fat Free Honey Mustard	60	0	14
Light Italian Dressing	15	0.5	2
Spicy Dressing	135	14	2
Thousand Island	145	14	5
Strips, Nuggets: Nuggets (8-pack)	260	12	12
Chick-n-Strips® (4-count)	290	13	14
Dipping Sauces: Polynesian, 1 oz	105	6	13
Barbecue; Honey Mustard, avg.,1 oz	45	0	10
Buffalo Sce, ¾ oz	20	1.5	1
Sides: Carrot & Raisin Salad, small	170	6	28
Fresh Fruit Cups, 4 oz	60	0	16
Coleslaw, small	260	21	17
Garlic and Butter Croutons, ½ oz	50	3	6
Side Salad, 3.8 oz	60	3	4
Tortilla Strips, 1 pkt, ½ oz	70	3.5	9
Waffle Potato Fries, 3.9 oz	345	17	44
Desserts: Cheesecake, 3.3 oz slice	340	21	30
Icedream® Cup, small	230	6	38
Icedream® Cone, small	160	4	28
Lemon Pie, 4 oz slice	320	10	51
Fudge Nut Brownie (1), 2.6 oz	330	15	45

Chili's®

Starters	C	F	Cb
Awesome Blossom w. Sauce	2880	222	191
¼ Whole w. Blossom Sauce	720	55	48
Boneless Buffalo Wings + Sauce	1140	74	64
Boneless Shanghai Wings	1390	84	90
Fajita Nachos: Chicken	995	36	94
Beef	1130	50	100
Buffalo Wings w. Dressing	790	66	5
Guiltless Grill®: Chicken Platter	565	9	83
Chicken Grill Pita	545	9	77
Chicken Sandwich	535	9	70
Tomato Basil Pasta	670	15	106
Burgers: (No Fries): Ranch Burger	1070	66	64
Chipotle Bleu Chse Bacon Burger	1120	75	54
Grnd Peppercorn w. Strings, Dr.	1200	79	78
Bunless Burgers: Old Timer	575	38	11
Mushroom Swiss w. Mayo	600	38	14
Meals: Chili's Filet	1215	78	69
Bottomless Tostada Chips w. Salsa	910	46	109
Cajun Chicken Pasta	1190	56	103
Cajun Chicken Sandwich	850	41	77
Cheese Steak Sandwich (no Fries)	740	29	67
Chicken Caesar Pita (no Fries)	520	19	33
Citrus Fire Chicken & Shrimp	660	12	73
Country Fried Steak	1335	70	126
Flame Grilled Rib Eye	1080	66	70
Ginger Citrus Glazed Salmon	710	22	70
Grilled Baby Back Ribs	1130	54	109
Grilled Shrimp Alfredo	1290	53	142
Hawaiian Steak	685	13	88
Margarita Grilled Chicken	725	25	72
Margarita Grilled Tuna	875	25	97
South Western Egg Rolls	830	40	86
Veggie & Smoked Chse Quesadilla	1160	67	95
Fajitas: Includes 3 Tortillas & Garnishes			
Mushroom Jack	1270	60	103
Chicken	1020	41	99
Steak	1070	51	93
Knife & Fork Fajitas: (w. veggies, sour cream, pico de gallo, guacamole)			
Beef Chkn Fajita Combo, no tortilla	600	32	17
Chicken Fajitas, no tortilla	555	25	17
Salads: Includes Dressing			
Chicken Fajita Caesar Salad	515	24	11
Dinner Caesar Salad	180	15	5
Dinner House Salad w. Ranch	320	27	8
Quesadilla Explosion	1240	84	68
Desserts: Choc Chip Paradise Pie	1250	47	188
Molten Choc Cake	1505	67	207

For Complete Nutritional Data ~ see CalorieKing.com

197

Chipotle®

Bol Salad: Per Bowl (no Rice or Tortilla)

	C	F	Cb
Burrito w. Beans: Meat & Chse	475	22	24
Meat & Corn Salsa	475	14	45
Meat & Sour Cream or Cheese	470	23	25
Meat & Tomato Salsa	395	13	29
Fajita w. Vege: Meat & Corn Salsa	435	21	28
Meat & Sour Cream or Cheese	435	30	8.5
Meat & Tomato Salsa	355	20	12
Vegetarian: w. Guacamole			
w. Beans/Corn Salsa	420	17	52
w. Beans, Tomato Salsa	340	16	36
Burrito Bol: with Rice & Beans			
Meat & Cheese	710	29	63.5
Meat & Corn Salsa	710	21	85
Meat & Sour Cream or Cheese	705	30	65
Meat & Tomato Salsa	630	20	69
Vegetarian w. Guacamole:			
Rice & Beans	545	23	70
Tomato Salsa	575	23	76
Corn Salsa	655	24	92
Fajita Burrito Bol: with Rice & Beans			
Meat & Corn Salsa	1040	30	139
Meat & Sour Cream	1040	39	119
Meat & Tomato Salsa	960	29	123
Vegetables: Meat & Cheese	675	36	46
Meat & Corn Salsa	670	28	68
Meat & Sour Cream or Cheese	670	37	48
Vegetables & Meat: & Tom. Salsa	590	27	52
& Cheese or Sour Cream	1005	45	100
& Corn Salsa	1005	37	122
& Tomato Salsa	925	36	106
Taco w. 4 Crispy Shells: Per Serving			
Meat, Corn Salsa: & Cheese	705	31	57
& Sour Cream	675	32	58
Meat, Tomato Salsa: & Cheese	600	30	41
& Sour Cream	595	31	42
Vegetarian Burrito: w. Rice, Beans & Guacamole			
Black Beans	880	32	124
Corn Salsa	990	33	146
Sour Cream	985	42	126
Tomato Salsa	910	32	130

CinnaMonster®

Cinnamon Roll: Per Roll

	C	F	Cb
Caramel Pecan	840	32	120
Original	880	24	100

Chuck E. Cheese®

Appetizers: Per Serving

	C	F	Cb
Buffalo Wings	660	45	3
French Fries	240	9	37
French Fries ala Carte,	480	17	37
Italian Bread Sticks (1)	195	8	27
Sargento Mozzarella Sticks (1)	105	6	7
Pizzas: Per Slice (Medium)			
BBQ Chicken	270	8	43
Cheese	235	7	33
Pepperoni	265	10	33
Vegetarian	235	7	36
Sandwiches: Ham & Cheese	620	28	70
Grilled Chicken Sub	650	31	70
Italian Sub	730	40	69
Hot Dog	170	17	27
w. Cheese	335	30	28
Cakes: Per Serving (⅒ Cake)			
Birthday Cakes: 8" Chocolate White	310	13	45
8" White White	310	13	44

Church's Chicken®

Fried Chicken

	C	F	Cb
Breast w. Skin, 1 pce	200	12	4
Leg w. Skin, 1 piece	140	9	2
Thigh w. Skin, 1 piece	230	16	5
Crunchy Tenders (1)	135	5	11
Wing w. Skin, 1 piece	250	16	8
Tender Crunchers™, 6-8 pces	410	15	32
Side Items: Apple Pie, 3 oz	280	12	41
Honey Butter Biscuits (1)	250	16	26
Cajun Rice, regular, 3 oz	130	7	16
Chicken Fried Steak w. Gravy	470	28	36
Cole Slaw, regular, 3 oz	90	6	8
Corn on the Cob, 1 ear	140	3	24
French Fries, regular	210	11	29
Mashed Potatoes & Gravy, reg.	90	3	14

Cinnabon®

	C	F	Cb
Classic	815	32	117
Caramel Pecanbon, 1 roll	1090	56	141
Minibon, 1 roll	340	13	49
MiniBon, Strawberry	250	5	45
CinnaPretzel	755	6	156
CinnaPoppers (3)	370	21	41
Cinnabon Stix (5)	350	11	54
Drinks			
Frusia, 12 fl.oz	170	0	38
Mochalata Chill, 12 fl.oz	390	12	62

For Complete Nutritional Data ~ see CalorieKing.com

198

Cici's Pizza®

Buffet Pizza (12"): Per Slice (½)	C	F	Cb
Alfredo; Ham & Pineapple	235	7	31
Beef	280	11	30
Cheese	255	8	34
Pepperoni	290	11	34
Sausage	330	11	32
Zesty Ham & Cheddar	255	10	30

Cosi®

	C	F	Cb
Pasta: Penne Marinara	930	9	180
Penne Pesto w. Chicken	1285	36	178
Penne a la Cosi	1300	37	189
Thai Chicken & Peanut Noodles	1600	28	276
Pizza: Four Cheese	980	35	124
Meatlovers	1315	60	124
Spinach & Fresh Tomato	915	30	129
Sandwiches: Buffalo Blue	650	30	57
Cosi Club	680	34	59
Country Ham & Brie	790	39	69
Grilled Chicken TBM	665	34	57
Hummus & Fresh Veggies	435	8	77
Sesame Ginger Chicken	510	11	70
Tandoori Chicken	635	26	58
Tuna & Cheddar	960	54	56
Turkey Light	475	9	73
Melts: Bacon Turkey Cheddar	855	21	74
Grilled Chicken Parmesan	635	20	57
Salads (No Dressing): Bombay	175	3	13
Caesar	180	8	20
Chicken Caesar	340	16	21
Cobb	420	28	8
Greek	235	17	9
Mixed Greens	45	1	9
Shanghai Chicken	220	9	16
Signature	375	21	40
Regular Dressings: Per Serving (2 oz)			
Regular: Cosi Vinaigrette	355	39	2
Other varieties, average	300	30	2
Fat-Free, Balsamic Vinaigrette	45	0	11
Low-Fat, Ginger Soy	75	2	13
Desserts: Apple Pie	990	40	147
Caramel Coated Bread Pudding	640	31	84
Cheesecake	735	46	73
Double Trouble Brownie Sundae	1585	77	198
Ice Cream, Double Scoop	225	14	22
Mud Pie	900	49	109
Sundae, medium, 8 oz	410	24	43

For Complete Nutritional Data ~ see CalorieKing.com

Cousins Subs®

Ciabatta Sandwiches	C	F	Cb
Classic Cubano Pork	590	34	38
Spicy Chicken Sedona	480	23	36
Tuscan Market Club	440	23	33
Salads: Chef Salad	280	15	15
Garden Salad	195	13	14
Garden Salad w. Chicken Breast	335	17	15
Italian Salad	360	25	15
Oriental Sesame Chicken	265	8	20
Seafood Salad	440	35	19
Side Salad	105	7	7
Tuna Salad	370	28	14
French Fries: Medium	400	19	55
Large	525	24	72
Soups: Per Regular Serving			
Cheese	240	16	18
Chicken Dumpling	170	5.5	19
Chicken w. Rice	230	12	21
Chili	250	9.5	26
Cream of Broccoli w. Cheese	190	12	15
Cream of Potato	190	9.5	24
New England Clam Chowder	150	5.5	19
Subs 7½": Per Sandwich (With Dressing)			
BLT	615	42	45
Balsamic Garden Turkey	500	18	50
Cappacola & Cheese	635	39	48
Cappacola & Genoa	630	40	48
Cheese Steak	540	24	46
Cheese Steak Double	850	46	46
Chicken Breast	620	34	46
Chicken Breast Lower Fat	365	6	46
Club Sub	705	40	48
Garden Veggie	365	11	49
Genoa & Provolone	730	49	48
Gyro	680	40	55
Hot Veggie	490	23	49
Italian Special	795	53	48
Meatball & Provolone	585	27	50
Pepperoni Melt	785	52	47
Philly Cheese Steak	600	29	49
Provolone	685	45	46
Roast Beef	620	36	46
Seafood w. Crab	555	32	53
Tuna	830	60	46
Turkey Breast	560	32	48

For Complete Nutritional Data ~ see CalorieKing.com

Cold Stone Creamery®

	C	F	Cb
Sweet Cream Ice Cream			
Like It, average all flavors	400	24	40
Love It, average all flavors	660	40	67
Gotta Have It, average all flavors	920	56	93
Cake Batter, Like It	420	23	48
Oreo Cookie, Like It	430	25	46
Low-Fat Frozen Yogurt (Choc)			
Like It	230	1.5	48
Love It	380	3	79
Non-Fat Frozen Yogurt: Like It	230	0	48
Love It, average all flavors	380	0.5	80
Gotta Have It, average all flavors	540	1	113
Sinless Sorbet: Like It	200	0	50
Love It	335	0	84
Gotta Have It	470	0	118
Ice Cream Cake: Per Slice (⅛ Cake)			
Butterfinger Bonanza	450	22	58
Celebration Sensation	350	17	46
Cheesecake Named Desire	410	19	57
Chocolate Chipper	450	26	50
Midnight Delight	510	28	61
Peanut Butter Playground	490	29	54
Strawberry Passion	380	19	50
Zebra Stripes Dark	480	29	54
Waffle Cone or Bowl	160	4	29

For Complete Nutritional Data ~ see CalorieKing.com

Culver's®

	C	F	Cb
Butterburgers: Cheese, Double	580	32	37
Bacon Deluxe	765	51	34
Deluxe Single	505	32	34
Deluxe, Double	685	44	34
Low-Carb	445	32	1
Favorite Sandwiches: Chkn Filet	615	27	57
Beef Pot Roast	305	10	33
Chicken Salad	665	38	38
Grilled Chicken Breast	370	8	49
Grilled Ham & Swiss	455	22	35
Philly Steak	485	19	45
Pork Tenderloin	705	29	87
Smoked Turkey	315	21	44
Turkey Sourdough BLT	595	34	39
Garden Fresh Salads: Club	455	24	17
Chicken Caesar	310	12	17
Chicken Cashew	485	27	25
Taco Salad	690	47	46
Side Salad	100	6	7
Fish & Chicken: Shrimp Basket	1250	63	119
Chicken Dinner, 2 pieces	1660	89	129
Chicken Tenders, 4 pieces	390	20	22
Norwegian Cod, 2 pce Basket	1155	58	120

Culver's® cont...

	C	F	Cb
Sides			
Cheese Curds	710	43	54
Chili Cheese Fries, regular	635	35	65
French Fries, regular, 5 oz	365	18	47
Mashed Potatoes & Gravy, small	150	3	27
Onion Rings, breaded, 6.7 oz	380	29	73
Desserts: Lemon Ice, 9 oz	210	0	46
Lemon Smoothie, 18 oz	670	28	94
Root Beer Float	650	18	116
Frozen Van. Custard: Dish, Single	310	18	32
Cake Cone, Single	340	18	38
Waffle Cone, Single	410	21	53
Sundaes: Turtle, 15.4 oz	1245	68	141
Caramel Cashew, small	1185	55	152
Hot Fudge Sundae, small	1015	65	91

For Complete Nutritional Data ~ see CalorieKing.com

D'Angelo's®

	C	F	Cb
Sandwiches			
Cheeseburger: Pokket	480	25	37
Sub	525	26	44
Wrap	570	26	52
Chicken Stir Fry: D'Lite Pokket	385	8.5	43
Sub	450	11	53
Wrap	490	10	61
Classic Veggie: D'Lite Pokket	360	7	64
Wrap	485	13	68
Grilled Chkn Breast D'Lite Pokket	390	7	52
Italian: Sub	550	27	54
Number 9 Steak Sandwich: Pokket	435	18	36
Roast Beef: D'Lite Pokket	355	5	51
Sub	320	5	48
Steak: D'Lite Pokket	480	26	16
Wrap	400	13	41
Turkey: D'Lite Pokket	365	4	51
Sub	315	4	45
Salads: No Dressing Unless Indicated			
Caesar Salad w. Dressing	480	39	25
Chef Salad	275	12	18
Chicken Stir Fry	165	3	10
Greek Salad	315	23	17
Roast Beef	145	3	10
Lobster	385	26	12
Turkey	155	2	9

For Complete Nutritional Data ~ see CalorieKing.com

Dairy Queen®

Burgers/Sandwiches	C	F	Cb
GrillBurger: ½ lb Burger, no cheese	800	50	41
Classic, no cheese	540	30	41
Bacon Cheeseburger	710	45	40
Crispy Chicken Sandwich	690	37	64
DQ Homestyle: Hamburger	290	12	29
Bacon Double Cheeseburger	610	36	31
Cheeseburger	340	17	29
Double Cheeseburger	540	31	30
Ultimate Burger	670	43	29
Grilled Chicken Sandwich	520	26	44
Hot Dog, regular	330	21	22
Chili 'n' Cheese Dog, regular	330	21	22
Entrees/Sides: Chicken Strips (4)	400	24	21
Onion Rings, small, 4 oz	470	30	45
French Fries, small, 5 oz	380	15	56
Chicken Quesadilla, no dressing	550	31	35
Salads: No Dressing			
Crispy Chicken Salad	350	20	21
Grilled Chicken Salad	240	10	12
Ice Cream Cones/Soft Serve			
DQ Vanilla Soft Serve, ½ cup	140	4.5	22
DQ Choc. Soft Serve, ½ cup	150	5	22
Chocolate Cone, medium	335	11	51
Dipped Cone, medium	480	24	59
Vanilla Cone, medium	320	10	53
Novelties: Buster Bar	500	28	45
Chocolate Dilly Bar	220	13	25
DQ Fudge Bar, No Sugar Added	50	0	13
DQ Sandwich	200	6	31
DQ Vanilla Orange Bar, NAS	60	0	17
Lemon DQ Freez'r; Starkiss, avg.	80	0	20
Blizzards® & Sundaes			
Choc. Chip Cookie Dough, med.	1005	39	147
Oreo Cookie, medium	675	25	98
Chocolate Sundae, medium	400	10	70
DQ Treatzza Cake ⅛ cake	370	13	56
DQ Treatzza Pizza ⅛ pizza	180	7	28
Royal Treats: Banana Split	510	12	96
Peanut Buster Parfait	730	31	99
Strawberry Shortcake	430	14	70
Drinks: Chocolate Shake, medium	760	20	129
Malts, medium	870	22	153
Misty Slushes, medium	290	0	74
MooLatte: Cappuccino	490	18	68
Mocha	590	23	80

For Complete Nutritional Data ~ see CalorieKing.com

Daphne's®

Meals: Per Plate	C	F	Cb
Chicken: Combo	530	36	9
Kabob Plate	350	10	5.5
White Meat	370	16	6
Hummus & Pita	230	12	45
Kabob Lunch w. Chicken	210	9	2
Sandwich: Pita w. Gyros	650	45	37
w. Chicken Breast	565	22	34
Salads			
Greek Chicken	415	18	9
Spicy Greek Chicken w. 1 oz Fire Feta	510	24	12
Soups			
Avgolemono, 1 cup	100	8	7
Extras			
Fire Feta, 2 Tbsp	100	9	2
Gyros, 4 oz	380	33	6
Pita Bread, whole	190	4	33
Rice Pilaf, 6 oz	275	7.5	46
Salad Dressing, 2 Tbsp	30	3	1
Tzatziki Sauce, 1.5 oz	60	6	3

Davanni's®

Hoagies: Per Half Hoagie (6") w. Mayonnaise			
Assorted	405	31	21
Cheese	400	29	21
Chicken Breast	495	33	23
Chicken Parmigana	385	19	22
Club	400	27	22
Italian Sausage	520	37	28
Meatball	465	31	31
Mediterranean	510	38	22
Pastrami	460	27	22
Pizza	315	18	23
Roast Beef	385	25	21
Salami	485	38	21
Tuna	565	44	24
Turkey	370	24	22
Vegie	445	29	29
Without Cheese ~ Deduct	40	3	0
Without Mayo ~ Deduct	100	11	1
Calzones Average all varieties	700	35	66
Pizzas			
Pepperoni & Vegie Works:			
Thin, 1 slice	245	12	18
Traditional, 1 slice	295	12	28
Solo	775	35	70
The Works: Thin, 1 slice	250	13	18
Traditional, 1 slice	300	14	28
Solo	735	32	70
Vegie Works: Thin, 1 slice	210	9	18
Traditional, 1 slice	260	9	28
Solo	635	22	70

Deep Dish ~ Similar to Traditional slice

Fast - Foods & *Restaurants*

Del Taco®

Breakfast	C	F	Cb
Breakfast Burrito	250	11	24
Bacon & Egg Quesadilla	450	23	40
Egg & Cheese Burrito	450	24	39
Macho Bacon & Egg Burrito	1030	60	82
Steak & Egg Burrito	580	34	41
Hash Brown Sticks (5)	250	19	20
Tacos: Big Fat Chicken Taco	340	13	38
Big Fat Steak Taco	390	19	38
Big Fat Taco	320	11	39
Chicken Del Carbon	170	5	19
Steak Taco Del Carbon	220	11	19
Taco; Soft Taco, average	160	10	13
Ultimate Taco	260	17	13
Burritos: Combo Burrito	530	22	61
Bean & Cheese Red/Green Burrito	270	8	38
Chicken Works Burrito	520	23	57
Del Beef Burrito	550	30	42
Del Classic Chicken Burrito	560	36	41
Deluxe Combo Burrito	570	25	64
Deluxe Del Beef Burrito	590	33	45
Half Pound Red/Green Burrito, average	430	12	63
Macho Beef Burrito	1170	62	89
Macho Combo Burrito	1050	44	113
Spicy Chicken/Veggie Works, avg.	480	17	68
Steak Works Burrito	590	31	58
Quesadillas: Cheddar	490	27	39
Chicken Cheddar	575	31	41
Spicy Jack Chicken	560	30	40
Spicy Jack	480	26	38
Salads: Deluxe Chicken Salad	745	34	77
Deluxe Taco Salad	795	40	76
Taco Salad	350	30	10
Burgers: Cheeseburger	330	13	37
Double Del Cheeseburger	560	35	35
Del Cheeseburger	430	25	35
Nachos: Regular	395	24	40
Macho Nachos	1145	63	113
Sides: Rice Cup, 4 oz	140	2	27
Beans 'n Cheese Cup, 7.7 oz	265	3	44
Fries: Chili Cheese, 10.5 oz	670	46	51
Deluxe Chili Cheese, 12 oz	710	49	53
Medium	490	32	47
Macho	690	46	68
Shakes: Chocolate, 15 fl.oz	680	16	117
Vanilla; Strawbrttu. 15 fl.oz	545	9	97

Denny's®

Breakfast	C	F	Cb
Corned Beef Hash Slam, no bread	670	55	11
Pancakes (3), no syrup/marg.	225	4	47
Country Scramble, no syrup/marg.	1040	62	79
Two Egg Breakfast w. hash browns	680	55	20
All American Slam, no toast	815	65	3
French Slam, no syrup/marg.	1195	83	74
Grand Slam Slugger, no brd/pot.	925	55	74
Lumberjack Slam, w. hash browns	1035	58	73
Moons Over My Hammy	840	51	42
Original Grand Slam, no toast	665	49	33
w. Syrup & Margarine	1030	60	101
Extra Breakfast Items ~ See CalorieKing.com			
Soup: Chicken Noodle, 8 fl.oz	120	5	14
Vegetable Beef, 8 fl.oz	80	1	11
Sandwiches (No Fries/Sauces)			
Albacore Tuna Melt	640	39	42
BBQ Chicken	1090	62	86
BLT	610	38	50
Bacon Cheddar Burger	910	52	58
Boca Burger	450	11	64
Buffalo Chicken Sandwich	710	28	80
Chicken Ranch Melt	840	47	57
Classic Burger	695	35	56
Club Sandwich	600	38	45
Grilled Chicken, no dressing	475	14	56
Hoagie Chicken Melt	750	44	43
Hoagie Philly Melt	875	50	58
Mushroom Swiss Burger	880	49	63
The Super Bird Sandwich	480	29	32
Grilled Tilapia Dinner	465	18	31
Appetizers/Entrees: No Sides/Condiments			
Buffalo Wings (9)	975	72	11
Buffalo Chicken Strips (5)	735	42	43
Chicken Strips (5)	720	33	56
Country Fried Steak	645	46	30
Fish & Chips	960	54	83
Fried Shrimp Dinner	220	10	18
Fried Shrimp & Shrimp Scampi	345	20	15
Grilled Chicken Dinner	200	5	15
Grilled Tilapia Dinner	465	18	31
Mozzarella Sticks (8)	710	41	49
Roast Turkey & Stuffing w. Gravy	435	10	62
Sampler, no condiments	1405	80	124
Shrimp Scampi Skillet Dinner	290	19	3
Sirloin Steak Dinner	335	28	1
Smothered Cheese Fries	765	48	69
Steak & Shrimp Dinner	645	42	31
T-Bone Steak Dinner	860	65	0

Denny's® cont...

Sides	C	F	Cb
Garlic Bread, 2 pces	170	11	5
Corn in Butter Sauce, 3 oz	105	2	23
Onion Rings, 4 oz	380	23	38
Fries: Unsalted, 6 oz	420	20	57
Seasoned, 4 oz	260	12	35
Gravy, all types, average	15	0.5	2
Green Beans in Sauce, 3 oz	40	1	8
Potato: Baked, plain with skin	220	0	51
Mashed, 5 oz	170	7	23

Salads (No Dressing/Bread Unless Indicated)

	C	F	Cb
Albacore Tuna Salad	570	30	22
Fried Chicken Strips Salad	470	26	26
Grilled Chkn Caesar w. Dressing	600	41	20
Grilled Chicken Breast Salad	270	11	10
Side Caesar with Dressing	360	26	20
Side Garden Salad, no Dressing	115	4	16

Dressings & Sauces

	C	F	Cb
BBQ Sce, 1.5 oz	45	1	11
Blue Cheese, 1 oz	165	18	1
Caesar; Ranch, 1 oz	135	14	1
French, regular, 1 oz	105	10	3
Honey Mustard, 1 oz	160	15	20
Italian Dressing, Low Calorie; Salsa	15	0.5	3
Marinara Sauce, 1.5 oz	50	2	7
Sour Cream, 1.5 oz	90	9	2
Tartar Sauce, 1.5 oz	225	23	3
Thousand Island, 1 oz	120	11	5

Desserts:

	C	F	Cb
Carrot Cake, 8 oz	800	45	99
Hot Fudge Brownie, 10 oz	345	16	49
Pies (⅙ Whole): Apple, 7 oz	470	24	64
Cheesecake, no topping, 4 oz	580	38	51
Chocolate Peanut Butter, 6 oz	655	39	64
Sundaes: Banana Split	895	43	121
Single Scoop, no topping	190	14	14
Double Scoop, no topping	380	27	29
Dessert Toppings: Choc., 2 oz	135	0.5	34
Blueberry, 3 oz	105	0	26
Fudge, 2 oz	200	10	30
Strawberry, 3 oz	155	1	26

Drinks:

	C	F	Cb
Cappuccino, 8 fl.oz	100	2	28
Floats, Rootbeer/Cola, 12 fl.oz	280	10	47
Milkshake, Van/Choc., 12 fl.oz	560	26	76
Ruby Red Grapefruit Juice, 10 oz	160	0	41
Raspberry Iced Tea, 16 fl.oz	80	0	21

For Complete Nutritional Data ~ see CalorieKing.com

Dippin' Dots®

Ices	C	F	Cb
Ices: All flavors	90	0	23
Frozen Yogurt: All flavors, ½ cup	110	0	23
Ice Creams: Per Serving (½ Cup)			
All flavors	190	9	22
Fat-Free, Fudge, No Sugar Added	60	0	14
Low-Fat, Vanilla, No Sugar Added	120	6	17
Sherbet: Per Serving (½ Cup)			
All flavors	100	1	21

Donato's® Pizza

14" Traditional Pizza: Per Slice (⅛ Large)	C	F	Cb
Chicken Vegy Medley	330	10	41
Founders Fav.; The Works, avg.	460	20	43
Hawaiian; Serious Cheese, avg.	410	16	45
Mariachi Beef/Mariachi Chkn, avg.	825	18	44
Serious Meat	480	23	42
Vegy	400	15	45
Vegy (without Cheese)	270	5.5	45
Salads: Tuscan Chicken, no dress.	200	8	6.5
Tuscan Side Salad, no dressing	85	6	3
Tortilla Subs: Big Ham & Cheese	400	23	19
Big Don: Italian	500	34	18
Original	435	26	20
Sausage Italian	780	56	19
Sausage Original	715	48	21
Big Steak Hoagy w. Sauce	580	39	19
Grilled Chicken Club	575	33	22
Low Fat Chicken Vegy	260	6	23
Roasted Vegy; Turkey	405	26	24
Steak & Cheese	450	23	20

Individual No Dough Pizza: (Whole Pizza)	C	F	Cb
Chicken Vegy Medley	495	29	20
Classic Trio	530	37	18
Founder's Favorite	560	38	18
Hawaiian	435	26	22
Mariachi Beef	530	34	23
Mariachi Chicken	495	30	21
Pepperoni	500	35	17
Philly Cheese Steak	520	33	19
Serious Cheese	455	30	17
Serious Meat	655	46	19
Spinach	455	29	21
Vegy	420	25	23
White	385	26	15
Works	545	37	21

For Complete Nutritional Data ~ see CalorieKing.com

Fast - Foods & *Restaurants*

Domino's® Pizza

	C	F	Cb
Carb Cruncher			
14" Large (Thin Crust): *Per Slice (⅛ Pizza)*			
Extravaganzza Feast	315	21	16
Hawaiian Feast	190	10	16
Mushroom & Green Pepper	150	7	15
Pepperoni	175	11	12
Sausage & Onion	190	11	15
Cheese	150	8	13
Classic Hand-Tossed			
14" Large: *Per Slice (⅛ Pizza)*			
Beef; Pepperoni, average	310	12	38
Cheese	255	8	38
Green Pepper, Onion & Mushroom	265	8	39
Ham	270	8.5	38
Ham & Pineapple	275	8.5	40
Pepperoni & Sausage	350	16	39
Sausage	330	13	39
Crunchy Thin Crust			
14" Large: *Per Slice (⅛ Pizza)*			
Beef; Sausage, average	245	15	19
Cheese	190	10	19
Green Pepper, Onion & Mushroom	200	10	21
Ham	205	10	19
Ham & Pineapple	205	10	21
Pepperoni	235	14	19
Pepperoni & Sausage	280	18	19
Feast Pizza Classic Hand-Tossed			
14" Large: *Per Slice (⅛ Pizza)*			
America's Favorite	355	16	39
Bacon Cheeseburger; MeatZZa	380	18	38
Barbecue	345	13	43
Deluxe	315	12	39
ExtravaganZZa	390	18	40
Hawaiian	310	11	41
Pepperoni	365	17	39
Vegi	300	11	40
Feast Pizza Crunchy Thin Crust			
14" Large: *Per Slice (⅛ Pizza)*			
America's Favorite	285	18	20
Bacon Cheeseburger	310	20	19
Barbecue	275	15	24
Deluxe	255	15	20
ExtravaganZZa	320	20	20
Hawaiian	240	13	21
MeatZZa	310	20	20
Pepperoni	295	19	20
Vegi	230	13	21

Domino's® Pizza cont...

	C	F	Cb
Feast Pizza Ultimate Deep Dish			
14" Large: *Per Slice (⅛ Pizza)*			
America's Favorite	435	23	42
Bacon Cheeseburger	460	25	41
Barbecue	425	20	46
Deluxe	395	20	42
ExtravaganZZa	470	25	43
Hawaiian	390	18	43
MeatZZa	460	25	42
Pepperoni	445	24	42
Vegi	380	18	43
Ultimate Deep Dish			
14" Large: *Per Slice (⅛ Pizza)*			
Beef	390	20	41
Cheese	335	15	41
Green Pepper, Onion & Mushroom	345	15	42
Ham	350	15	41
Ham & Pineapple	355	15	42
Pepperoni	385	19	41
Pepperoni & Sausage	430	23	41
Sausage	400	20	42
Personal Pizza			
6" Cheese, 100g	245	6.5	36
6" Pepperoni, 100g	260	9.5	34
Philly Cheese Steak Pizza			
1 slice, ⅛ medium	235	9	27
1 slice, ⅛ large	310	12	36
Salads: *Per Serving*			
Croutons, Garlic & Butter,	35	1.5	4
Garden Fresh, ½ container	65	3.5	4.5
Grilled Chicken Caesar	100	4	4
Salad Dressing: Blue Cheese	230	24	2
Creamy Caesar	210	22	2
Italian	210	23	2
Lite	20	1	2
Ranch	220	24	2
Side Dishes: Breadsticks (1), 1 oz	115	6.5	12
Buffalo Chicken Kickers (1), 0.8 oz	45	2	3
Buffalo Wings: Barbecue (1)	55	2.5	2
Hot (1), 0.8 oz	45	2.5	1
Cheesy Bread (1), 1.2 oz	125	6.5	13
Cinna Stix (1), 1 oz	125	6	15
Dipping Sauce: Blue Cheese	225	23	2
Hot	15	0	4
Marinara	25	0	5
Ranch	195	20	2
Garlic Sauce	440	49	0
Sweet Icing	250	2.5	57

For Complete Nutritional Data ~ see CalorieKing.com

Restaurants & Fast - Foods

Don Pablos®

Appetizers: Per Serving	C	F	Cb
Beef Taquito (1), no garnish	65	3	5
Buffalo Chicken Wings (8)	1035	78	43
Chicken Flauta (1), no garnish	65	4	6
Nachos: Taco Beef	1625	113	85
Beef Fajita	1430	99	71
Chicken Fajita	1395	87	73
Quesadillas: Incl. Sour Cream & Guacamole (Whole)			
Cheese Quesadilla	1595	99	105
Mesquite Grilled Chicken	1330	65	110
Mesquite Grilled Steak	1560	91	122
Portabello Mushroom & Veges	1505	83	136
Primo Club	1745	100	114
Dips: Per Cup (No Chips)			
Queso Blanco	340	27	13
Prairie Fire Bean w. Cheese	380	25	23
Spinach	315	28	8
Burritos (No Sides): Chicken	880	48	70
Beef & Bean	1390	73	123
Chimichangas: Includes Rice & Refritos			
Spicy Beef Chimi De Oro	1190	63	109
Chicken Chimi	815	44	71
Rellenos: Beef	300	17	20
Cheese	395	26	19
Chicken	295	11	21
Salads (No Dress.): Steak Fajita	620	35	27
Chicken Fajita	565	30	28
Traditional Taco Salad, average	1290	80	94
Salad Dressing: Per 3 oz			
Blue Cheese	450	48	3
House Vinaigrette	355	31	10
Honey Mustard	315	27	17
Low Fat French	150	4	30
Ranch	320	34	3
Sides: Chips & Salsa, 1 order	340	17	43
Guacamole, 1.5 oz	50	5	2
Mexican Rice, 3 oz	105	1	21
Refritos, 5 oz	180	6	23
Salsa, 1 oz	5	0	1
Side Salad	110	7	8
Sour Cream, 1.25 oz	80	7	2
Sour Crema, 1 oz	60	5	1
Flour Tortilla , 7"	125	4	20

For Complete Nutritional Data ~ see CalorieKing.com

Dunkin Donuts®

Donuts	C	F	Cb
Apple/Blueberry Crumb Donut	240	10	36
Apple N' Spice Donut	200	8	29
Black Raspberry/Strawberry Donut	210	8	32
Blueberry Cake Donut	290	16	35
Boston Kreme Donut	240	9	36
Chocolate Coconut Cake Donut	300	19	31
Chocolate Frosted Cake Donut	360	20	40
Chocolate Frosted Donut	200	9	29
Chocolate Glazed Cake Donut	290	16	33
Cinnamon Cake Donut	330	20	34
Glazed Cake Donut	350	19	41
Jelly Filled Donut	210	8	32
Kreme Filled (Choc./Vanilla)Donut	270	13	35
Lemon Cake Donut	240	14	28
Maple/Marble Frosted Donut, avg.	210	9	29
Old Fashioned Cake Donut	300	19	28
Powdered Cake Donut	330	19	36
Strawb./Van. Frosted; Bavarian	210	9	30
Sugar Raised Donut	170	8	22
Whole Wheat Glazed Cake Donut	310	19	32
Muffins: Banana Walnut	540	25	69
Blueberry: Regular	470	17	73
Reduced Fat	440	12	75
Chocolate Chip	630	26	89
Coffee Cake Muffin, 6.5 oz	580	19	78
Corn	510	18	77
Cranberry Orange	440	17	66
Honey Raisin Bran	480	15	79
Danishes: Apple	250	10	36
Cheese	270	14	32
Strawberry Cheese	250	12	33
Crullers: Plain Cruller	240	15	25
French Cruller	150	8	17
Sandwiches: Per Sandwich			
Biscuit Sandwiches:			
Egg/Cheese Sandwich	370	20	32
Sausage/Egg/Cheese Sandwich	570	39	32
Croissant: Egg & Cheese	440	26	39
Sausage, Egg & Cheese	650	45	39
Eng. Muffin S'wich: Ham/Egg/Chse	310	10	34

Continued Next Page ...

Fast - Foods & *Restaurants*

Dunkin Donuts® cont...

Bagels: Per Bagel	C	F	Cb
Reduced Carb	380	12	45
Everything	370	6	67
Onion	320	3.5	61
Sesame	380	8	64
Salt; Plain	320	2.5	62
Cream Cheese (Per Packet): Lite	130	11	3
Average of other flavors	180	17	3
Cake Munchkins: Plain (4)	270	16	27
Cinnamon; Powdered, (4)	250	14	29
Glazed (5)	200	9	27
Lemon Filled (4)	170	8	23
Sugar Raised (7)	220	12	26
Cake Sticks: Per Stick			
Cinnamon	450	30	42
Glazed/Chocolate	470	29	50
Jelly	530	29	61
Plain	420	29	35
Powdered	450	29	42
Cookies: Chocolate varieties, avg. (1)	220	11	27
Oatmeal Raisin Pecan	220	10	29
Drinks: Dunkacinno, 10 fl.oz	230	10	35
Hot Chocolate, 10 fl.oz	220	8	38
Iced Coffee: 16 fl.oz	15	0	4
w. Cream, 16 fl.oz	70	6	4
w. Milk, 16 fl.oz	35	1	4
Choc Dipped Iced Lattes: Per 16 fl.oz			
Chocolate Banana: Whole Milk	300	10	50
Non-Fat Milk	250	4	50
Chocolate Strawberry Whole	290	10	50
Non-Fat Milk	240	4	40
Vanilla Chai, 10 fl.oz	230	8	40
Coolatta: Per 16 fl.oz			
Coffee Coolatta®: w. Cream	350	22	40
w. Milk	210	4	42
w. 2% Milk	190	2	41
Orange Mango Fruit Coolatta®	270	0	66
Strawberry Fruit Coolatta®	290	0	72
Vanilla Bean Coolatta®	440	17	70

For Extra Menu Items + Full Nutritional Data
~ See Author's Website
www.CalorieKing.com

Eat 'N Park®

Breakfast	C	F	Cb
Apple Waffles	960	44	125
Cornbeef Hash, 7.5 oz	340	23	16
Egg Beaters® Breakfast	75	0	5
Fruit Cup	60	0.5	14
Hash Browns, 6 oz	235	12	28
Homefries, 6 oz	210	12	24
Omelette: Cheese	390	30	2.5
Ham & Cheese	465	33	3
Supreme	420	30	9
Pancake, Plain (1)	225	3	42
Burgers: American Grill	790	50	31
Bacon & Cheddar	1035	69	50
Black Bean Burger	790	48	62
Cheeseburger	540	30	32
Classic Burger	815	50	40
Hamburger 1/3 lb	495	26	32
Mushroom & Onion	885	56	44
Superburger	705	49	37
Swiss Burger	580	32	34
Swiss, Mushroom & Bacon	880	55	45
Turkey Burger	500	22	37
Sandwiches: Tuna Melt	610	40	35
Bacon Turkey Swiss	525	37	16
Chicken Bacon Deluxe	565	23	50
Chicken (Breaded)	515	20	50
Chicken Chargrill/Spicy, 4 oz	320	6	32
Chicken Fiesta, 4 oz	325	11	21
Dutch Ham & Swiss	570	30	35
Grilled Cheese	505	35	26
Hot Roast Beef	310	6.5	32
Hot Turkey	260	5	27
Reuben	720	49	31
Steak'n Cheese	765	50	42
Tuna Melt	610	40	35
Turkey Club	775	46	50
Turkey Pastrami	715	46	40
Croissants, Chicken Salad; Tuna	595	39	36
Pita: Chicken Fajita	620	18	68
Tuna	640	25	72
Turkey	445	5	67
Appetizers: Cheese Fries	880	50	93
Cheese Sticks	410	24	17
Onion Rings	210	13	20
Wings	400	28	0.5

Eat 'N Park® cont...

	C	F	Cb
Dinners: Chicken Breast, stuffed	370	16	27
Chicken Fillets (5)	530	26	28
Chicken Naturelle, 6 oz	210	5.5	4
Chicken Parmigiana	900	38	86
Chicken Stir-Fry	555	24	47
Country Fried Chicken Steak	790	41	43
Floridian Scrod, 4 oz	120	1.5	4
Rib Eye	615	42	1
Spaghetti Marinara	620	8	120
Veal Parmigiana w. Meat Sauce	820	27	108
Ziti w. Meat Balls & Meat Sauce	960	42	102
Salads & Dressings			
Buffalo Chicken Salad	605	42	42
Chicken Caesar Salad	270	9	15
Chicken Portabella Salad	330	12	21
Garden Salad	100	3	16
Steak Salad	640	39	35
Taco Salad	805	40	70
Dressings: Bleu Cheese, 2 Tbsp	90	7	7
French Fat Free	70	0	17
Italian Fat Free	10	0	3
House, 2 Tbsp	115	11	2.5
Thousand Island , 2 Tbsp	95	9	3
Desserts: Cheesecake	505	36	40
Banana Fudge Sensation	975	44	147
Grilled Sticky Loaf	485	28	53
Ice Cream, 2 scoops	285	16	33
Pies: Apple (Reduced Fat)	340	10	62
Peach Lite	300	10	50
Pudding (Sugar Free)	90	2.5	13
Strawberry Shortcake	685	26	114

Edo Japan®

Meals: Per Regular Serving	C	F	Cb
Beef Yakisoba	575	26	54
Chicken & Beef	560	17	68
Chicken Yakisoba, serving	430	6	52
Curry Chicken	395	5	87
Ginger Pork	520	10	71
Grilled Vegetables	325	1	71
Hawaiian Chicken	500	7.5	71
Seafood Grill	495	8	73
Sukiyaki Beef	635	26	68
Teriyaki Chicken	490	7.5	68
Teriyaki Shrimp	465	6	72

Einstein Bros®/Noahs®

	C	F	Cb
Bagels: Average, 4.2 oz	350	1	75
Chocolate Chip Bagel, 4 oz	370	3	76
Egg Bagel	340	3	69
Sesame Dip	380	5	75
Gourmet, average	440	6	78
Lower Carb 9 Grain	210	3.5	28
Cream Cheese Shmear: Plain, 2 T.	70	7	1
Plain Reduced Fat, 2 Tbsp	60	5	2
Smoked Salmon, 2 Tbsp	65	6	2
Flavors, average, 2 Tbsp	70	5	5
Spreads: Fruit, 2 Tbsp	75	0	19
Honey Butter, 1 Tbsp	90	8	4
Peanut Butter, 2 Tbsp	190	15	8
Sandwiches: Per Sandwich			
Classic: Albacore Tuna Salad Low-Fat	400	9	49
Black Forest Ham	570	23	61
Roasted Turkey	590	28	50
Tasty Turkey	600	18	81
Veg Out	500	13	82
Culinary: Club Mex	730	38	60
Cobbie	620	29	59
Einstein Club	670	29	54
Hummus & Feta	450	10	77
Lower Carb 9 Grain Bagel:			
w. 100% Albacore Tuna Salad	360	9	34
w. Egg & Bacon Frittata	570	29	32
w. Plain Cream Cheese	310	13	29
Dog a la Carte	560	33	35
Panini: Cali Club	750	34	68
Ham & Cheese	620	22	68
Italian Chicken	690	27	68
Low-Fat: Rsted Turkey Deli Bagel	420	2.5	73
Salads: Asiago Chicken Caesar	740	54	25
Bros Bistro	810	69	37
Chicken Chipotle	630	40	38
Kickin' Jerk Chicken			
w. Spicy Mango Vinaigrette	510	28	43
Soups: Per Bowl (14 oz)			
Broccoli Sharp Cheddar	540	35	31
Caribbean Crab Chowder,	520	38	30
Chicken & Wild Rice	440	9	67
Chicken Noodle	510	21	39
New England Clam Chowder	370	25	25
Turkey Chili,	330	11	34
Low-Fat: Vegetarian Minestrone	360	10	62
Cookies: Chocolate Chip	520	24	68
Trail Mix	480	19	70
Coffee: Cafe Latte, 12 fl.oz	135	5	13
Cappuccino, 12 fl.oz	90	3.5	9

Fast - Foods & *Restaurants*

El Pollo Loco®

	C	F	Cb
Flame-Grilled Chicken			
Chicken Breast w. Skin	185	7	0
Leg	85	3	0
Thigh	120	7	0
Wing	85	3	0
Burritos: Chicken Guacamole	525	17	59
Classic: BRC	530	15	79
Chicken Lovers	525	18	55
Classic Chicken	635	19	81
Spicy Chicken	555	19	64
Grilled Signature: Grilled Fiesta	1070	54	91
Twice Grilled	855	41	62
Ultimate Chicken	700	24	84
Bowls: Chicken Caesar Salad	535	29	47
Pollo	545	10	84
Loco Favorites			
Cheese Quesadilla	545	26	51
Chicken Nachos	1300	77	90
Chicken Quesadilla	655	30	53
Chicken Soft Taco	235	11	18
Chicken Taquitos	370	17	43
Taco Al Carbon	135	3	18
Salads: Per Serving (With Dressing)			
Chicken Caesar	535	42	17
Chicken Fiesta	745	57	29
Chicken Monterrey	260	11	17
Chicken Tostada	740	33	83
Tostada Salad no Shell	415	16	42
Tamales (1)	185	8	21
Side Dishes: Per Individual Serving			
Cole Slaw, 5 oz	205	16	12
Corn Cobbette, 3 oz	40	0	10
French Fries, 5.5 oz	445	19	61
Fresh Vegetables, 4 oz	70	4	6
Garden Salad, 4.8 oz	110	7	8
Pinto Beans, 6 oz	155	4	24
Spanish Rice, 4 oz	160	1	33
Tortilla Chips, small, 2 oz	305	17	34
Tortillas: 6" Corn, 3 oz	210	3	42
6½" Flour, 3 oz	330	12	48
Condiments			
Dressings: Creamy Chipotle	270	28	3
Creamy Cilantro	275	29	1
Guacamole, 1.7 oz	50	3	5
Jalapeno Hot Sauce, pkt, 0.3 oz	5	0	0
Sour Cream	105	10	2
Salsa: Avocado	20	1	1
Chipotle; House	5	0	1
Pico de Gallo	10	0	1
Desserts: Churro (1)	180	11	24
Flan, 5.5 oz	305	12	43
Soft Serve, Regular, 5 oz	180	5	30

For Complete Nutritional Data ~ see CalorieKing.com

Fatburger®

	C	F	Cb
Burgers: Baby Fat	295	13	25
Bacon & Egg Sandwich	440	27	31
Chicken Sandwich	400	15	32
Chili Dog	510	26	45
Fatburger	600	34	39
Fatburger w. Cheese	625	36	38
Kingburger	825	46	56
Kingburger w. Cheese	1020	58	65
Turkey Burger	590	33	41
Shakes (21 fl.oz): Vanilla	810	44	85
Chocolate, Strawberry, average	900	42	110
Fries & Sides: Chili Cup, 7.2 oz	345	23	14
Fat Fries, 7.6 oz	540	26	70
Skinny Fries, 5 oz	515	26	65
Onion Rings, 6.1 oz	235	23	56

For Complete Nutritional Data ~ see CalorieKing.com

Fazoli's® Italian Food

	C	F	Cb
Pasta: Per Serving			
Classic: Classic Sampler Platter	780	18	119
Classic Ziti w. Meat Sce: Regular	670	25	73
Small	430	16	47
Fettucine Alfredo: Regular	740	15	122
Small	490	10	81
Peppery Chicken Alfredo, small	570	11	81
Ravioli Marinara	580	17	86
Six Layer Lasagna	610	22	74
Spaghetti Marinara: Regular	650	3	121
Small	440	2.5	84
Spaghetti w. Meat Sauce: Reg.	690	6	125
Small	460	4	84
Spaghetti w. Meatballs: Regular	980	27	135
Small	680	20	91
Ultimate Sampler Platter	980	26	140
Oven-Baked: Chicken Parmesan	760	17	110
Spaghetti	700	24	84
Spaghetti w. Meatballs	950	41	91
Twice Baked Ziti	810	36	73
Paninis: Four Cheese & Tomato	820	52	51
Grilled Chicken	420	7	51
Smoked Turkey	710	40	51
Pizza (9"): Italian Meat	970	46	92
Mediterranean	890	43	85
Pepperoni	870	39	89
Ultimate Cheese	800	32	89

Fazoli's® cont...

	C	F	Cb
Submarinos: Club	1040	44	117
Ham n' Swiss	980	38	117
Original	1390	78	116
Meatball	1070	41	124
Turkey	940	36	114
Three Meatballs, no bread	250	18	7
Salads: Dressing Not Included			
Garden Side Salad	25	0	4
Caesar Side Salad	110	5	12
Chicken Caesar Salad	200	7	14
Chicken and Pasta Caesar Salad	360	17	27
Grilled Chicken Salad	100	2	6
Italian Market Salad	620	41	32
Pasta Side Salad	230	13	22
Salad Dressing: Italian Dressing	160	14	7
Fat Free Honey Mustard	60	0	15
Caesar Dressing	230	25	1
Honey French	220	18	14
Thousand Island	210	20	6
Ranch Dressing	220	24	2
Lite Ranch Dressing	120	12	2
Breadsticks, Soup, Meatballs			
Breadstick, dry	100	1.5	18
Minestrone Soup, small bowl	90	1.5	19
Desserts: Chocolate Chunk Cookie	590	28	77
Cheesecake: Plain	290	22	17
Turtle	450	16	43
Freezi's, average all flavors	360	3.5	85
Kids Meals: Lasagna	310	11	37
Fettuccine Alfredo	290	5	50
Cheese Ravioli w. Meat Sauce	300	8	42
Pizza: Cheese	380	15	43
Pepperoni	450	21	43
Spaghetti: w. Meatballs	340	7	53
w. Marinara or Meat Sauce, avg.	270	2	51

For Complete Nutritional Data ~ see CalorieKing.com

Fox's Pizza Den®

12" Pizzas: Per Slice (⅛ Pizza)	C	F	Cb
Cheese	155	5	21
Pepperoni	180	7	21
16" Pizzas: Per Slice (¹⁄₁₀ pizza)			
Cheese	220	7	30
Pepperoni	250	9	30

Firehouse Subs®

Subs: Per Medium	C	F	Cb
Chicken Salad,	550	29	65
Engine Co	405	11	57
Engineer	375	14	61
Ham	420	7	62
Hero	475	12	61
Hook & Ladder	395	10	60
Italian	655	33	60
NY Steamer	520	20	56
Roast Beef	440	8	56
Tuna Salad	615	28	62
Turkey	370	14	58
Veggie	365	11	60

Frisch's Big Boy®

Same Menu & Data as Big Boy

Freshens®

	C	F	Cb
Frozen Yogurt			
Yogurt, average, 1 fl.oz	105	0	6
Ice Cream			
Hand Dipped Ice Cream, avg., ½ cup	215	12	22
Smoothies: Per Container (21 fl.oz)			
Berry Berry	260	0.5	66
Blueberry Breeze	325	1	69
Caribbean Craze	315	0	79
Cayman Cooler	320	0	82
Club Trim	290	0	72
Fitness Fuel	520	5	81
Immune Support	375	3	84
Jamaican Jammer	380	0.5	69
Maui Mango	355	0	90
Mocha Coffee	385	3	74
Mystic Mango	405	3	93
Orange Shooter	340	3	76
Orange Sunrise	365	3	82
Peach Sunset	390	0	96
Peachy Pineapple	415	1	78
Peanut Butter Choc	310	20	14
Pina Collider	450	4.5	79
Pineapple Passion	390	4	90
Raspberry Royale	345	0.5	86
Rockin' Raspberry	330	1	58
Strawberry Shooter	250	0	65
Strawberry Squeeze	315	0.5	55
Vanilla Coffee	440	3	90
Vanilla Fudge	275	16	13
Snacks: Per Serving (3 oz)			
Pretzel Logic: Gourmet Bites	115	9	4
Gourmet Pretzels, ½ pretzel	255	3	49

Fast - Foods & *Restaurants*

Gino's East®

	C	F	Cb
Deep Dish Pizza: Medium 11" ~ Per Slice (⅙ Pizza)			
Cheese	410	11	58
Crumbled Sausage	420	21	38
Pepperoni	445	15	57
Spinach	405	11	59
Deep Dish Pizza: Small 6" ~ Per Whole Pizza			
Cheese	360	8	58
Crumbled Sausage	420	21	38
Pepperoni	380	10	58

Gold Star Chili®

Meals	C	F	Cb
Bowls: Low Carb Coney, 10.4 oz	570	47	7
Veggie Chili, 9 oz	160	2	29
Cheese Coney, 5.1 oz	285	14	30
Chili, 8 oz	215	12	8
Chili Bean, 8 oz	275	10	22
Chili Cheese Nachos	410	25	30
Chili Cheese Sandwich	285	12	30
Chili Sandwich	210	5	32
Coney	285	13	30
Regular 2-Way	420	11	58
Bean	490	12	71
Onion	260	11	62
Onion Bean	505	12	75
Regular 3-Way	650	30	59
Regular 4-Way	665	30	63
Regular 5-Way	735	30	76
Super 5-Way	1140	51	109
Tex Mex	210	9	17
Sides: Fries, 5 oz	365	19	44
Garlic Bread: Without Cheese	215	13	19
w. Cheese	270	18	19
Side Salad	70	5	2

Golden Corral®

Meals	C	F	Cb
Bourbon Str Chkn, 3.5 oz	210	11	5
Fish Fillet Cajun style, 2 pces	210	9.5	18
Fresh Fried Chkn, Leg or Thigh (1)	245	19	2
Meatloaf, 3.5 oz	190	10	10
Sirloin Steak, Buffet, 3 oz	220	13	0
Steakburgers, Lunch, 6 oz	860	55	0
Turkey Breast w. Wing, 2 oz	70	3	1
Whitefish Cajun, 3 oz	110	7	0
Sides: Baked Potato, plain (1)	110	0	25
Carrot & Raisin Salad, ½ cup	115	5	17
Macaroni Salad, ½ cup	190	8	26

Godfather's™ Pizza

Golden Pizza: Per Slice	C	F	Cb
Cheese: Medium, ⅛ pizza	215	8	26
Large, ¹⁄₁₀ pizza	235	9	28
Combo: Medium, ⅛ pizza	275	13	27
Large, slice, ¹⁄₁₀ pizza	315	15	30
Original Pizza			
Cheese: Mini, ¼ pizza	145	4	20
Medium, ⅛ pizza	245	7	34
Jumbo, ¹⁄₁₀ pizza	410	13	53
Combo: Mini, ¼ pizza	195	8	21
Medium, ⅛ pizza	340	14	36
Jumbo, ¹⁄₁₀ pizza	555	24	57
Thin Pizza			
Cheese: Medium, ⅛ pizza	190	9	19
Large, ¹⁄₁₀ pizza	200	10	19
Combo: Medium, ⅛ pizza	260	14	21
Large, ¹⁄₁₀ pizza	285	16	21
Sides			
Breadstick (1)	80	2	14
Cheesestick,1 piece, ⅙ whole	130	4	18
Chocolate Chip Cookie, slice	200	8	30
Potato Wedges, 4 oz	190	9	24

*F*or full nutritional data and product updates
check the food database of the author's
website www.CalorieKing.com

(The) Great American Bagel Co®

	C	F	Cb
Bagels: Plain	390	1.5	85
4-Grain Honey; Cinn. Raisin	420	1.5	88
Apple/Blueberry Crumb, average	570	8	106
Banana Nut; Cheddar Herb, avg.	410	5	82
Blueberry; Onion; Strawberry	380	1	83
Cheddar Salsa	430	11	63
Cheese Twist	740	20	107
Chocolate Chip	390	4	75
Cinnamon Sugar; Egg	390	2	83
Cranb. Nut; P'nut Butter Choc Chip	400	6	72
Jalapeno Cheddar	330	4.5	58
Pumpernickel; Pumpkin, average	330	1.5	72
Pumpkin Chocolate Chip	350	3.5	67
Spinach Herb	300	1	60
Stuffed Pepperoni	500	12	74
Stuffed Spinach	720	22	98
Sun-Dried Tomato Basil	390	1.5	77
Other varieties, average	370	2	75

Green Burrito

	C	F	Cb
Burritos: Bean & Cheese	760	36	87
Grilled Chicken	1030	52	91
Meat Bean & Cheese: Chicken	660	28	67
Ground Beef	820	43	71
Steak	700	31	68
The Green w. Steak	920	34	117
Sides: Chips, 2 oz	300	15	75
Chips & Cheese, 5 oz	690	40	133
Guacamole, 1.4 oz	50	3	6
Make Any Burrito Wet (Green Sauce)	400	27	43
Make Any Entree a Plate			
Beans Rice & Tortilla Chips	440	17	85
Pinto Beans & Cheese,	330	16	43
Rice, 5 oz	220	3.5	43
Sour Cream, 1.4 oz	50	3.5	3
Specialties: Enchiladas w. Cheese	420	26	31
Super Nachos: Chicken; Steak	1020	56	165
Ground Beef	1170	70	167
Taco Salad: Chicken	790	45	68
Ground Beef	950	59	71
Steak	830	47	68
Taquitos: Chicken, 2 taquitos	160	8	18
Chicken, 5 taquitos	370	17	42
Tacos: Fish, 6 oz	290	14	34
Hard: Chicken; Steak	200	11	14
Ground Beef	300	19	16
Soft: Chicken	200	8	19
Ground Beef	270	14	20

(The) Great Steak & Potato Company®

	C	F	Cb
Sandwiches			
Cheeseburger, Kids	340	19	20
Chicken Philly	715	34	64
Chicken Teriyaki	760	34	74
Ham Delight	675	31	64
Ham Explosion	530	15	63
Phillyburger	610	41	23
Rueben Philly	670	32	64
Super Steak	710	34	60
Turkey Philly	640	28	60
Veggie Delight	700	38	62
Sides: Bacon Bits, 15g	35	1.5	2
Cheese: Average all types, 1 oz	110	9	0
Chicken Nuggets, Kids	185	10	11
Fries: Kids, 11.5 oz	960	44	128
Small	1125	55	142
Regular	1265	62	159
Large	2230	109	281
Potato Skins, 7 oz	755	57	54
Potato, Plain, 10.5 oz	240	0	52
Meat: Per Serving (Sides Not Included)			
Chicken, 4 oz	165	7	6
Corned Beef, 3 oz	75	2.5	0
Gyro, 4 oz	345	29	14
Ham, 3 oz	115	4	4
Salami, 2 oz	135	11	1
Steak, 4.5 oz	65	7	0
Turkey, 4 oz	90	1	4
Salad: Chef	310	12	12
Tossed	40	0	8
Sour Cream	80	7	3
Vegetables: Broccoli, 3 oz	25	0	4
Other Vegetables, avg., 1 serving	10	0	2
Salad Dressings: Per Serving			
1000 Island, 1½ Tbsp	185	18	6
Lo-Fat Mayo, 1 Tbsp	40	1.5	6
Mayonnaise, 1 Tbsp	145	16	0
Sauces: Cheese, 2 oz	75	5	6
Red Pepper, 1 oz	90	7	6
Teriyaki Glaze, 1.3 oz	45	0	10
Tzatziki, 1 oz	90	9	1
Bun: Regular, 3.5 oz	290	3	55
Wheat Bun, 4 oz	310	4	56
Pita, 3 oz	185	2	36
Wrap, Tortilla, 2 oz	125	3	17
Drinks: Medium, 16 fl.oz			
Lemonade	225	0	56
Cherry ; Root Beer	250	0	62
Mountain Dew	265	0	66
Pepsi; Sierra Mist	220	0	55

Haagen-Dazs®

Ice Cream: Per ½ Cup

	C	F	Cb
Almond Hazelnut Swirl	320	22	26
Baileys Irish Cream	270	17	23
Banana Split	280	16	31
Bananas Foster	260	15	28
Black Walnut	300	22	21
Butter Pecan	310	23	21
Caramel Cone	320	19	32
Cherry Vanilla	240	15	23
Chocolate	270	18	22
Chocolate Chip Cookie Dough	310	20	29
Chocolate Chocolate Chip	300	20	26
Chocolate Peanut Butter	360	24	27
Coffee	270	18	21
Cookies & Cream	270	17	23
Creme Brulee	280	19	23
Dulce De Leche	290	17	28
Eggnog	300	18	30
Macadamia Brittle	300	20	25
Mango	250	14	28
Mint Chip	300	19	26
Mocha Almond Fudge	340	23	28
Peaches & Cream	240	12	29
Pineapple Coconut	230	13	25
Pistachio	290	20	22
Rocky Road	300	18	29
Rum Raisin	270	17	22
Strawberry,	250	16	23
Strawberry Cheesecake	270	16	28
Strawberry Shortcake	260	14	29
Triple Chocolate,	330	21	31
Vanilla	270	18	21
Vanilla Bean	290	18	26
Vanilla Chocolate Chip	310	20	26
Vanilla Fudge	290	18	26
Vanilla Fudge Brownie	300	19	28
Vanilla Swiss Almond	300	20	24
White Chocolate Raspberry Truffle	310	18	32
Light Ice Cream: Dutch Chocolate	190	5	33
S'mores	240	6	42
Other varieties, average	220	7	33
Sorbet: Tropical	150	0	38
Other varieties, average	120	0	33

Frozen Yogurt: Per ½ Cup

	C	F	Cb
Choc. Fudge Brownie	200	2.5	35
Coffee; Vanilla; avg.	200	4.5	31
Dulce De Leche	190	2.5	35
Strawberry Fat Free	140	0	31
Strawberry Banana	160	2	32
Vanilla Raspberry Swirl	170	2.5	32

Ice Cream Bars: See Page 37

Hardee's®

Sandwiches

	C	F	Cb
Bacon Cheese Thickburger ⅓ lb	910	63	50
Bacon Cheese Thickburger ⅔ lb	1300	96	51
Big Chicken Sandwich	770	36	73
Big Hot Ham N Cheese	485	20	40
Big Roast Beef	470	23	38
Charbroiled BBQ Chicken S'wich	310	3.5	47
Charbroiled Chicken	590	26	53
Cheeseburger ⅓ lb	680	39	52
Chili Cheese Thickburger ⅓ lb	870	54	55
Double Thickburger ⅔ lb	1230	90	53
Grilled Sourdough Thickburger ½ lb	1040	73	49
Hot Dog	420	30	22
Hot Ham N Cheese	285	13	30
Mushroom N Swiss Thickburger ⅓ lb	720	42	48
Regular Roast Beef	330	16	29
Six Dollar Burger ½ lb	1060	72	60
Slammer	240	12	19
Slammer w. Cheese	280	16	20
Spicy BBQ Thickburger	860	48	74
Spicy Chicken	470	26	46
Thickburger ⅓ lb	850	57	54
Monster Thickburger ⅔ lb	1420	107	49
Low Carb: Thickburger ⅓ lb	420	32	5
Chicken Club Sandwich	420	24	11

Fried Chicken: Per Portion (edible portion, no bone)

	C	F	Cb
Breast portion	370	15	29
Leg portion	170	7	15
Thigh portion	330	15	30
Wing portion	200	8	23

Sides: Per Serving

	C	F	Cb
American Cheese Slice, ½ oz	65	5.5	1
Chicken Strips (3), 5 oz	380	21	27
Chicken Strips (5), 8.5 oz	630	34	45
Chili Cheese Fries	700	39	67
Coleslaw, small, 4 oz	170	10	20
French Fries: Small, 4.4 oz	390	19	51
Medium, 5.2 oz	515	25	67
Large, 6 oz	595	29	78
Mashed Potato & Gravy, small	90	2	17
Breakfast Platters: Bacon	980	56	90
Low Carb Breakfast Bowl	620	50	6
Breakfast Ham	970	52	90
Chicken	1140	61	105
Country Ham	970	53	90
Country Steak	1150	68	98
Dessert: Apple Turnover	290	15	36
Chocolate Chip Cookie	290	11	44

For Complete Nutritional Data ~ see CalorieKing.com

212

Harvey's®

Main Menu

	C	F	Cb
Angus Burger	375	16	34
Angus Burger w. Cheese	430	20	35
Original Hamburger	405	20	36
Original Cheeseburger	460	24	36
Value Burger	335	15	32
w. Cheese	390	19	33
Hot Dog, 4.2 oz	315	14	34
Grilled Salmon Burger	335	8	32
Harvey's Grilled Chicken	335	6	32
Harvey's Crispy Chicken	455	15	56
Veggie Burger	345	12	46
Chicken Nuggets, 2.3 oz	170	9	11
Crispy Fries: Junior, 3.2 oz	290	15	34
Regular, 4.3 oz	380	20	45
Large, 5.3 oz	475	25	56
Onion Rings: Regular, 2.9 oz	280	14	34
Large, 4.3 oz	420	21	51
Side Orders: Per Serving			
Poutine, 10 oz	640	40	67
Gravy, 3 oz	35	1	5
Salads: Dressing Not Included			
Garden Salad	130	6	11
Caesar Salad	80	4	5
Chicken Caesar Sala	280	14	5
Grilled Chicken BLT	290	12	11
Soup: Harvest Vegetable, 1 cup	120	1	26
Cream of Mushroom, 1 cup	150	5	24
Chicken Noodle, 1 cup	90	1	14
Breakfast: Bagel, 4 oz	290	2	58
Breakfast Club Sandwich	400	20	35
Eggs (2): Fried	170	13	0
Scrambled Eggs	165	12	0
Hashbrowns, 2 oz	180	9	23
Home Fries, 4.6 oz	300	19	29
Pancakes (2), 4 oz	150	2	29
Pancake Syrup, 1.4 fl.oz	180	0	44
Sausage Patty, 1½ oz	130	9	3
Toasted Western Sandwich	370	20	37
Dressings: Light Caesar/Italian	35	2.5	3
Other flavors, average	70	7	1
Desserts & Shakes			
Apple Turnover, 3 oz	260	13	34
Shakes: Choc.; Vanilla, 14.5 fl.oz	540	13	88
Strawberry, 14.5 fl.oz	550	12	99

Hogi Yogi®

Frozen Yogurt: Per ½ Cup

	C	F	Cb
Chocolate Base, 2.5 oz	80	0	17
Vanilla (No Sugar Added): Base, 2.6 oz	100	0	22
Vanilla Base, 2.5 oz	85	0	18
Regular Sandwiches: Club	340	5	47
BBQ Chicken	360	4.5	59
Roast Beef	300	4.5	46
Smokey Turkey	320	3	46
Turkey	290	3	57
Vegetarian	240	2.5	45
Smoothies: Per 24 oz			
Berry Blast	310	0	70
Fruit Safari	370	3.5	84
Jungle Mist	430	4	101
Peach Treat	430	0	105
Pina Collision	450	4.5	105
Pure Passion	430	4	105
Ragin Rasberry	370	3.5	84
Strawberry Kist	420	0.5	98

Hot Dog on a Stick®

Menu Items

	C	F	Cb
Hot Dog on a Bun	470	26	41
Hot Dog on a Stick	255	14	23
Veggie Dog	175	3	24
American Cheese on a Stick	240	13	22
Pepper Jack Cheese on a Stick	235	13	21
French Fries, 7 oz	700	37	83
Lemonade (12 fl.oz): Original	135	0	34
Cherry/Lime, average	170	0	42
Sugar Free Lemonade	10	0	2

Hot Stuff Pizza®

Pizza: Per Slice (⅛ Medium or ¹⁄₁₀ Large)

	C	F	Cb
Beef	380	15	39
Breakfast Pizza	350	21	36
Canadian Bacon	320	17	38
Cheese	310	9	38
Double Pepperoni	390	20	43
Garden Style	330	20	40
Italian Sausage	380	24	39
Masterpiece Supreme	380	19	40
Pepperoni	350	19	40
Pork Sausage	410	15	39
Western Omelet	370	21	37

Fast - Foods & *Restaurants*

Hungry Howie's Pizza®

Pizzas: *Per Slice (Cheese Only)*

	C	F	Cb
Small, ⅛ pizza	160	3.5	20
Medium, ⅛ pizza	190	5.5	23
Large, ¹⁄₁₀ pizza	210	5	25
X-Large, ⅛ pizza	395	9.5	42
Low-Carb: Medium ⅛ pizza	110	5	9.5
Large, ¹⁄₁₀ pizza	125	5.5	10

Sides

Chicken Tenders, 2 pieces	140	4.5	11
Howie Wings, 5 wings	180	13	0

Toppings: *Per Slice (For Medium or Large Pizza)*

Anchovies	55	3	0
Bacon	40	0.5	0.5
Banana Peppers	10	0	1.5
Beef; Pepperoni; Sausage	30	2	0.5
Black Olives; Green Olives	10	0.5	0.5
Green Peppers; Mushroom	0	0	0.5
Ham	5	0.5	0
Onions	5	1	0.5
Pineapple	5	0.5	1.5

I Can't Believe It's Yogurt®

	C	F	Cb
Original Frozen Yogurt: *Regular Serving (9 fl.oz)*			
Awesome Amaretto	280	6	51
Cookies 'N Cream	260	3	54
French Vanilla	260	6	47
Peanut Butter Bliss	310	12	46
White Chocolate Mousse	280	7	49
Nonfat Frozen Yogurt: *Regular*	220	0.5	48
Small, 6.2 fl.oz	160	0.5	32
Nonfat *(with NutraSweet):* *Regular*	190	0.5	40
Small, 6.2 fl.oz	140	0.5	29

In-N-Out Burger®

	C	F	Cb
Burgers: Hamburger w. Onion	390	19	39
w. Mustard/Ketchup, no Spread	310	10	41
Protein Style, no Bun	240	17	11
Cheeseburger w. Onion	480	27	39
w. Mustard/Ketchup, no Spread	400	18	41
Protein Style, no Bun	330	25	11
Double Double® (2 patty/2 sl. chse)	670	41	39
w. Mustard/Ketchup, no Spread	590	32	41
Protein Style, no Bun	520	39	11
French Fries, 4.4 oz	400	18	54
Drinks: Milk, 10 fl.oz	180	6	18
Coca-Cola®; Dr. Pepper, 16 fl.oz	200	0	54
Lemonade, 16 fl.oz	180	0	40
Root Beer; Seven-Up® 16 fl.oz	220	0	54
Shakes, average all flavors, 15 fl.oz	690	36	83

For Complete Nutritional Data ~ see CalorieKing.com

IHOP®

Pancakes: (Syrup/Butter extra)

	C	F	Cb
Buttermilk (1), 1.7 oz	110	3	17
Short Stack, 3	330	9	51
Full Stack, 5	550	15	85
Country Griddle Cakes (1), 2 oz	120	3.5	19
Harvest Grain 'N Nut (1) 2¼ oz	180	9	20
Crepe-Style, 2 oz	120	6	14
Syrup: 1 Tbsp	50	0	12
Whipped Butter, 1 Tbsp	80	9	0
Waffles (Plain): Regular (1), 3 oz	310	15	37
Belgian, Regular (1), 4 oz	390	19	48

Breakfast: *Per Serving*

Classic Combos: Cntry Fried Steak/Eggs	1530	105	73
Fruity Country Griddle Cakes Combo	960	56	83
Harvest Grain 'N Nut Combo	1035	65	80
T-Bone Steak & Eggs	1310	86	63
Signature, Rooty Tooty Fresh & Fruity, average all flavors	855	45	84

Omlette Feast

Colorado Omelette: No pancakes	790	68	5
with 3 buttermilk pancakes	1205	83	66
The Big Steak Omelette: No pancakes	910	72	14
with 3 buttermilk pancakes	1325	87	75

Burgers

Sourdough Bacon Burger Melt:			
Burger Only	690	41	37
with French Fries	1265	74	104
with Onion Rings	1230	88	64
with Salad & 2 ½ T. Reg. Dress.	870	56	47
Entrees: Old Fashioned Pot Roast	765	48	30
with Mashed Potatoes	965	53	65
Salad: Southwestern Chicken Fajita,			
with Tortilla Shell	1110	85	48
no Tortilla Shell	890	67	35

Jack's®

	C	F	Cb
Sandwiches: Big Bacon	700	42	45
Big Jack	505	27	40
Cheeseburger	380	17	35
Chicken Fillet	635	31	69
Double Big Jack Cheese	935	60	43
Double Cheeseburger	595	33	37
Grilled Chicken	410	15	44
Hamburger	270	8	35
Sides: Brown Gravy, 1 oz	10	0	2
Coleslaw, 4 oz	215	16	14
Green Beans, 4 oz	20	0	5
Mashed Potatoes, 4 oz	65	0.5	15

For Complete Nutritional Data ~ see CalorieKing.com

Restaurants & Fast - Foods

Jack in the Box®

Breakfast	C	F	Cb
Biscuit: Bacon, Egg & Cheese,	430	25	34
Sausage	440	29	32
Sausage, Egg & Cheese,	740	55	35
Spicy Chicken	460	22	44
Breakfast Jack: Regular	285	11	28
w. Sausage	450	28	30
Sourdough	425	24	31
Ultimate	575	27	49
Croissant: Sausage	580	39	36
Supreme	455	26	36
Extreme Sausage Sandwich	675	48	31
Hash Browns (1)	150	10	13
Meaty Breakfast Burrito: w. Salsa	490	29	30
No Salsa	480	29	29

Sandwiches & Burgers			
Bacon Bacon Cheeseburger	840	56	51
Bacon Ultimate Cheeseburger	1095	77	53
Junior Bacon Cheeseburger	430	25	30
Ultimate Cheeseburger	1010	71	52
Hamburger	310	14	30
Hamburger w. cheese	355	17	31
Deluxe Hamburger: No Cheese	375	21	31
w. Cheese	465	28	31
Jumbo Jack: Regular	595	34	51
w. cheese	685	41	54
Sourdough Jack	715	51	36
Pannido: Deli Trio	665	35	56
Ham & Turkey	690	34	57
Zesty Turkey	835	48	55

Chicken & Fish			
Bacon Chicken Sandwich	440	24	39
Chicken Breast Strips, 8 oz	630	37	38
Chicken Fajita Pita	305	10	32
Chicken Sandwich	400	21	39
Ciabatta: Bruschetta Chicken	660	26	36
Classic Chicken	510	13	69
Fish & Chips	890	63	62
Jack's Spicy Chicken Sandwich	615	31	61
w. Cheese	695	37	62
Sourdough Grilled Chicken Club	535	28	34
Southwest Pita	260	4.5	35

Tacos & Snacks			
Bacon Cheddar Potato Wedges	620	41	45
Egg Rolls (3)	445	19	55
Monster Taco (1)	240	14	20
Stuffed Jalapenos (3)	230	13	22
Taco (1)	160	8	15

Fries & Rings	C	F	Cb
Natural Cut Fries, medium, 4.7 oz	365	16	47
Seasoned Curly Fries, med., 4.4 oz	400	22	44
Onion Rings, 4.2 oz	500	30	51

Salads: With Dressing			
Asian Chicken	590	33	55
Chicken Caesar	630	44	26
Chicken Club	820	63	31
Side Salad	155	8	16
Southwest Chicken	730	45	54

Sauces & Dressings			
Dipping Sauce: Barbecue	45	0	11
Buttermilk House	130	13	3
Frank's Red Hot Buffalo	10	0	2
Sweet & Sour	45	0	11
Tartar,	210	22	2
Sauce: Mayo-Onion, ½ oz	95	10	1
Soy, 0.3 oz	5	0	1
Taco, 0.3 oz	0	0	1
Reduced-Fat: Herb Mayo, 1 oz	45	1	3

Condiments			
Cheese: American; Swiss	45	3.5	1
Provolone	70	6	0
Ketchup	10	0	2
Mustard	5	0	1
Salsa	5	0	1
Sour Cream	60	5	2

Desserts			
Cheesecake	310	16	34
Double Fudge Cake	310	11	49

Ice Cream Shakes: Per Medium (14.5 oz)			
Chocolate Ice Cream	860	37	116
Choc. Malted Crunch Ice Cream	940	42	122
Oreo Cookie Ice Cream	830	36	112
Strawberry Banana Ice Cream	905	36	128
Strawberry Ice Cream	835	37	109
Vanilla Ice Cream	745	38	84

For Complete Nutritional Data ~ see CalorieKing.com

Fast - Foods & *Restaurants*

Jamba Juice®

Juices: Per Original	C	F	Cb
Carrot	160	1	34
Lemonade	455	0	112
Orange Banana	370	1.5	84
Orange Carrot	260	1.5	56
Orange	340	1.5	77
Vibrant C	395	1	92
Shots: Average all, 4 fl.oz	70	0	14
Wheatgrass, 1 fl.oz	10	0	1
Yogurt Blend:			
Bright Eyed & Blueberry	380	1	76
Sunrise Strawberry	400	1	83
Smoothies: Per Original			
Aloha Pineapple	500	1.5	117
Banana Berry	475	1	112
Berry Lime Sublime	460	2	106
Caribbean Passion	440	2	102
Chocolate Moo'd	720	8	148
Citrus Squeeze	480	2	110
Coldbuster	430	2.5	100
Cranberry Craze	460	0.5	104
Jamba Powerboost	440	1.5	103
Kiwi Berry Burner	470	0.5	112
Mango A Go-Go	440	1.5	104
Orange A Peel	455	1.5	102
Orange Berry Blitz	410	2.5	94
Orange Dream Machine	540	2.5	118
Peach Pleasure	460	2	108
Peanut Butter Moo'd	880	22	149
Peenya Kowlada	690	5	152
Protein Berry Pizzazz	440	1.5	92
Razzmatazz	480	2	112
Strawberries Wild	450	0.5	105
Energy: Acai Supercharger	570	1	86
Matcha Green Tea Blas	480	0.5	106
Turbo Tropic	470	1.5	112
Enlightened:			
Berry Fulfilling	290	1	62
Mango Mantra	310	1	72
Strawberry Nirvana	280	1	64
Tropical Awakening	320	1	73
Baked Goods			
Pretzels: Apple Cinnamon	410	5	78
Savory: Cheddar Jalapeno Twist	250	5	41
Grin n' Carrot	250	10	36
Pizza Protein Stick	230	6	33
Sweet: Blueberry Cinnamon Swirl	320	6	55
Honey Berry Bran	320	12	48
Lemon Poppyseed Bundt	300	12	44

Jimmy John's®

Club Sandwiches	C	F	Cb
Beach Club	785	40	72
Billy Club	870	43	72
Bootlegger's Club	745	32	69
Club Lulu	935	46	71
Country Club	815	40	70
Gourmet Smoked HamClub	825	42	71
Gourmet Veggie Club	1035	63	74
Hunter's Club	885	42	71
Italian Night Club	965	56	72
Tuna Club w. cheese	645	21	70
Gargantuan™ Sandwich			
Regular	890	56	75
Subs: Figures based on 8" French Bread, Mayo, Chse, Sce			
Beach Club	765	35	77
Billy Club	850	38	77
Bootlegger's Club	725	28	74
Club Lulu	915	42	76
Country Club	815	38	84
Gourmet Smoked Ham Club	805	37	76
Gourmet Veggie Club	1015	59	79
Hunter's Club	865	37	76
Italian Night Club	945	51	77
Slim Bacon	320	20	55
Slim John	340	2	52
Slim Pepe	410	10	53
Slim Tom	300	1	51
Slim Tuna	310	1	50
Slim Veggie	450	16	52
Slim Vito	510	20	52
Tuna Club	625	17	75
Unwich Wraps: Including Mayo, Cheese & Sauce			
Beach Club	430	35	10
Big John	340	27	6
Billy Club	515	38	10
Bootlegger's Club	390	28	7
Club Lulu	580	42	9
Country Club	460	36	8
Gourmet Smoked Ham Club	470	37	9
Gourmet Veggie Club	680	59	12
Hunter's Club	530	37	9
Italian Night Club	610	51	9
JJBLT	320	45	9
The JJ Gargantuan	750	54	12
The Pepe	410	35	7
Tuna Club	470	36	12
Turkey Tom	305	26	5
Vegetarian	380	35	9
Vito	320	24	7
Sides: Jimmy Chips, average, 1 oz	160	8	18
Cookies, average	420	17	63

Johnny Rockets®

Original Hamburgers	C	F	Cb
#12	905	60	54
Chili Size	920	56	59
Original Burger	620	35	44
Patty Melt	945	60	51
Rocket Double	1240	84	57
Rocket Single	880	57	56
Route 66	890	61	45
Smoke House	990	59	70
St Louis	960	61	53
Streamliner	420	16	50
Sandwiches: Chicken Club	870	50	62
Bacon, Lettuce and Tomato	530	33	44
Egg Salad	700	49	40
Grilled Breast of Chicken	600	29	54
Grilled Cheese	520	31	42
Grilled Ham & Cheese	450	17	48
Tuna Melt	830	54	42
Tuna Salad	720	46	41
Other Favorites: Hot Dog	430	23	39
Chicken Club Salad			
with Chicken Tenders	670	40	37
with Grilled Chicken Breast	440	25	8
Chicken Tenders	520	22	47
Chili Dog	570	33	46
Garden Salad	250	20	5
Extras: Bacon, 0.7 oz	100	7	0
Extra Patty, 3 oz	270	20	1
Chili, 2½ oz	170	15	3
Grilled Onions or Mushrooms, 1 oz	20	2	2
Starters: American Fries, 8 oz	530	23	77
½ Fries & ½ Rings, 9.3 oz	720	36	92
Cheese Fries, 10 oz	760	43	77
Chili Bowl, 10 oz	660	59	12
Chili Fries, 12 oz	710	40	76
Onion Rings, 6.8 o z	500	34	22
Desserts: Apple Pie	930	59	88
Hot Fudge Sundae	830	47	93
a la mode	260	16	26
Drinks (Medium): Rootbeer	170	0	43
Coke; Sprite	170	0	43
Lemonade	190	0	49
Float	410	25	41
Shakes: Chocolate, 20 oz	1100	60	120
Strawberry, 20 oz	815	48	82
Vanilla, 20 oz	1120	60	130
Extra for Malt	65	2	10

Kenny Rogers Roasters®

Chicken	C	F	Cb
½ Chicken, No Skin or Wing	315	10	1
with Skin	515	28	2
¼ Dark Meat, No Skin	170	7	1
with Skin	270	17	1
¼ White Meat, No Skin or Wing	145	2	1
with Skin, serving	245	11	1
Grilled Breast Platter	990	52	100
Tenders (3)	510	37	24
Tenders Platter	1315	79	119
Pies: Chicken Pot Pie	710	33	78
Pitas: BBQ Chicken	400	7	51
Chicken Caesar	605	35	34
Roasted Chicken	685	35	42
Turkey: Sliced Breast	160	2	0
Salads (No Dressing): Side Salad	25	0	5
Chicken Caesar	285	9	18
Pasta	230	12	18
Roasted Chicken	290	10	19
Sour Cream & Dill Pasta	230	16	20
Tomato Cucumber	125	2	10
Sandwiches			
Chicken Tender	695	46	45
Chicken Tender Pita	610	38	45
Grilled Chicken	525	29	32
Turkey	385	12	30
Side Dishes: Cinnamon Apples	200	5	41
Cole Slaw	225	16	18
Cornbread Stuffing	325	19	34
Corn Cob	70	0.5	14
Corn Muffin	165	6	25
Sweet Corn Niblets	115	0.5	28
Creamy Parmesan Spinach	120	6	10
Honey Baked Beans	150	1	32
Italian Green Beans	115	8	10
Macaroni & Cheese	200	6	24
Potatoes: Baked Sweet	265	0	62
Garlic Parsley	260	12	37
Potato Salad	390	27	34
Real Mashed	295	14	39
Rice Pilaf	175	5	43
Steamed Vegetables	50	0	8
Zucchini & Squash Santa Fe	70	5	8
Soups: Chicken Noodle, 1 bowl	90	2	12
Chicken Noodle, 1 cup	55	1	7

KFC®

	C	F	Cb
Extra Crispy™: Breast, 5.7 oz	460	28	19
Drumstick, 2.1 oz	160	10	5
Thigh, 4 oz	370	26	12
Whole Wing, 1.8 oz	190	12	10
Hot & Spicy: Breast, 6.3 oz	450	27	20
Drumstick, 2.1 oz	140	9	4
Thigh, 4.5 oz	390	28	14
Whole Wing, 1.9 oz	180	11	9
Original Recipe®: Breast, 5.7 oz	380	19	11
Breast, no skin or breading	140	3	0
Drumstick, 2 oz	140	8	4
Thigh, 4.4 oz	360	25	12
Whole Wing, 1.6 oz	150	9	5
Crispy Strips, 3 pieces	400	24	17
Sandwiches: Honey BBQ	300	6	41
Original Recipe Chicken: w. Sce	445	27	22
without Sauce	360	13	21
Snacker Sandwich: Regular	320	16	31
Honey BBQ	220	3.5	32
Tender Roast Chicken: w. Sauce	390	19	24
without Sauce	270	5	23
Tender Roast Twister	510	22	50
Triple Crunch Chkn, no Sauce	540	26	41
Twister Wrap	670	38	55
Zinger: w. Sauce	675	41	42
without Sauce	540	26	41
Entrees: Chicken Pot Pie, 13 oz	770	40	70
Boneless Wings (7)	600	28	49
Honey BBQ Wings, 6 pces	540	33	36
Hot Wings, 6 pieces	450	29	23
Kentucky Nuggets, 6 pieces	285	18	15
Popcorn Chicken: Large, 6 oz	660	44	37
Individual, 4 oz	450	30	25
Tender Roast Plated Meal	360	7	41
Caesar Salad, no Dressing	220	9	6
BLT Salad, no Dressing	210	7	8
Side Dishes: BBQ Beans, 4.8 oz	230	1	46
Biscuit, 2 oz	190	10	23
Coleslaw, 4.6 oz	190	11	22
Corn on the Cob (3") 2.9 oz	70	1.5	13
Green Beans, 4 oz	50	1.5	7
Macaroni & Cheese, 10 oz	135	6	15
Mashed Potatoes: w. Gravy, 4.8 oz	120	4.5	18
without Gravy, 3.8 oz	110	4	16
Potato Salad, 4.5 oz	180	9	22
Potato Wedges, small, 3.6 oz	240	12	30
Desserts: Apple Pie Slice, 4 oz	290	11	44
Pecan Pie Slice, 4 oz	480	21	68
Sweet Potato Pie Slice, 4 oz	340	16	44
Double Choc. Chip Cake, 2.7 oz	400	29	31
Little Bucket™ Parfaits:			
Chocolate Cream, 4 oz	270	13	37
Fudge Brownie, 3.5 oz	270	9	44
Lemon Creme, 4.5 oz	400	14	65

Koo•Koo•Koo®

Rotisserie Chicken	C	F	Cb
Leg & Thigh, 4.8 oz	300	18	1
Breast & Wing, 6.5 oz	345	16	1
Half Rotisserie Chicken, 11.3 oz	635	34	2
Original Skinless Flame Broiled Chicken™			
3 Piece Original Dark, 5 oz	320	16	5
Original Breast, 4.1 oz	190	5.5	0
Roasted Turkey: Breast, sliced, 4 oz	180	8	0
Hand-Carved Turkey Sandwich	600	31	31
Traditional Turkey Dinner	690	29	67
Turkey Pot Pie (1)	885	43	83
Salads: Per Regular (no Dressing)			
BBQ Chicken Salad	365	14	22
Chicken Caesar Salad	285	11	12
Chinese Chicken Salad	550	28	39
Koo Koo Roo House Salad	115	4	16
Chicken Bowls (No Sce): Chargrill	570	18	57
Southwest	570	18	66
Spicy Ginger Garlic	485	6	62
Tostada (no shell)	530	22	45
Soup: Ten Vegetable, 5 oz	95	2	16
Sandwiches: BBQ Chicken w. Sce	560	11	71
Original Chkn Breast w. Dressing	660	28	62
Chicken Caesar w. Dressing	780	35	62
Wraps: Caesar Chicken	755	39	60
Chipotle Chicken	925	43	88
Sides: Baked French Fries, 5 oz	250	7.5	42
Baked Yams, 6 oz	195	0	47
Black Beans, 6 oz	125	2.5	24
Buffalo Wings (no sauce), 6 wings	605	27	42
Creamed Spinach, 5 oz	110	6.5	10
Mashed Potatoes, 6.5 oz	185	5	32
Macaroni & Cheese, 6 oz	340	16	32
Roasted Garlic Potatoes, 5 oz	135	4.5	21
Extras/Dressings			
Lahvash (flatbread), each	60	0	12
BBQ Vinaigrette, 2oz	100	4	14
Caesar Dressing, 1½ oz	235	26	1.5
Chinese Salad Dressing, 3 oz	325	26	26
Chipotle Sauce, 1 oz	130	14	0.5
Cranberry Sauce, 1 oz	45	0	11

For Complete Nutritional Data ~ see CalorieKing.com

Kilwin's® ~ see CalorieKing.com

Kohr Bros® ~ see CalorieKing.com

Kolache® ~ see CalorieKing.com

Restaurants & Fast - Foods

Krispy Kreme®

Doughnuts

	C	F	Cb
Caramel Kreme Crunch	360	19	43
Chocolate Brownie Deluxe	300	17	33
Chocolate Glazed Cruller	290	15	37
Chocolate Iced Cake	280	14	36
Chocolate Iced Custard Filled	305	17	35
Chocolate Iced Glazed	250	12	33
Chocolate Iced Kreme Filled	345	20	38
Chocolate Iced w. Sprinkles	270	12	38
Cinnamon Apple Filled	285	16	32
Cinnamon Bun	270	16	28
Cinnamon Twist	225	9	33
Dulce de Leche	295	18	30
Glazed Blueberry	335	17	43
Glazed Chocolate Cake	310	15	41
Glazed Cinnamon	210	12	24
Glazed Cruller	240	14	26
Glazed Kreme Filled	345	20	38
Glazed Lemon Filled	295	16	35
Glazed Raspberry Filled	310	16	39
Glazed Sour Cream	340	18	42
Key Lime Pie	325	17	40
Maple Iced Cake	270	13	35
Maple Iced Glazed	245	12	32
New York Cheesecake	325	19	35
Original Glazed	205	12	22
Powdered Blueberry Filled	290	16	33
Powdered Cake	285	14	37
Powdered Strawberry Filled	290	16	33
Pumpkin Spice Cake	340	18	42
Sugar Coated	200	12	21
Traditional Cake Doughnut	230	13	25
Doughnut Holes, 4 pieces	210	10	29

Beverages: Per Container

	C	F	Cb
Frozen Double Chocolate Blend/w. Coffee:			
large, 20 fl.oz	740	26	116
medium, 16 fl.oz	595	21	93
Frozen Latte Blend: large, 20 fl.oz	740	26	114
medium, 16 fl.oz	595	21	91
Frozen Original Kreme Blend:			
large, 20 fl.oz	750	27	119
medium, 16 fl.oz	600	21	95
Frozen Original Kreme w. Coffee Blend:			
large, 20 fl.oz	725	24	117
medium, 16 fl.oz	580	19	94
Frozen Raspberry Blend:			
large, 20 fl.oz	720	22	123
medium, 16 fl.oz	580	18	99

For Complete Nutritional Data ~ see CalorieKing.com

Krystal®

Burgers/Sandwiches

	C	F	Cb
B.A. Burger	470	27	39
w. Cheese	530	32	40
Double B.A. Burger	800	53	41
Krystal, Regular	160	7	17
Krystal Chik	240	11	24
Bacon Cheese Krystal	190	10	16
Cheese Krystal	180	9	17
Double Krystal	260	13	24
Double Cheese Krystal	310	16	26
Chili Cheese Pup	210	12	17
Corn Pup	260	19	19
Plain Pup	170	9	15
Sampler Combo (Krystal, Chik, Chili Cheese Pup, Fries, 24 oz drink)	1320	50	171
French Fries: Medium, 4.2 oz	540	28	59
Chili Cheese Fries, 7.3 oz	470	20	53
Sides: Krystal Chili	200	7	22
Chik'n Bites, Small	310	19	16
Chik'n Bites & Salad	290	20	12
Kryspers	190	13	17

Breakfast Items

	C	F	Cb
Krystal Sunriser	240	14	14
Biscuit & Gravy	280	14	34
Biscuit: Bacon, Egg & Cheese	390	23	33
Chik Biscuit	360	15	40
Plain Biscuit	270	13	33
Sausage Biscuit	480	33	33
Country Breakfast	660	42	46
Scrambler, 11 oz	440	26	33
4-Carb Scrambler: Bacon	370	29	4
Sausage	600	51	3
Desserts: Apple Turnover, fried	220	10	31
Lemon Icebox Pie	260	9	41

Drinks: Per Small Serving (16 fl.oz w. ¼ ice)

	C	F	Cb
Coca-Cola Classic	160	0	40
Coca-Cola Classic, frozen	145	0	36
Diet Coke	0	0	0
Sprite	155	0	39

For Complete Nutritional Data ~ see CalorieKing.com

**More extensive menu listings
in website database
www.calorieking.com**

219

La Rosa's Pizzeria®

Pan Crust Medium Pizza: Per Slice	C	F	Cb
Blanca, 1/10 pizza	350	22	28
Cheese	300	15	30
Deluxe/Pepperoni Topper	370	21	31
Meat Topper	400	23	30
Veggie Topper	320	16	32
Traditional Crust Medium Pizza: Per Slice			
Blanca, 1/10 pizza	260	16	17
Cheese	200	10	19
Deluxe/Pepperoni Topper	280	16	20
Meat Topper	300	18	20
Veggie Topper	220	11	21
Calzones: Per Calzone			
3 Meat & 3 Cheese	1080	55	102
3 Veggie & 3 Cheese	860	34	105
Cheese	840	34	101
Cheese & Pepperoni	960	45	101
Philly Cheese Steak	865	39	90
Hoagy: No Cheese/Dressing/Sauce			
Baked Buddy, 8.7 oz	765	40	62
Baked Royal, 9 oz	595	22	62
Meatball, 11.7 oz	685	26	77
Original Steak, 11.3 oz	730	35	65
Philly Steak, 9.2 oz	615	25	64
Hoagy Dressing: Chse on Hoagy	220	18	0
Italian Dressing, 2 oz	320	34	3
Mayonnaise, 2 oz	400	11	0
Mushroom Sauce, 2 oz	20	0.5	3
Pizza Sauce, 2 oz	50	2	7
Tartar Sauce, 2 oz	260	24	11
Lite & Low Fat Menu			
Grilled Chicken Hoagy, low fat	520	9	56
Grilled Chicken Salad, low fat	380	10	40
Lite Deluxe Pizza, Medium, 1 slice	190	6	27
Minestrone Soup, 1 bowl	80	1	15
Pasta Dinner: No Sides			
Cheese Ravioli	675	26	80
Lasagna w. Meat Sauce	745	38	61
Meat Ravioli	725	22	102
Spaghetti: w. Meat Sauce	680	18	104
w. Meatballs	870	28	119
w. Traditional Sauce	640	12	113
Chicken Wings: BBQ Wings (12)	1295	77	48
Special Recipe Wings (12)	1270	87	21
Spicy Hot Wings (12)	1275	85	26

For Complete Nutritional Data ~ see CalorieKing.com

La Salsa Fresh Mexican Grill®

Appetizers	C	F	Cb
Chips: Guacamole & Salsa	970	56	103
Nachos: w. Chicken	1515	84	133
w. Steak	1530	86	129
Burritos			
Baja Fish	875	54	59
Bean & Cheese: w. Black Beans	595	19	82
w. Pinto Beans	565	19	78
w. Chicken, no Beans	550	22	57
w. Steak, no Beans	710	25	81
California: w. Chicken	750	35	81
w. Steak	760	37	77
w. Veggie	620	31	74
El Champion: w. Chicken	1285	54	148
w. Steak	1315	58	139
Fire-Roasted Bowl: w. Chicken	650	34	60
w. Steak	720	39	59
Grande: w. Chicken	750	36	83
w. Steak	765	38	76
Los Cabos Shrimp	720	36	78
Original Gourmet: w. Chicken	630	27	68
w. Steak	645	29	64
Sonora Fish	575	21	56
The No Rice No Bean: w. Chicken	765	36	69
w. Steak	780	38	65
Three Pepper Fajita: w. Chicken	810	37	86
w. Shrimp	740	36	80
w. Steak	825	39	82
Veracruz Grilled Fish	1035	54	93
Meal Platters			
Burrito Ranchero: w. Chicken	850	37	98
w. Steak	865	39	94
Enchilada: w. Chicken	925	51	64
w. Steak	945	54	58
Taquitos & Quesadilla: w. Chkn	1620	91	130
w. Steak	1930	93	126
Three Pepper Fajita:			
w. Chicken & Corn Tortillas	760	33	88
w. Chicken & Flour Tortillas	850	39	91
w. Steak & Corn Tortillas	785	36	80
w. Steak & Flour Tortillas	875	42	83
Two Soft Tacos: w. Chicken	655	24	89
w. Steak	675	26	83
w. Veggie	685	34	99

La Salsa Fresh cont...

Quesadillas: No Beans	C	F	Cb
Classic: w. Chicken	985	59	63
w. Steak	1000	61	59
Grande: w. Chicken	1075	62	81
w. Steak	1090	64	77
Stuffed Fajita: w. Chicken	920	55	59
w. Steak	995	61	58
Salads			
Chile Lime: w. Chicken	765	50	52
w. Steak	780	52	48
Taco: w. Chicken	860	44	94
w. Steak	875	46	90
Sides			
Black Beans	500	5	109
Pinto Beans	425	5	97
Rice	155	5	30
½ Rice & ½ Black Beans	440	8	78
½ Rice & ½ Pinto Beans	395	8	70
Tacos			
Baja Fish	395	25	30
Baja Style Shrimp	370	25	45
Fajita: w. Chicken	260	13	26
w. Steak	270	14	23
La Salsa: w. Chicken	265	10	33
w. Steak	275	11	30
Mexico City: w. Chicken	205	5	31
w. Steak	215	6	28
Sonora Fish	220	10	24
Taquitos	895	54	73

For Complete Nutritional Data ~ see CalorieKing.com

LaMar's®

Bars: Caramel Iced, Unfilled	430	18	59
Chocolate Iced: Unfilled	540	22	81
Bavarian Cream Filled	600	22	96
Chocolate/White Fluff Filled	810	35	120
Bizmarks: Bavarian Cream	620	22	101
Blueberry/Lemon Filled	530	21	80
Cherry Filled	550	19	88
Donuts: Apple Spice Cake	340	17	44
Bluberry Cake	350	18	37
Chocolate Iced Cake	330	18	37
Old Fashioned Sour Cream	420	18	60
Ray's Chocolate Glazed	290	11	44
Ray's Original Glazed	220	10	31
White Iced Cake	320	17	38
Other Items: Apple Fritter	650	26	91
German Chocolate Knot	480	27	54
Cinnamon Roll	690	25	106
Cinnamon Twist	770	26	120
Raisin Nut Cinnamon Roll	850	27	137

Little Caesar®

Pizza: Per Slice	C	F	Cb
12" Round: Cheese, ⅛ pizza	180	6	23
Pepperoni, ⅛ pizza	210	7.5	23
12" Thin Crust: Cheese, ⅛ pizza	140	7	13
Pepperoni, ⅛ pizza	150	8.5	13
14" Round: Cheese, ⅒ pizza	200	6.5	25
Meatsa, ⅒ pizza	280	13	26
Pepperoni, ⅒ pizza	230	8	25
Supreme, ⅒ pizza	270	10	31
Veggie, ⅒ pizza	240	7.5	32
14" Thin Crust: Cheese, ⅒ pizza	160	7.5	14
Pepperoni, ⅒ pizza	180	9	14
16" Round: Cheese, ¹⁄₁₂ pizza	220	7	27
Pepperoni, ¹⁄₁₂ pizza	240	8.5	27
18" Round: Cheese, ¹⁄₁₄ pizza	230	7	30
Pepperoni, ¹⁄₁₄ pizza	260	9	30
Large Deep Dish: Cheese, ⅛ pizza	320	12	37
Pepperoni, ⅛ pizza	350	14	38
Medium Deep Dish: Cheese, ⅛ pizza	230	9	27
Extras			
Baby Pan! Pan!, 1 piece, 5.1 oz	360	16	34
Chicken Wings (1)	70	5	0
Crazy Bread: 1 stick	90	2.5	15
Cinnamon, 2 sticks	100	2	19
Crazy Sauce, 4 oz	45	0	9
Italian Cheese Bread, 1 piece	130	6	13
Sandwiches			
Deli: Ham & Cheese	640	29	66
Italian	800	44	66
Veggie	600	27	67
Side Salads			
Antipasto	140	7.5	6
Caesar	90	3	12
Greek	120	6.5	11
Tossed	100	3	15
Salad Dressings: Per Serving			
Caesar	230	25	1
Greek	270	29	0
Italian	220	23	2
Ranch	230	24	2
Fat-Free: Italian	25	0	5

For Complete Nutritional Data ~ see CalorieKing.com

Lone Star Steakhouse®

Meals

	C	F	Cb
Grilled Chicken	185	2.5	0
Grilled Pork Chop	1430	100	0
Mesquite Grilled Steaks:			
Cajun Ribeye, 16 oz	1250	101	0
Chopped Steak, 12 oz	900	71	0
Delmonico, 11 oz	860	69	0
Five Star Filet, 9 oz	740	60	0
New York Strip, 14 oz	1035	80	0
San Antonio Sirloin, 12 oz	770	55	0
T-Bone, 20 oz	1540	124	0
Texas Ribeye, 14 oz	1090	88	0
Ribs, 12 oz	970	80	0
Shrimp Dinner, 3.45 oz	105	1.5	1
Smoked Prime Rib, 16 oz	1250	101	0
Sweet Bourbon Salmon, 6 oz	240	11	0
Texas Teasers Ribs, 6 oz	485	40	0

Sides: Per Serving

	C	F	Cb
Baked Potato	665	18	114
Baked Sweet Potato	635	8	137
Lone Star Chili, 6 fl.oz	230	15	8
Sauteed Mushrooms	115	9	6
Sauteed Onions	95	7	8
Steamed Vegetables	70	1	14
Texas Rice	80	2	12

Soups

	C	F	Cb
Black Bean, 6 fl.oz	190	4	31

Desserts

	C	F	Cb
Homemade Cobbler	240	8	43

Long John Silver's®

	C	F	Cb
Sandwiches: Ultimate Fish	500	25	48
Fish Sandwich	440	20	48
Chicken Sandwich	360	15	41
Sides: Fries: Regular	230	10	34
Large, 5 oz	390	17	56
Cheese Sticks (3)	140	8	12
Coleslaw, 4 oz	200	15	15
Corn Cobbette, no butter	90	3	14
Crumblies, 1 oz	170	12	14
Hushpuppy (1)	60	2.5	9
Rice, 4 oz	180	3.5	34
Soup: Clam Chowder, 1 bowl	220	10	23
Chicken: Battered Plank, 1 piece	140	8	9
Seafood: Battered Fish, 1 piece	230	13	16
Battered Shrimp, 1 piece	45	2.5	3
Breaded Clams, 1 order	240	13	22
Desserts: Per Serving			
Chocolate Cream Pie	310	22	24
Pecan Pie	370	15	55
Pineapple Cream Pie	290	13	39

For Complete Nutritional Data ~ see CalorieKing.com

Luby's®

Entrees: (Without Sides)

	C	F	Cb
Blackened Chicken Breast	350	15	5
Blackened Tilapia	270	11	5
Carved Ham	300	11	6
Grilled Chicken Breast w. skin	400	20	1
Lemon Basil Salmon	355	20	1
Pan Grilled Fillet	330	12	19
Parmesan Chicken Alfredo	435	22	22
Parmesan Crusted Tilapia	300	14	6
Roasted Chicken, ½, no skin	460	23	0
Roasted Turkey, no skin, no Gravy	280	3	0

Sides

	C	F	Cb
Bread Rolls: White	130	3	23
Whole Wheat	170	5	23
Black-eyed Peas	220	5	33
Blue Lake Green Beans	85	5	9
Broccoli	80	4	9
Cabbage	70	5	6
Carrots	95	4	15
Cauliflower Peas & Carrots	65	4	7
Corn	190	5	38
Fresh Green Beans	90	5	10
Holiday Rice	165	3	30
Mixed Vegetables, Roasted,	135	8	16
Pinto Beans	190	5	28
Spinach	65	4	5

Salads: Grapefruit

	C	F	Cb
Salads: Grapefruit	45	0	12
Grilled Chicken Caesar	535	30	17
Grilled Chicken Caesar no Dressing	370	13	16
Jello	100	0	24
Marinated Cumumbers	115	8	13
Mediterranean Vegetables	140	10	9
Mixed Field Greens no Dressing	35	0	7
Mixed Melons	65	0	20
Pineapple	50	0	12
Spinach Salad no Dressing	45	2	5

Sauces & Dressings: Per 2 Tablespoons (1 fl.oz)

	C	F	Cb
Dressings: Blue Cheese	175	18	0
Caesar	145	16	0
French	160	14	10
Greek	65	6	0
Honey Mustard; Italian	160	14	8
Ranch	115	12	2
Thousand Island	105	10	4
Soups: Chicken Noodle, 1 bowl	235	9	21

For Complete Nutritional Data ~ see CalorieKing.com

McDonald's®

Burgers/Sandwiches	C	F	Cb
BBQ Chicken Sandwich	340	8	48
Big Mac Burger	560	30	46
Big N' Tasty Burger: no Cheese	520	29	41
with Cheese	570	33	43
Cheeseburger	310	12	35
Double Cheeseburger	460	23	37
Chicken McGrill	400	16	38
no Mayo	300	5	37
Crispy Chicken	500	23	50
Deli Trio	415	7	61
Filet-O-Fish	400	18	42
Grilled Chicken Flatbread, no dress.	355	6	50
Hamburger	260	9	33
McChicken	430	22	41
McChicken Hot & Spicy	440	24	42
McVeggie Burger	355	8	48
New York Corned Beef Reuben	565	23	58
New York Turkey Reuben	540	19	60
Quarter Pounder Burger	420	18	40
w. Cheese	510	25	43
Double Quarter Pounder w. Cheese	730	40	46
Turkey Club Flatbread	595	29	52
Turkey McDeli Wrap	775	50	54
Premium			
Chicken Ranch BLT, Crispy	560	20	63
Chicken Ranch BLT, Grilled	460	13	53
Chicken Club, Crispy	650	29	63
Chicken Club, Grilled	560	21	53
Chicken Classic, Crispy	480	16	62
Chicken Classic, Grilled	380	9	52
Extra Value Meals			
Large Fries & Large Soda, add	825	25	141
French Fries			
Small, 2.6 oz	230	11	30
Medium, 4 oz	350	16	47
Large, 6 oz	520	25	70

McDonald's® cont...

Chicken McNuggets®/Sauces	C	F	Cb
Chicken McNuggets: 4 pieces	170	10	10
6 pieces	250	15	15
10 pieces	420	24	26
Sauce: Barbeque, 1 oz	45	0	11
Honey, ½ oz	50	0	12
Hot Mustard, 1 oz	50	2	9
Sweet 'N Sour, 1 oz	50	0	11
Chicken Selects® Breast Strips			
Strips: 3 pieces	380	20	28
5 pieces	630	33	46
10 pieces	1270	66	92
Sauces (1.5 oz pkg): Creamy Ranch	200	21	3
Spicy Buffalo	60	6	1
Tangy Honey Mustard	70	2	13
Chipotle Barbeque	70	0	16
Mozzarella Sticks w. Marinara Sce, 4 oz	290	18	21
Breakfast Menu			
Bagel: Plain	260	1	54
Ham, Egg & Cheese	550	21	62
Spanish Omelete	710	38	64
Steak, Egg & Cheese	640	29	61
Big Breakfast Platter	730	46	53
Bacon, Egg & Cheese Biscuit	440	24	36
Cinnamon Roll: Regular	420	18	57
Deluxe	590	24	86
Deluxe Breakfast Platter	1220	60	136
English Muffin, 2 oz	150	2	27
Grape/Strawberry Jam	35	0	9
Hash Browns (1), 2 oz	140	8	15
Hotcakes: Plain (3)	340	8	58
w. Margarine (2 pats)	420	17	56
w. Margarine (2 pats) & Syrup (1)	600	17	102
Hotcakes with Sausage Platter	770	33	104
McGriddles: Bacon, Egg & Chse	450	21	46
Sausage	420	22	44
Sausage, Egg & Cheese	560	32	48
McMuffin: Egg	290	11	30
Sausage	370	21	31
Sausage w. Egg	450	26	31
Sausage, 1.5 oz patty	170	15	2
Sausage Biscuit	410	26	34
w. Egg	500	32	36
Sausage Breakfast Burrito	300	16	26
Scrambled Eggs (2)	180	11	5
Breakfast Value Meal (Extras)			
If Hash Browns & Coffee (black/no sugar,) add	140	8	15
If Hash Browns & Orange Juice, add	270	8	47

Salads/Desserts/Drinks ~ Next Page ...

McDonald's® cont...

Salads: (No Dressing)	C	F	Cb
Chef Salad	150	8	5
Bacon Ranch Salad: No Chicken	130	7	9
w. Crispy Chicken	350	17	23
w. Grilled Chicken	250	9	12
Caesar Salad: No Chicken	90	4	8
w. Crispy Chicken	310	14	23
w. Grilled Chicken	210	6	10
California Cobb Salad: No Chicken	150	9	8
w. Crispy Chicken	370	18	23
w. Grilled Chicken	270	11	10
Fruit & Walnut Salad w. Yogurt	310	13	44
Side Salad, 3.1 oz	15	0	3
Butter Garlic Croutons, ½ oz	60	1	10
Salad Dressings: Per Package			
Newman's Own: Cobb Dressing	120	9	9
Low-Fat Balsamic Vinaigrette	40	3	4
Creamy Caesar Dressing	190	18	4
Italian Dressing	50	2.5	7
Ranch Dressing	170	15	9
Desserts/Cookies/Shakes			
Apple Dippers w. Caramel Dip	100	1	22
Apple Dippers, 1 pkg	35	0	8
Caramel Dip, 0.8 oz	70	1	14
Baked Apple Pie, 2.7oz	250	11	34
Cookies: Oatmeal Raisin (1)	140	5	22
Chocolate Chip Cookie (1)	160	7	22
Sugar Cookie	150	6	22
McDonaldland® Cookies, 2 oz	250	8	42
Chocolate Chip Cookies, 2 oz	270	11	39
Fruit 'n Yogurt Parfait: Regular	160	2	31
without Granola	130	2	25
Ice Cream: Kiddie Cone	45	1	8
Vanilla Reduced Fat Cone	150	3.5	24
McFlurry™: M&M®, 12 fl.oz cup	620	20	96
Oreo®, 12 fl.oz cup	560	16	88
Sundaes: Nuts (Topping)	50	3.5	2
Hot Caramel Sundae	340	7	62
Hot Fudge Sundae	330	9	55
Strawberry Sundae	280	6	51
Triple Thick Shakes, average all flavors:			
12 fl.oz cup	430	12	70
16 fl.oz cup	580	17	94
21 fl.oz cup	750	22	123
32 fl.oz cup	1150	33	187

McDonald's® cont...

	C	F	Cb
Drinks: 1% Low Fat Milk, 8 fl.oz	100	2.5	12
Coffee (black), 16 fl.oz	10	0	2
Half & Half Creamer, 1 pkg	15	1.5	0
Cappuccino: Per 12 fl.oz			
French Vanilla	215	6	38
Original; Swiss Mocha	205	4	39
White Choc. Raspberry	225	9	34
Coca-Cola or Sprite (with ⅓ Ice):			
Childs, 12 fl.oz cup	110	0	29
Small, 16 fl.oz cup	150	0	40
Medium, 21 fl.oz cup	210	0	58
Large, 32 fl.oz cup	310	0	86
Diet Coke	0	0	0
Hi-C Orange Drink (with ⅓ Ice):			
Childs, 12 fl.oz cup	120	0	32
Small, 16 fl.oz cup	160	0	44
Medium, 21 fl.oz cup	240	0	64
Large, 32 fl.oz cup	350	0	94
Iced Tea	0	0	0
Orange Juice: 12 fl.oz cup	140	0	33
16 fl.oz cup	180	0	42
Powerade Mountain Blast (with ⅓ Ice):			
Childs, 12 fl.oz	70	0	20
Small, 16 fl.oz	100	0	27
Medium, 21 fl.oz	150	0	39
Large, 32 fl.oz	220	0	58
Whipped Hot Chocolate, 12 fl.oz	195	1	43

For Complete Nutritional Data ~ see CalorieKing.com

Manhattan Bagel®

Bagel: Per Bagel (4 oz)

	C	F	Cb
Blueberry	370	1	81
Cheddar Cheese	330	4	72
Chocolate Chip	370	3	76
Cinnamon Raisin	340	1	74
Cranberry Orange	350	1	76
Egg, 4 oz	330	1.5	72
Jalapeno Cheddar	330	1.5	72
Marble Rye	330	1	72
Oat Bran	330	3	71
Plain, 4 oz	330	1	72
Pumpernickel; Rye	340	1	73
Spinach	330	1	73
Sundried Tomato	330	1	73
Whole Wheat	320	1	69
Cream Cheese: Reduced Fat, 2 Tbsp	60	5	1

For Complete Nutritional Data ~ see CalorieKing.com

Max & Erma's®

Appetizers

	C	F	Cb
Black Bean Roll-Ups	575	10	94
Entrees			
Bleu Cheese NY Strip			
w. Broccoli & Salad, no dress.	1340	107	9
Chicken Cordon Bleu w. Broccoli	920	52	10
Salads: No Breadstick			
Half Hula Bowl w. Dressing	405	6	62
Small Low-Carb Salad, no dressing	150	11	3
Sandwiches & Hamburgers			
Burger Stack w. Broccoli	1105	81	6.5
Chicken Stack w. Broccoli	825	51	6.5
Garden Grill			
w. Dressing & Fruit Salad	430	7	75
Sides			
Black Bean Salsa, ½ cup	215	14	17
Buttered Broccoli, 3.5 oz	105	9	4.5
Fruit Salad, 4.5 oz	55	0	16
Garlic Breadstick (1)	155	6	21
Soups: Hearty Beef Chili	390	15	39
Beverages: Fruit Smoothie	125	0.5	28
Dressings: Per Serving (2 Tbsp., 1 fl.oz)			
Bleu Cheese	200	21	0.5
Italian	110	12	1
Ranch	120	12	0.5
Fat Free: French	125	0	31
Honey Mustard	60	0	14
Low-Fat Tex Mex Dressing	20	0	1.5

For Complete Nutritional Data ~ see CalorieKing.com

Mazzio's® Pizza

Appetizers: Per Serving

	C	F	Cb
Breadsticks, ¼ order	130	3	22
Cheese Dippers, ⅓ order	410	18	47
Cinnamon Sticks, ¼ order	640	37	69
Spicy Chicken Wings, 2 wings	110	7.5	0.5
Nachos: Beef w. Jalapenos, ½ order	495	36	19
Cheddar w. Jalapenos, ½ order	435	31	18
Calzones: Per Slice (⅒ Whole)			
Ham Bacon & Cheddar	245	7.5	32
Pepperoni	265	10	32
Low Carb Bakes: Per Serving			
Chicken: California	390	26	8
Ham & Swiss	415	23	7
Philly	290	16	9.5
Supreme: Italian Meat	540	47	9
Pepperoni Chicken	415	29	8
Pastas			
Fettuccine: Alfredo	1065	56	105
Lasagna: w. Meat Sauce	940	52	60
w. Marinara	695	4.5	127
w. Meat Sauce & 4 Meatballs	1160	51	116
Sandwiches: Ham & Cheddar	975	51	87
Mazzio's Sub	1000	53	86
Turkey & Swiss	940	40	88
Tuscan Smash	860	37	87
Pizzas: Per Slice (⅛ Medium Pizza)			
Cheese: Original Crust	215	9	29
Thin Crust	160	9	17
Chicken Club: Original Crust	235	8.5	30
Thin Crust	185	9	18
Mazzio's Works: Original Crust	290	15	30
Thin Crust	240	15	18
Meatbuster: Original Crust	270	13	29
Thin Crust	220	13	17
Mexican: Original Crust	300	14	33
Thin Crust	245	15	22
Pepperoni: Original Crust	235	11	30
Thin Crust	185	11	17
Sausage: Original Crust	260	12	29
Thin Crust	205	13	17
Supreme Buster: Original Crust	245	11	29
Thin Crust	190	11	17
Veggie: Original Crust	215	8	30
Thin Crust	165	9	18
Sides: Kosher Pickle Spear	5	0	1
Potato Chips	150	10	15

For Complete Nutritional Data ~ see CalorieKing.com

Fast - Foods & *Restaurants*

Mimi's Cafe®

Menu Items: Per Serving	C	F	Cb
Broiled 10 oz Halibut Steak	800	16	94
Chicken and Fruit	545	9	59
EggBeater Fitness Omelette	655	8	110
Half-A-Turkey Sandwich	410	6	55
Roasted Turkey Breast	540	8	52
Spaghettini w. Tomatoes & Basil	680	8	130
Two "AA" Large Eggs	395	8	62

Miami Subs®

Burgers	C	F	Cb
Deluxe Burger	785	59	31
Deluxe Cheeseburger	860	65	32
Deluxe Bacon Cheeseburger	920	69	32
Platters: Chicken Breast	745	41	57
Gyros	1420	93	81
10 Wings w. Fries & Blue Cheese	1020	67	50
Salads: Caesar w. Dressing	460	34	26
Chicken Caesar w. Dressing	610	39	28
Chicken Club	490	25	23
Garden	310	18	21
Greek	285	15	24
Side Greek w. Dressing	80	5	4
Cheesesteaks (6"): Original	410	11	45
Classic	420	11	47
Chicken Philly Classic	550	27	46
Works	530	22	51
Pitas: Gyros	660	39	46
Chicken	390	13	33
Subs(6"): Ham & Cheese	450	18	79
Italian Deli	515	24	49
Meatball	490	22	49
Tuna	470	19	44
Turkey	485	18	51
Sides: Mozzarella Sticks	755	56	34
Onion Rings	870	68	55
Spicy Fries: Regular	530	39	39
Large	1040	72	85

Mr. Goodcents®

	C	F	Cb
Cold Sub: Per Half Sandwich on Wheat Bread			
Centsable Sub	495	20	57
Cheese Mix	570	26	57
Ham & Cheese	410	10	57
Italian Sub	630	35	57
Mr. Goodcents Original	520	24	56
Oven Roasted Chicken Breast	370	5	57
Penny Club	375	7	57
Pepperoni & Cheese	745	46	57
Roast Beef	385	6	57
Hot Sub: Per Half Sandwich on Wheat Bread (w. Cheese)			
Chicken Bacon Ranch	620	28	55
Chicken Parmesan	455	10	60
Meatball	710	38	65
Pasta: Chicken Parmesan	630	9	94
Red Sauce	225	2	47

Mr. Hero®

Sandwiches: Per 7" Sub	C	F	Cb
Hot Subs: Grilled Chkn Philly	440	14	48
Cheesesteak: Grilled Steak Philly	450	14	48
Hot Buttered Deluxe	565	33	48
Cold Subs: Classic Italian	585	36	49
Tuna & Cheese	665	47	47
Turkey & Cheese	455	20	46
Ultimate Italian	610	33	51
Meatball	620	32	53
Romanburger	715	47	49
Round: Bacon Cheeseburger	350	23	23
Chicken	420	22	23
Fish	410	23	31
Tuna	430	33	22
Pasta: Breadsticks w. Sauce, 5 oz	290	9	47
Spaghetti Dinner, 16.8 oz	610	8	110
Spaghetti w. Meatballs, 19.8 oz	845	26	116
Salads: Garden Salad	35	0.5	7
Grilled Chicken	225	10	7
Seafood Crab	450	37	17
Side Salad	30	0.5	6
Tuna Salad	740	69	8
Dressings: Buttermilk, 2 oz	290	29	6
Creamy Italian, 2 oz	190	17	11
Croutons, ½ oz	60	2	8
Fat-Free: French ; Ranch	70	0	18
Side Orders: Onion Rings, 6 oz	565	32	64
Cheddar Cheese Sauce, 1.5 oz	60	4.5	5
Potato Waffers, 3.7 oz	335	17	42
Desserts: Cheesecake, plain, 3.5 oz	350	26	26
Cheesecake w. Cherries, 4.7 oz	385	26	35

Mrs Fields Cookies®

Brownies: Per Brownie (3 oz)	C	F	Cb
Butterscotch Blondie	260	11	29
Double Fudge	230	12	32
Mint Fudge	260	14	35
Pecan Fudge	280	17	31
Pecan Pie	230	14	8
Pecan Pie Chocolate Chip	230	14	24
Special Walnut Fudge & Blondie	260	13	35
Toffee Fudge	260	14	35
Walnut Fudge	270	16	31
Cakes			
Blueberry, 3 oz	270	12	36
Carrot Cake, 3 oz	280	13	37
Chocolate, 3 oz	350	21	35
Chocolate Chip, 3 oz	350	17	45
Cinnamon Sugar Pecan, slice, 2.1 oz	270	14	32
Lemon Bundt, slice, 2.1 oz	300	14	40
Raspberry, 3 oz	270	12	36
Raspberry Chocolate Chip, 2.1 oz	260	12	36
Cookies			
Bite Size Nibblers: Cinn. Sugar (2)	120	4.5	17
Debra's Special (2)	100	4.5	13
Peanut Butter (2)	110	6	13
Semi-Sweet Chocolate (2)	110	5	15
Triple Chocolate (2)	110	6	15
White Chunk Macadamia (2)	120	7	13
Cinnamon Sugar (1)	300	12	41
Coconut & Macadamia (1)	280	13	39
Debra's Special (1)	280	12	39
Milk Chocolate & Walnuts (1)	320	17	37
Milk Chocolate Macadamia (1)	320	18	36
Milk Chocolate, no nuts (1)	280	13	38
Oatmeal Chocolate Chip (1)	280	13	40
Oatmeal Raisin (1)	180	7	29
Peanut Butter (1)	310	16	34
Semi-Sweet Chocolate (1)	280	14	40
w. Walnuts (1)	310	16	38
Triple Chocolate (1)	220	10	31
White Chunk Macadamia (1)	310	17	37

For Complete Nutritional Data ~ see CalorieKing.com

My Favorite Muffin®

~ Same Menu & Data as
Big Apple Bagel (See Page 189) ~

Nathan's Famous®

Burgers	C	F	Cb
¼ lb Burger	535	30	42
¼ lb Burger w. Cheese	850	61	45
Bacon Cheeseburger	705	44	43
Super Burger	865	61	42
Cheesesteaks: Chicken	565	19	62
Original	740	43	50
Supreme	785	43	61
Fish Sandwich	465	20	41
Hot Dogs: Nathan's Famous (1)	310	20	22
Sides:			
French Fries: Regular, 9.6 oz	545	37	46
Large, 13.4 oz	760	52	65
Super, 21 oz	1190	82	101
Nuggets (6), 3.5 oz	350	27	20
Onion Rings, 5.6 oz	560	44	36

For Complete Nutritional Data ~ see CalorieKing.com

Noodles & Company®

Classics: Buttered Noodles & Parm.	1010	36	134
Chicken Noodle Soup	290	9	37
Mushroom Stroganoff	1000	45	116
Pad Thai	720	9	147
Pesto Cavatappi	760	30	89
Tomato Marinara	560	13	87
Wisconsin Mac & Cheese	970	44	99
Noodle-Less: Chicken Rustica	530	26	11
Mediterranean Mixed Grill	530	27	12
Shrimp Curry Saute	190	6	20
Sweet Chili Chicken	470	14	29
Specialties: Bangkok Curry	400	10	71
Indonesian Peanut Saute	820	21	128
Japanese Pan Noodle	630	8	128
Pasta Fresca	660	19	93
Penne Rosa	670	32	70
Thai Curry Soup	360	15	49
Whole Grain Tuscan Fettuccine	500	17	70
Salads			
Caesar Salad	440	35	28
Chinese Chop Salad	305	19	33
Market Salad w. Fat Free Dressing	190	2	43
Mediterranean Salad	220	19	11
Spicy Peanut Noodle Salad	480	9	83
Spicy Thai Caesar Salad	220	19	11
Sides: Potstickers (3)	490	22	55
Cucumber Tomato Salad	100	0	21
Grilled Chicken Breast	160	6	0
Sauteed Organic Tofu	100	6	3
Sauteed Shrimp, 8 pieces	60	2	1
Thin-Cut Grilled Steak, 4 oz	250	16	1
Veggie Trio, 5 oz	40	0	7

O'Charley's®

Appetizers: Per Serving	C	F	Cb
Chicken Quesadilla, ½ order	490	30	26
Chicken O'Tenders, ½ order	580	15	74
Chips & Salsa, ½ order	470	23	62
Fried Cheese Wedges, ½ order	270	23	62
Over-Loaded Potato Skins, ½ order	570	40	19
Spinach & Artichoke Dip, ½ order	700	44	69
Brunch: Per Order (w. Brunch Potatoes & Bread)			
Cajun Chicken Omelette	1150	80	48
Spanish Omelette	960	70	47
Ultimate Omelette	970	66	50
Strawberry Waffle	975	33	158
Chicken: Per Order			
Chicken Parmesan w. Vegetables	835	27	90
Chicken O'Tenders	1310	34	178
Chicken Teriyaki on Rice	690	17	69
Grilled Chicken Dinner	560	17	36
Salad: Black & Bleu Caesar	1010	66	15
O'Charley's Caesar Salad	465	36	11
Cajun Chicken w. Ranch Dressing	975	78	21
Island Chicken Salad w. dressing	1465	30	225
Southern Fried Chkn w. Dressing	1805	85	173
Sandwiches: No Sides			
Bacon & Cheese Trio Chicken	760	45	36
Buffalo Chicken	720	32	65
Cajun Chicken	480	21	38
French Dip	945	41	77
Grilled Chicken Sandwich	470	21	35
Half Pound Cheeseburger	1130	73	35
Three Cheese Bacon Burger	1305	88	36
Seafood: Per Order (w. Sides & Salad)			
Fisherman's Platter	1890	95	180
Fried Shrimp Platter, 8 shrimp	550	28	26
Sides: Baked Potato, plain	205	0.5	46
Cole Slaw	220	14	21
French Fries	410	21	50
Rice Pilaf	220	6	38
Smashed Potatoes	365	12	44
Vegetable Medley	135	8	13
Steak & Ribs: Per Serving (No Sides or Fries)			
Steak Tips Monterey, 1 order	1140	82	46
Choice Sirloin, 10 oz	450	18	1
Filet Mignon, 9 oz	755	53	1
Flame Grilled Sirloin: 7 oz	320	13	1
10 oz	480	18	1
Prime Rib: 8 oz	920	80	0
10 oz	1165	100	0
16 oz	1865	159	0
Full Rack of Ribs w. Fries/Slaw	2925	193	164
Ribeye Steak, 12 oz	905	71	1

Old Country Buffet®

	C	F	Cb
Entrees: BBQ Beef Ribs, 5 oz	300	23	7
BBQ Smoked Sausage, 2.8 oz	140	10	9
Beef Patties w. Mushr. Gravy (1)	110	7	2
Carved: Beef Brisket, 3 oz	200	11	1
Ham, 3 oz	140	9	0
Peppered Pork Loin, 3 oz	160	8	0
Roast Beef, 3 oz	230	15	0
Roast Turkey, 3 oz	170	8	0
Salmon Filet, 3 oz	190	12	0
Cheese Enchiladas, 1 piece, 4.1 oz	200	13	13
Chicken Wings: Hot, Drummies (1)	35	2	0
Hot, Wing (1), 1.5 oz	25	1.5	0
Teriyaki, Drummie (1), 0.9 oz	50	2.5	2
Teriyaki, Wing (1), 0.45 oz	50	2.5	2
Chicken Hand Breaded Fried:			
Breast, 5 oz	310	16	3
Drumstick (1), 1.4 oz	90	6	-
Thigh (1), 3.1 oz	210	14	4
Chicken, Traditional Baked: Breast	280	17	0
Drumstick (1), 1.4 oz	90	6	0
Thigh (1), 3.2 oz	160	11	0
Fish: Patties, 1 piece, 2.5 oz	160	9	13
Baked, 1 piece, 3 oz	120	4	0
Fried, 1 piece, 1.3 oz	80	3.5	9
Meatloaf, 1 piece, 3.2 oz	220	12	9
Shrimp, fried, 6 shrimp, 1.9 oz	110	5	11
Smoked Sausage & Sauerkraut	195	17	3
Spanish Rice, 3 oz	140	9	9
Salads: California Coleslaw, 3.5 oz	90	0.5	22
Macaroni Vegetable Salad, 3.5 oz	230	15	20
Marinated Vegetables, 3.5 oz	60	3.5	6
Seven Layer Salad, 2.6 oz	180	17	4
Tosses Green Salad, 1 cup, 1.6 oz	5	0	1
Sides: Potato: Baked (1), 6.3 oz	160	0	39
Mashed, 5 oz	150	2.5	30
Soups: Chili Bean, 4 fl.oz	100	3.5	9
Corn Chowder, 4 fl.oz	140	8	15
Navy Bean Soup w. Ham, 4 fl.oz	50	0	10
Desserts			
Cheesecake, plain, 1 piece, 2.8 oz	220	10	29
Chocolate Decadence Cake, 1 piece	200	9	27
Cookie, Sugar Free Ranger (1)	100	5	11
Hot Fudge Sundae Cake, 3 oz	160	3.5	32
Pumpkin Pie, reduced sugar, 4.2 oz	270	9	31
Pudding: Chocolate, 1 spoon, 3 oz	150	7	19
Reduced Sugar/Calorie, 3 oz	70	1	14
Vanilla, 1 spoon (3 oz), 86g	140	6	19
Soft Serve Ice Cream, avg., 4 oz	140	4.5	24

Restaurants & Fast - Foods

Olive Garden®

Appetizers	C	F	Cb
Bruschetta	440	21	57
Sicilian Scampi (4)	460	31	16
Stuffed Mushrooms (2)	385	31	12
Entrees (Includes Vegetables):			
Lunch: Lasagna Classico (4"x4½")	860	47	54
Eggplant Parmigiana	900	39	78
Fettuccine Alfredo	850	58	70
Sausage & Peppers Rustica	885	51	71
Dinner: Pork Fillettino	1010	58	116
Mixed Grill, 21.4 oz	840	43	65
Manicotti Formaggio	800	38	57
Chicken Castellina	895	46	78
Stuffed Chicken Marsala	1315	87	72
Garden Fare Selections (Lower Fat)			
Lunch: Capellini Pomodora, 13 oz	410	9	52
Chicken Giardino, 15.5 oz	410	12	40
Linguine alla Marinara, 10.6 oz	340	6	48
Shrimp Primavera, 19 oz	485	12	65
Dinner: Chicken Giardino, 21.5 oz	560	15	59
Capellini Pomodora, 21 oz	645	14	84
Linguine alla Marinara, 17 oz	550	8	79
Shrimp Primavera, 26 oz	705	24	84
Extras: Minestrone Soup, 6 fl.oz	160	1	30
Breadstick, plain, 1 stick	140	1.5	24
Dressing (Low Fat): Italian	37	2	4
Parmesan Peppercorn, 2 fl.oz	45	2	5

(The) Old Spaghetti Factory®

	C	F	Cb
Lunch Entrees: Fettuccine Alfredo	1130	83	71
Pot Pourri, 10 oz	1140	49	137
Garlic Cheese Bread Starter, 13.5 oz	1220	85	105
Lasagna, 16 oz	630	33	36
Chicken Marsala, 18 oz	960	44	55
Chicken Parmigiana, 19 oz	840	34	84
Spinach & Cheese Ravioli, 12 oz	480	15	59
Spinach Tortellini w. Alfredo, 12 z	930	56	82
Spaghetti: w. Clam Sauce, 10 oz	460	19	56
w. Meat Sauce, 10 oz	310	3.5	55
w. Meatballs, 13.5 oz	610	24	62
w. Meat Sauce & Mizithra, 9.2 oz	450	19	53
w. Mizithra/Mushr./Tom. Sauce	450	19	54
w. Sausage & Meat Sce, 13.7 oz	620	29	57
w. Tomato & Meat Sauce, 10 oz	300	3.5	56

On the Border®

Salads: With Dressing Unless Indicated	C	F	Cb
Chicken Chopped Salad, w. dressing	1330	89	54
Chicken Fiesta: Blackened	1150	75	54
Grilled	1140	74	52
Grande Taco Salad, Beef, no dress.	1450	102	78
House Salad, no dressing	170	10	15
Sizzling Beef Fajita, no dressing	910	65	24
Sizzling Chicken Fajita, no dressing	760	48	23
Dressings: Per Serving (2 fl.oz)			
Chipotle Honey Mustard	310	29	11
Jalapeno Caesar	300	31	3
Ranch Dressing	220	23	2
Smoked Jalapeno Vinaigrette	230	22	8
Sweet Pepper Vinaigrette	270	25	10
Fat-Free: Balsamic Vinaigrette	50	0	10
Low-Fat: Ranch	110	6	11
Soups: Chicken Tortilla, 1 bowl	350	22	24
For Complete Nutritional Data ~ see CalorieKing.com			

Orange Julius®

Original (Orange, Strawberry):	C	F	Cb
Small, average, 16 fl.oz	220	0	55
Medium, average, 20 fl.oz	275	0.5	68
Large, average, 32 fl.oz	450	1	109
Classic Smoothy® Drinks: Per 16 fl.oz			
Bananarilla; Tropical, average	300	7	56
Cool Cappuccino	390	10	69
Pina Colada; Tripleberry, average	360	7	70
Strrawberry Banana	400	7	77
20 fl.oz Size ~ Add 25% to above figures			
32 fl.oz Size ~ Double the above figures			
Premium: Per 20 fl.oz			
Berry Lively; Blackberry Toner	450	1	100
Blackberry Storm	630	8	130
Blueberrathon	350	1.5	90
Chai Tea Dragon	470	3	110
Cocoa Latte Swirl	640	9	122
Fruitasia	395	3	90
Orange Swirl	400	10	96
Raspberry Crush	330	2	83
Strawb. Treasure; Raspb. Creme	540	8	103
Strawberry Xtreme	410	0.5	87
Tart 'N' Berry	450	1	102
Tropi-Colada	560	8	110
Add Banana, 1 medium	110	0.5	27
Nutrifiers: Avg. all types, ¼ oz	15	0	4

Fast - Foods & *Restaurants*

Outback Steakhouse®

Aussie-Tizers	C	F	Cb
Aussie Cheese Fries, 28 oz	2900	182	240
Bloomin Onion, w. dressing	2210	134	241
¼ serving	550	33	60
Gold Coast Coconut Shrimp	690	30	97
Grilled Shrimp on the Barbie	660	42	32
Kookaburra Wings w. Sauce (10)	1160	75	65
Lobster-Crab Cakes w. Sauce (2)	840	72	33
Steaks: *Meat Only ~ Add Extra for Sides*			
Michael J. "Crocodile" Dundee:			
New York Strip, 14 oz	900	60	0
Outback Special, 12 oz Sirloin	810	50	0
Prime Minister's Prime Ribs:			
8 oz cut	450	38	0
12 oz cut	675	57	0
16 oz cut	905	77	0
Rockhampton Rib-Eye, 14 oz	730	40	0
The Melbourne, P/house, 20 oz	1365	110	0
Lean meat only	700	37	0
Victoria's Filet, Tenderloin, 9 oz	570	44	0
Sides: Aussie Chips w Ketchup	725	32	100
Fresh Veggies	80	1	14
Grilled Onions, 7.5 oz	180	11	19
Jacket Potato, Plain	270	0	63
Jacket Potato, w. Butter/Cheese	400	14	63
Mushrooms, Sauteed	150	11	12
Desserts: Cheesecake Olivia	700	38	79
Choc. Thunder from Down Under	1220	78	134

Panda Express®

Chicken: Black Pepper, 5.5 oz	180	10	10
Orange Chicken, 5.5 oz	480	21	50
w. Mushrooms, 5.5 oz	130	7	7
Spicy w. Peanuts, 5.5 oz	200	7	17
BBQ Pork, 4.5 oz	350	19	13
Beef & Broccoli, 5.5 oz	150	8	9
Sweet & Sour Pork, 4 oz	410	30	17
Mixed Veges, 5 oz	70	3	8
Fried Tofu w. Beans, 5.5 oz	180	11	11
Rice & Noodles: *Serving (8 oz)*			
Steamed Rice	330	0.5	74
Vegetable Chow Mein	330	11	48
Vegetable Fried Rice	390	12	61
Appetizers: Chkn Egg Roll (1)	190	8	21
Fried Shrimp, 6 pieces	260	12	26
Veggie Spring Roll (1)	80	2.5	14

Panera Bread®

Bagels: Asiago Cheese	C	F	Cb
Bagels: Asiago Cheese	330	5	58
Blueberry	320	1.5	67
Chocolate Raspberry	380	7	69
Cinnamon Crunch	420	7	78
Dutch Apple & Raisin	340	2.5	70
Everything; Sesame Seed, avg.	300	1.5	60
Plain	280	1	57
Lower Carb: Plain	200	2	25
Asiago Cheese	240	9	20
Spreads: *Per 2 oz*			
Plain Cream Cheese	190	18	2
Reduced Fat, average	130	12	2
Salad: Asian Sesame Chicken	430	19	33
Caesar	440	32	25
Classic Cafe	400	37	18
Greek	520	48	17
Grilled Chicken Caesar	560	34	26
Sandwiches: Asiago Roast Beef	730	35	54
Bacon Turkey Bravo	770	28	84
Chicken Salad on Nine Grain	640	29	56
Frontega Chicken Panini	860	42	71
Garden Veggie	570	23	74
Italian Combo	1050	54	80
Peanut Butter & Jelly on French	450	15	63
Sierra Turkey	950	55	71
Smoked Ham & Swiss on Rye	650	34	47
Smoked Turkey Brst on Sourdough	440	15	44
Smokehouse Turkey on Artisan	670	23	68
Tuna Salad on Honey Wheat	720	43	50
Turkey Artichoke Panini	810	38	76
Tuscan Chicken	950	56	75
Soup (8 oz): Baked Potato	260	16	23
Boston Clam Chowder	210	11	19
Broccoli Cheddar	230	16	13
Chicken Noodle, Low Fat	100	2	15
Cream of Chicken & Wild Rice	200	12	19
French Onion	220	10	23
Vegetarian:Tomato	110	3	17
Black Bean	160	1	31
Garden Vegetable	90	0.5	17
Muffins: Banana Nut Muffie	260	12	34
Chocolate Chip Muffie	240	10	36
Pumpkin Muffie	270	6	43
Low Fat Tripleberry Muffin	300	3	63

For Complete Nutritional Data ~ see CalorieKing.com

..
Restaurants & Fast - Foods

Papa Gino's®

	C	F	Cb
Appetizers: Per Serving			
Buffalo Chkn Tenders, small, 4.2 oz	200	7	20
Cheese Breadsticks, small, 5.8 oz	450	19	52
Cheese Garlic Bread, large, 3.8 oz	215	5	36
Chicken Tender, small, 3.3 oz	190	7	18
Cinnamon Sticks, small, 7.2 oz	620	18	105
French Fries, small, 12.7 oz	665	37	76
Mozzarella Sticks, large, 3.3 oz	300	15	27
Pastas: Entree Size			
Papa Platter			
Penne or Spaghetti, plain	650	11	118
Ravioli	445	20	49
Spaghetti & Meatballs	885	19	123
Spaghetti Chicken Parmigiana	1035	34	129
Pizzas: Per Slice			
Large Thin Crust: BBQ Chicken	285	6	41
Buffalo Chicken	255	6	35
Cheese	240	6	36
Cheeseburger	330	13	38
Chicken Pepper	295	9	36
Fenway	325	12	40
Garlic Chicken	300	9	38
Hawaiian	295	8	38
Meat Combo; PapaRoni	335	15	36
Pepperoni	285	10	36
Super Veggie	260	7	39
Works	315	12	38
Subs			
BLT: small, 11 oz	680	30	75
Italian: small, 11 oz	775	36	74
Meatball: small, 11 oz	750	16	81
Meatball Parmesan: small, 11.5 oz	830	35	81
Seafood Salad: small, 10 oz	685	34	72
Steak & Cheese: small, 7.5 oz	625	35	47
Steak: small, 6.7 oz	560	31	45
Super Steak: small, 11.2 oz	565	24	53
Tuna: small, 9.9 oz	745	38	70
Turkey: small, 7.5 oz	410	1	70
Salads			
Buffalo Chicken Tender	320	15	32
Caesar	190	8	21
Chicken Bacon Cheddar	480	21	26
Chicken Tender	280	10	30
Garden	175	6	27
Italian Chopped	575	50	12
Side: Caesar	70	3	7
Garden	65	2	10
Dressings: Bleu Cheese	150	15	3
Caesar	395	43	0
Ranch	285	31	3
Fat-Free, Honey Dijon	60	0	13

Papa John's®

	C	F	Cb
Original Crust (14"): Per Slice (⅛ Whole)			
All the Meats w. Beef	370	17	38
BBQ Chicken & Bacon	340	11	44
Cheese	310	12	39
Garden Fresh	280	9	40
Hawaiian BBQ Chicken	340	11	46
Pepperoni	320	13	38
Sausage	330	15	38
Spinach Alfredo/Chicken	290	11	36
The Works	330	11	40
Thin Crust (14"): Per Slice (⅙ Pizza)			
All the Meats: w. Beef	320	20	23
BBQ Chicken & Bacon	290	14	29
Cheese	260	14	24
Garden Fresh	230	12	25
Grilled Chicken Alfredo	250	13	21
Grilled Chicken Club	270	14	25
Hawaiian BBQ Chicken	290	14	31
Pepperoni	270	15	23
Sausage	280	18	23
Spicy Italian	320	24	24
Spinach Alfredo/Chicken	240	14	21
The Works	280	14	25
Side Orders: Bread Sticks, 1 stick	140	2	26
Cheese Sticks, 2 sticks	360	16	42
Papa's Chickenstrips, 2 strips	160	8	10
Papa's Cinnapie, 2 slices, 2 oz	200	8	29
Sauce: Garlic, 1 oz	150	17	0
Honey Mustard, 1 oz	150	15	5
Pizza, 1 oz	20	0	3

Papa Murphy's®

	C	F	Cb
Pizzas: Per Slice (Family Size)			
Deeper Dish, Traditional, ⅛ pizza	440	24	34
Gourmet: Chicken Garlic, 1/12 pizza	320	15	30
Classic Italian, 1/12 pizza	360	19	30
Veggie, 1/12 pizza	300	14	31
Papa's: BBQ Chicken, 1/12 pizza	320	13	32
Cheese, 1/12 pizza	270	10	29
All Meat; Cowboy, 1/12 pizza	370	19	31
Hawaiian, 1/12 pizza	290	11	34
Murphy's Combo, 1/12 pizza	380	20	32
Pepperoni, 1/12 pizza	310	15	29
Specialty; Perfect, 1/12 pizza	300	13	32
Rancher, 1/12 pizza	330	15	31
Veggie Combo, 1/12 pizza	300	13	32

Continued Next Page ...

Fast - Foods & *Restaurants*

Papa Murphy's® cont...

Pizzas: Per Slice (Cont)	C	F	Cb
Stuffed: Big Murphy, 1/16 pizza	380	17	39
Other varieties, 1/16 pizza	370	16	39
Thin Crust deLITEs: Cheese, 1/10	130	6	11
Hawaiian, 1/10 pizza	140	7	14
Meat, 1/10 pizza	190	12	11
Pepperoni, 1/10 pizza	160	9	11
Veggie, 1/10 pizza	150	8	11
Salads: Club	290	21	11
Garden	160	11	9
Italian	220	17	7

Pepe's Mexican®

Burritos: Beef & Bean	510	24	52
Beef & Bean Suizo	640	34	55
Chicken & Bean	480	21	51
Chicken & Bean Suizo	610	31	54
Pork & Bean	470	19	51
Pork & Bean Suizo	600	29	54
Flauta: Beef, plain	160	9	10
Beef, w. cheese & sauce	190	12	11
Chicken, plain	190	10	16
Chicken, w. cheese & sauce	230	13	17
Taco Salad			
Beef w. 4 oz salsa	550	26	52
Chicken w. 4 oz salsa	520	23	51
Pork w. 4 oz salsa	505	20	52
Without Taco Shell, deduct	210	7	32
Tacos: Beef Crisp	210	11	16
Beef Soft Corn	250	10	28
Beef Soft Flour	250	11	24
Chicken Crisp	190	9	15
Chicken Soft Corn	230	8	27
Chicken Soft Flour	230	9	23
Pork Crisp	170	6	16
Pork Soft Corn	220	6	27
Pork Soft Flour	220	7	24
Tostada			
Beef & Bean	380	23	26
Beef & Bean Suiza	440	29	26
Chicken & Bean	360	21	21
Chicken & Bean Suiza	410	26	25
Pork & Bean	350	20	26
Pork & Bean Suiza	410	25	26

Perkin's® Family Restaurant

Entrees	C	F	Cb
Chicken Dinner	620	13	60
Fish Dinner	470	7	60
Fruit Cup	50	0.5	12
'Lite & Healthy'	105	2	15
Omelettes: Country Club	930	79	6
Deli Ham & Cheese	960	79	8
'Everything' Omelette	695	54	9
Granny's Country Omelette	940	82	7
w. 9 oz Hash Browns	1245	90	57
Salads: Chef's, Mini	215	11	7
Muffins: Banana	650	33	78
Blueberry; Pumpkin	550	26	78
Bran Muffin	550	16	94
Carrot	455	26	55
Chocolate Chips	620	26	81
Cranberry Nut	585	29	75
Lemon Poppyseed	685	33	88
Oat Bran	455	15	68
Peaches & Cream; Apple, avg.	520	23	72
Raspberry & Cream	585	26	81
Reduced Fat: Banana	520	6.5	0
Blueberry; Honey Bran	425	6.5	0
Plain	490	8	0
Pancakes: Buttermilk (1), no syrup	140	4.5	20
Short Stack (3), no syrup	425	14	60
Regular Stack (5), no syrup	705	24	100
Pies (Per Slice): Apple Pie, 1/6 pie	375	15	56
Brownie, Low Fat, no icing	160	0.5	0
Wildberry, 1/6 pie	390	16	66
Bundt Cake, w. Icing (sugar free)	385	17	70

Penn Station®

Subs (6")	C	F	Cb
Artichoke: w. mayo	360	18	37
No mayo	260	7	37
Cheese Bread	250	6	41
Chicken Salad	360	15	41
Chicken Teriyaki	435	13	48
Grilled Vegetarian	245	4	46
Ham Dagwood, no cheese	260	6.5	35
Philadelphia Cheesesteak	500	25	45
Philadelphia Cheesesteak, no mayo	395	14	45
Reuben	500	21	40
Reuben, no 1000 Island Dressing	390	12	37
Tuna Salad	365	15	41
Turkey Dagwood	420	18	36
Turkey Dagwood, no Cheese/Mayo	240	4	34

232

Petro's®

Petro: Per Serving	C	F	Cb
Chicken: small	465	24	43
medium	665	36	59
large	970	52	88
Lite: small	380	12	48
medium	530	16	66
large	785	24	99
Original: small	515	30	43
medium	735	43	58
large	1075	63	87
Pasta Lite: small	335	2.5	52
medium	495	3.5	79
large	680	4.5	107
Pasta: small	405	16	45
medium	625	26	67
large	850	36	91
Veggie: small	525	28	52
medium	745	41	70
large	1090	60	105

Chili: Per Serving (Medium Container)			
Chicken	275	4	43
Original	370	14	42
Veggie	385	11	58

Baked Potato: #1 Lite (1)	365	0.5	74
#2 Butter Sour Cream (1)	480	18	74
#3 Loaded (1)	680	33	78
#4 Loaded w. Chili (1)	780	37	90
#5 Broccoli 3 Cheese, (1)	655	30	77

Hot Dogs			
Chili	315	17	28
Chili & Cheese	345	19	29
Loaded	350	19	30
Plain	265	14	22
Slaw	350	16	23

Tostitos Chips: Per Serving			
Loaded Ultimate Nachos	880	51	79
Tostitos Chips: Queso	500	27	60
Ransalsa	560	35	61
Salsa	415	18	62

Salads			
Garden, small	45	0.5	8
Petro, Original	570	36	42
Petrol, Grilled Chicken	740	41	42

For Complete Nutritional Data ~ see CalorieKing.com

Peter Piper® Pizza

Cheese Pizza: Per Slice	C	F	Cb
Personal Slice	110	3.5	13
Personal Pizza (7")	430	14	51
Small Pizza (10"): ½ pizza	160	5	19
Whole Pizza	960	31	114
Medium Pizza (12"): ⅛ pizza	175	5.5	20
Whole Pizza	1385	45	164
Large Pizza (14"): ⅛ pizza	235	8	28
Whole Pizza	1885	61	223
Extra Large Pizza (16"): ¹⁄₁₂ pizza	205	6.5	24
Whole Pizza	2460	79	291

Pepperoni Pizza			
Personal Slice	150	6.5	15
Personal Pizza (7")	600	25	60
Small Pizza (10"): ⅙ pizza	185	8	18
Whole Pizza	1105	47	111
Medium Pizza (12"): ⅛ pizza	200	8	20
Whole Pizza	1600	68	160
Large Pizza (14"): ⅛ pizza	270	12	27
Whole Pizza	2170	92	218
Extra Large Pizza (16"): ¹⁄₁₂ pizza	235	10	24
Sides: Chicken Wings (4)	210	16	1
Breadsticks (1)	120	4.5	17

For Complete Nutritional Data ~ see CalorieKing.com

P F Chang's®

Appetizers			
Crab Wontons w. Plum Sauce	520	26	51
Harvest Spring Rolls	640	17	106
Lettuce Wraps: Soothing Chicken	630	8	92
Vegetarian	370	3.5	71
Peking Dumplings: Pan-Fried	420	22	31
Steamed	400	20	31
Seared Ahi Tuna w. Mustard	220	5	18
Shanghai Street Dumplings	860	46	90
Shrimp Dumplings: Pan-Fried	360	17	26
Steamed w. Ginger Sauce	320	12	26
Spare Ribs: w. Barbecue Sauce	1410	109	47
Northern Style	1090	95	6
Vegetable Dumplings: Pan-Fried	340	12	47
Steamed	300	8	47
Desserts: Banana Spring Rolls	1860	97	235
New York Style Cheesecake	870	58	72
The Great Wall of Chocolate	1885	71	325

Meals			
Beef: A La Sichuan	990	55	55
Mongolian	1080	72	18
Orange Peel	1330	82	69

Continued Next Page ...

P F Chang's® cont...

Meals (Cont)

	C	F	Cb
Chicken: Chang's Spicy	990	51	70
Ginger Chicken and Broccoli	620	21	43
Kung Pao	1230	78	51
Mango	730	19	68
Mu Shu	750	31	55
Orange Peel	1090	60	73
Philip's Better Lemon Chicken	810	21	94
Spicy Ground Chkn w. Eggplant	890	43	70
Sweet & Sour	800	31	89
Duck: Cantonese Roasted	1160	59	109
Lamb: Wok Seared	1270	95	22
Pork: Mu Shu	780	38	53
Sichuan Style	910	47	43
Sweet & Sour	910	43	89
Seafood: Alaskan Sockeye Salmon	740	36	49
Cantonese Scallops	370	13	20
Cantonese Shrimp	380	15	17
Crispy Honey Shrimp	860	37	85
Hot Fish (Catfish)	960	42	86
Kung Pao Scallops	1180	76	56
Kung Pao Shrimp	1230	79	52
Lemon Pepper Shrimp	520	25	31
Lemon Scallops	720	18	96
Oolong Marinated Sea Bass	740	30	39
Orange Peel Shrimp	1070	60	74
Sichuan From The Sea: Calamari	720	21	88
Scallops	630	19	66
Shrimp	630	21	52
Spicy Salt & Pepper Prawns	770	50	28
Wild Alaskan Salmon Lem. Pepper	670	36	32
Vegetarian Plates: Ma Po Tofu	760	52	40
Buddha's Feast, Steamed	200	1.5	44
Stir-Fried	370	7	64
Coconut-Curry Vegetables	950	63	79
Garlic Snap Peas	220	7	20
Shanghai Cucumbers	120	6	8
Sichuan Style Asparagus	170	4	29
Sichuan Style Long Beans	190	3.5	36
Spinach Stir-Fried with Garlic	110	3.5	15
Stir-Fried Spicy Eggplant	510	29	60

Salads

	C	F	Cb
Oriental Chicken w. Vinaigrette	940	56	49
Peanut Chicken			
w. Peanut Lime Dress. & Noodles	1080	69	47
Warm Duck Spinach Salad	940	66	44
Wild Alaskan Sockeye Salmon Salad	470	30	18

Soups: Hot & Sour | 55 | 4 | 2

Pin Rice Noodle	270	2	55
Wonton	50	3	4

For Complete Nutritional Data ~ see CalorieKing.com

Philly Connection®

Sandwiches: Regular Serving

	C	F	Cb
Cheesesteak: Hoagie	490	23	42
Mushroom	460	19	43
Pizza Steak	470	19	44
Steak	350	11	40
The Original	460	20	41
The Works	490	19	52
Hoagie: Chicken	430	19	42
Chicken Parmesan	440	14	45
Chicken Works	440	14	54
Italian	500	26	40
Tuna	580	35	39
Turkey	420	20	41
Veggie Delite	410	16	55
Philly Lite: Chicken Hoagie	290	3.5	42
Chicken Parmesan	330	6	45
Chicken Works	330	5	54
Grilled Chicken	290	3.5	42
Turkey Hoagie	280	4	41
Veggie Hoagie	260	2.5	54
Specialty: Cheese Chicken	400	12	43
Meatball Parmesan	590	33	46

Sides

	C	F	Cb
Chicken Tenders, 9.5 oz	600	28	44

Salads

	C	F	Cb
Cheesesteak	330	18	15
Chicken Tenders	360	15	33
Grilled Chicken Salad	150	2	15
Grilled Chicken Caesar	190	5	13
Philly Lite: Garden	40	0.5	8
Grilled Chicken	150	2	15
Turkey	130	2.5	11
Tuna	290	18	9
Turkey	130	2.5	11
Veggie Delite	230	10	27

Piccadilly Cafeteria®

Meals: No Sides Included

	C	F	Cb
Beef: Chopped Steak Fried, 4.5 oz	415	33	6
Roast Leg, 4 oz	350	22	2
Steak: Filet Mignon, 6 oz	340	20	1
New York Strip, 10 oz	875	71	1
Ribeye, 10 oz	1040	91	2
Chicken: Breast, Mesquite Smoked	210	8	1
Baked Cajun, Boneless Breast	430	27	9
Fish: Catfish Cajun Baked	405	28	6
Catfish Filet Stuffed	550	40	9
Tilapia Baked	210	11	10
Trout Almondine Baked	490	22	11
Trout Cajun Baked	520	27	7
Trout Filets Baked	465	19	10
Pork Loin: Bone in Roast, 5 oz	375	13	10
Shrimp, Fried	460	19	34
Turkey Breast, Carved, 5.5 oz	265	10	5

Salads

	C	F	Cb
Caesar	145	11	7
Chef's	145	9	4
Italian Coleslaw	165	16	5
Louisianne Bowl	45	3	2
Mexican	60	3	8
Piccadilly Bowl	25	0	6
Shrimp Remoulade	515	28	33

Dressings

	C	F	Cb
Au Jus, 3 fl.oz	5	0	1
Blue Cheese, 2 Tbsp	160	18	1
Cheese Sauce, 2 fl.oz	35	1	5
French, 2 Tbsp	130	13	5
Italian, 2 Tbsp	160	17	1
Ranch, 2 Tbsp	150	17	1
Thousand Island, 2 Tbsp	170	18	2
Fat-Free: Ranch Fat-Free	35	0	7

Soups: Per Serving (9.5 oz, No Rice)

	C	F	Cb
Gumbo: Chicken, no rice	100	2	11
& Sausage	225	15	10

Extras

	C	F	Cb
Broccoli w. Cheese Sauce	105	7	9
Cabbage: Buttered, Steamed	70	5	6
Bacon Seasoned	105	8	6
Cauliflower, Buttered	90	6	8
Fried Okra	240	13	26
Greens: Collard Mustard & Turnip	135	10	3
Turnip w. Diced Turnips, 3.2 oz	150	12	4

Pick-Up-Stix®

	C	F	Cb
California Rolls	200	8	27
Beef Dishes: Beef and Broccoli	510	27	37
House Special	875	27	48
Mongolian	350	20	20
Szechwan	340	20	20

Bowls

	C	F	Cb
Teriyaki Chicken	1155	22	148
Teriyaki Vegetable	450	1.5	96
Buddah's Feast: Dark	105	0.5	16
Light	80	0.5	16
Chicken Dishes (Per Cup): Cashew	360	16	33
Garlic	285	12	24
House	755	34	58
Kung Pao	440	22	33
Lemon Twisted	260	3	37
Orange Peel	535	15	76
Sweet n Sour	475	22	60
w. Vegetables	195	3	20

Chow Mein: Per Cup

	C	F	Cb
Beef	350	10	50
Chicken	355	9	52
House Special	360	9	52
Shrimp	310	5.5	51
Vegetable	270	3.5	49
Fried Rice (Per Cup): Beef	505	16	68
Chicken	475	13	70
Egg	420	8	74
House	480	14	69
Shrimp	430	10	68
Vegetable	390	8	67
Rice: White, 1 cup	205	0.5	45

Salad: Per Serving

	C	F	Cb
Chicken Salad w/out Dressing	470	20	35
Chinese Chicken Salad w. Lime Dressing	675	20	35
Chinese Chicken Salad w. Original Dressing	650	22	75

Shrimp: Per Cup

	C	F	Cb
Black Bean	190	5	23
Garlic	185	5	23
Orange Peel	310	5	54
Szechwan	180	5	21
w/Vegetables	170	5	19

Soup: Per 2 Cup Bowl

	C	F	Cb
Hot & Sour	290	5	38
Wonton	290	13	27
Vegetables: Szechwan, 1 cup	105	1	21

Fast - Foods & *Restaurants*

Pizza Hut®

	C	F	Cb
Lower Fat Pizzas: *Per Slice (⅛ Medium Pizza)*			
Diced Chkn, Red Onion, Peppers	170	4.5	23
Diced Chkn, Mushroom, Jalapeno	170	5	23
Ham, Red Onion, Mushroom	160	4.5	22
Ham, Pineapple, Diced Red Tomato	160	4	24
Peppers, Red Onion, Diced Tom.	150	4	24
Tomato, Mushroom, Jalapeno	150	4	22
Carb Tracker: *Per 6" Pizza*			
Pepperoni	520	29	37
Pepperoni & Mushroom	490	25	39
Meat Lovers	740	46	41
Pan Pizza: *Per Slice (⅛ Medium Pizza)*			
Cheese	280	13	29
Chicken Supreme	280	12	30
Ham	260	11	29
Sausage Lover's	330	17	29
Meat Lover's	340	19	29
Pepperoni	290	15	29
Pepperoni Lover's	340	19	29
Pepperoni Trio	320	17	29
Super Supreme	340	18	30
Supreme	320	16	30
Veggie Lover's	270	12	30
Personal Pan Pizza: *Per Pizza*			
Cheese	640	28	72
Ham	600	24	72
Pepperoni	680	32	72
Sausage Lover's	760	40	72
Supreme	760	36	76
Veggie Lover's	600	24	76
Thin 'n Crispy: *Per Slice (⅛ Medium Pizza)*			
Cheese	200	8	21
Chicken Supreme	200	7	22
Ham	180	6	21
Meat Lover's	270	14	21
Pepperoni	210	10	21
Pepperoni Lover's	260	14	21
Pepperoni Trio	240	12	21
Sausage Lover's	240	13	21
Supreme	240	11	22
Super Supreme	260	13	23
Veggie Lover's	180	7	23
P'zone Pizza: *Per ½ Pizza*			
Classic	610	21	71
Meat Lover's	680	28	70
Pepperoni	610	22	69

Pizza Hut® cont...

	C	F	Cb
Hand Tossed: *Per Slice (⅛ Medium Pizza)*			
Cheese	240	8	30
Chicken Supreme	230	6	30
Ham	220	6	29
Sausage Lover's	280	12	30
Meat Lover's	300	13	29
Pepperoni	250	9	29
Pepperoni Lover's	300	13	30
Pepperoni Trio	280	11	29
Super Supreme	300	13	31
Supreme	270	11	30
Veggie Lover's	220	6	31
3 Cheese Stuffed Crust: *Per Slice (½ Large Pizza)*			
Cheese	350	13	43
Chicken Supreme	370	13	44
Ham	330	11	42
Meat Lover's	440	20	43
Pepperoni	360	14	42
Pepperoni Lover's	420	18	43
Super Supreme	430	19	45
Supreme	360	16	43
Veggie Lover's	360	13	45
The Full House XL: *Per Slice*			
Cheese Only	280	12	30
Chicken Supreme	270	10	31
Meat Lover's	380	21	30
Pepperoni	290	13	30
Pepperoni Lover's	310	15	30
Pepperoni Trio	320	15	30
Quartered Ham	260	10	30
Sausage Lover's	510	23	51
Super Supreme	330	16	32
Supreme	310	15	31
Veggie Lover's	260	11	32
Dessert Pizza: Apple Dessert	260	3.5	53
Cherry Dessert Pizza	240	3.5	47
Pasta: Cavatini Pasta	420	15	55
Cavatini Supreme Pasta	460	18	56
Spaghetti: w. Marinara	490	8	90
w. Meat Sauce	640	20	92
Meatballs	630	19	92
Sides: Breadsticks, 1.3 oz	150	6	20
Buffalo Wings, Hot (1)	55	3	1
Buffalo Wings, Mild (1)	55	2.5	0
Ranch Dipping Cup, 1½ oz	210	22	4
Garlic Bread, 1 piece	170	12	13

Pizza Pizza® (Canada)

Pizza: Per Slice (⅛ Classic Pizza)	C	F	Cb
Bacon Dble Cheeseburger	230	8	29
Big Bacon Bonanza	240	9	29
Big Cheese	200	6	29
Canadian Eh!	240	8	30
Garden Veggie	200	5	30
Harvest Medley	210	5	32
New York Style Pepperoni	230	9	29
Pepperoni & Mushroom,	220	7	29
Pepperoni	220	7	29
Sicilian	260	10	31
Spicy BBQ Chicken	220	5	33
Super	220	7	30
Tropical Hawaiian	220	6	30
Medium Pizza: Per Slice			
Deduct 10% fewer calories/fat/carbs from figures for			
large pizza			
Extra Large Pizza: Per Slice			
Add 10% more calories/fat/carbs from figures for			
large pizza			
Classic Slice: Big Bacon, 1 slice	710	26	88
Other varieties, average, 1 sl.	640	19	88
Signature Slice: Bacon Chkn, 1 sl.	830	39	88
Other varieties, avg., 1 slice	620	22	85
Oven Toasted Sandwiches			
BBQ Chicken	530	8	78
BBQ Chicken, no cheese	475	3	78
Deli Classic	645	20	81
Honey Mustard Club	575	12	86
Meatball	600	18	78
Mediterranean Vegetable	550	15	79
Roast Beef Supreme	540	14	73
Stuffed S'wich: Classic Super	530	8	78
Mediterranean Vegetable	550	15	79
Chicken			
Classic Wings, 6 wings	420	30	0.5
Crispy Wings, 6 wings	680	46	22
Nuggets, 6 nuggets	315	22	29
Strips, 4 pieces	345	22	26
Fries: Regular, 5 oz	340	47	15
Large, 7 oz	470	66	20
Garlic Stix: Regular (3)	390	13	54
X-treme Cheese (3) w. 1 oz cheese	480	21	54
Garlic Bread: Regular bun	710	38	74
X-treme with Cheese	880	52	74
Drinks			
Lipton's Brisk, 11.8 fl.oz	120	0	31
Mug Root Beer, 11.8 fl.oz	160	0	41
Orange Crush, 11.8 fl.oz	180	0	48
7-UP, 11.8 fl.oz	160	0	43

Pizza Ranch®

Pizzas, 12 ": Per Slice (⅛ Pizza)	C	F	Cb
Original: BBQ Beef	220	8	28
BBQ Chicken	210	6	27
Bacon Cheeseburger	220	9	26
Beef; Canadian Bacon	210	7	25
California Chicken	250	12	26
Cheese; Chicken Broccoli, avg.	220	8	26
Garlic Cheese	230	11	25
Italian Sausage; Pepperoni	220	9	25
Prairie; Sweet Swine	210	7	26
Roundup; Tabasco Pepperoni	230	10	26
Stampede	250	10	27
Texan	240	9	31
Skillet: BBQ Beef	230	8	30
BBQ Chicken	220	6	29
Bacon Cheeseburger	230	9	28
Beef; Canadian Bacon	220	7	27
Bronco; California Chicken	270	12	27
Cheese; Chicken Broccoli	230	8	28
Garlic Cheese	240	11	27
Italian Sausage; Pepperoni	230	9	27
Prairie; Sweet Swine	220	7	28
Roundup; Tabasco Pepperoni	240	10	28
Stampede	260	11	29
Texan	250	9	33
Thin: BBQ Beef	170	7	17
BBQ Chicken	150	6	16
Bacon Chesseburger	170	8	15
Beef; Canadian Bacon	150	7	14
California Chicken; Bronco, avg.	200	11	15
Cheese; Chicken Broccoli	160	8	14
Garlic Cheese	170	10	14
Italian Sausage; Pepperoni	160	8	14
Prairie; Sweet Seine	150	7	15
Roundup; Tabasco Pepperoni	180	9	15
Stampede	190	10	16
Texan	190	9	20
Broasted Chicken: Breast, 1 pce	440	23	4
Leg, 1 piece	190	12	2
Thigh, 1 piece	370	26	4
Wing, 1 piece	190	13	2
Sides: Potato Wedges (1)	60	0	13

For Complete Nutritional Data ~ see CalorieKing.com

Planet Smoothie®

Cool Blended Smoothies	C	F	Cb
Per 22 fl.oz Unless Otherwise Stated			
Captain Kid, 12 fl oz	195	1.5	47
PBJ	560	17	97
Shag-a-delic	430	1	104
The Last Mango	355	3.5	83
Twig & Berries	300	0.5	74
Vinnie del Rocco	385	3.5	92
Energy Smoothies: Per 22 fl.oz			
Berry Bada-Bing	360	0.5	88
Chocolate Elvis	520	9	109
Frozen Goat	360	0.5	85
Grape Ape	305	0.5	78
Road Runner	280	0.5	72
Spazz	265	0.5	68
Protein Smoothies: Per 22 fl.oz			
Big Bang	350	0.5	80
Chocolate Chimp	400	1	94
Merlin's Planet Living Pineapple	345	1	35
Strawberry	415	1.5	55

Pollo Tropical®

Chicken			
Boneless Chicken Breast, 2 pieces	240	3	0
Quarter Chicken: Dark Meat w. skin	290	18	0
no skin	190	10	0
White Meat w. skin	325	15	0
no skin	205	6	0
TropiChop: Shrimp Creole	505	10	75
Chicken w. Rice & Black Bean	565	10	95
Chicken w. Yellow Rice & Vege.	340	5	50
Grilled Chicken Deluxe	410	6	51
Pork w. Rice & Black Beans	715	23	97
Pork w. Yellow Rice & Vegetables	480	21	90
Ropa Vieja (shredded beef)	620	17	98
Shrimp Creole	505	10	75
Vegetarian	580	13	109
Salads: With Dressing			
Balsamic Tomato & Chicken Salad	325	6.5	19
Chicken Caesar Salad w. dressing	560	40	13.5
Sandwiches			
Chicken Caesar	880	34	71
Grilled Chicken	825	25	84
Sides: Corn Combo, 4 oz	120	4	19
Black Beans: Combo, 4 oz	90	2.5	18
Small, 9 oz	205	5.5	40
Boiled Yucca, Combo, 7.5 oz	190	0	51
Tropical Favorites: Bananas	435	11	89
Yucatan Fries	495	24	69
White Rice, Combo, 4.5 oz	205	3.5	40

For Complete Nutritional Data ~ see CalorieKing.com

Popeye's®

	C	F	Cb
Chicken: Chkn Breast, Mild/Spicy	530	31	18
Chicken Leg, Mild/Spicy	200	12	7
Chicken Thigh, Mild/Spicy	390	29	12
Chicken Wing, Mild/Spicy	220	15	10
Sides: Biscuit, 2 oz	240	14	25
Cajun Rice, regular	180	7	23
Cinnamon Apple Turnover	250	10	37
Coleslaw, regular	230	17	20
Corn on the Cob (1)	260	4	48
French Fries, 3 oz	260	12	34
Mashed Potatoes: no Gravy, reg.	100	3	17
w. Gravy, regular	120	4	18
Red Beans & Rice, regular	340	19	33

Port of Subs®

Salads: Includes Dressing	C	F	Cb
Caesar	335	30	7
Chef	390	25	13
Garden	95	5	10
Grilled Chicken Caesar	540	34	15
Grilled Chicken	300	10	16
Macaroni	440	30	36
Potato	360	26	54
Tun	310	23	12
Sandwiches: Per 5" Sub (No Mayonnaise)			
#1 Ham Salami Capicolla & Pepperoni w. Provolone	530	26	45
#2 Ham & Turkey w. Provolone	435	15	46
#3 Salami & Turkey w. Provolone	455	20	46
#4 Ham & Salami w. Provolone	470	21	45
#5 Smkd Ham & Turkey w. Cheddar	430	15	47
#6 Vegetarian w. Avocado & Olives	355	15	48
#7 Roast Beef w. Provolone,	420	14	43
#8 Turkey w. Provolone	420	14	47
#9 Peppered Pastrami w. Swiss	440	17	44
#10 Rstd Chicken Brst w. Provolone	410	13	45
#11 Ham w. American	380	20	45
#12 Salami w. Provolone	480	25	45
#13 Combination of Cheeses	510	26	44
#14 Smoked Ham w. Swiss	445	17	45
#15 Salami & Pepperoni w. Prov.	510	27	45
#16 BLT no Cheese	400	19	43
#17 Tuna no Cheese	420	18	45
#18 Rst Beef & Turkey w. Provolone	420	14	45

Port of Subs® cont...

Hot Subs: Per 8" Sub	C	F	Cb
Grilled Chicken	565	11	68
Hot Pastrami	760	17	62
Meatball	655	25	76
Tortilla (1)	200	7	27
Tortilla Wrap: Per Wrap (12" Tortilla)			
Chicken Caesar	630	34	35
Hot Grilled Chkn & Smokey Cheddar	485	18	35
Turkey & Bacon Ranch	590	38	34
Sauces & Dressings: Per 2 Tablespoons			
Mayo & Mustard Mix	110	12	0
Mayonnaise	130	14	0
Mustard	0	0	0
Soups: Medium Bowl (6 oz)			
Campbell's: Boston Clam Chowder	105	4	13
Broccoli Cheese	120	6	13
Minestrone	55	1	8
Roasted Chicken Noodle	85	2	9

Pret A Manger®

Bakery: Per Serving			
Almond Croissant	365	21	35
Carrot Card Box Cake	400	22	46
Elephant Poo	110	4	17
Ham, Cheese & Tomato Croissant	400	22	32
Orange & Lemon Muffin	605	28	61
Brownie Pret Pot	200	10	21
Pretzel	370	8	62
Pecan Pie	295	20	26
Sandwiches			
Big BLT	495	29	38
Chicken Avocado w. Half Fat Mayo	520	32	37
More Than Mozzarella	510	30	38
Smoked Salmon & Egg	440	18	38
Super Club	580	34	39
Sushi: Deluxe Sushi	365	3.5	65
Wraps: Avocado	325	38	35
Chicken Salad	360	17	34
Salads: Alfresco Chicken	440	34	14
Tuna Salad Bowl	370	26	11

For Complete Menu ~ See CalorieKing.com

Pretzelmaker®

Pretzels	C	F	Cb
Caramel Crunch (1), 4.7oz	390	6	74
Cinnamon (1), 4.6 oz	380	5	74
Garlic (1), 4.7 oz	380	6	72
Iced Cinnamon Swirl, 5.3 oz	470	9	87
Original: (1), 4.4 oz	340	2	70
Butter Flavor & Salt (1), 4.6 oz	370	5	71
Parmesan (1), 4.7oz), 134g	390	6	72
Poppy Seed (1), 4.6 oz), 130g	380	6	71
Pretzel Dog (1, 5.6 oz), 159g	490	30	38
Sesame (1), 4.6 oz), 130g	380	6	71
Sour Cream & Onion (1), 4.7 oz	390	7	72
Stix: Plain (1), 4.6 oz	360	2.5	73
Butter Flavored & Salt (1), 4.9 oz	390	6	73
Wrapzel: Ham & Swiss	540	15	73
Pepperoni	510	14	78
Turkey & Swiss	580	17	71
Sauces: Per Serving (2 oz)			
Caramel	140	0	35
Cheddar Cheese	130	10	6
Chili Spice	360	5	72
Cream Cheese	200	20	2
Honey Mustard	80	0	20
Mustard	10	0	1
Nachos Cheese	105	0	4
Pizza Sauce	20	0.5	6
Drinks			
Mrs Fields Lemonade: Small, 20 fl oz	160	0	39
Regular, 32 fl oz	280	0	65
Large, 44 fl oz	390	0	91

Pretzel Time®

Pretzels			
Bites: Plain, small, 3 oz	210	0.5	45
medium, 4 oz	280	1	59
large, 3.5 oz	250	1	52
Whirl & Salt, small, 3.2 oz	240	3.5	45
medium, 4.2 oz	310	4	59
large, 4 oz	270	3.5	52
Caramel Crunch (1), 4.7 oz	335	4	66
Cinnamon Sugar (1), 4.1 oz	330	4	65
Italian Parmesan (1), 4.2 oz	310	3.5	60
Plain, 3.8 oz	280	1	59
Sour Cream & Onion (1), 4.2 oz	310	3.5	60

Pretzel Time® cont...

Pretzels	C	F	Cb
Stuffers: Cheese, regular, 13 oz	1200	69	95
small, 7.6 oz	700	36	82
Jalapeno, regular, 13.6 oz	1210	69	97
small, 8 oz	700	38	64
Whirl & Salt (1), 4 oz	310	4	59
Pretzel Dog, 5.5 oz	480	29	38
Sauces & Dressings: Per Serving (2 oz)			
Caramel	140	0	35
Cheddar Cheese	80	5	4
Cream Cheese	200	20	2
Honey Mustard	80	0	20
Ketchup	20	0	4
Mustard	10	0	1
Nacho Cheese	80	5	4
Pizza Sauce	20	0.5	6
Vanilla Glaze	180	0	45
Drinks: Mrs Fields Lemonade,			
20 fl.oz	160	0	39
32 fl.oz	280	0	65
44 fl.oz	390	0	91

Quizno's Subs®

Signature Subs	C	F	Cb
Classic Italian Sub: (No Dressing)			
Small, 9 oz	645	30	60
Regular, 11½ oz	730	33	69
Large, 19½ oz	1200	58	102
Honey Mustard Chicken w. bacon,			
large, 22½ oz	1355	40	137
Philly Cheese Steak, large, 10½ oz	720	16	92
Steakhouse Sub (6"), 6½ oz	510	21	52
Traditional (no dressing) (8"), 15 oz	800	24	94
Turkey Ranch Swiss (no dress.), 8"	690	18	89
Low-Fat Sandwiches (Small)			
Honey Bourbon Chicken	330	6	45
Sierra Smoked Turkey			
w. Raspberry Chipotle Sauce	360	6	53
Turkey Lite	360	6	52
Dressings: Beef Au Jus, 4 oz	20	0.5	3
Honey Mustard, 2 oz	140	6	22
Italian Vinagarette, 1 oz	130	14	3
Ranch Dressing, 2 oz	285	30	3
Potato Chips			
Classic Potato Chips: Trad., 1.5 oz	240	14	25
Kettle Cooked, 1.375 oz	200	11	23
Jalapeno, 1.375 oz	210	12	22
Salt & Vinegar, 1.375 oz	185	9	23
Sour Cream & Onion, 1.5 oz	250	15	25
Cookies			
Peanut Butter, 3 oz	380	21	42
Other cookies, average	360	18	48

Rally's Hamburgers®

Burgers/Sandwiches	C	F	Cb
Rallyburger	435	22	35
with Cheese	490	27	35
Big Buford	745	48	35
Chicken Fillet Sandwich	400	15	43
Chili w. Cheese & Onion: 7 oz	360	22	20
13 oz size	670	41	37
Super Barbecue Bacon	595	31	49
Super Double Cheeseburger	760	48	37
French Fries: Regular	210	11	26
Large	320	16	39
X-Large	425	21	52
Shakes: Vanilla, small	320	11	49
Other flavors, small	410	12	73

Ranch 1®

	C	F	Cb
Salads: Gourmet Greens, 12½ oz	225	7	31
Chicken on Gourmet Greens, 15 oz	350	11	31
Zesty Caesar Salad, 7 oz	185	3	31
Zesty Chicken Caesar Salad, 9 oz	280	6	31
Sandwiches: American Rancher	390	10	51
Club Sandwich	470	16	53
Grilled Chicken Philly	450	14	53
Ranch Classic	370	5	53
Spicy Grilled Chicken	420	11	58
Side Kicks: Fruit Cup, 8.3 oz	90	0.5	18
Ranch Fries, regular, 4.5 oz	350	14	51
Specialties: Chicken Tenders	370	15	7
Baked Potato: w. Broccoli	520	0.5	117
w. Cheese	790	25	118
w. Chicken	610	4	114
Grilled Chkn & Vegetable Platter	790	7	129
Grilled Chicken Fajita	330	16	25
Grilled Chicken Hot Pasta	580	10	86

Rax®

Sandwiches	C	F	Cb
Regular Rax	390	22	32
Deluxe	520	35	35
BBC	715	51	37
Grilled Chicken: Philly Melt	535	32	35
Jr. Deluxe	365	25	25
BBQ Beef	400	20	43
Mushroom Melt	600	38	35
Turkey/Bacon Club	680	47	37
Turkey	485	32	33
Cheddar Melt	345	23	26
Potatoes: Cheese/Broccoli	285	0	72
Plain: No Topping	205	0	60
w. Butter	305	12	60
w. Sour Topping	255	4	62
Soups: Cream of Broccoli	95	4	14
Chicken Noodle	115	1	21
Chili	160	9	12
Salads: Grilled Chicken	160	5	6
Side Salad	40	4	2
Garden	220	9	12
Salad Dressings: Fat Free Italian	10	0	2
Fat Free Catalina; Ranch	30	0	6
1000 Island	130	13	5
Buttermilk Ranch	175	20	1
Blue Cheese; Creamy Caesar	145	16	1
Honey French	140	5	9
Vinaigrette	30	2	4

Red Lobster®

Fresh Fish: *Dinner Entree*	C	F	Cb
Atlantic Salmon	580	33	0
Rainbow Trout	510	25	6
Tilapia	345	10	0
Tilapia in a Bag	565	16	30
Fresh Fish: *Lunch Entree*			
Atlantic Salmon	260	12	0
Rainbow Trout	275	14	2
Tilapia	185	6	0
Tilapia in a Bag	295	9	15
Specialties: Broiled Flounder	240	5	0
Grilled Chicken	315	8.5	0
Grilled Shrimp	140	3	1
Signature Shellfish			
Jumbo Shrimp Cocktail	230	4	2
King Crab Legs	490	9	0
Live Maine Lobster	145	1	2
Lobster Chops	320	8.5	0
Rock Lobster Tail	260	3	2
Snow Crab Legs	260	4.5	0

Red Lobster® cont...

Lighthouse Menu	C	F	Cb
Awesome Additions:			
100% Pure Melted Butter	185	21	0
Baked Potato, no topping	180	2	36
w. Pico de Gallo topping	185	2	37
Cheddar Bay Biscuits	160	9	17
Cocktail Sauce	45	1	9
Fresh Buttered Vegetables	145	11	9
Garden Salad	50	2	9
Jumbo Shrimp Cocktail	140	2	1
King Crab Legs	165	3	0
Lemon Wedge	10	0	2
Maine Lobster Tail	105	5	2
Petite Shrimp Topping	30	1	1
Red Wine Vinaigrette Dressing	50	3	5
Seasoned Fresh Broccoli	55	0	10
Snow Crab Legs	130	2	0
Wild Rice Pilaf	205	5	36

For Complete Nutritional Data ~ see CalorieKing.com

Rita's®

Ice: Kids, 7.5 oz	C	F	Cb
Ice: Kids, 7.5 oz	165	0	43
Regular, 12 oz	265	0	69
Large, 19 oz	415	0	109
Quart, 32 oz	705	0	185
Cream Ice: Kids, 7.5 oz	195	2	44
Regular, 12 oz	310	4	70
Large, 19 oz	495	6	109
Quart, 32 oz	830	11	187
Custard: Kids, 5 oz	285	15	32
Regular, 6.75 oz	555	30	62
Large, 9.75 oz	555	30	62
Gelati w. Custard: Vanilla, Reg., 10 oz	365	13	59
Vanilla, large, 17 oz	560	17	102
Chocolate, regular, 10 oz	350	11	60
Chocolate, large, 17 oz	535	14	101
Misto w. Custard: Van., reg., 15 oz	420	7	90
Vanilla, large, 23 oz	620	10	135
Chocolate, regular, 15 oz	410	7	90
Chocolate, large, 23 oz	605	9	135
Sugar Free: (w. Sorbitol)			
Ice: Kids, 7.5 oz	60	0	24
Regular, 12 oz	100	0	39
Gelati w. Van. Custard, reg., 10 oz	285	13	45
Misto w. Van. Custard, reg., 15 oz	245	8	57

For Complete Nutritional Data ~ see CalorieKing.com

Fast - Foods & *Restaurants*

Rocky Rococo®

Pastas: *Per Serving*	C	F	Cb
Can't Decide, 14 oz	465	9	77
Fettuccine w. Alfredo Sauce:			
Regular, 14 oz	460	14	66
Light, 7 oz	230	7	33
Spaghetti with Meat Sauce: Reg.	485	7	87
Light, 7 oz	250	3	44
Spaghetti w. Meatballs: Reg., 15 oz	630	16	89
Light, 7.5 oz	315	8	45
Spaghetti w. Tomato Sauce: Reg.	470	4	87
Light, 7 oz	235	2	44
Pizzas: *Per Regular Slice*			
Cheese	380	9	54
Garden	390	10	56
Pepperoni	425	13	54
Sausage	495	19	54
Sausage Mushroom	500	19	55
Sides			
Breadsticks: w. Marinara Sce (6)	420	7	72
w. Jalapeno Cheese Sauce (6)	530	18	72
Wheat Muffin (1)	210	4	38

Roly Poly®

Sandwiches: *Per ½ Sandwich (White Bread)*	C	F	Cb
Baked Ham & Roast Pork:			
BarBQ Pork Melt	315	10	27
Italian Classic	340	12	30
Key West Cuban Mix	310	9.5	28
Peachtree Melt	340	12	29
Porky's Nightmare	325	12	28
Chicken: Basil Cashew Chicken	300	11	28
Catalina Chicken Salad	320	13	28
Chicken Caesar	325	12	30
Chicken Cordon Bleu	320	11	28
Chicken Fajita	290	8	28
Chicken Popper	260	7	31
Cobb Salad	330	14	30
Delhi Chicken	330	13	33
Hickory Chicken	350	11	29
Oriental Chicken	275	6	32
Santa Fe Chicken	285	8	29
Seafood: Salmon Club	310	14	30
Salmon Roll	295	11	27
Texas Tuna Melt	320	14	27
Thai Hot Tuna	340	13	29
Tuna Luau	325	15	30

Round Table® Pizza

Large Pizza (14") *Per Slice (½ Whole)*	C	F	Cb
Chicken & Garlic Gourmet: Pan Crust	320	11	39
Skinny Crust	200	9	19
Chicken Rostadoro: Pan Crust	330	12	40
Skinny Crust	220	10	20
Gourmet Veggie: Pan Crust	310	11	40
Skinny Crust	190	8	20
Hawaiian: Pan Crust	290	9	39
Skinny Crust	180	7	20
Hearty Bacon Supreme: Pan Crust	360	17	38
Skinny Crust	260	15	17
Italian Garlic Supreme: Pan Crust	360	16	39
Skinny Crust	240	14	18
Maui Zaui, Polynesian Sauce:			
Pan Crust	330	11	40
Skinny Crust	210	9	20
Maui Zaui, Zesty Red Sauce:			
Pan Crust	320	11	40
Skinny Crust	20	1	2.5
Montague's All Meat Marvel:			
Pan Crust	350	16	37
Skinny Crust	260	16	18
Pepperoni Rostadoro: Pan Crust	350	14	40
Skinny Crust	240	12	21
Roastin' Toastin' Chicken Club:			
Pan Crust	350	14	39
Skinny Crust	230	12	18
Western BBQ Chicken: Pan Crust	320	11	36
Skinny Crust	200	9	17
Sandwiches			
Chicken Club	820	39	75
Ham Club	810	37	76
RT Pizza Sandwich	690	34	65
RT Veggie Sandwich	680	29	79
Turkey Club	800	37	75
Sides			
Buffalo Wings, 6 pieces	420	28	2
Garlic Bread, 4.6 oz	470	21	59
Garlic Bread with Cheese, 6.6 oz	630	33	59
Honey BBQ Wings, 6 pieces	390	25	8

For Complete Nutritional Data ~ see CalorieKing.com

Roy Rogers®

Breakfast Itrems	C	F	Cb
Big Country Breakfast: w. Bacon	740	43	61
w. Sausage	920	60	61
w. Ham	710	39	67

Burgers	C	F	Cb
Hamburger	260	9	33
Cheeseburger	300	13	34
¼ lb Hamburger	430	18	41
¼ lb Cheeseburger	470	22	42
Sourdough Grilled Chicken	500	21	46
Sandwiches: Roast Beef	260	4	30
Chicken Fillet	500	24	49
Grilled Chicken	340	11	32
Fries: Regular	350	15	49
Large	430	18	59
Desserts: Hot Fudge Sundae	320	10	50

Rubio's Fresh Mexican Grill®

Burritos	C	F	Cb
Baja Gourmet Seafood: Fish	740	40	70
Lobster	670	32	79
Mahi Mahi	700	38	56
Shrimp	630	25	75
Baja Grill: Carne Asada	680	32	58
Chicken	630	24	58
Cheesy Bean	820	36	88
Especial: Carne Asada	940	37	117
Chicken	890	29	117
HealthMex: Veggie	520	8	98
Chicken	530	10	77
Street: Carnitas	300	11	35

Quesadillas	C	F	Cb
Favorites: Carne Asada	990	61	58
Cheese	830	52	56
Chicken	950	54	58

Tacos	C	F	Cb
Carne Asada	250	10	24
Chicken	300	15	24
Fish: Especial	370	21	30
Original	300	16	28
HealthMex Chicken	170	2	23
Mahi Mahi	310	16	24
Street: Carne Asada	130	6.5	10
Carnitas	110	5	11
Chicken	110	3.5	10

Rubio's cont...

Meals	C	F	Cb
Burrito Deals: Fish w. Chips	960	51	98
Especial Chicken w. Chips	1100	41	137
Shrimp w. Chips	840	36	100
Classic Plates: Carne Asada Dos Tacos	770	28	96
Chicken Dos Tacos	940	43	97
Original No. 1	940	45	105
Pesky	1070	56	109
Favorites: Chicken Taquitos (3)	290	11	34
Nachos Grande	1270	78	111
Nachos Grande Carne Asada	1420	87	113
Nachos Grande w. Chicken	1380	80	113
Grilled Grande Bowl, Chicken	720	30	73
Street Deals: Carnitas	830	33	85
Chicken	840	27	83
Carne Asada w. Sides	710	22	106
Chicken w. Sides	790	30	107
Fish w. Sides	800	31	111
Tres Taco Deals:			
3 Carne Asada & Chips	600	29	58
3 Carnitas Street & Chips	530	25	59
3 Chicken Street & Chips	550	21	34
3 Fish & Chips	1130	59	111

Sandwiches	C	F	Cb
Tortas: Carne Asada	390	26	23
Carnitas	370	24	23
Chicken	370	23	23

Sides: Per Serving	C	F	Cb
Cheese, 1 oz	100	8	1
Guacamole, 1 oz	45	4	2
Sour Cream, 1 oz	60	6	1
Fries: Beer Battered, 4.5 oz	260	15	29
Black Beans, 7 oz	170	2	28
Carne Asada, 3 oz	160	8	2
Carnitas, 3 oz	120	6	3
Chicken, 3 oz	120	2	2
Chips, 1.5 oz	220	11	28
Chips, 3 oz	435	21	55
Churro, 1.6 oz	170	8	22
Guacamole: Small, 3.7 oz	170	16	8
Large, 7.7 oz	340	32	16
Original & Pinto Beans, 9.3 oz	420	18	50
Pinto Beans, 7 oz	190	3	37
Rice, 4 oz	160	2	28

Salads	C	F	Cb
Chicken Low-Carb	470	33	11
Grilled Chicken Chopped	570	33	34
HealthMex Chicken	250	2	31
Dressings: Serrano Grape, 1.3 oz	40	0	9

For Complete Nutritional Data ~ see CalorieKing.com

Fast - Foods & *Restaurants*

Ruby Tuesday®

	C	F	Cb
Burgers: *(No Sides or Sauces Incl.)*			
Bacon Cheeseburger	1010	67	52
Classic Burger	830	53	51
Colossal Burger	1680	114	78
Turkey Burger Club	780	41	52
Veggie Burger	805	41	69
Gourmet Sandwiches: *(No Sides or Sauces Included)*			
Ruby's Chicken Sandwich	640	25	58
Ultimate Roasted Turkey BLT	1120	66	71
Low-Carb: Roasted Turkey Wrap	275	7	25
Grilled Chicken/Caesar Wrap	395	18	21
Panini: Cuban/Ham, average	1170	82	56
Turkey & Bacon	1320	87	52
Steaks & More: *(No Sides or Sauces Included)*			
Top Sirloin	285	11	1
Petite Sirloin	220	8	1
Ruby's Ribeye	635	44	4
Smothered Sirloin Tips	990	52	53
Grilled BBQ Chicken: Single Breast	210	5	3
Platters: *(No Sides or Sauces Included)*			
Louisiana Fried Shrimp	1000	52	103
Chicken Tenders: Original	965	47	86
Spicy Buffalo	1190	70	92
Ribs, Half Rack: average all types	940	51	73
Full Rack	1430	84	87
Pasta: *(Garlic Toast Not Included)*			
Chicken Parmesan	1465	95	89
Pasta Marinara	660	10	115
Shrimp Alfredo; Roma Chkn, avg.	1180	50	107
Sonora Chicken	1170	41	121
Specialties: *(No Sides or Sauces Included)*			
Creole Catch	665	31	44
New Orleans Seafood	860	46	47
Oven Roasted Turkey Dinner	730	30	60
Low-Carb: New Orleans Seafood	800	50	28
Church Street Chicken	790	51	26
Creole Catch	610	35	23
Peppercorn Salmon	585	32	29
Oven Roasted Turkey Dinner	630	24	27
Appetizers: *Per ¼ Order (Sauces not Included)*			
Asian Pot Stickers	120	5	13
Chicken Quesadilla	190	11	12
Fried Cheese	170	11	13
Loaded Cheese Fries	290	18	21
Low-Carb Chicken Quesadilla	155	10	4
Low-Carb Spicy Buffalo Wings	230	16	1
Original Chicken Tenders	130	7	7
Queso Dip	320	22	23
Signature Sampler	280	17	19
Southwestern Spring Rolls	175	10	15
Spicy Buffalo Chicken Tenders	190	13	9
Spicy Honey BBQ Chicken Tenders	160	7	15
Spinach Dip	290	20	19
Tuesday Sampler	200	12	14

	C	F	Cb
Salads (Entree)			
Dressing Not Included Unless Indicated			
Carolina Chicken Salad	880	62	37
Low-Carb: Chicken Cobb	620	41	12
Chicken Caesar w. Dressing	500	35	16
Peppercorn Salmon w. Dress.	655	46	16
Spring Chicken Salad	400	24	10
Signature Sauces & Dressings: *Per 2 Tbsp (1 oz)*			
Barbecue Sauce	50	0	13
Cocktail Sauce	23	0	6
Marinara Sauce	15	1	2
Remoulade Sauce	160	17	1
Salsa	10	0	2
Sour Cream; Turkey Gravy	30	2	2
Steak Butter, 1 Tbsp, ½ oz	90	10	0
Thai Peanut Sauce	65	3	8
Dressings: Ranch	100	11	1
Light Balsamic Vinaigrette	35	2	4
Bleu Cheese Dressing	175	19	1
Honey Mustard Dressing	90	8	5
Caesar Dressing	100	10	2
Smoky Honey Dijon	100	8	7
Signature Soups: Onion Soup	200	13	20
Baked French Onion	550	39	30
Low-Carb Broccoli & Cheese	330	27	15
Side Items: Baked Beans	130	3	22
Baked Pot. w. Butter & Sour Crm	460	19	62
Broccoli, Fresh Steamed	130	8	8
Brown Rice & Black Beans	275	6	45
Brown Rice Pilaf	220	6	35
Cole Slaw	130	8	12
Creamed Spinach	205	17	11
Creamy Mashed Cauliflower	165	11	15
Fresh Sauteed Zucchini	55	3	5
Garlic Toast	220	12	24
Mashed Potatoes	330	15	46
Onion Straws	320	23	25
Ruby's Fries	185	9	24
Sugar Snap Peas	130	6	14
Desserts: Blueberry D'lite	215	5	37
Brownie	1000	46	129
Candy Bar Ice Cream Pie	830	42	102
Low-Carb: Cheesecake	400	32	6
Chocolate Lava Cake	630	40	24
Chocolate Sauce	75	2	9

For Complete Menu ~ See CalorieKing.com

Runza®

Sandwiches

	C	F	Cb
Original Runza Sandwich	495	17	65
Cheese Runza Sandwich	555	21	66
BBQ Chicken Sandwich, grilled	335	10	34
Fish Sandwich	485	23	49
Polish Dog	425	26	30
Smothered Chicken, grilled	350	11	36
Special Deluxe Chicken, grilled	300	10	27
Burgers			
Junior: Cheeseburger Deluxe	325	17	28
Cheeseburger	305	14	30
Swiss Mushroom	380	21	26
Legendary: ¼ lb Cheeseburger	430	21	32
½ lb Double Cheeseburger	640	32	37
¼ lb Bacon Cheeseburger Deluxe	515	29	36
¼ lb Legend Supreme	765	37	62
¼ lb Swiss Cheese Mushroom	450	25	36
Sides			
French Fries: Small, 3.1 oz	280	15	31
Medium	410	23	46
Large	625	35	70
Frings, 6.3 oz	540	28	64
Onion Rings: Medium, 4 oz	370	20	41
Large, 6.5 oz	590	32	66
Onion Ring Dip, 2.1 oz	90	6	4
Salads & Dressings			
Tossed Salad w. Crispy Chicken	435	27	29
Tossed Salad w. Grilled Chicken	275	13	13
Dressing: Ranch, 2.6 oz	300	32	5
Reduced Calorie Ranch, 2.6 oz	170	11	17
Lite Italian, 2.6 oz	85	5	10
Raspberry Vinaigrette	25	0	6
Soups: Per Bowl			
Boston Clam Chowder	320	23	33
Broccoli Cheese,	360	27	35
Cauliflower Cheese	335	26	32
Chicken Noodle	170	5	21
Homemade Chili	310	10	26
Potato w. Bacon	305	20	40
Vegetable Cheese	330	22	28
Wisconsin Cheese	425	35	36
Kids-Size: Mini Corn Dogs (5)	275	17	25
Chicken Strips (2)	185	10	11
Desserts & Drinks			
Chocolate Chip Cookie (1)	310	16	34
Vanilla Shake, regular, 12 fl.oz	465	16	69
Oreo Shake, regular, 12 fl.oz	605	24	84
Pepsi Slushie, medium, 18 fl.oz	225	0	60

Ryan's® Family Steakhouse

Main Courses: Sides Not Included

	C	F	Cb
Baked Whole Salmon, 7 oz	245	10	0
BBQ Beef, 6 oz	220	12	9
BBQ Chicken, ¼, 5 oz	225	15	5
Carved Turkey Breast, 6 oz	275	12	0
Chkn Fried Beef Steak (1), no gravy	180	9	16
Chkn Fried Beef Steak (1), w. gravy	220	11	24
Chicken Pot Pie, 8 oz	345	16	48
Grilled Chicken Breast, plain, 6 oz	280	18	0
Grilled Pork Chop: Plain, 1 chop	240	14	1
BBQ; Teriyaki, avg., 1 chop	160	8	8
Grilled Salmon, 7 oz entree	240	9	0
Grilled Sliced Sausage: BBQ Sce, 6 oz	545	48	8
in Peppers and Onions, 6 oz	445	42	6.5
Grilled Teriyaki Chicken Thighs, 6 oz	210	6	6
Macaroni and Cheese, 8 oz	345	16	40
Meat Lasagne, 8 oz	370	16	30
Meat Loaf, 4 oz	215	12	9
Mexican Casserole, 8 oz	400	16	45
Pizza: Cheese, 1 slice, 3½ oz	200	10	11
Pepperoni, 1 slice, 3½ oz	230	13	10
Rotisserie Chicken, ¼, 5 oz	250	15	0
Salisbury Steak w. gravy, 1 patty	200	11	11
Sirloin Steak: 8 oz	480	33	0
10½ oz	640	44	0
16 oz	970	67	0
Sirloin Tips, 5.5 oz	330	23	0
Stuffed Alaskan Pollock Fillet, 6 oz	360	30	18
Taco Beef, 4 oz	180	10	8
Vegetable Lasagne, 8 oz	350	16	30
White Turkey w. gravy, 6 oz	140	4	6.5
Sides: Baked Potato, plain, 8 oz	250	0	56
Bowtie Pasta and Veges, 8 oz	210	0	38
Chicken Salad, 8 oz	480	36	24
Coleslaw, 4 oz	180	12	12
Corn Cobbet (1) 4 oz	90	6	11
Garlic Mashed Potatoes, 4 oz	120	4	16
Glazed Baby Carrots w. Sauce, 4 oz	125	8	12
Low Carb Grilled Veges, 8 oz	40	0	8
Marinated 7-Bean Salad, 6 oz	300	0	66
Pinto Beans, 4 oz	125	2	16
Potato Salad, 6 oz	275	12	33
Sweet Pot. w. M'mallows, 4 oz	240	18	16
Yellow Squash w. Onions, 4 oz	50	2	7
Desserts: Cheesecake, plain, 1 sl.	190	15	11
Ice Cream Cone (flat bottom)	20	0	4
Key Lime Pie, 1 slice	410	17	58
Lemon Creme Cake, 1 slice	170	15	9
Cookies: Oatmeal Raisin (1)	110	3.5	18
Sugar Cookie (1)	120	5	18

Fast - Foods & *Restaurants*

7-Eleven®

Breakfast Sandwiches	**C**	**F**	**Cb**
Big Bite: Breakfast Sandwich	330	19	23
⅓ lb Cheeseburger	410	33	71
Croissant: w. Bacon, Egg & Chse	420	26	34
w. Ham, Egg & Chse	390	22	34
Engl. Muffin w. Saus., Egg, Chse	450	24	37
Sausage, Egg & Cheese Biscuit	500	31	34

Hot Dogs (Big Bite)			
¼ Pound Hot Dog, no bun	360	34	6
⅓ Pound Hot Dog, no bun	480	45	11
Burritos: The Bomb (14 oz)	940	42	116
The Bomb w. Green Chillies	910	42	114
Reynoldos Jumbo Burritos (10 oz):			
Beef & Bean	680	22	93
Beef & Potato	590	20	82
Red Hot Burrito	640	20	88
Green Burrito	710	26	93

Sandwiches (7-Eleven)			
Big Eats Deli Sandwiches:			
Chicken Salad, 7.3 oz	630	35	47
Classic Chicken Caesar, 8.3 oz	590	27	45
Hearty Ham, 8.3 oz	570	30	48
Smoked Turkey w. Chse/Mayo	560	15	45
Stacked Turkey & Ham, 7.8 oz	630	34	46
Tuna Salad, 7.5 oz	550	22	56
Hot Pockets: Ham 'n' Cheese, 7 oz	480	19	55
Meatballs w. Mozzarella	490	18	59

Bakery Stix™ Treats: Per Stick (3.5 oz)			
BBQ Chicken	230	6	34
Pepperoni & Cheese	340	18	30
Other flavors, average	290	12	33

Sushi			
California Rolls, 8-Pack	560	8	80

Donuts & Muffins (World Ovens)			
Donuts: Boston Creme (1)	290	9	47
Blueberry Cake (1)	330	22	31
Chocolate Iced (1)	250	17	23
Glazed (1)	250	16	24
Jelly (1)	420	16	66
Muffins: Apple Spice, 7.5 oz	520	4	114
Banana Nut, 7 oz	660	26	97
Blueberry, 5.6 oz	450	14	73

7-Eleven® cont...

Go-Go Taquitos	**C**	**F**	**Cb**
Beef Taco & Cheese, 3 oz (1)	250	11	30
Fiesta Chicken, 3 oz (1)	220	12	22
Jalapeno & Cream cheese, 3 oz	240	13	27
Monterey Jack Chkn, 3 oz (1)	280	14	30

Fountain Drinks (Figures Assume ⅓ Ice)			
Coca-Cola/Pepsi/Dr.Pepper/7Up:			
Gulp, 20 oz	190	0	48
Big Gulp, 32 oz	300	0	75
Super Gulp, 44 oz	410	0	102
Double Gulp, 64 oz	600	0	150
Diet Coke/Diet Pepsi, 16 oz	1	0	0
Slurpees: Average All Flavors,			
12 oz size	165	0	41
22 oz size	300	0	75
28 oz size	385	0	96
40 oz size	545	0	136
Crystal Light, 12 fl.oz	60	0	12
Slurp & Gulp Combo,			
32 oz Big Gulp & 22 oz Slurpee	600	0	150
Café Coolers: Mocha, 12 oz	350	12	63
French Vanilla, 12 oz	380	16	58
Fruit Coolers			
Orange/Strawb. Creme, 12 fl.oz	280	1	68
16 fl.oz size	370	1	90
20 fl.oz size	470	2	113
Arizona Rasp. Green Tea, 12 fl.oz	230	0	56
Cafe Select Coffee: 12 fl.oz	7	0	2
16 fl.oz size	10	0	2
20 fl.oz size	12	0	3
24 fl.oz size	15	0	4
Hot Drinks: Hot Chocolate, 8 fl.oz	130	2	24
French Vanilla Cappuccino, 8 fl.oz	100	6	25

Restaurants & Fast - Foods

Sammy's®
Woodfired Pizza

Healthy Dining Meals	C	F	Cb
Chinese Chicken Salad	480	13	49
Chopped Chicken Salad	385	11	20
Grilled Shrimp Wrap	560	19	57
Grilled Vegetable Penne	620	21	84
Tomato Angel Hair Pasta	670	18	105
Vegetarian Pizza, ½ Pizza	860	21	130

Samurai Sam's®

Appetizers: Per Serving	C	F	Cb
California Rolls	240	1	53
Grilled Egg Rolls	120	5	20
Bowls: Per Regular Bowl			
Teriyaki Chicken	605	11	94
Teriyaki Chicken & Steak	610	10	94
Teriyaki Chicken & Steak, All White	565	7	91
Teriyaki Chicken, All White	530	3	89
Teriyaki Steak	510	9	93
Teriyaki Veggie	405	1	88
Salads			
Oriental Chicken	495	8	89
Specialties			
Chicken & Prawns	755	9	92
Chicken & Prawns, All White	700	4	92
Steak & Prawns	780	8	92
Teriyaki Prawns	645	2	88
YakiSoba	530	9	96

Sbarro's®

Entrees: Per Serving	C	F	Cb
Baked Ziti w. Sauce	700	41	43
Chicken Parmigiana	520	22	16
Meat Lasagne	650	37	36
Spaghetti w. Sauce	820	28	120
Pizza: Per Slice			
Cheese	460	13	60
Pepperoni	730	37	61
Sausage	670	31	60
Supreme	630	27	63
Stuffed Pizza: Per Slice			
Spinach & Broccoli	790	34	89
Pepperoni	960	42	89

Schlotzsky's®

Bread/Buns	C	F	Cb
Dark Rye, regular	330	2	68
Sourdough, regular	335	2	68
Wheat, regular	340	3	66
Jalapeno Cheese, regular	350	4	66
Pizza Crust	335	2	68
Original Sandwiches: Per Sandwich			
The Original, regular	730	31	79
Large Original, family size	1390	58	152
Deluxe Original, regular	925	42	84
Ham & Cheese Original, regular	745	27	82
Turkey Original, regular	815	32	81
Sandwiches: Per Regular Sandwich			
Albacore Tuna	520	10	77
Albacore Tuna Melt	770	29	83
BLT	580	24	70
Chicken Breast	500	4	80
Chicken Club	685	23	75
Corned Beef	595	12	78
Corned Beef Reuben	840	33	82
Dijon Chicken	500	6	74
Fiesta Chicken	840	36	79
Pastrami & Swiss	890	36	81
Pastrami Reuben	935	41	83
Pesto Chicken	520	9	73
Roast Beef	620	15	78
Roast Beef & Cheese	850	32	83
Santa Fe Chicken	620	14	81
Smoked Turkey Breast	500	7	75
Texas Schlotzsky's	765	32	76
The Philly	840	29	86
The Vegetarian	480	11	79
Turkey & Bacon Club	835	35	79
Turkey Guacamole	645	19	84
Turkey Reuben	825	34	80
Vegetable Club	540	18	76
Western Vegetarian	630	28	76
Wraps: Asian Almond Chicken	445	7	72
Chicken Caesar	505	27	40
Salsa Chicken w. Cheddar	435	17	44
Zesty Albacore Tuna	315	7	45
Soups: Per Cup (8 oz)			
Boston Clam Chowder	235	15	24
Broccoli Cheese w. Florets	250	17	23
Chicken Gumbo	110	5	13
Chicken Tortilla	165	3	13
Chicken w. Wild Rice	380	19	36
Minestrone	90	1	17
Old-Fashioned Chicken Noodle	120	2	18

Continued Next Page ...

247

Schlotzsky's® cont...

Deli Salads: Per 5 oz Container	C	F	Cb
Albacore Tuna, small, 4.4 oz	170	9	2
California Pasta	60	3	10
Elbow Macaroni	275	19	23
Homestyle Cole Slaw	190	10	24
Mustard Potato	250	13	31
Potato	290	15	35

Leaf Salads: w/out Dressing/Croutons/Noodles			
Chicken Caesar	105	3	4
Chinese Chicken	130	3	10
Garden Salad	50	1	7
Greek Salad	175	11	10
Ham & Turkey Chef's	225	11	13
Smoked Turkey Chef's	180	10	3

8" Pizzas: Bacon, Tom. & Mushr.	620	22	78
Barbeque Chicken	655	15	93
Chicken & Pesto; New Orleans	650	19	78
Double Cheese	580	19	76
Double Cheese & Pepperoni	730	27	77
Fresh Tomato & Pesto	540	16	76
Mediterranean	535	18	72
Smoked Turkey & Jalapeno	625	17	80
Thai Chicken	665	17	89
The Original Combination	625	23	79
Vegetarian Special	555	17	76

Salad Extras: Chow Mein Noodles	75	4	9
Garlic Chinese Croutons, ½ oz, pkg	40	2	5
Greek Balsamic Vinaigrette, 1.5 oz	160	17	2
Light Italian Dressing, 1.5 oz	90	8	3
Olde World Caesar Dress., 1.5 oz	260	27	1
Ranch Dressing: Traditional, 1.5 oz	270	29	1
Spicy, 1.5 oz	230	25	2
Light Spicy, 1.5 oz	140	11	9
Schlotzsky's Deli Chips, 1.5 oz bag	210	11	26
Sesame Ginger Vinaigrette, 1.5 oz	170	15	8
Thousand Island Dressing, 1.5 oz	220	21	6

Kid's Deals: without Cookie/Drink			
Cheese Pizza	460	11	72
Cheese Sandwich	400	15	49
PBJ Sandwich	490	16	71
Pepperoni Pizza	510	16	72

Desserts/Cookies: Fudge Brownie	430	25	46
Cookies: Oatmeal Raisin	145	5	24
Cookies w. Real M&M's	135	5	20
Other varieties, average	165	7	23
Cheesecake: Cookies & Creme	330	18	36
New York; Strawberry Swirl	310	18	31

Second Cup® ~ see CalorieKing.com

Shakey's®

Pizzas (12"): Per Slice (¹/₁₀ Pizza)	C	F	Cb
Cheese only:			
Thin Crust	135	5	13
Thick Crust	170	5	22
Homestyle Pan	305	14	31
Onion/Olives/Mushrooms:			
Thin Crust	125	5	14
Thick Crust	160	4	22
Homestyle Pan	320	15	32
Sausage Pepperoni:			
Thin Crust	165	8	13
Thick Crust	205	8	22
Homestyle Pan	375	20	31
Sausage Mushroom			
Thin Crust	140	6	13
Thick Crust	180	6	22
Homestyle Pan	340	17	31
Pepperoni:			
Thin Crust	150	7	13
Thick Crust	185	6	22
Homestyle Pan	345	15	31
Shakey's Special:			
Thin Crust	170	9	13
Thick Crust	210	8	22
Homestyle Pan	385	21	32

Other Items			
3-Piece Chicken & Potato	945	56	51
5-Piece Fried Chicken & Potato	1700	90	130
Hot Ham & Cheese Sandwich	550	21	56
Potato Wedges, 15 pieces	950	36	120
Shakey's Super Hot Hero	810	44	67
Spagh. w. Meat Sce/Garlic Bread	940	33	134

Sheetz®

Coffeez™: Per 16 fl.oz	C	F	Cb
Hot Chocolate, medium	195	3	39

Cupo'ccino®: Per Medium (16 fl.oz)			
Almond Amaretto; French Vanilla	220	8	34
Fat Free French Vanilla	225	0	47

M.T.O® Cold Subs:			
Per 6" Sub (No Cheese Unless Indicated)			
Cheese Sub w. American Cheese	410	11	75
Chicken Salad	405	12	51
Club Combo Sub	335	5	42
Cold Cut Sub	400	17	43
Cooked Ham Sub; Roast Beef	300	5	42
Egg Sub	270	7	42
Italian Sub	345	10	43
Tuna Salad	420	12	50
Turkey Sub	275	4	42
Veggie Sub	330	3	41

Sheetz® cont...

M.T.O® Hot Subs: Per 6" Sub	C	F	Cb
Buffalo/Rstd Chicken, no Cheese	355	6	42
Meatball, no Cheese	410	18	46
Pepperoni Sub	605	29	41
Steak, no Cheese, 10 oz	380	10	43
M.T.O® Bagelz: No Cheese Unless Indicated			
Cheese Bagel w. American Cheese	385	11	60
Chicken Salad	475	11	71
Club Combo	425	5	62
Cold Cut	490	17	63
Cooked Ham; Roast Beef, avg.	380	5	62
Egg	360	6	62
Italian	435	9	63
Tuna Salad	510	12	70
Turkey	565	3	62
Veggie	300	2	61
M.T.O® Hot Dogs: No Cheese			
Big Deli Dog, 7 oz	550	34	43
Hot Dog, 2 oz	270	15	23
M.T.O® Nachos: Per Serving			
Nachos Bueno/Grande w. Cheese	520	32	42
Nachos Grande, no Cheese	260	12	36
M.T.O® Salads: No Cheese			
Caesar Salad	15	0	3
Chef Salad	100	3	5
Chicken Caesar; Roasted Chicken	200	4	3
Chicken Salad	215	9	14
Garden Salad	20	0	4
Oriental Chicken	430	12	37
Steak Salad	190	7	6
Taco Salad	210	9	27
Tuna Salad	230	10	13
M.T.O® Breakfast			
Shmagels: Bacon & Egg Breakfast	410	10	62
Egg	470	15	62
Ham & Egg	560	18	64
Shmiscuits (Includes Cheese):			
Egg	320	15	26
Ham & Egg	410	18	28
Sausage & Egg	460	28	26
Shmuffins (Includes Chse): Egg	320	15	28
Bacon & Egg	370	19	28
Ham & Egg	380	18	30
Italian Meats & Egg	365	17	29

Shoney's®

Breakfast	C	F	Cb
All Star Breakfast, no extras	185	14	1
Deluxe Pancake Platter	1610	32	300
Half Stack Pancake Platter	930	14	187
Big Eater Steak Brkfast, no extras	630	41	1
Country Fried Steak Breakfast	990	66	49
Sunrise Breakfast	975	60	88
Sausage Biscuit (1)	540	34	42
Burgers			
All-American: Burger	690	32	44
Bacon Cheeseburger	890	44	44
Mushroom Swiss Burger	970	57	49
Famous Patty Melt	945	60	40
Half O-Pound Burger	1350	52	130
Sandwiches			
Blackened Chicken	885	21	122
Charbroiled Chicken Sandwich	895	22	122
Chicken Parmesan Sandwich	750	30	80
Corned Beef Reuben	795	53	37
Fish Sandwich	830	16	126
Fried Chicken Sandwich	565	14	76
Original Slim Jim Sandwich	1010	33	122
Raymond's French Dip	510	14	53
Turkey Club/Whole Wheat	945	52	46
Ultimate Grilled Cheese S'wich	890	46	77
Steaks			
BBQ Ribs	1520	78	124
Choice Sirloin, 6 oz	1225	51	127
Half-O-Pound w. Grilled Onions	1335	52	133
Half-O-Pound w. Grilled Mushr.	1320	52	127
Ribeye, 8 oz	1475	75	127
Southwest Half-O-Pound	1305	69	83
T-Bone, 12 oz	1810	100	127
Surf & Turf:			
Ribeye & 5 Fried Shrimp	1640	82	138
Ribeye & 6 Grilled Shrimp	1590	81	128
Sirloin & 5 Fried Shrimp	1380	58	138
Sirloin & 6 Grilled Shrimp	1330	57	128
T-Bone & 5 Fried Shrimp	1965	107	138
T-Bone & 6 Grilled Shrimp	1920	105	128
Rib Combos, w. Fries:			
¼ Rack & BBQ Chicken	1230	54	103
¼ Rack & Tenderloins	1370	70	120
¼ Rack & Fried Shrimp	1145	50	113
¼ Rack & Grilled Shrimp	1125	52	103

Continued Next Page ...

Fast - Foods & *Restaurants*

Shoney's® cont...

Blue Plate Specials	C	F	Cb
Cajun Whitefish	475	10	56
Baked Whitefish	500	8.5	58
Grandma's Meatloaf w. Glaze	1080	46	92
Grandma's Meatloaf w. Gravy	1075	48	87
Original Country Fried Steak	1160	62	103
Grilled Liver & Onions	710	22	79
Ham Steak Dinner (no veges)	665	25	60
Roast Beef Platter (no veges)	885	30	96
Pasta: Per Serving			
Chicken Alfredo	1705	78	170
Italian Feast	1435	45	204
Pasta Ya-Ya	1875	81	176
Shrimp Alfredo	1780	85	171
Spaghetti	495	16	63
Seafood: Fish 'n' Shrimp	1100	39	159
Fried Fish Platter	1050	38	122
Grilled Cod/Salmon Lite	200	4	0
Grilled Salmon	750	19	95
Grilled Shrimp	720	20	95
Grilled Shrimp Lite	305	8	30
Shrimper's Feast	1035	39	127
Shrimp Stir Fry	875	19	131
Sides: Baked Potato, Plain	350	6	67
French Fries, 4 oz	215	10	25
Onion Rings, 1 order (7 rings)	510	14	83
Chicken: Chicken Stir Fry	1200	35	172
Charbroiled Blackened Chicken	830	26	100
Charbroiled Chicken Breast	800	22	99
Fried Chicken Tenderloins	1160	60	121
Monterey Chicken	905	40	83
Smothered Chicken	890	34	90
Junior Meals: Fish 'N Chips	300	11	29
Chicken Dinner	190	10	12
Desserts, Ice cream, Sundaes			
Apple Pie: a la Mode	1200	53	173
w. NutraSweet	455	18	64
Cheesecake, 1 slice, 4 oz	365	25	23
Hot Fudge Sundae	600	30	75
Original Strawberry Pie, 1 slice	330	17	45
Ultimate Hot Fudge Sundae	605	30	75
Cherry/Peach Pie w. Nutrasweet	480	20	68
Caramel Sundae	625	27	83
Chocolate Milk Shake	1080	51	141
Strawberry Sundae	610	27	85
Walnut Brownie a la Mode	575	33	60

Sizzler®

Hot Entrees: (No Sides)	C	F	Cb
Hamburger	625	33	36
Dakota Ranch Steak: 6 oz	315	20	0
8 oz	420	27	0
9½ oz	500	32	0
Hibachi Chicken Breast,			
w. Pineapple	195	3	13
Lemon-Herb Chicken Breast	140	3	0
Malibu Chicken Patty, each	310	19	11
Salmon	250	12	0
Santa Fe Chicken Breast	150	3	0
Shrimp: Broiled	150	6	0
Fried, 4 only	225	2	35
Mini	150	1	24
Shrimp Scampi	145	3	0
Swordfish	315	14	0
Low Carb Grill Menu			
Grilled Salmon w. Broccoli	405	19	14
Hibachi Chicken w. Broccoli	295	6	15
Petite Sizzler Steak w. Broccoli	520	26	11
Hot Bar			
Broccoli Chse Soup, 4 oz	140	9	10
Chicken Noodle Soup, 4 oz	30	1	4
Chicken Wings, 1 oz	75	4	4
Clam Chowder, 4 oz	120	6	11
Focaccia Bread, 2 pces	110	7	9
Meatballs, 4 balls	155	11	5
Minestrone Soup, 4 oz	35	0	7
Pasta: Fettucine, 2 oz	80	1	15
Spaghetti, 2 oz	80	0	16
Potato Skins, 2 oz	160	8	22
Refried Beans, ¼ cup	60	1	11
Saltine Crackers, 2 crackers	25	1	4
Taco Filling, 2 oz	105	9	3
Taco Shells, each	50	2	7
Dessert Bar: Chocolate Syrup, 1 oz	90	0	21
Choc/Vanilla Soft Serve, 4 oz	135	4	24
Strawberry Topping, 1 oz	70	0	18
Whipped Topping, 1 Tbsp	10	1	1
Salads & Toppings			
Prepared Salads: *Per 2 oz*			
Carrot & Raisin	130	10	10
Chinese Chicken; Teriyaki Beef	55	2	6
Mediterranean Minted Fruit	30	0	7
Mexican Fiesta	55	1	10
Old Fashioned Potato	85	5	10
Red Herb Potato	120	5	9
Seafood	55	3	4
Seafood Louis Pasta	65	2	9
Spicy Jicama	15	0	4
Tuna Pasta	135	10	6

Sizzler® cont...

Sides	C	F	Cb
Baked Potato, plain	220	0	50
Cottage Cheese, 2 oz	50	1	2
Eggs, 1 oz	45	3	0
Garbanzo Beans, ¼ cup	65	1	11
Kidney Beans, ¼ cup	50	0	10
Olives, 1 oz	60	6	1
Peaches, ¼ cup	35	0	9
Peas, ¼ cup	30	0	6
Real Bacon Bits, 1 Tbsp	30	2	2
Turkey Ham, 1 oz	60	5	0
Dressings: Per 2 Tbsp (1 oz)			
Blue Cheese	110	12	1
Honey Mustard	160	16	4
Italian, Lite	15	0	2
Japanese Rice Vinegar, Fat Free	10	0	2
Parmesan Italian	100	10	2
Ranch	120	12	2
Ranch, Reduced-Calorie	90	8	4
Thousand Island	145	15	3

Skyline Chili®

Menu Items: *Per Serving*	C	F	Cb
Chili (Regular): Plain, ½ pint	250	15	4
Burritos			
Deluxe	640	34	47
Regular	570	30	42
Chili: Per Regular Serving			
Plain, regular	250	15	4
Plain w. Beans	260	12	17
3 Way, Spaghetti, Chili & Cheese	710	42	39
4-Way w. Beans	780	42	52
5-Way	790	42	54
Spaghetti: Spaghetti	400	14	44
w. Beans	480	14	57
w. Onions	410	14	47
w. Beans & Onions	490	14	60
Meals			
Blackbeans & Rice	330	12	44
Coney: Regular	240	14	23
Cheese	350	24	23
Lo-Carb Coney Bowl	780	62	4
Salads: With Dressing			
Classic Chicken	330	27	8
Garden Salad	80	5	4
Greek Chicken Salad	440	37	10
Greek Salad	370	36	9
Nacho	450	25	40
Southwestern Chicken Salad-Chili	890	64	51
Southwestern Taco Salad-Bean	840	59	50

Skyline Chili® cont...

Sandwiches	C	F	Cb
Chili Plain	190	9	25
Chili w. Cheese	300	24	18
Wrap: *With Dressing*			
Classic Chicken	670	37	52
Greek Chicken	740	47	54
Southwestern Chicken	670	29	67
SkyFries: Regular	430	20	50
Cheese	660	39	51
Chili Cheese	810	48	53

Smoothie King®

Weight Gain Smoothies: *Per 20 oz*	C	F	Cb
Hulk™: Chocolate/Vanilla	845	29	129
Strawberry	955	29	156
Malts	755	37	86
Peanut Power	500	21	72
Peanut Power Plus: Grape	705	21	119
Strawberry	630	21	104
Shakes	740	37	83
Lowfat Smoothies: Per 20 oz			
Angel Food; Mangofest, avg.	330	0.5	79
Blackberry Dream	345	0.5	86
Blueberry Heaven	260	1	58
Celestial Cherry High	285	0.5	69
Cherry Picker	360	0.5	98
Cranberry Cooler	540	0	132
Cranberry Supreme	575	0.5	138
Grape Expectations	350	0.5	84
Grape Expectations II	420	0.5	129
Hearty Apple	380	2	91
Immune Builder; Island Treat	335	1	80
Instant Vigor	360	1	87
Lemon Twist Banana	340	0.5	82
Lemon Twist Strawberry	400	0.5	97
Light & Fluffy	390	0.5	98
Muscle Punch/Plus	340	1.5	80
Orange Ka-Bam	320	0	104
Peach Slice	340	0	80
Peach Slice Plus	470	0	113
Pep Upper	335	1	80
Pineapple Pleasure	315	0.5	76
Pineapple Surf	440	1	104
Raspberry Sunrise	335	0.5	85
Slim & Trim: Chocolate	270	1.5	55
Strawberry	355	1	79
Orange-Vanilla	200	0.5	43
Vanilla	225	1	51

Continued Next Page ...

Smoothie King® cont...

Lowfat Smoothies (Cont): 20 fl.oz	C	F	Cb
Strawberry Kiwi Breeze	300	0	70
Strawberry X-Treme	370	0	91
Youth Fountain	265	0.5	65
Specialty Smoothies: Per 20 fl.oz			
Banana Boat	520	14	93
Coconut Surprise	455	6	99
Mo'cuccino	420	12	71
Pina Colada Island	550	11	102
Yogurt D-Lite®	345	4	67
Workout Smoothies: Per 20 oz			
Activator: Chocolate	420	1.5	93
Strawberry	580	1.5	130
Vanilla	435	1.5	94
Power Punch	430	1.5	102
Power Punch Plus	500	2	113
Super Punch	425	0.5	95
Super Punch Plus	515	0.5	118
High Protein Smoothies: Per 20 fl.oz			
Almond Mocha; Chocolate	400	13	45
Banana	410	14	44
Lemon/Pineapple	385	13	41

Snappy Tomato®

Large Pizza: Per Slice (¹/₁₂ Pizza)			
Cheese Pizza	160	5	21
Sausage	190	8	22
Pepperoni	200	9	21
Snappy Supreme	425	28	24
Sides: Snappy Wings, 3 pces	160	11	0
Chicken Snappers, 2 pces	150	5	12

Sonic Drive-In®

Burgers	C	F	Cb
#1. Burger w. Mayonnaise	575	36	43
#2. Burger w. Mustard	480	25	43
#1. Cheeseburger w. Mayonnaise	625	42	44
#2. Cheeseburger w. Mustard	550	31	44
Bacon Cheeseburger	730	49	44
Super Sonic #1 w. Mayonnaise	930	66	45
Super Sonic #2 w. Mustard	840	55	46
Junior Burger	355	21	27
Toaster Sandwiches:			
Bacon Cheddar Burger	675	38	60
Chicken Club	675	29	75
Sandwiches			
Breaded Chicken	585	23	66
Grilled Chicken	345	13	31
Wraps			
Chicken Strip, w. Ranch Dressing	575	29	55
Grilled Chicken w. Ranch Dressing	540	27	40
Chicken			
Chicken Strip Dinner	750	32	86
Chicken Strip Snack	270	13	22
Jumbo Popcorn Chicken: Large	520	29	36
Snack	350	20	24
Salads: Grilled Chicken, no dressing	355	17	20
Jumbo Popcorn Chicken, no dress.	475	26	39
Santa FeGrilled Chkn, no dress.	425	18	33
Coneys			
Plain: Regular	260	17	23
Extra Long	485	27	44
Cheese: Regular	365	24	24
Extra-Long	665	42	47
Corn Dog	260	17	23
Breakfast			
Breakfast Burrito	505	33	36
Bacon Egg & Cheese Toaster	500	29	40
Sausage Egg & Cheese Toaster	570	36	44
Ham Egg & Cheese Toaster	435	19	41
Sonic Sunrise Breakfast: Regular	225	0	60
Large	370	0	100

Sonic Drive-In®cont...

Faves & Craves	C	F	Cb
French Fries: Regular, 3.7 oz	195	11	22
Large, 4.9 oz	250	13	30
Super Sonic, 7.2 oz	360	18	44
Ched 'R' Peppers (4)	255	12	29
Cheese Fries: Regular, 4.3 oz	265	17	23
Large, 5.5 oz	320	20	31
Chili Cheese Fries: Regular, 5.1 oz	300	19	24
Mozzarella Sticks, 5.4 oz	380	19	35
Onion Rings: Regular	330	5	66
Large, 19 oz	510	7	102
Super Sonic, 20.6 oz	705	10	141
Tater Tots: Regular, 4.2 oz	260	16	27
Large, 6.1 oz	365	21	40
Supersonic, 8.1 oz	485	28	53
Cheese Tater Tots: Regular	330	22	28
Large, 6.8 oz	435	27	41
Chili Cheese Tater Tots: Regular	365	25	28
Large, 9 oz	550	36	43
Blasts: Regular, all types, avg.	520	27	58
Large, all types, average	765	39	89
Slushes: Small, average	230	0	58
Regular, average all flavors	325	0	81
Large, average all flavors	510	0	127
Wacky Pack, average	210	0	50
Route 44, average	490	0	123
Slush Floats/CreamSlush			
Regular, average	340	12	52
Large	485	17	74
Desserts: Banana Split, 12 ½ oz	425	11	75
Chocolate Sundae, 8½ oz	290	11	41
Dish of Vanilla, 7 oz	195	11	19
Hot Fudge Sundae, 8½ oz	320	15	40
Ice cream Cone	215	11	23
Pineapple Sundae, 9 oz	330	11	53
Strawberry Sundae	250	11	32
Drinks: Barq's Root Beer, large	360	0	90
Coca-Cola, large	325	0	81
Coca-Cola Float, large	425	17	59

For Complete Nutritional Data ~ see CalorieKing.com

Souper Salad®

Soups: Per Serving (5 oz)	C	F	Cb
Beef Stroganoff	130	6	14
Chicken Creole	100	3.5	13
Chicken Tetrazini	120	5	12
Cream of Cauliflower	60	2.5	10
Cream of Spinach	70	3	9
German Potato; Potato Corn	100	5	11
Hungarian Mushroom	120	8	10
Mac and Cheese	140	4	19
New England Clam Chowder	100	3	12
Santa Fe Chicken	100	4	11
Other varieties, average	80	2	10
Bread: Blueberry, 1.3 oz	150	3	27
Corn Bread, 1.3	140	2.5	27
Focaccia Bread, 1.7 oz	110	2.5	18
Garlic Bread Stick (2)	120	2	23
Gingerbread, 3.4 oz	130	3.5	29
Focaccia, all varieties, 1.7 oz	110	2.5	18

For Complete Nutritional Data ~ see CalorieKing.com

Souplantation®

Soups: Per Cup	C	F	Cb
Low Fat: Chicken Tortilla	100	3	5
Minestrone	120	2	20
Vegetable Medley	90	1	14
Regular Soup: *Per Cup*			
Chesapeake Corn Chowder	280	16	30
Cream of Mushroom	290	21	15
Irish Potato Leek	250	15	23
Manhattan Clam Chowder	130	4	16
Minestrone w. Italian Sausage	210	11	14
Navy Bean w. Ham	340	10	30
Vegetarian Harvest	190	8	23
Chili: Low-Fat Kettle House, 1 cup	230	3	26
Breads: Sourdough	150	0.5	27
Buttermilk Cornbread, 1 pce	140	2	27
Focaccia: Garlic Parmesan	100	3	15
Pizza /Tomatillo	140	6	16
Fresh Tossed Salads: Per Cup			
Antipasto Salad; BBQ, average	140	10	6
Caesar Salad Asiago	190	14	10
Won Ton Chicken Happiness	150	8	12

Continued Next Page ...

Feedback Welcome
Please send comments and suggestions to the author.
Email: feedback@calorieking.com

Souplantation® cont...

Prepared Salads: Per 1/2 Cup	C	F	Cb
Aunt Doris' Red Pepper Slaw	70	0	18
Baja Bean & Cilantro	180	3	29
BBQ Potato	160	8	20
Carrot Raisin	90	3	17
Dijon Potato w. Garlic Dill Vinegar	150	12	9
Greek Couscous w. Feta Cheese	170	9	19
Oriental Ginger Slaw w. Krab	70	3	9
Southern Dill Potato	120	3	20
Thai Noodle w. Peanut Sauce	170	8	17
Zesty Tortellini	190	15	18
Dressing & Croutons: Per 2 Tbsp			
Blue Cheese Dressing	140	14	3
Balsamic Vinaigrette	180	19	1
Italian Dressing	120	13	1
Fat Free	20	0	5
Honey Mustard Dressing	150	13	8
Fat Free	45	0	10
Ranch Dressing	130	13	1
Fat Free	10	0	2
Thousand Island Dressing	110	11	3
Croutons, Garlic Parmesan, 5 pces	40	3	2
Hot Tossed Pastas: Per Cup			
Bruschetta	260	4	41
Creamy Bruschetta	360	16	43
Garden Vegetable: w. Meatballs	270	7	42
w. Italian Sausage	300	10	42
Italian Vegetable Beef	270	6	43
Vegetarian Marinara w. Basil	260	4	44
Muffins: Chocolate Brownie	170	8	22
Georgia Peach Poppyseed	150	6	20
Tangy Lemon	140	4	24
Wildly Blue Blueberry, small	140	5	22
Fruit Medley Bran	80	0.5	17
Desserts:			
Apple Cobbler, 1/2 Cup	350	10	64
Apple Medley (fat-free), 1/2 cup	70	0	18
Banana Royale (fat-free), 1/2 cup	80	0	20
Chocolate Chip Cookie, small	70	3	10
Chocolate Lava Cake, 1/2 cup	295	8	56
Jello, flavored, 1/2 cup	85	0	20
Rice Pudding, 1/2 cup	110	2	20
Vanilla Pudding, 1/2 cup	140	4	24
Chocolate Syrup, 2 Tbsp	70	0	18
Granola Topping, 2 Tbsp	110	4	16
Soft Serve: Chocolate, 1/2 cup	95	0	21
Vanilla Soft Serve (reduced fat)	140	4	22

For Complete Nutritional Data ~ see CalorieKing.com

Southern Tsunami®

Sushi: Per Pack	C	F	Cb
California Roll, 12 pieces	360	6	66
California Roll & Inari, 9 pieces	505	11	87
California Roll Plus	495	10	87
Cream Cheese Roll w. Salmon (12)	515	20	59
Crunchy Shrimp Roll, 12 pieces	510	21	64
Dragon Roll, 12 pieces	645	18	66
Eel Roll (Freshwater Eel), 12 pieces	495	16	65
Eel Roll (Sea Eel), 12 pieces	435	12	66
Futomaki	505	1	96
Inari, 4 pieces	420	9	73
Inari & Futomaki	560	9	102
M&M Roll: Shrimp & Avocado (16)	330	5	59
Tuna & Cucumber, 16 pieces	305	1	57
Nigiri: Cuttlefish, 1 piece	40	0	8.5
Egg Cake, 1 piece	75	1	13
Fish Roe, 1 piece	60	0.5	9
Fresh Salmon, 1 piece	70	1	9
Fresh Water Eel, 1 piece	110	5	11
Octopus, 1 piece	55	1	9
Sea Eel, 1 piece	90	3	11
Shrimp, 1 piece	45	0	8
Smoke Salmon, 1 piece	70	1	9
Tilapia, 1 piece	50	0.5	8
Tuna, 1 piece	60	0	8
Yellowtail, 1 piece	55	0.5	8
Ocean Crab Roll, 12 pieces	390	7	60
Orange Roll, 12 pieces	395	8	65
Rainbow Roll, 12 pieces	490	9	66
Snack Pack: Cucumber, 16 pieces	265	0	57
Imitation Crab & Cucumber (16)	290	1	61
Spicy Roll: Salmon, 12 pieces	485	16	59
Shrimp, 12 pieces	395	11	57
Tuna, 12 pieces	450	11	57
Tempura Roll, 12 pieces	530	11	82
Tofu Roll, 12 pieces	320	3	62
Tsunami Roll, 12 pieces	470	13	71
Vegetable Combo: 12 pieces	350	7	65
24 pieces	445	4	92
Combinations: Fullmoon, 12 pcs	425	13	64
Marina Plate, 6 pcs	380	8	52
Meteor Special, 14 pieces	385	3	69
Seaside, Tuna & Salmon, 16 pcs	360	3	58
Seaside, Tuna, Salmon, Shrimp, Eel	355	4	7
Shoreline, 12 pieces	480	8	78
Stardust, 16 pieces	540	8	78

Spaghetti Warehouse®

Lunch	**C**	**F**	**Cb**
Minestrone Soup	80	1.5	12
Grilled Chicken Marinara	530	8	65
Seafood Marinara	385	5	65
Spaghetti: w. Tomato Sauce	425	5	82
w. Marinara Sauce #12	440	5	84
Spicy Marinara Sce Spaghetti	280	4	52
Vegetable Primavera	340	4	65
Dinner			
Minestrone, 1 bowl	110	2	18
Grilled Chicken Marinara	640	10	85
Grilled Halibut Dinner	880	14	106
Grilled Marinated Chicken Breast	910	17	116
Marinara Sauce #12	520	6	99
Seafood Marinara	520	8	86
Spaghetti w. Tomato Sauce	525	6	101
Spicy Marinara Sce Spaghetti	330	6	60
Vegetable Primavera	610	8	116

Feedback Welcome

Please contact the author with comments and suggestions.

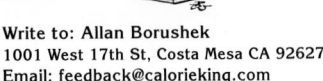

Write to: Allan Borushek
1001 West 17th St, Costa Mesa CA 92627
Email: feedback@calorieking.com

Starbuck's®

Figures Based on Grande (16 fl.oz)
Without Whip Unless Indicated

Drinks: Per 16 fl.oz	**C**	**F**	**Cb**
Apple Juice	230	0	57
Caramel Apple Cider	290	0	72
Chocolate Milk, Whole Milk	365	15	42
Hot Chocolate, Whole Milk	340	15	42
Steamed Apple Cider	230	10	57
Vanilla Creme	340	14	40
White Hot Chocolate, Whole Milk	480	18	63
Steamed Milk, Whole	280	15	21
w. Nonfat Milk	160	0	23
w. Soy Milk	210	6	28
Cafe Misto/Au Lait, Whole Milk	150	8	11
Caffe Americano	15	0	3
Caffe Latte, Whole Milk	265	14	21
w. Nonfat Milk	160	0	24
w. Soy Milk	210	6	28
Breve	555	47	20
Caffe Mocha, Whole Milk	325	12	41
w. Nonfat Milk	245	2	43
w. Soy Milk	280	6	46
Breve	540	37	40
Hot Drinks: Per Grande (16 fl.oz)			
Cappuccino: w. Whole Milk	150	8	13
w Nonfat Milk	90	0	14
w. Soy Milk	120	3	17
Breve	325	27	12
Caramel Macchiato: w. Whole Milk	320	14	37
w. Nonfat Milk	230	2	40
w. Soy Milk	300	8	49
Breve	565	42	36
Caramel Mocha w. Whole Milk	395	11	61
White Choc. Mocha: w. Whole Milk	410	15	56
w. Nonfat Milk	340	5	58
w. Soy Milk	420	14	62
Breve	630	40	55
Espresso (Hot): Per Serving			
Espresso: Doppio	10	0	2
Solo	5	0	1
Espresso con Panna: Doppio	40	3	2
Solo	35	3	1
Espresso Macchiato: Doppio	15	0	2
Solo	10	0	1
Iced Shaken Drinks: Per 16 fl.oz			
Iced Shaken Coffee	80	0	20
Tazo® Iced Tea/Tea	80	0	20
Lemonade	125	0	31

Continued Next Page ...

255

Starbuck's® cont...

Figures Based on Grande (16 fl.oz)
Without Whip Unless Indicated

Iced Drinks: *Per 16 fl.oz*	C	F	Cb
Caffe Americano	15	0	3
Caffe Latte: w. Whole Milk	155	8	13
w. Nonfat Milk	90	0	14
w. Soy Milk	125	3.5	17
Caffe Mocha: w. Whole Milk	250	8	35
w. Nonfat Milk	200	2	36
w. Soy Milk	220	4.5	38
Caramel Macchiato, Whole Milk	270	10	34
Syrup Flavored Latte; Vanilla Latte	210	7	31
White Choc. Mocha, Whole Milk	360	11	56

Frappuccino® Blended Tea: *Per 16 fl.oz*			
Tazo® Chai Creme	385	5	72

Frappuccino® Blended Coffee: *Per 16 fl.oz*			
Caffe Vanilla	345	3.5	72
Caramel	280	3.5	57
Coffee	260	3.5	52
Espresso	230	3	46
Mocha varieties, average	310	4	58

Frappuccino® Light Blended Coffees: *Per 16 fl.oz*			
Caffe Vanilla	235	1	49
Caramel; Mocha	185	1.5	36
Caramel Mocha	230	2	46
Coffee	155	1	30
Espresso	140	1	27
Java Chip	280	7	46
Mint Mocha Chip	290	7	52
White Chocolate Mocha	215	2.5	40

Frappuccino® Blended Cremes: *Per 16 fl.oz*			
Caramel Chocolate	460	7	87
Double Chocolate Chip	490	12	79
Green Tea w. syrup	380	5	71
Mint Chocolate Chip	510	12	94
Strawberries & Creme	455	5	90
Toffee Nut	360	4.5	65
Vanilla Bean	390	5	73

Tazo® Tea: *Per 16 fl.oz*			
Iced Tazo® Chai, Whole Milk	285	7	48
Tazo® Chai, Whole Milk	285	7	48

Drink Extras: *Per Serving*			
Flav. Sugar Free Syrup, 1 pump	0	0	0
Flavored Syrup, 1 pump	20	0	5
Mocha Syrup, 1 pump	30	0.5	6
Toppings: Chocolate, 4g	5	0	1
Caramel, 15g	10	0.5	2
Sprinkles	0	0	0
Whipped Cream Topping:			
Tall, 25g	85	8.5	1.5
Grande/Venti, 35g	115	12	2
Hot Beverage, 27g	90	9	2

Bottled Drinks: *Per Bottle/Can*	C	F	Cb
Double Shot, 6.5 fl.oz can	140	6	18
Frappuccino: Caramel, 9.5 fl.oz	200	3	36
Coffee; Vanilla, 9.5 fl.oz	200	3	37
Mocha, 9.5 fl.oz	180	3	33
Mocha Lite, 9.5 fl.oz bottle	100	3	12

Bagels			
Sesame	460	3	92
Other types, average	440	1	92

Bars: Caramel Apple	310	16	38
Lemon Bar	320	14	44
Peanut Butter Brownie	465	29	45
Raspberry Sammy	300	14	44
Carrot Cake; Enrobed Brownie	430	25	48

Cakes: Apple Walnut Coffee	335	17	41
Banana Pound; Coffee Cake	360	18	48
Choc. Big Baby Bundt	335	15	45
Iced Carrot Pound Cake	540	13	101
Pumpkin Pullman	375	17	51
Low-Fat Cinnamon Coffee Cake	360	8	65
Reduced Fat Lemon Zucchini Cake	310	6	58

Cookies & Biscotti			
Biscotti, all types, 1 oz	115	5	15
Black & White	440	17	68
Crisp Cinnamon Twist	55	2	9
Madeline	80	3.5	11
Double Chocolate Chunk	440	21	58
Milk Chocolate Graham	150	8	17

Croissants: Almond, 3¼ oz	330	18	39
Butter w. Apricot Glaze, 3 oz	320	17	37
Chocolate Filled	360	19	43
Raspberry & Cream Cheese, 3¼ oz	260	12	34

Muffins: Blueberry	385	19	49
Chocolate Cream Cheese	450	24	53
Cranberry Orange	410	20	53
Morning Sunrise	345	12	54

Scones: Apricot Currant; Blueberry	455	17	67
Butterscotch Pecan	525	27	64
Cinnamon Chip w. Icing	515	23	71
Maple Oat w. Icing	500	22	69
Raspberry	450	18	65

Sweet Rolls: Cinnamon	615	29	80
Caramel Pecan Sticky Roll	700	40	75
Cinnamon	615	29	80
Cinnamon Flavored Twist	320	17	37

Ice Cream & Ice Cream Bars ~ See Page 35, 38
For Complete Nutritional Data ~ see CalorieKing.com

Restaurants & Fast - Foods

Steak Escape®

	C	F	Cb
Small Sandwiches (7"): No Cheese or Condiments			
Grand Gobbler	380	2	67
Grand Escape	435	6	64
Grandest Chicken	425	5	64
Great Escape	430	6	63
Hambrosia	380	2	69
Ragin' Cajun	420	5	63
Turkey Club	390	2	65
Vegetarian	300	1	64
Wild West BBQ	470	6	72
Large Sandwiches (12"): No Cheese or Condiments			
Grand Gobbler	680	4	116
Grandest Chicken	770	10	110
Great Escape; Grand Escape	775	12	108
Hambrosia	685	4	119
Ragin' Cajun	755	10	108
Turkey Club	675	4	111
Vegetarian	525	2	109
Wild West BBQ	840	12	126
Fresh Salads: No Cheese or Condiments			
Side Salad	40	0.5	8
Grilled Salad: w. Chicken	175	5	11
w. Ham	130	2	8
w. Steak	185	6	11
w. Turkey	130	2	8
Smashed Potatoes: Plain, 14 oz	245	0	53
w. Chicken	380	4	56
w. Ham	335	2	59
w. Steak	390	4	56
w. Turkey	340	2	59
Loaded: Bacon & Cheddar	635	26	91
Ranch & Bacon	690	34	87
Fresh Cut Fries: Per Serving			
Small, 6 oz	500	26	67
Medium, 7.8 oz	650	34	87
Large, 11.3 oz	920	48	123
Loaded: Bacon & Cheddar	905	44	88
Ranch & Bacon	1045	71	84
Condiments			
Mayonnaise, 1 oz	100	11	0
BBQ Sauce, 1 oz	40	0	9
Cheddar Cheese, 1 oz	115	9	1

For Complete Nutritional Data ~ see CalorieKing.com

Steak 'n Shake®

	C	F	Cb
Meals			
All-American Melt Sandwich	1300	103	53
Chicken Fingers, no fries	615	46	22
Chili 3-Way	660	36	63
Chili 5-Way	1035	67	66
Chili Deluxe, 6 oz cup	480	38	17
Fish Fillet Sandwich w. Cheese	825	58	54
Frisco Melt Sandwich	1175	93	43
Grilled Cheese Sandwich	680	51	40
Grilled Chicken Breast Sandwich	470	26	33
Original Dbl Steakburger w. Cheese	580	38	29
Original Single w. Cheese	400	23	29
Philadelphia Sandwich	850	52	63
Triple Steakburger	690	47	29
Tuna Melt Sandwich	920	77	27
Fries: French, reg., 5 oz	625	35	70
French, large, 7.25 oz	910	51	101
Cheddar Cheese, reg., 5 oz	470	23	62
Salads: Beef Taco Salad w. dress.	940	59	75
Chicken Chef Salad w. dressing	470	32	10
Fried Chicken Salad w. dress.	1060	81	47
Soups: Chicken Gumbo, 6 fl.oz cup	95	2.5	10
Chicken Noodle, 6 fl.oz cup	70	1	9.5
Cream of Broccoli, 6 fl.oz cup	125	8	11
Vegetable Beef, 6 fl.oz cup	125	6.5	10
Breakfast: Bacon 'n Egg (1) Works	875	70	38
Biscuits, Gravy 'n Hash Browns	1585	99	154
Classic Stack 'O Cakes (2)	240	4	47
Country Scrambler (1)	1030	78	51
Cinnamon Swirl French Tst, 3 sl.	265	7	44
One Egg, cooked w. Margarine	140	13	1
Hash Browns	370	25	35
Steak 'n Eggs Breakfast	1015	80	36
Sandwich on Bagel: Egg & Chse	365	20	30
Egg, Cheese & Bacon	475	30	31
Desserts: Apple Cobbler	505	22	76
Hot Fudge Brownie	490	23	69
Hot Fudge Sundae	510	26	64
Outrageous Parfait, no cream	770	40	95
Pumpkin Pie, ⅛ w. topping	395	14	61
Beverages: Root Beer Float	570	22	87
Hot Chocolate, 7 fl.oz, no topping	180	6.5	29
Orange Freeze, regular	630	19	101
Shake: Chocolate, no Cream reg.	710	22	110
Banana; Vanilla, regular	670	21	106

Subway®

6" Sandwiches w. 6g Fat or Less

Figures based on Italian bread and toppings: lettuce, tomato, onion, green peppers, olives and pickles.

	C	F	Cb
Ham; Roast Beef, average	300	5	46
Honey Mustard Ham	320	5	53
Oven Roasted Chicken Breast	330	5	47
Savory Turkey Breast & Ham	290	5	47
Savory Turkey Breast	280	4.5	46
Subway Club	330	6	47
Sweet Onion Chicken Teriyaki	370	5	59
Veggie Delite	230	3	44

Cold Sandwiches (6")

Figures based on Italian bread and following toppings: lettuce, tomato, onion, green peppers, olives, pickles, cheese, oil, vinegar, salt and pepper.

Classic Tuna	530	31	45
Cold Cut Combo	410	17	47
Italian BMT	450	21	47
Subway Seafood Sensation	450	22	51

Hot Sandwiches (6")

Figures based on Italian bread and following toppings: lettuce, tomato, onion, green peppers, olives, pickles, cheese, oil, vinegar, salt and pepper.

Cheese Steak	360	10	47
Chicken & Bacon Ranch	530	25	47
Chipotle Southwest Steak & Chse	470	20	48
Meatball Marinara	560	24	63
Turkey Breast, Ham & Bacon Melt	380	12	48

Deli Style Sandwich: Classic Tuna | 360 | 18 | 35 |

Ham	225	4	36
Roast Beef	235	4.5	36
Savory Turkey Breast	230	3.5	36

Double Meat Subs (6"): Ham | 380 | 7 | 57 |

Cheese Steak	450	14	50
Chipotle Southwest Steak & Chse	540	24	51
Cold Cut Combo	550	28	49
Italian BMT	630	35	49
Meatball Marinara	960	42	82
Oven Roasted Chicken	430	8	50
Roast Beef	360	7	46
Seafood Sensation	640	38	58
Subway Club	420	8	50

Double Meat Subs (6") (Cont)

	C	F	Cb
Sweet Onion Chicken Teriyaki	490	7	68
Turkey Breast & Ham	360	7	50
Turkey Breast	340	6	48
Turkey Breast, Ham & Bacon Melt	450	14	51
Turkey Breast, Ham & Roast Beef	425	8	49

Wraps

Chicken & Bacon Ranch w. Cheese	440	27	18
Tuna w. Cheese	440	32	16
Turkey Breast	190	6	18
Turkey & Bacon w. Chipotle Sce	440	28	20

Breads: 6" Hearty Italian | 210 | 2.5 | 41 |

6" Honey Oat	250	3.5	48
6" Italian Herbs & Cheese	240	6	40
6" Italian White	200	2.5	38
6" Monterey Cheddar	240	6	39
6" Parmesan Oregano	210	3.5	40
6" Wheat	200	2.5	40
Carb Conscious Wrap	120	4.5	13
Deli Style Roll	170	2.5	32

Breakfast Sandwiches (6")

Subs, Italian or Wheat Bread, avg.	440	18	42
Deli Style (Round), average	320	13	35

Breakfasts: French Toast w. Syrup | 355 | 8 | 57 |

Omelets, average all types	235	17	2

Personal Pizza: Per Pizza

Cheese Pizza	630	19	96
Pepperoni Pizza	730	28	97
Veggie Pizza	660	20	101

Salads: No Dressing Unless Indicated

Garden Fresh, no dressing	65	1	11
Grilled Chicken & Baby Spinach	140	3	11
Subway Club, no dressing	160	4	15
Tuna w. Cheese, no dressing	360	29	12
Veggie Delight	60	1	12

Salad Dressings: Per Package (2 oz)

Atkins Honey Mustard	200	22	1
Greek Vinaigrette	200	21	3
Kraft Fat Free Italian	30	0	7
Ranch	200	22	1

Sauces: Per 1 ½ Tablespoons

Chipotle Southwest	100	10	1
Dijon Horseradish	95	10	1

Fat-Free: Red Wine Vinaigrette | 25 | 0 | 6 |

Honey Mustard	30	0	7
Sweet Onion	40	0	9

Subway® cont...

Soups: Per Cup	C	F	Cb
Brown & Wild Rice w. Chicken	190	11	17
Cheese w. Ham & Bacon	240	15	17
Chicken & Dumpling	130	4.5	16
Chili Con Carne	240	10	23
Cream of Broccoli	135	6	15
Cream of Potato w. Bacon	200	11	21
Golden Broccoli & Cheese	180	11	16
Minestrone	90	4	7
New England Style Clam Chowder	110	3.5	16
Roasted Chicken Noodle	60	1.5	7
Spanish Style Chicken w. Rice	90	2	13
Tomato Garden Vegetable w. Rotini	100	0.5	20
Vegetable Beef	90	1	15

Condiments & Vegetables			
Bacon, 2 strips	45	3.5	0
Cheese (slices for 6"): Avg., ½ oz	45	3.5	1
Feta, ½ oz	25	2	0
Shredded Monterey/Swiss, 1 oz	110	9	1
Cucumber, Lettuce, Pickles, Peppers	0	0	0
Tomato (3 slices), Onion, Olives	5	0	1
Mayonnaise: Reg., 1 Tbsp, ½ oz	110	12	0
Light, 1 Tbsp, ½ oz	50	5	1
Mustard, Yellow or Brown, 2 tsp	5	0	1
Olive Oil Blend, 1 teaspoon	45	5	0
Vinegar, 1 tsp, ½ oz	0	0	0

Cookies & Desserts			
Apple Pie, 2.5 oz	245	10	37
Cookies: Oatmeal Raisin (1)	200	8	30
Peanut Butter (1); Sugar (1)	230	12	26
Other varieties, avg. (1)	220	10	30
Fruit Roll Up (1) ½ oz	50	1	12

Fruizle Express: Per Small Cup			
Berry Lishus, 13 oz	110	0	28
Berry Lishus w. Banana, 14 oz	140	0	35
Peach Pizzazz, 12 oz	100	0	26
Pineapple Delight, 13 oz	130	0	33
Pineapple Delight w. Banana, 14 oz	160	0	40
Sunrise Refresher, 12 oz	120	0	29

Sub Station®

Sandwiches	C	F	Cb
Per ½ Sub (Incl. Oil, Vinegar, Salad)			
Ham & Cheese	580	36	48
Ham, Turkey & Cheese	605	37	49
Turkey & Cheese	600	37	48
Roast Beef & Cheese	630	40	44
Ham, Salami, Pepperoni, Cappicola, Bologna, Turkey & Cheese	825	57	43

Sweet Tomatoes®

~ Same Menu & Data as Souplantation (See Page 253) ~

Swiss Chalet®

Burgers: Includes Garnishes	C	F	Cb
Bacon Cheese Burger	870	46	45
Swiss Burger	730	49	44
Veggie Burger	440	14	51

Rotisserie Chicken: Meat Only			
Double Leg	630	34	2
Half Chicken, no Skin	455	18	0
w. Skin	615	31	2
Quarter Chicken: Dark, no Skin	235	11	1
Dark meat w. Skin	315	17	1
White meat, no Skin	215	7	0
White meat w. Skin	300	12	1

Starters: Per Serving			
Baked Garlic Cheese Loaf, 9 oz	730	31	83
Chalet Chicken Wings, 8 wings	1030	59	38
Chicken Fingers, 4 strips	560	32	40
Perogies w. Cajun Sauce, 6.5 oz	420	10	69
Soup: Chalet Chicken, 1 cup	160	4	17

Side Salads: Garden	30	0	6
Caesar Salad	365	32	15

Meals: Chicken Pot Pie, 1 pie	640	33	53

From The Grill: No Flatbread			
BBQ Ribs: Regular Cut	630	38	4
Large Cut BBQ Ribs	1270	77	9
Feature Cut BBQ Ribs	420	26	3
Entree Salad: w. Chicken	410	25	13
Vegetable	270	21	14
Grilled Chicken Breast	130	1.5	41
Grilled Chicken Caesar	495	34	16

Lighter Favorites: Includes Salad & Vegetables			
Quarter Chicken Breast Dinner	415	12	11
Quarter Chicken Leg Dinner	410	18	12
Santa Fe Grilled Chicken Salad	210	7	13
Vegetables Stir-Fry	270	2.5	54
w. Grilled. Chickn Breast	400	4	55

Continued Next Page ...

For Extra Menu Items + Full Nutritional Data
~ See Author's Website
www.CalorieKing.com

Swiss Chalet®cont...

	C	F	Cb
Sides: Baked Potato	220	0	48
Flatbread	240	2.5	46
Butter, ½ oz	100	11	0
Coleslaw	70	4	6
Corn, 3.5 oz	140	3	24
French Fries, 6 oz	470	25	56
Gravy, 4 oz	40	1	7
Mashed Potatoes	140	5	21
Rice Pilaf	280	3.5	57
Sour Cream & Chives, 1 oz	70	5	3
Vegetables, 6 oz	75	0	15
Sandwiches: Chicken Club Wrap	680	32	51
Chicken on Kaiser, white meat	515	13	43
Grilled Santa Fe Chicken	430	10	49
Messy Chicken, white meat	485	12	40
Salad Dressings: Per Serving			
1000 Isle Dressing, 15ml	55	6	2
Famous Chalet Sauce, 125ml	35	1	6
French Dressing, 15ml	65	6	2
Light Italian, 15ml	30	3	3
Mayonnaise, 15ml	100	11	1
Raspberry Vinaigrette, 15ml	15	0	1
Dipping Sauce: BBQ, 33ml	55	0	13
Honey Mustard, 33ml	75	1	19
Plum, 28ml	50	0	13
Salsa, 50ml	20	0	13
Desserts: Apple Blossom	490	25	62
Apple Pie	330	14	49
Carrot Cake	700	45	70
Chocolate Eruption Cheesecake	820	55	72
Coconut Cream Pie	310	16	39
Colossal Caramel Fudge Chsecake	700	39	78
Cranberry, Raspberry Yogurt	120	2	23
Lemon Meringue Pie	280	9	66
Pecan Pie	530	28	63
Swiss Alps Choc Layer Cake	590	39	55
Ice Cream: Butter Pecan	150	7	21
Chocolate	115	5	17
Vanilla	125	6	17
Sauce: Butterscotch	105	0	26
Chocolate	85	0	20
Strawberry	40	0	9

For Complete Nutritional Data ~ see CalorieKing.com

Taco Bell®

Burritos	C	F	Cb
7-Layer Burrito	530	21	66
Bean Burrito	370	10	55
Burrito Supreme Beef, avg	430	17	50
Chili Cheese Burrito	390	18	40
Fiesta Burrito Beef	390	15	50
Fiesta Burrito Chicken; Steak	370	13	48
Grilled Stuft Beef	720	33	79
Grilled Stuft Chicken; Steak, avg.	680	27	76
Tacos: Taco, regular/Crispy	170	10	13
Taco Supreme	220	14	14
Soft Taco Ranchero Chicken	270	15	21
Soft Taco Steak	280	17	21
Soft Taco Supreme Beef	260	14	23
Crunch Wrap Supreme	560	24	70
Big Bell Value Menu: Per Serving			
Burrito, ½ lb Bean, Especial	600	21	82
Burrito, ½ lb Beef & Potato	530	24	65
Burrito, ½ lb Beef Combo	470	19	52
Burrito, Spicy Chicken	430	19	50
Caramel Apple Empanada	290	15	37
Cheesy Fiesta Potato	280	18	27
Double Decker Taco	340	14	39
Double Decker Taco Supreme	380	18	40
Taco, Grande Soft	450	21	44
Taco, Spicy Chicken	180	7	21
Gorditas: Gordita Baja Beef	350	19	31
Gordita Baja Chicken; Steak	320	16	29
Gordita Supreme Beef	310	16	30
Gordita Supreme Chicken; Steak	300	12	28
Gordita Nacho Cheese Beef	300	13	32
Gordita Nacho Cheese Chkn; Steak	270	10	30
Chalupas: Chalupa Baja Beef	430	27	32
Chalupa Baja Chicken; Steak	400	25	30
Chalupa Supreme Beef	390	24	31
Chalupa Supreme Chicken	370	20	30
Chalupa Supreme Steak	370	22	29
Chalupa Nacho Cheese Beef	380	22	33
Chalupa Nacho Cheese Chkn; Steak	350	19	31
Fresco Style (Less Than 15g Fat)			
Burritos: Bean	350	8	56
Fiesta Chicken	350	9	49
Supreme Chicken/Steak	350	9	50
Enchiritos: Beef	270	9	35
Chicken	250	5	34
Steak	250	7	34
Gordita Baja: Beef	250	9	31
Chicken; Steak, average	230	7	29
Tacos: Regular/Crunchy, average	145	7	14
Soft Taco Beef	190	8	22
Soft Beef Chicken/Steak	170	5	21
Tostada	200	6	30

Taco Bell® cont...

	C	F	Cb
Nachos and Sides: Nachos, 3.5 oz	320	19	33
Nachos Supreme	470	26	42
Nachos BellGrande	760	43	80
Pintos 'n Cheese, 4.5 oz	180	7	20
Mexican Rice, 4.6 oz	210	10	23
Cinnamon Twists, 1.25 oz	160	5	28
Specialities			
Cheese Quesadilla	490	28	39
Chicken Quesadilla	540	30	40
Chicken Fiesta Taco Salad	820	39	79
Enchirito Beef	380	18	35
Enchirito Chicken; Steak, avg.	350	16	33
Express Taco Salad w. Chips	630	33	58
MexiMelt	290	16	23
Mexican Pizza, 7½ oz	550	31	46
Southwest Steak Bowl	700	32	73
Tostada	250	10	29
Zesty Chicken Border Bowl	730	42	65
w/out Dressing	500	19	60

For Complete Nutritional Data ~ see CalorieKing.com

Taco Cabana®

	C	F	Cb
Grilled Chicken: Per Serving			
¼ Chicken White, 5 oz	300	14	1
No Skin, 4 oz	170	3	0
¼ Chicken Dark, 4.5 oz	300	18	0.5
No Skin, 3.5 oz	170	9	0
Fajitas: Beef, 4 oz	245	12	4
Chicken White, 4 oz	190	6	3
Chicken Dark, 4 oz	235	11	2
Sides: Black Beans, 4 oz	110	0.5	21
Borracho Beans, 4 oz	110	2.5	17
Chips, 2 oz	290	14	36
Guacamole, 1 oz; Sour Cream, 1 oz	50	4	2
Queso, 3 oz	170	12	7
Refried Beans, 4 oz	170	6	21
Salsa, all types, 1 oz	10	0	2
Spanish Rice, 4 oz	180	5	30
Tortillas: 6" Flour	130	3.5	22
6" Table Corn	60	1	11
Tortilla Soup: Small, 8.5 oz	250	8.5	31
Large, 19 oz	375	13	32
Tacos: Bean & Cheese	295	12	35
Black Bean	225	5	37
Carne Guisada	210	8	20
Crispy Beef	150	7	13
Soft Chicken	220	9	21

Taco Cabana® cont...

	C	F	Cb
Burritos			
Bean & Cheese	545	27	85
Beef/Chicken, average	485	24	76
Black Bean	465	11	95
Breakfast Tacos: Barbacoa	310	15	2
Chorizo & Egg	250	12	22

Taco John's®

	C	F	Cb
Tacos: Taco Bravo	340	14	39
Taco Burger	280	12	28
Crispy Taco	180	10	13
Softshell Taco	220	10	21
Softshell Chicken	190	6	19
Burritos: Bean Burrito	380	12	53
Beef/Chicken Grilled, avg.	590	32	49
Beefy Burrito; Super Burrito, avg.	445	20	44
Combination Burrito	400	16	47
Meat and Potato Burrito	490	23	55
Favorites: Bean Tostada	160	6	19
Cheese Crisp	210	14	11
Chilito	430	22	38
Double Enchilada	720	40	54
Mexi Rolls®	480	30	33
Tostada	180	10	14
Specialities			
Chicken Festiva Salad, no dressing	580	24	60
Chicken Super Nachos	780	45	62
Chicken Taco Salad, no dressing	530	27	45
Potato Oles Bravo	580	36	55
Cheese Quesadilla	480	26	39
Super Nachos	830	51	73
Super Potato Oles	980	62	82
Taco Salad, no dressing	580	32	46
Platters: Beef and Bean Chimi	760	34	88
Beef Enchilada	780	37	80
Chicken Enchilada	700	32	73
Smothered Burrito	830	33	102
Sides: Mexican Rice	240	8	35
Nachos	380	23	38
Potato Oles, Medium, 7 oz	620	36	67
Refried Beans	400	14	50
Crunchy Chicken Side, 5 oz	450	27	24
Desserts: Apple Grande, 3 oz	240	9	36
Choco Taco, 4 oz	300	15	38
Churros, 2 oz	230	11	13

For Complete Nutritional Data ~ see CalorieKing.com

Taco Mayo®

Beans	C	F	Cb
Refried w. Cheese	315	9	43
No cheese	285	6.5	42
Burritos: Bean w. Cheese	500	15	71
No cheese	445	11	70
Chicken Supreme Burrito	410	18	39
No cheese & sour cream	345	12	38
Fajita Steak Grilled Burrito	490	24	41
No cheese	435	19	41
Taco: Crispy, with cheese	160	9.5	10
No cheese	135	7	10
Soft Taco: with cheese	230	11	17
No cheese	200	9	16
Chicken Soft Taco: with cheese	185	8	16
No cheese	160	5.5	16
Extreme Fajita Chicken Soft Taco	265	13	19
No cheese & sour cream	195	7	18
Rice: Mexicalli	165	1	35
Salads			
Fiesta Acapulco	725	53	33
No cheese, guacamole & corn stix	410	32	7.5
Fiesta Monterey	510	31	32
No corn stix	295	19	9
Fiesta Santa Fe	590	36	38
No cheese & corn stix	320	19	14

Target Food Court

Breakfast:	C	F	Cb
Breakfast: Pancakes (3) + Syrup	490	4	104
Breakfast Sandwich w. Bacon	380	20	29
Cinnamon Swirl French Toast, 2 slices	230	5	36
Pretzels (Cinnabon): Cinnamon, 5¾ oz	550	12	105
Mega Cinnamon, 6½ oz	650	15	115
Salted Pretzel, 5½ oz	435	3.5	89
Meals: Bowl of Chili, 9 oz cup	300	10	32
Chicken Breast Sandwich, 4 oz	280	9	31
Chicken Tenders, 5 strips, 3 oz	280	19	14
Hot Dog Meal: w. Chips & Soda	570	12	84
w. Apple Sauce & Soda	520	12	93
Hot Dog: Plain, 3½ oz	260	12	28
All Beef Meat, 5 oz	350	20	30
Cheddar, 4 oz	310	16	38
Macaroni & Cheese: 8 oz	340	13	41
w. Apple Sauce & Soda Meal	600	13	106
w. Chips & Soda, Meal	650	23	97
Mini Pizza (6"), 5½ oz	360	14	42
Nachos w. Cheese, 40 chips, 4 oz	1100	59	132
Spaghetti O's Meal: w. Chips & Soda	490	11	93
w. Apple Sauce & Soda	440	1	102

For Complete Nutritional Data ~ see CalorieKing.com

Taco Time®

Burritos	C	F	Cb
Beef, Bean & Cheese	615	23	66
Big Juan Beef Burrito	640	25	71
Big Juan Chicken Burrito	620	24	69
Casita Burrito, Beef	645	31	54
Chicken & Black Bean	400	18	45
Chicken BLT	580	39	38
Crisp Burrito: Bean	425	18	53
Meat	560	30	39
Chicken	420	25	32
Soft Bean Burrito	380	10	58
Soft Meat Burrito	490	21	48
Veggie Burrito	490	16	70
Tacos: Cheeseburger Taco	640	36	48
Crisp Taco	295	17	16
½ lb Chicken Soft Taco	385	16	41
½ lb Soft Taco	510	23	46
Soft Taco	315	15	23
Super Soft Taco	510	23	50
Specialties			
Cheddar Fries, Medium, 7 oz	520	35	40
Cheddar Melt	210	11	17
Mexi Fries®, Medium, 6 oz	400	25	40
Mexi-Rice, 4 oz	160	2	30
Nachos: Regular, 10.5 oz	680	38	61
Deluxe, 15.25 oz	1050	57	91
Stuffed Fries, Medium, 6.2 oz	725	54	50
Refritos, 7 oz	325	10	44
Salads: Per Serving			
Chicken Fiesta, 12 oz	390	19	35
Chicken Taco	370	21	27
Taco Salad, regular	480	28	30
Tostada Salad	630	33	48
Sauces & Dressings: Per 1 oz			
Green Sauce	10	0	2
Original Hot Sauce	10	0	2
Salsa Fresca	65	0	16
1000 Island Dressing	120	12	3
Desserts: Cinnamon Crustos	375	15	47
Fruit Filled Empanadas	250	9	37

For Complete Nutritional Data ~ see CalorieKing.com

Tacone®

Gourmet Wrapped Sandwiches	C	F	Cb
Campfire, ½ wrap	340	12	41
Pilgrim, ½ wrap	260	14	21
Samurai, ½ wrap	310	3.5	51
Thai Cone, ½ wrap	300	9	35

For Complete Nutritional Data ~ see CalorieKing.com

Restaurants & Fast - Foods

TCBY®

Frozen Yogurt: Per Serving (½ Cup), No Toppings	C	F	Cb
96% Fat-Free Yogurt	140	3	23
Low Carb Yogurt	110	7	16
(Note: Carb figures do not include fiber or sugar alcohols)			
Non-Fat Yogurt	110	0	23
Non-Fat No Sugar Added	90	0	20
Ice Creams: Per Serving (2.5 oz), No Toppings			
Hand-Dipped: Butter Pecan	170	12	14
Chocolate	150	9	15
Chocolate Chip	160	10	15
Chunck	150	9	16
Cookie Dough; Pralines & Cream	160	9	17
Mint Chocolate Chip	160	10	15
Pistachio	160	9	13
Rocky Road	170	9	20
Strawberry	140	8	13
Vanilla; White Chocolate Caramel	150	9	13
Arthur's Favorites, 1 scoop (½ cup)	150	9	16
Cones: Sugar or Jnr Waffle	70	1	15
Waffle Cone	110	2	22
Sorbet: Per Serving (½ Cup)			
NonFat & NonDairy Sorbet	100	0	24
Smoothies: Per Small (20 fl.oz)			
A Lotta Colada	380	12	69
w. yogurt	550	17	99
Berry Slim	300	0	75
w. yogurt	410	3	95
Healthy Balance	300	0	75
w. yogurt	410	3	95
Holy-Cal	360	0	94
w. yogurt	470	3	114
Peachy Lean	360	0	96
w. yogurt	470	3	116
Raspberry DeLITE	240	0	59
w. yogurt	360	3	85
Raspberry Revitalizer	300	0	79
w. yogurt	370	3	84
Tropical Replenisher	240	0	61
w. yogurt	370	3	87
Workout Whey	340	0	92
w. yogurt	460	3	112

Teriyaki Stix®

Bowls: Beef Bowl	620	7	102
Chicken Bowl; Hot & Spicy	730	15	101
Chicken Curry	680	17	92
Teriyaki Chicken Salad	360	13	26
Teriyaki Special	740	13	111
Veggie Bowl	440	1	99
Yakisoba	360	4.5	56

The Taco Maker®

Burritos	C	F	Cb
Bean	295	9	44
Beef	445	16	43
Chicken	375	12	44
Crisp Bean; Crisp Beef, avg.	420	27	30
Enchiladas: Beef	375	20	23
Cheese	585	38	25
Chicken	315	13	21
Nachos: Cheese	605	35	49
Chips 'n Beans	290	16	32
Macho Nacho w. Beef	815	50	57
Macho Nacho w. Guacamole	845	55	62
Salad: Chicken Fiesta	625	35	38
Taco	685	42	39
Tacos: Crisp	185	9	16
Crisp Super	310	15	24
Soft	180	6.5	20
Soft Super	390	13	27
Tater Gem Fries, Regular	485	30	48

The Wrap®

Breakfast Wraps: Per Wrap	C	F	Cb
Bacon & Egg	475	23	46
Egg & Cheese	435	20	46
Huevos Rancheros	505	20	58
Truck Stop	525	24	56
Special Wraps: Buffalo Chkn, 12"	1040	53	90
Bangkok w. Chicken, 12"	885	29	104
Teriyaki Tofu, 12"	750	25	108
Burritos: Per 12" Burrito			
Cajun Chicken	1070	34	132
Classic Chicken	1015	37	104
Classic Tofu	970	34	134
The Big Green w. Steak	870	38	67
Bowls: Per Large Bowl			
Bangkok Chicken	545	19	53
Cajun Chicken	730	24	82
Classic Chicken	675	27	54
Classic Roasted Vegetables	480	18	58
Classic Tofu	575	27	55
The Big Green w. Steak	530	28	17
Teriyaki Tofu	410	15	58
Salads: Per Large Bowl			
Caesar Salad	515	36	9
Chicken Caesar	735	45	10
Greek Salad	290	26	7.5
House Salad	75	3	11

Tim Hortons®

Sandwiches	C	F	Cb
Tim's Own: Chicken Salad	420	12	54
Garden Vegetable			
w. Lt Cream Cheese & Dressing	400	14	57
Ham & Swiss w. Tim's Own Dress.	420	12	55
Tuna Salad	380	9	54
Turkey Bacon Club w. Mustard	440	8	63
Turkey Breast w. Tim's Own Dress.	350	5	54

Soup: Per Bowl (10 fl.oz)	C	F	Cb
Beef Noodle	135	2	23
Clam Chowder	185	4	31
Cream of Broccoli	190	7	30
Cream of Mushroom	170	7	25
Hearty Vegetable	125	1	27
Italian Florentine	165	4	26
Minestrone	120	2	24
Tim's Own, Chicken Noodle	115	3	18
Turkey & Wild Rice	125	2	24

Cookies	C	F	Cb
Chocolate Chip	155	7	21
Double Chocolate Fudge	160	7	22
M&M w. Chocolate Chips	160	7	21
Oatmeal Raisin	150	6	22
Peanut Butter	165	9	18
Chocolate Chunk	170	9	19

Donuts: Per Donut	C	F	Cb
Cake: Chocolate Glazed	240	8	40
Old Fashion Plain	180	7	27
Sour Cream Plain	250	15	27
Filled: Blueberry	220	5	37
Boston Cream	220	6	37
Canadian Maple	240	6	41
Strawberry	210	5	36
Honey Stick	280	13	38
Sugar Twist	220	7	34
Yeast: Apple Fritter	310	9	50
Dutchie	230	6	40
Other varieties	200	7	30

Baked Goods: Per Serving	C	F	Cb
Croissant: Butter	330	19	36
Cheese	360	22	34
Cherry Cheese Danish	320	14	43
Southern Country Biscuits, avg. (1)	470	19	68
Tea Biscuit: Plain, 3 oz	220	6	36
Raisin, 3 oz	230	6	38
Bagels: Average all types	305	3	59

Cream Cheese: Per 1 ½ oz	C	F	Cb
Plain	140	14	1
Plain Light	90	7	3
Garden Vegetable; Strawberry	150	13	3

Muffins: Per Muffin	C	F	Cb
Blueberry Bran	350	12	54
Carrot Whole Wheat	440	23	52
Cranberry Fruit	360	12	59
Chocolate Chip Plain	440	16	68
Fruit Explosion	360	11	61
Raisin Bran	390	12	65
Strawberry Sensation	380	12	61
Low Fat: Cranberry; Blueberry	290	2.5	62
Raspberry	290	2.5	63

Timbits, Low-Fat	C	F	Cb
Cake: Choc. Glazed	60	2	10
Old Fashion Plain	50	2	8
Filled, all varieties	60	2	10
Yeast: Dutchie	50	1.5	10
Honey Dip	60	2	10
Walnut Crunch	350	20	39

Desserts	C	F	Cb
Cheesecake: Apple, 1 slice, ¼ pie	370	12	57
Blueberry, 1 slice, ¼ pie	380	12	60
Cherry, 1 slice, ¼ pie	380	12	60
Mini Blueberry/Strawberry	610	36	61
Mini Triple Chocolate Fudge	580	29	71
Chocolate Danish	430	24	51
Yogurt & Berries Cup	160	2.5	30

Beverages: Per Serving	C	F	Cb
Cafe Mocha, 10 fl.oz	150	6	23
Cappuccino: Eng. Toffee, 10 fl.oz	235	7	40
French Vanilla, 10 fl.oz	255	9	39
Iced w. 2% Milk, 12 fl.oz	295	14	39
Coffee w. sugar/cream, 10 fl.oz	80	4	10
Fruit Punch, 10 fl.oz	150	0	38
Hot Chocolate, 10 fl.oz	240	6	44
Iced Tea, 12 fl.oz	135	0	34

T.J. Cinnamons®

Bakery	C	F	Cb
Chocolate Twist	250	12	34
Cinnachips			
50/50 blend of Pecan Chips, 10 oz	1130	50	157
Cinnamon Twist, 1 roll, 2.5 oz	260	13	33
Icing w. Twists, 1 oz	120	5	18
Original Roll: no icing, 5.2 oz	510	10	73
w. Cream Cheese Icing	650	17	95
Pecan Sticky Roll, 1 roll, 6.5 oz	690	22	91

Beverages: Per Serving (12 fl.oz)	C	F	Cb
Coffee	0	0	0
Mocha Chill: no Whipped Cream	260	4	46
w. Whipped Cream	310	7	49

Restaurants & Fast - Foods

Togo's Eatery®

Sandwiches: Regular 6" Roll	C	F	Cb
Albacore Tuna	455	10	69
Avocado & Cucumber	615	26	79
Avocado & Turkey	690	27	78
BBQ Beef	525	13	64
California Chicken	620	15	68
Cheese	670	30	70
Chunky Chicken Salad	1087	63	93
Hot Pastrami	810	42	72
Hummus	807	31	104
Meatball,	690	23	80
Philly Cheesesteak	720	21	102
Reuben	660	25	69
Roast Beef	670	22	68
The Italian	745	37	68
Turkey & Cheese	600	18	71
Turkey, Ham & Cheese	600	19	70
Turkey, Roast Beef & Cheese	670	23	70
Large Size: Add 50% to Regular Size			
Salads: Per Serving			
Chicken Caesar, 9 oz	315	13	13
Farmers Market, 9 oz	120	3	18
Oriental Salad, 21.3 oz	390	7	53
Taco, 24.5 oz	1050	66	79
Dressings: Caesar Dressing	125	9	9
Ranch Dressing	100	9	3
Low Fat Balsamic Vinaigrette	55	2	9
Oriental Sesame Salad Dressing	140	9	15
Sesame Orange Ginger	330	28	19
Soup: Black Bean	200	7	27
Chicken Noodle; Chili, avg.	150	3.5	20
New England Clam Chowder	105	6	6

Topz®

Burger: Ahi Fillet Burger	360	8	42
Cheeseburger	490	23	38
Chicken Breast	320	5	37
Double Cheeseburger	720	36	45
Garden Cheeseburger	490	17	62
Grilled Cheese Burger	440	20	50
Spicy Chicken Breast	350	6	43
Topz Burger	420	15	44
Topz Jr Burger	230	9	21
Turkey Burger	390	11	38
Chili: Half Order, 4 oz	110	5	4
Fries: Aero, 5.6 oz	380	14	58
Chili Cheese, 9 oz	660	35	68
French Fries, 6 oz	500	22	68

Tropical Smoothie Cafe®

Tortizzas: BBQ Chicken	C	F	Cb
Tortizzas: BBQ Chicken	595	13	88
Cheese	530	19	66
Hawaiiwan	590	19	81
Pepperoni	760	40	68
Sandwiches: Per Sandwich (no Cheese)			
BBQ Chicken	395	2	63
Blazin Buffalo	395	3	57
Golden Roasted Chicken	395	2	63
Half Hoagie: BLT	285	16	21
Pastrami	245	6	21
Turkey	250	2	26
Wraps: Blazin BBQ	590	13	87
Buffalo Chicken	625	28	59
Totally Turkey	655	27	57
Veggie Veggie	615	26	72
Salads: Per Salad			
Specialty: Chef, no chse or dress.	245	8	12
Garden Salad w. chse, no dress.	140	8.5	6
Chicken Caesar w. cheese, no dr.	160	4.5	8
Sesame Chicken, no chse/dress.	535	11	77
Tuna, no cheese/dressing	215	7	15
Dressings: Blue Cheese, 1 Tbsp	80	8.5	0.5
Caesar, 1 Tbsp	80	8.5	0.5
Sesame, 1 Tbsp	45	2.5	5.5
Vinaigrette, 1 Tbsp	45	3	1.5
Dessert Smoothies (with Turbinado)			
Beach Bum (Chocolate)	565	5	125
Beach Bum (Vanilla)	570	5.5	126
Chocolate Chiller	555	7	117
Coffee Cooler	450	7.5	90
Mocha Madness	645	12	126
Strawberry Cheesecake	405	4	90
Tropi-colada	300	5.5	61
With Splenda, deduct 200 calories & 50g carbs			
Kids Smoothies (with Turbinado):			
Chocolate Chimp,	260	2.5	57
Groovy Grape	290	0	71
Jetty Jr	85	0.5	19
With Splenda, deduct 100 calories & 25g carbs			
Low-Fat Smoothies (with Turbinado):			
Berry Blast	345	0.5	84
Blimey Limey	410	0	102
Blue Lagoon	330	1	79
Cool Breeze	410	0	99
Cranberry Cove	445	0.5	109
Grape Gumbo, w. Turbinado	470	0.5	115

Tubby's®

Subs: Per 6" Sandwich

	C	F	Cb
Burger Subs: Big Tub	665	45	41
Cheeseburger	615	41	37
Pizza Burger	630	41	39
Taco Burger	575	31	48
Deli Style Subs: Ham & Cheese	455	24	39
Turkey & Cheese	425	23	37
Turkey Club Sub	480	27	38
Specialty Subs: BLT	530	36	35
Tuna Salad	385	20	35
Veggie Stir Fry	410	20	46
Tubby's Subs: Tubby's Famous	500	29	40
Grilled Chicken Subs: *Per 6" Sub*			
Chicken & Broccoli	460	20	40
Chicken & Cheddar	390	16	38
Chicken Club Sub	445	21	36
Chicken Fajita Sub	350	9	40
Grilled Chicken	240	2	35
Grilled Steak Subs: *Per 6" Sub*			
Mushroom Steak & Cheese	630	42	39
Pepper Steak & Cheese	625	42	38
Pizza Steak & Cheese	620	41	39
Steak & Cheese	610	41	37
Salads: Side, no dressing	50	1	8
Antipasto Salad, no dressing	455	30	18
Chicken Salad	410	23	16
Taco Salad	655	46	25
Tuna Salad	340	26	11

Una Mas®

Burritos

	C	F	Cb
El Cheapo	635	7	118
Fajita Burrito: Chicken	980	40	113
Steak	960	37	111
Gallito	990	60	53
Thai Chicken Burrito	625	22	79
Vegetariano Burrito	690	27	91
Una Mas Burrito: Chicken	705	20	96
Steak	735	21	96
Low Carb Burrito: Steak	700	34	41
Chicken Breast	680	33	41
Tofu	490	16	61
Tacos: Crispy Chicken Taco	375	24	24
Pescado Cabo Style	345	21	24
Una Mas Taco: Chicken; Steak, avg.	340	13	37
Veggie	335	13	46
Favoritos: Chicken Enchiladas (2)	560	24	54
Nachos (no Meat)	1390	86	107

Uno Chicago Grill®

	C	F	Cb
Entrees			
Veggie Burger Meal	610	15	104
Tomato Basil Chicken	570	8	83
Zesty Pasta Marinara	380	3.5	75
Thin Crust Pizza: 9" Individual			
Vegetarian: w. Cheese	850	22	127
No Cheese	620	5	124
Soup: Light Lunch w. Soup	745	6	150
Tomato Garden Vegetable	125	1	25
Salads: Special House	90	1	17
Light Lunch w. Salad	710	6	141
Pasta Green Salad	410	9	69
Veggie Dip Platter	460	11	77

For Complete Nutritional Data ~ see CalorieKing.com

Wahoo's Fish Taco®

Bowls			
Carne Asada, Steak	760	22	90
Chicken, Skinless Breast	750	18	90
Fish of the Day	705	16	90
Classic Burrito			
Fish, average	455	14	51
Chicken, average	545	17	50
Carne Asada	515	20	49
Carnitas	595	26	49
Shrimp	470	14	51
Veggie	600	14	98
Mushroom	415	17	57
Tacos: Carne Asada, Steak	195	7	16
Carnitas, Pork	230	10	18
Chicken, Skinless Breast	210	6	18
Fish of the Day	175	4	19
Veggie	200	4	33
Sides: Beans	445	2	80
Rice	475	6	94
Salads: Chips Not Included			
Carne Asada, Steak	555	33	13
Chicken, average	560	28	15
Fish, average	520	23	15

For Complete Nutritional Data ~ see CalorieKing.com

**For Extra Menu Items
+ Full Nutritional Data**
~ See Author's Website
www.CalorieKing.com

WAWA®

Breakfast & Baked Goods

	C	F	Cb
Bagel: Plain	295	1	61
w. Butter	505	23	64
w. Cream Cheese	390	8	66
Avg. other varieties	320	2	66
Bagel Melts: Ham & Cheese	500	13	67
Pepperoni & Cheese	705	31	67
Turkey Club w. Mayo	720	32	70
Breakfast Bowls: *Per Bowl*			
Crmd Chipped Beef on a Biscuit	425	21	45
Sausage Gravy on a Biscuit	455	25	43
Croissant: Regular, 2 oz	300	15	35
Hash Brown: (1), 1.7 oz	90	5	10
Muffins: Banana Walnut, 4 oz	435	24	48
Blueberry, 4.2 oz	420	19	55
Chocolate Chip, 4 oz	425	21	52
Corn, 4 oz	395	17	55
Sizzli Bagels: Bacon Egg & Chse	470	19	53
Sausage Egg & Cheese	500	22	54
Sizzli Biscuits: Bacon Egg & Chse	500	31	37
Sausage Egg & Cheese	525	34	37
Sizzli Muffins: Bacon Egg & Chse	385	21	31
Sausage & Egg	410	24	31
Hot Sandwiches: No Cheese Unless Indicated			
BBQ Pork Kaiser	560	20	61
Chicken Breaded Club	715	36	56
Classics: BBQ Pork w. Cheese	1090	48	112
Chicken Grilled, no Dressing	470	16	40
Meatball w. Cheese	660	37	49
Roast Beef Homestyle w. Cheese	665	21	67
Cold Sandwiches: No Cheese Unless Indicated			
Italian w. Pesto & Rstd Peppers	900	64	40
Pepper Turkey w. Rstd Tomato	705	44	41
Roast Beef & Horseradish	460	18	26
Healthy Choice: Chkn on White	220	3	27
Ham on White	255	5	28
Smoked Turkey on White	270	4	31
Roast Beef on White	255	4	31
Turkey Carolina on White, avg.	250	2	30
Turkey on White	440	6	67
Roast Beef	375	7	37
Seafood Salad	450	21	46
Tuna Salad	465	22	43
Veggie	200	2	37
Veggie Supreme	325	11	43

WAWA® cont...

	C	F	Cb
Cold Shortis: American	425	18	40
BLT; Cheese, average	500	28	37
Chicken Salad	480	22	41
Egg Salad w. Cheese	630	40	43
Healthy Choice: Ham; Roast Beef	320	6	40
Honey Smoked Turkey	335	5	42
Hot Shortis: Chicken Grilled	325	3	42
Meatball w. Cheese	660	37	49
Roast Beef Homestyle w. Cheese	425	14	40
Wraps: Buffalo Blue Chicken	340	16	33
Roast Beef & Pepper Jack	430	17	42
Roasted Chicken Caesar	390	20	33
Smoked Turkey Supreme	325	7	44
Turkey Bacon & Colby Jack	455	22	37
Hot Dogs: ¼ lb Beef Frank	390	28	20
All Beef Hot Dog	270	17	20
Big Bacon Cheese Dog	730	50	37
Hot Sausage	300	17	21
Kielbasa	215	17	21
Bowls: Per 12 oz Bowl			
Chicken Teriyaki	535	9	94
Chili	550	13	86
Steak & Vegetable	480	6	46
Southwest Chicken Bowl	455	5	82
Sides: Per Medium (11 oz)			
Beef Stew	265	13	24
Chili, 11 oz	275	9	31
Homestyle Chicken & Noodles	325	16	26
Macaroni & Cheese	430	20	45
Mashed Potatoes	520	33	49
Meatballs in a Cup	375	27	14
Shepherd's Pie	400	24	37
Soups: Per Medium (11 oz)			
Boston Clam Chowder	290	15	26
Chicken Corn Chowder	370	24	29
Potato Au Gratin	465	28	40
Potato w. Bacon	260	15	25
Drinks: Cappuccino, 12 fl.oz	170	7	27
French Vanilla, 12 fl.oz	195	7	30
Fat Free Cappuccino, 12 fl.oz	160	0	37
Frozen Cappuccino, 12 fl.oz	250	7	47

Wendy's®

Sandwiches	C	F	Cb
Big Bacon Classic, w. Mayo	580	29	46
Classic Single w. Mayo	430	20	37
Classic Double w. Cheese, Mayo	700	39	38
Classic Triple w. Cheese, Mayo	970	59	38
¼ lb Double Stack	420	20	34
¼ lb Deluxe Double Stack	470	24	36
Chicken Temptations: Ultimate	360	7	44
Spicy Fillet w. mayo	510	19	57
Homestyle Fillet	540	22	57
French Fries: Medium, 5 oz	440	21	58
Biggie, 5.6 oz	490	24	65
Great Biggie, 6.7 oz	590	29	77
Kid's Meal, 3.2 oz	280	14	37
Chicken: Crispy Nuggets, 5 pce	220	14	13
Homestyle Strips (3), no sauce	410	18	33
Sauce: Heartland Ranch, 1 pkt	200	21	1
Other varieties, avg., 1 pkt	175	17	5
Garden Sensations Salads			
Caesar Side Salad, no toppings	70	4.5	3
Chicken BLT Salad: no toppings	330	18	10
w. Croutons/Dressing	680	46	30
Mandarin Chicken: no toppings	170	2	17
w. Dressing/Nuts/Noodles	550	26	52
Side Salad, no Dressing	35	0	7
Homestyle Chicken Strips: no Dress.	440	22	33
w. Creamy Dressing	670	45	38
Spring Mix Salad: no Dress./Pecans	180	11	11
w. Dressing/Pecans	500	42	24
Taco Supremo: no toppings	380	17	31
w. Chips/Sour Cream/Salsa	660	30	69
Kids Meal: Hamburger only	270	9	33
Cheeseburger only	320	13	34
Chicken Nuggets, 4 pieces	180	11	10
Frosty, 6 oz	160	4	28
Baked Potatoes: Plain	270	0	61
Bacon & Cheese	560	25	69
Broccoli & Cheese	440	15	70
Sour Cream & Chives	320	4	63
Country Crock Spread, 1 pkg	65	7	0
Sides: Chili, small, 8 oz	220	6	23
Chili, large, 12 oz	330	9	35
Hot Chili Seasoning, 1 pkg	10	0	2
Cheddar Cheese, shredded, 2 Tbsp	70	6	1
Saltine Crackers (2)	30	0.5	5
Fresh Fruit Cup, 6 oz	80	0	20
Mandarin Oranges, 5 oz	80	0	20
Yogurt w. Granola Cup	300	6	10
Chocolate Chip Cookie, 2 oz	280	14	34
Frosty: Medium, 16 oz	435	11	73

For Complete Nutritional Data ~ see CalorieKing.com

WesterN SizzliN®

Steaks (Meat Only, Raw Wts)	C	F	Cb
New York Strip, 14 oz	900	60	0
Ribeye, 10 oz	520	28	0
Sirloin: 8 oz Steak	540	33	0
16 oz Steak	1080	66	0
T-Bone, 20 oz	1230	99	0
Baked Potato, plain, 8 oz	245	0	58

Wienerschnitzel®

Breakfast: Per Serving	C	F	Cb
Biscuit: w. Egg	285	18	20
Egg, Sausage & Bacon	410	29	22
Egg, Sausage, Bacon & Cheese	465	34	22
Sausage & Bacon, 3.7 oz	325	23	21
Burrito: Breakfast, 9 oz	575	33	41
Chili Cheese, 9.2 oz	500	24	44
Country Breakfast, 10.1 oz	630	45	31
Croissant, 6.5 oz	580	36	41
French Toast, 5.2 oz	495	30	50
Hash Browns, 2.8 oz	285	25	14
Platter, 9.8 oz	700	48	42
Burgers: Chili Cheeseburger	345	13	32
Deluxe Cheeseburger	430	23	33
Deluxe Hamburger	385	19	33
Double Chili Cheeseburger	535	24	35
Tamale: Chili Cheese	445	27	33
Fries: Regular, 4.6 oz	350	25	28
Large, 6.4 oz	480	34	39
Chili Cheese, 8.1 oz	545	38	39
Hot Dogs: BBQ Bacon Dog	370	20	33
Chili Dog	285	13	31
Chili Cheese Dog	335	17	31
Deluxe; Kraut; Mustard; Relish	270	12	30
All Beef: BBQ Bacon Dog	470	28	35
Chili Cheese Dog	435	25	33
Other varieties, avg.	385	21	33
Healthy Choice: BBQ Bacon Dog	320	12	38
Chili Cheese Dog	295	10	36
Other varieties, avg.	235	5	36
For Pretzel Bun add extra	140	3	26
Sandwiches: Bacon Ranch Chkn	540	31	41
Cheddar Sausage Melt	670	38	58
Fish	390	17	48
Italian Sausage; Bratwurst	345	17	31
Polish Sausage	495	28	39
Southwest Smoky Sausage	460	27	35
Sides: Jalapeno Poppers	485	32	37
Onion Rings	475	25	56
Ranch Dressing	120	12	2

Restaurants & Fast - Foods

Whataburger®

Burgers/Sandwiches	C	F	Cb
Whataburger	605	30	53
No Bun	270	18	4
Double Meat Whataburger	850	48	53
Whataburger w. Bacon/Cheese	810	45	53
Triple Meat Whataburger	1105	66	53
Justaburger	310	15	28
Whatacatch	475	26	44
Whatachick'n	525	21	63
Whataburger Jr.	315	15	29
Grilled Chicken S'wich: w. Dressing	495	20	49
No Bun	190	7	10
Grilled Chicken Fajita Taco	365	12	35
Whatameals: Includes Drink & Fries			
Whataburger Meal	1275	50	169
Whataburger w. Bacon & Chse	1420	62	170
Chicken Strips w. Toast & Gravy	1055	49	127
Double Meat Whataburger	1515	67	169
Grilled Chicken S'wich Meal	1115	39	165
WhataChick'N S'wich Meal	1240	51	172
French Fries: Small	255	13	33
Medium	385	20	50
Large	515	26	66
Onion Rings: Medium	200	10	23
Large	305	16	35
Chicken & Salads			
Chicken Strips (2)	380	24	22
Chicken Strips Salad	425	25	29
w. Cheddar Cheese, no Bacon	600	39	32
Garden Salad	50	0	10
w. Cheddar Cheese	220	14	10
Grilled Chicken Salad	230	7	18
w. Cheddar Cheese	400	21	18
Dressings: Ranch, 2 oz	310	33	3
Reduced-Fat Ranch, 2 oz	230	22	6
Low-Fat Vinaigrette, 2 oz	40	1.5	6
Thousand Island, 2 oz	150	13	11
Shakes			
Chocolate; Strawberry:			
Small, 20 fl oz	615	16	100
Medium, 32 fl oz	905	25	146
Vanilla: Small, 20 fl oz	535	17	81
Medium, 32 fl oz	800	26	122
Breakfast			
Bacon, 2 slices	75	5.5	0
Cinnamon Roll	860	34	126
Hashbrown Sticks (4)	140	8	16
Texas Toast, 1 slice	330	14	42

Whataburger® cont...

Breakfast (Cont)	C	F	Cb
Biscuit: Buttermilk	300	16	34
w. Bacon	375	22	34
w. Bacon, Egg, Cheese	475	29	35
w. Egg & Cheese	445	27	35
w. Sausage	515	35	34
w. Sausage Gravy	490	33	47
w. Sausage, Egg, Cheese	665	46	35
Breakfast-On-A-Bun: w. Bacon	400	23	28
w. Sausage	540	36	28
Ranchero: w. Bacon	405	23	29
w. Sausage	545	36	29
Breakfast Platters (Biscuit/Eggs/Hash Brown):			
w. Bacon, 2 slices	700	43	52
w. Sausage, 1 patty	840	56	51
Pancakes: Plain (3)	610	7.5	117
w. Bacon, 2 slices	690	13	118
w. Sausage, 1 patty	830	26	118
Taquito: Bacon & Egg	385	22	25
Potato & Egg	380	20	33
Sausage & Egg	390	23	25
Desserts: Hot Apple Pie	240	12	31
Chocolate Chunk Cookie, 2 oz	210	8	33
White Choc Macadamia Cookie	230	11	30

White Castle®

Sandwiches & Hamburgers	C	F	Cb
Bacon Cheeseburger	200	12	13
Cheeseburger	160	9	13
Chicken Ring Sandwich	170	8	17
Double Bacon Cheeseburge	360	23	20
Double Cheeseburger	290	18	19
Double White Castle	250	14	19
Fish w. Cheese	180	8	18
White Castle Burger	140	7	13
Sides			
Chicken Rings, 6 rings	335	24	16
French Fries, small, 3.6 oz	300	14	37
Mozzarella Cheese Sticks, 3 sticks	250	14	22
Onion Rings, small, 1.9 oz	230	12	28
Drinks: Coca-Cola, 16 fl.oz	215	0	54
Chocolate/Vanilla Shake, 16 fl.oz	270	8	40
Iced Tea, 16 fl.oz	95	0	24

269

Winchell's®

Baked Products	C	F	Cb
Bagel	130	1	22
Croissant	285	17	28
Muffins: Banana Nut	560	28	63
Blueberry	480	25	54
Bran	405	20	48
Cheese	485	25	51
Chocolate Chip	450	22	54
Low-Fat varieties, average	225	3	43
Cake Donuts: Glazed Old Fashion (1)	290	18	28
Buttermilk Bar Glazed (1)	275	16	29
Cinnamon Crumb Cake (1)	290	18	30
Iced Cake (1)	255	15	28
Iced French (1)	230	13	24
Iced Old Fashion (1)	300	19	28
Iced Donut Holes (4)	255	15	28
Plain Donut Holes (4)	235	14	26
Raised Donuts: Apple Fritter	615	41	55
Bear Claw	480	30	47
Chocolate Bavarian	330	18	36
Chocolate Rounds/Twist/Bar	275	16	29
Glazed Cinnamon Roll	290	24	12
Glazed Jelly; Sugar Jelly	320	17	36
Glazed Rounds/Sugar Rounds/Twist	250	15	27
Iced Bar	240	16	29
Drinks: Frozen Orange Chilla	340	8	66
Frozen Mocha Cappuccino	490	19	74

Yoshinoya®

Bowls	C	F	Cb
Beef Bowl: Regular, 15 oz	840	30	109
Large, 21 oz	1160	41	153
Chicken Bowl: Regular, 19 oz	760	15	125
Large, 30 oz	1110	22	180
Combo Bowl: Regular, 17 oz	750	19	117
Large, 27 oz	1120	36	171
Vegetable Beef Bowl: Reg.,18 oz	770	23	114
Large, 28 oz	1090	32	163
Vegetable Bowl: Regular 19 oz	530	3.5	116
Large, 32 oz	780	5	169
Tempura: Fish Tempura, 22 oz	990	24	168
Fish & Beef Tempura, 30 oz	1450	45	194
Fish & Chicken Tempura, 31 oz	1450	37	225
Shrimp Tempura, 20 oz	890	19	160
Shrimp & Beef Tempura, 28 oz	1350	40	206
Shrimp & Chicken Tempura, 29 oz	1340	32	217
Extras			
Beef, 5½ oz	370	28	6
Chicken & Vegetables, 9½ oz	300	12	21
Rice, 10 oz	460	2.5	104
Vegetable, 9 oz	60	0.5	12

Note: Yoshinoya Beef Bowl Restaurants are based in California.

Zoup!®

Soups: Per Cup (8 fl.oz)	C	F	Cb
Chicken & Dumplings	130	3	21
Corn Chowder	280	18	20
Gazpacho (chilled)	70	1	13
Ginger Butternut Squash	240	15	27
Jamaican Bay Gumbo	140	2.5	18
New England Clam Chowder	200	5	20
Old Fashion Chicken Noodle	90	2	16
Potato Cheddar	210	13	15
Spicy Black Bean Chili	150	1	24
Turkey Chili	120	2	16
Vegetarian Split Pea	60	0.5	7
Paninis: Per ½ Sandwich			
Italian Chicken	370	21	22
Smoked Ham and Swiss	190	8	17
Turkey Club	470	28	21
Bread: Per Piece (2 oz)			
Extra Low-Carb French, 2 oz	130	2	7
Extra Multigrain, 2 oz	190	4	30
Extra Sourdough, 2 oz	170	1.5	31

Zero's Subs®

Oven Baked Subs (6")	C	F	Cb
(Includes cheese, lettuce, tomato, onions,			
oil & vinegar)			
BLT	410	19	48
BLT, no Mayo	330	12	43
Cosmo Vegetarian	470	23	46
Cosmo Deluxe	490	25	48
Grinder	560	31	48
Grinder, Multigrain	560	32	50
Ham & Cheese	440	19	44
Meatball & Cheese	560	30	50
without Cheese	460	22	50
Pepperoni & Cheese	550	31	42
without Cheese	345	15	41
Roast Beef & Cheese	460	19	45
The Club	515	23	44
Tuna & Cheese	520	26	47
Turkey & Cheese	450	17	44
12" Size Subs: Double the figures for 6" size			
6" Subs From The Grill			
Grilled Veggie	395	14	52
Hot Italian Sausage & Cheese	665	37	45
Philly Chicken & Cheese	400	10	48
w. Mushrooms/Green Peppers	415	10	49
without Cheese	325	4	45
Philly Steak & Cheese	495	21	49
w. Mushrooms/Green Peppers	500	21	50
without Cheese	410	15	46

Notes on Cholesterol

- **Cholesterol** is a white waxy substance produced mainly by our liver. It is also found in animal food products. Plant foods have no cholesterol.

- **Cholesterol is essential to life.** It is a structural part of every body cell wall and is the building block for vitamin D, sex hormones, and bile acids which help in the digestion of dietary fats.

- **The body makes sufficient cholesterol** for its needs and does not rely on cholesterol in the diet. Dietary fats have a major influence on blood cholesterol levels - more so than dietary cholesterol.

- **A high blood cholesterol increases** the risk of atherosclerosis - the thickening of arteries that can reduce or block blood flow to the heart muscle, brain, eyes, kidneys, sex organs and other body parts.

  This in turn increases the risk of heart attack, stroke, blindness, kidney failure, impotence and other blood circulatory problems.

  Other risk factors which increase the risk of atherosclerosis include high blood pressure, tobacco smoking, obesity and diabetes (uncontrolled).

HEART ATTACK WARNING SIGNALS

Many victims die before reaching hospital by ignoring warning signals and delaying medical help.
Symptoms vary and commonly include:

- **Chest pain**, vice-like squeezing or burning sensation in centre of chest or between shoulder blades, or feeling of severe indigestion.

- **Pain** may spread to shoulders, neck, jaw or arms.

- **Sweating**, nausea, dizziness, shortness of breath, irregular pulse.

If you experience any of the above symptoms seek IMMEDIATE medical attention!

Every minute counts.

BLOOD CHOLESTEROL

Check Your Risk!

Cholesterol Level (mg/dL)	Risk of Heart Attack
240 and above ~	High Risk
200 - 239 ~	Borderline/High
Below 200 ~	Desirable

❤ Know your cholesterol level, particularly if there is a family history of heart disease or stroke. If high, see your doctor.

❤ All adults should have their cholesterol, HDL and triglycerides tested at least every 5 years.

▲ Atherosclerosis can clog arteries and impede blood flow to the heart muscle or other body organs.

▼ A thrombus (blood clot) can form on unstable, festering atherosclerotic plaque and rapidly block blood flow. A heart attack or stroke can result.

Fats & Cholesterol Guide

The amount and type of dietary fat has the greatest influence on blood cholesterol levels.

Fats in food are a mixture of 3 basic types: saturated, monounsaturated, and polyunsaturated. Animal fats are mainly saturated while plant oils and fish oils are mainly mono- and polyunsaturated.

Saturated fats have subgroups known as long chain, medium chain, and short chain fats. Most of the long chain fats raise blood cholesterol; and increase the risk of blood clots and thrombosis leading to artery blockage.

Long chain saturated fats are found mainly in full cream milk, cheese, butter, cream, fatty meats and sausages, and processed foods.

Monounsaturated fats tend to more selectively lower 'bad' LDL-cholesterol and maintain the protective 'good' HDL-cholesterol in the bloodstream - but only if they replace saturated fats in the diet.

Foods rich in monounsaturates include canola and olive oils, canola margarine, peanuts, and avocados.

Polyunsaturated fats consist of two main classes. **Omega-6** polyunsaturates tend to lower blood cholesterol. Rich sources include safflower, sunflower and corn oils.

Omega-3 polyunsaturated fats can lower blood cholesterol, and also confer extra benefits by lowering blood triglycerides, and reducing the risk of thrombosis, heart arrhythmias, and artery spasm.

Best practical omega-3 sources include canola oil and margarine, soybean oil and fish. (See adjoining chart)

A balanced intake of the two omega classes is important for optimal health. Increasing slightly omega-3 intake by Americans would help to attain a more ideal balance. Adequate vitamin E intake is also important.

> **All fats are high in calories and need to be limited for weight control.**

DIETARY FATS COMPARISON

■ Saturated Fat   ▫ Monounsaturated Fat
Polyunsaturated Fats:
▫ Linoleic (Omega-6)   ■ Alpha-Linolenic (Omega-3)

OILS	Saturated Fat	Monounsaturated Fat	Linoleic (Omega-6)	Alpha-Linolenic (Omega-3)
CANOLA OIL	7	63	20	10
LINSEED/FLAX OIL	9	19	17	55
SAFFLOWER OIL	9	14	77	
GRAPESEED OIL	10	22	68	
SUNFLOWER OIL	11	23	66	
CORN OIL	14	32	52	2
OLIVE OIL	14	76		10
SOYBEAN OIL	15	23	54	8
PEANUT OIL	19	45	34	2
COTTONSEED OIL	26	16	58	
PALM OIL	51	39		10

SPREADS & FATS
Saturated Fat includes 'Trans Fats'   ☐ WATER CONTENT

	Saturated Fat	Monounsaturated	Linoleic	Alpha-Linolenic	Water Content
LIGHT MARGARINE	14	14	21		51
CANOLA MARGARINE	18	45	12	6	19
POLYUNSATURATED MARG	24	20	36		20
BUTTER	57	18	2		24
LARD	41	47			12
BEEF FAT	44	37	4		15

GOOD SOURCES OF OMEGA-3 FATS

Plant Sources	Omega-3 Fats (Grams)
Canola Oil, 1 Tbsp, ½ fl.oz	1.5g
Flaxseed Oil, 1 Tbsp	8g
Soybean Oil, 1 Tbsp	1.2g
Canola Margarine, 1 Tbsp, ½ oz	1g
Soybeans, cooked, ½ cup, 4 oz	0.5g
Walnuts, ½ oz	0.5g

FISH - Per 4 oz Serving

High Content: Salmon (Chinook), Tuna, Trout (Lake), Sardines, Herring, Mackerel	3g / 3g
Medium Content: Salmon, (Pink/Red/Coho), 4 oz	2g
Fair Content: Per 4 oz Serving Bass, Catfish, Cod, Grouper, Hake, Halibut, Kingfish, Perch, Pollock, Shark, Trout (Rainbow), Tuna (Skipjack), Crab, Oysters, Blue Mussel, Shrimp, Squid	0.5-1g

How Much Is Needed?

As little as 1-2 grams daily of omega-3 fats may benefit general health. High doses of fish oil supplements should only be taken as directed by your doctor.

Cholesterol in Food

Dietary Cholesterol

Cholesterol in food varies in its effect on blood cholesterol level (BCL) from person to person. Much depends on the amount and type of fat, and fiber eaten at the same meal.

Any elevating effect of dietary cholesterol on BCL is more likely to occur when the diet is high in saturated fat. Little elevation, if any, generally occurs when dietary fats are balanced in favor of mono- and polyunsaturated fats (including omega-3 fats).

For example, while fish does contain cholesterol, the omega-3 fats can prevent any increase in BCL. Conversely, a meal containing no cholesterol but rich in saturated fat, may result in a significant increase in BCL.

Consequently, the need to be overly concerned about dietary cholesterol is being de-emphasized in favor of a stricter approach to limiting total fats, as well as saturated fat and trans fats in particular.

The liver usually cuts back its own cholesterol production in response to cholesterol in the diet. Many people can consume normal amounts of high cholesterol foods without concern.

However, it is difficult to identify just who is at risk - the so-called 'hyper-responders' - and because over 50% of Americans have a BCL above ideal levels, the **American Heart Association** advises all Americans to be prudent and limit their cholesterol intake to less than 300mg daily – as well as adopting a heart-healthy diet.

This limitation still allows the inclusion of most foods regularly eaten - even the overly maligned egg.

Note: Eggs contain a modest 5 grams of fat per large egg of which barely 2 grams are saturated, the rest being mono- and polyunsaturated.

By comparison, a cup of whole milk has almost 10g fat of which 6g are saturated.

CHOLESTEROL COUNTER

Cholesterol is found only in foods of animal origin. Plant foods contain no cholesterol.
AHA recommends limiting dietary cholesterol to less than 300mg/day.

	Chol mg
Meat - Average all types:	
Lean Meat, cooked, 4 oz	70
Fatty Meat, cooked, 4 oz	105
Fat, thick strip, 2 oz	35

(Note: While lean meat and fat have similar amounts of cholesterol, choose lean meat to limit fat intake.)

Chicken/Turkey, average, 4 oz	90
Organ Meats: Liver, fried, 4 oz	500
Brains, beef, pan fried, 3 oz	1700
Sausages: Frankfurter, 1.5 oz	25
Salami, 2 slices, 2 oz	40
Bacon: 3 slices, cooked, 1 oz	20
Fish: Fish fillets, average, ckd, 4 oz	70
Tuna/Salmon, canned, 3 oz	30
Scallops, 9 medium, 3 oz	30
Shrimp, 12 large, raw, 3 oz	130
Oysters, raw, 6 medium, 3 oz	45
Lobster, Crab, raw, 3 oz	80
Eggs (Chicken), 1 large	210
1 medium	180
Egg White, *Egg Beaters*	0
Milk/Yogurt: Whole, 1 cup, 8 fl.oz	35
1% Milk, 1 cup	10
Skim/Non-fat, 1 cup	5
Soy Milk, Tofu, Tempeh	0
Cheese: Natural/Hard/Cream, 1 oz	30
Cottage, lowfat, 4 oz	5
Ricotta, part skim, 4 oz	25
Fats: Butter, 2 Tbsp, 1 oz	60
Margarine, Oils (vegetable)	0
Mayonnaise, 1 Tbsp	10
Cream: Heavy, whipping, 2 T, 1 oz	40
Half & Half/Sour, 2 Tbsp, 1 oz	10
Icecream: Regular, ½ cup, 4 fl.oz	30
Fruit, Vegetables, Avocados	0
Nuts, Seeds, Grains	0
Coffee, Tea, Soda, Beer, Wine	0

For Comprehensive Food Listings ~ see CalorieKing.com

Blood Cholesterol ~ Diet Hints

1. **Maintain a healthy weight.**
   If overweight, lose weight with lowfat eating and daily exercise.

2. **Reduce saturated fat intake by:**
   (a) **eating less dairy fat.** Choose lowfat or fat-reduced varieties of milk, yogurt, cheese, and icecream. Enjoy soy drinks.

   (b) **replacing saturated fats** with fats and oils rich in mono- and polyunsaturated fats; and carbohydrate-rich foods. Choose vegetable oils such as canola, olive, sunflower and soybean. Avoid solid frying fats.
   Take Control and *Benecol* (spreads) contain plant stanol esters which can lower total and LDL cholesterol.

   (c) **eating less fat from meat** and poultry. Choose lean cuts of meat and skinless chicken. Go easy on luncheon meats, salamis and fatty sausages. Enjoy fish.

   (d) **eating less saturated and trans fats** from baked and fried fast-foods. Avoid deep-fried foods. Avoid donuts, cakes, pastries and cookies unless made with healthier fats and oils.

3. **Increase your 'soluble' fiber intake.**
   Foods rich in 'soluble' fiber include dried beans, baked beans, lentils, chick peas, hummus, nuts, seeds, psyllium seed husks and psyllium fiber supplements. Oat bran, rice bran and barley are also useful, as are fruit, veggies and avocados.

4. **Eat more soya bean products** such as: soy drinks, tofu, tempeh (cultured soya beans), soy flour and soy vegetarian foods. Soy protein in place of animal protein can significantly decrease high blood cholesterol levels - as well as 'bad' LDL-cholesterol and blood triglycerides. Good' HDL-cholesterol is maintained. For best results, eat at least 25g of soy protein per day (from 3-4 servings).

5. **Eat more fruit and vegetables in place of high-fat foods.**
   Aim for 2 fruits and 5 servings of vegetables per day. They also contain valuable antioxidants. The fat of avocados (and most nuts and seeds) is mainly unsaturated and lowers blood cholesterol levels.

6. **Limit cholesterol to 300mg per day.**
   (Extra Notes ~ See Previous Page)

7. **Avoid brewed unfiltered coffee** (espresso; plunger-style). It contains oil compounds (diterpenes) which can raise blood cholesterol. American style filtered coffee is fine.

8. **Spread your food intake over the day.**
   Have 5-6 small meals per day rather than just 2-3 large meals. Nibbling, versus gorging, favors lower blood cholesterol.

ALCOHOL - WINE

Alcohol is a mixed bag. Moderate amounts of 1-2 drinks daily appear to reduce the risk of heart attack and ischaemic stroke in older persons.

However, larger amounts increase the risk of high blood pressure, obesity, heart failure and hemorrhagic stroke; and can aggravate hypertriglyceridemia - in addition to many other health hazards.
(See Alcohol Guide - page 166)

The over-riding harmful effects of excess alcohol do not allow its recommendation for any aspects of health promotion.

Notes On Wine:
Red wine (more so than white) contains antioxidants which may help protect cholesterol in the blood from becoming oxidized.

Many fruits, vegetables and tea also contain protective antioxidants.

Fats in the diet not only affect blood cholesterol levels. They can also strongly influence blood clot formation and thrombosis, as well as blood flow and ultimate oxygen delivery to body parts and organs.

While advanced atherosclerosis can impede blood flow to the heart and other organs, it is thrombosis (complete blockage by blood clots) or arterial spasm which commonly result in a heart attack or stroke.

Plant and fish oils rich in omega-3 fats lessen the risk of blood clots, thrombus formation and artery spasm by reducing platelet stickiness and adhesion to artery walls. This reduces the risk of atherosclerotic plaque becoming unstable and reactive.

Omega-3 fats also improve blood flow by reducing blood viscosity; and increasing the flexibility of red blood cells (RBC) that need to flex and twist on themselves in order to squeeze through tiny narrow capillaries often half their diameter.

A diet high in saturated fats has the opposite effect by stiffening RBC membranes and increasing blood viscosity thereby hindering blood flow. The stiffening of the RBC membrane also reduces its ability to release vital oxygen to body cells and take up carbon dioxide.

Stiff red blood cells may also form aggregates like coin stacks. In narrow blood vessels, this further impedes blood flow and impairs oxygen release through the much lessened surface area of red blood cell membranes exposed to blood. (Smoking, lack of exercise, and stress can have similar adverse effects on thrombosis, red blood cell flexibility and blood flow.)

▲ **Picture of Healthy Blood Flow**

Flexible red blood cells twist and slide through tiny capillaries - often half the diameter of red blood cells.

▲ **A Not-So-Healthy Picture!**

Red blood cells have lost their flexibility and ability to twist and slip through capillaries. They are stacked up thereby impeding blood flow.

A diet high in saturated fats can contribute to this picture - as can smoking, lack of exercise and stress.

Fiber Guide

Introduction

Fiber is the general term for those parts of **plant** food that we cannot digest (although bacteria in the large bowel partly digests fiber through fermentation). It is not found in foods of animal origin (meats, dairy products).

Fiber promotes intestinal health, bowel regularity, can benefit diabetes and blood cholesterol levels, and may help prevent colon cancer. High fiber foods also assist weight control.

Most Americans don't eat enough fiber - less than 20 grams/day - instead of a healthier **25 to 35 grams/day.**

Fiber promotes good health, and better control of diabetes and cholesterol.

'An apple a day keeps the doctor away.' ... it just might!

Types of Fiber

Plant foods contain a mixture of different fibers in varying proportions. Insoluble and soluble fiber categories are based on their solubility in water. All types of fiber are beneficial to the body.

◆ **Insoluble fibers** (cellulose, hemi-celluloses, lignin) make up the structural parts of plant cell walls.

   Best food sources are wheat bran, corn bran, rice bran, wholegrain cereals and breads, dried beans and peas, nuts, seeds and the skins of fruits and vegetables.

These fibers absorb many times their own weight in water. They create a soft bulk and hasten the passage of waste products through the intestines.

They promote bowel regularity, and aid in the prevention and treatment of uncomplicated forms of **constipation, diverticulosis and haemorrhoids.**

The risk of colon cancer may also be reduced by fiber's diluting effect of potentially harmful substances.

◆ **Soluble fibers** (pectin, gums, mucilages) are found mainly within plant cells, soy milk (whole bean) and products.

Types of Fiber (Cont)

Best Sources of Soluble Fiber:
Fruits and vegetables, oat bran, barley, dried beans and peas, psyllium and flax seed.

These fibers form a gel which slows both stomach emptying and the absorption of sugars from the intestines. This helps to control **blood sugar** levels.

Weight control is also aided by the slower emptying of the stomach and the feeling of **fullness provided by soluble fiber.**

Some soluble fibers can lower **blood cholesterol** by binding bile acids and excreting them. More body cholesterol must then be broken down to supply bile acids for emulsification of dietary fats. **Rice bran, while not high in soluble fiber can also lower blood cholesterol.**

◆ **Resistant starch** is that part of starchy foods (approx. 10%) which is tightly bound by fiber and resists normal digestion. Friendly bacteria in the large bowel ferment and change the resistant starch into short-chain fatty acids which are important to bowel health and may protect against colon cancer.

Starchy foods include bread, cereals, rice, pasta, potatoes and legumes.

Fiber & Weight Control

Fiber can assist weight control in several ways. Fiber-rich foods such as fresh fruit and vegetables, potatoes and whole-grain bread contain few calories for their large volume (due to their lowfat, high water content).

Their bulk fills the stomach and satisfies appetite much earlier than fiber-depleted foods. The extra chewing time also contributes to satiety, and gives the stomach time to register a feeling of fullness. Excessive calories are less likely to be consumed.

Fiber-depleted foods and drinks are more concentrated in calories; e.g. fats, sugar, candy, soft drinks, fruit juices, alcohol. They require little or no chewing. Large amounts with excessive calories can be consumed before appetite is satisfied.

Example: Whereas one fresh apple might satisfy our appetite, an apple juice drink with the equivalent sugars and calories of 2-3 apples does little to satisfy appetite. (See illustration below.)

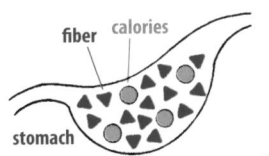

High Fiber Foods fill the stomach. Fewer calories are consumed.

fiber   calories

stomach

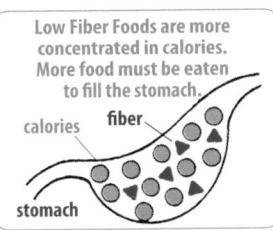

Low Fiber Foods are more concentrated in calories. More food must be eaten to fill the stomach.

calories   fiber

stomach

EFFECTS OF REMOVING FIBER FROM FOOD

2-3 pieces of fresh fruit produces 1 glass of fruit juice. The removal of fiber concentrates the sugar and calories.

FIBER REMOVED

Fresh Fruit	Fruit Juice
High Fiber	Negligible Fiber
Low Calorie Density	High Calorie Density
Long Eating Time	No Eating Time (Drink)
Satisfies Hunger	Does Not Satisfy Hunger
Sugar Slowly Absorbed	Sugar More Quickly Absorbed
Less Insulin Required	More Insulin Required

Guide - Constipation

...ation

Cons...ation can reasonably be defined as a failure to have a bowel movement at least every second day – and just as importantly, without straining or pain.

Typically, stools are too hard, too narrow and too small.

The **main cause** is simply a lack of dietary fiber. Other contributing factors include insufficient fluids, too little exercise, emotional stress, gastro-intestinal disease, lack of proper dentition to chew high-fiber foods, and some medications (e.g. some antacids, antidepressants, tranquilizers).

Note: Check with your doctor to rule out any underlying medical problem – especially if you have a change in bowel habits in middle-age or later years.

DESIRABLE FIBER INTAKE
Adults: 25-35gm per day
Children (under 18): Age + 5gm
Example: 6-year old (6 + 5)= 11gm

SAMPLE FOOD QUANTITIES
For 35 Grams of Fiber/Day

	Fiber
Breakfast Cereal (higher-fiber)	5g
plus 4 slices wholegrain Bread	6g
plus 3 servings fresh Fruit	9g
plus 1 medium Potato (w. skin)	
or 1 cup Brown Rice	4g
or ½ cup wholegrain Pasta	
plus 3-4 servings Veges/Salad	6g
plus 1 cup Bean Soup	
or ¼ cup Baked/Soy Beans	
or ½ cup Corn/Peas/Lentils	5g
or 1¼ oz Almonds (natural)	
or 3 medium Figs	

HINTS TO INCREASE FIBER AND AVOID CONSTIPATION

1. **Breakfast is an important** contributor to daily fiber intake. Eat high-fiber breakfast cereals (bran-based cereals, oatmeal etc.). Add 1-2 tablespoons of unprocessed bran (wheat/ barley/ rice) and wheat germ if required.

Dried fruits, chopped nuts, soy grits, and seeds are also excellent additions to cereals.

Note: A gradual increase in fiber will prevent bloating, gas or pain. People intolerant to bran may benefit from psyllium-based fiber supplements and cereals.

2. **Drink 6-8 glasses of water daily.** Fiber works by absorbing many times its own weight of water.

3. **Eat whole-grain breads**, or fiber-enriched breads. One slice of wholegrain bread has over double the fiber of regular white bread.

4. **Enjoy fruit as fresh fruit** with skins rather than as fruit juice. Enjoy wholegrain pasta, barley, brown rice, nuts and seeds.

5. **Eat more vegetables**, salads and legumes - especially dried beans, baked beans, lentils, potatoes with skins, avocado, broccoli, brussel sprouts, cabbage, carrots, celery, and peas.

6. **Add bran** (barley/rice/wheat) or soy grits to soups, casseroles, yogurt, desserts, cookies, cakes. Also use wholemeal flour or soy flour in place of white flour. Use nuts and seeds.

7. **Snack** on fresh or dried fruits, carrot or celery sticks, popcorn, nuts or seeds, wholegrain crackers, high-fiber bars (low-fat). Limit amounts if overweight.

8. **Exercise regularly** to strengthen abdominal muscles and stimulate the gut. Keep up fluids, especially in warm weather.

9. **Avoid** indiscriminate and regular use of harsh laxatives. They can overstimulate the intestinal muscles and may make normal bowel activity impossible. It may take several weeks to restore normal bowel function.

FOODS WITH ZERO FIBER
- Dairy Products (Milk, Cheese, etc)
- Meats, Poultry, Fish, Eggs
- Fats/Oils, Sugar/Syrups
  (Only foods of plant origin contain fiber.)

Fiber ~ Fiber (grams)

Breakfast Cereals

General Mills:	Fiber
Basic 4, 1 cup, 2 oz	3
Cheerios (Honey Nut; Multigrain), 1 c., 1 oz	3
Multi-Bran Chex, 1 cup, 2 oz	7
Oatmeal Crisp Almond, 1 cup, 2 oz	4
Raisin Nut Bran, 1¼ cup, 2 oz	5
Total, average all types, 1 oz	3
Wheat Chex; Wheaties, 1 cup	5
Wheaties Energy Crunch, 1 cup, 2 oz	4

Health Valley:	
Amaranth Flakes, ¾ cup, 1 oz	4
Fiber 7 Flakes, ¾ cup, 1 oz	4
Golden Flax, ¾ cup, 1.8 oz	6
Granola (Fat Free), ⅔ cup	6
Healthy Fiber Flakes, ¾ cup	4
Honey Crunches & Flakes, ¾ cup, 1 oz	4
Oat Bran Flakes, all types, ¾ cup, 1 oz	4
Oat Bran O's, ¾ cup, 1 oz	3
Real Oat Bran, ½ cup, 1.7 oz	5

Kellogg's:	
All-Bran, ½ cup, 1 oz	10
All-Bran w. Extra Fiber, ½ cup, 1 oz	13
All-Bran Bran Buds, ⅓ cup, 1 oz	13
Corn Flakes, Fruit Loops, Smacks, ¾ cup, 1 oz	1
Cocoa/Rice Krispies Treats, ¾ cup, 1 oz	0
Complete: Wheatbran Flakes, ¾ c., 1 oz	5
Oatbran Flakes, ¾ cup, 1.1 oz	4
Corn Pops, 1 cup, 1 oz	0
Cracklin' Oat Bran, ¾ cup, 1.8 oz	6
Crunchy Blends Granola w. Raisins, ⅔ cup	3
Frosted Mini Wheats, 24 bisc., 2 oz	5
Nutri-Grain, ¾ cup, 1 oz	4
Nutri-Grain Cereal Bars, 1 bar, 1.3 oz	1
Mueslix Crunchy Blends, ⅔ cup, 2 oz	4
Raisin Bran, 1 cup, 2 oz	7
Smart Start: Healthy Heart, 1¼ cups, 2 oz	5
Soy Protein, 1 cup, 2 oz	4
Special K; Product 19, 1 cup	1
Special K Red Berries, 1 cup	1

Breakfast Cereals (Cont)	Fiber
Kashi: GoLEAN Cereal, 1 cup, 1.8 oz	10
GoLEAN Crunch!, 1 cup, 1.8 oz	8
GoLEAN Bars, avg. (1)	4
Good Friends: 1 cup, 2 oz	12
Cinna-raisin Crunch, 1 cup, 1.8 oz	8
Heart to Heart, ¾ cup, 1.2 oz	5
Pilaf, ½ cup, cooked, 5 oz	6
Puffed Kashi, 1 cup, 0.7 oz	1
Quaker: Captain Crunch, 1 cup, 1 oz	1
100% Natural Granola, average, ⅔ cup	3
Crunchy Corn Bran, ¾ cup, 1 oz	5
Fruitangy Oh's, 1 cup, 1 oz	1
Honey Nut Oats, ¾ cup, 1 oz	1
Life Cereal (¾ cup), Oat Squares (½ c.)	2
Oat Bran, ¼ cup, 2 oz	6
Oatmeal, average, 1 packet	3
Puffed Rice, 1 cup, ½ oz	0
Puffed Wheat, 1 cup, ½ oz	1
Shredded Wheat, 3 biscuits	7
Post: 100% Bran, ⅓ cup, 1 oz	9
Alpha Bits, 1 cup, 1 oz	1
Blueberry Morning, 1 cup, 2 oz	2
Cocoa/Fruity Pebbles, 1 cup	0
Cranberry Almond Crunch, 1 cup, 2 oz	3
Fruit & Bran, 1 cup, 2 oz	6
Grape-Nuts, 1 cup, 2 oz	6
Great Grains, ⅔ cup, 1.8 oz	4
Honey Bunches of Oats, ¾ cup, 1 oz	2
Shredded Wheat'n Bran, ½ cup	3

Brans & Supplements

	Fiber
Oat Bran: 1 Tbsp (level)	1
⅓ cup, (5⅓ Tbsp), 1 oz	4.2
Rice Bran: ¼ cup, 1 oz	6
Wheat Bran: unprocessed: 1 Tbsp	1.5
2 Tbsp (level), ¼ oz	3
¼ cup, (4 Tbsp), ½ oz	6.5
½ cup, 1 oz	13
Corn Germ: ¼ cup, 1 oz	5
Wheat Germ: ¼ cup, 1 oz	3
Psyllium Seed Husks, 2 Tbsp	8
Metamucil, 1 dose	3.4

Hot Cereals, Oatmeal

	Fiber
Bulgur (cracked Wheat), ckd, 1 cup	8
Cream of Wheat, ckd, ⅔ cup	1
Hominy Grits, dry, 3 Tbsp, 1 oz	1.2
Oatmeal (uncooked ⅓ cup), ckd, ⅔ cup	2.7

Fiber Guide

Breads & Crackers	Fiber
Bread: White, 1 slice, 1 oz	0.7
Whole-wheat, 1 slice, 1 oz	1.5
Whole-grain, 1 slice, 1 oz	2
Rye, Pumpernickel, 1 oz	1.5
Bagel/Roll/Bun, 1 medium, 2 oz	1.5
Pita, whole wheat, 5" pocket	4.5
Crackers: Graham, average, 2	1.4
Saltine, 4 crackers	0.3
Crispbreads (Rye), average, 2	4
Matzo 1 board, 1 oz	1
Rice Cakes: Average, 1 cake	0.3
Tortilla: Regular, 6"	0.5
Whole-wheat, 6"	1.3

Barley, Pasta, Rice & Flours	
Barley, pearled, raw, ¼ cup, 1.7 oz	5
Rice: White, cooked, 1 cup, 7 oz	1.6
Brown, cooked, 1 cup	3.2
Rice-A-Roni, average, 1 cup, prepared	1.5
Spaghetti/Noodles: cooked, 1 cup	2
Whole-grain, cooked, 1 cup	7
Amaranth *(Health Valley)*, 1 cup	9
Flour: Wheat, All-purpose, 1 cup, 4½ oz	3.5
Whole-Wheat, 1 cup, 4½ oz	15
Cornmeal, stone ground, 1 cup, 4½ oz	13
Carob Flour, 1 cup, 3½ oz	13
Rye Flour, 1 cup, 3½ oz	15
Soy Flour: Defatted, 1 cup, 3½ oz	17
Full-fat, raw, 1 cup, 3 oz	8
Soy Meal, defatted, 1 cup, 4½ oz	14

Frozen Entrees & Dinners	
Average All Brands: Per Serving	
Beans/Chili base, average	6-10
Potato/Pasta base, average	4-6
Vegetable base, average	3
Meat/Chicken base, average	2-3
Pizzas, ¼ large, average	3
Vegetarian Soy Burgers, 1 pattie	5

Soups	
Chicken Noodle, 1 cup	0
Tomato Soup, average, 1 cup	0.5
Vegetable Soup, average, 1 cup	3
Health Valley: Per 1 Cup Serving	
Black Bean; Minestrone	5
Tomato	1
5-Bean Vegetable; Lentil & Carrots	10
Rotini & Veges; Mushroom Barley; Vegetable	4
Split Pea	4

Fast Foods & Restaurants	Fiber
Hamburgers: Small, average	1.5
Large/Whopper, average	2.5
Hot Dog, Regular	1.5
French Fries: Small serving, 2½ oz	2.5
Regular/Medium, 3½ oz	3.5
Chicken Nuggets, 6 pack	0.5
Chicken Sandwich, average	2
Taco, average	4
Sundaes, Shakes, Soft Drinks	0
Arby's: Baked Potato w. Broc. & Cheddar	6
Roast Beef Sandwich, regular	2
Denny's: Grilled Chicken Salad, no bread	4
Classic Burger, no fries	4
Club Sandwich, no fries	2
Grilled Chicken Sandwich, no fries	4
Domino's (Classic): Vegi Feast, 2 sl. (12")	2
Hawaiian Feast, 2 slices, (12")	2
Pepperoni Feast, 2 slices (12")	2
McDonald's: Big Mac; McChicken	3
Hamburger; Cheeseburger; Quarter Pounder	1
Egg McMuffin	2
Grilled Chicken Caesar Salad	3
McVeggie Burger	8
Pizza Hut: Per 2 Slices, Medium	
Pan Pizza: Cheese, Pepperoni	2
Supreme	4
Thin 'n Crispy, Supreme	4
Hand-Tossed, average	4
Personal Pan Pizza, 1 whole	5
Subway: Sandwich, white roll, avg.	4
w. Honey Wheat Roll, average	3.2
Footlong w. Wheat Roll, average	8
Salads, average	3

Cakes, Cookies, Snack Bars	
Apple/Fruit Pie, 1 serving	2
Cake: w. plain flour, 1 serving	1
w. whole-wheat flour, 1 serving	3
Carrot Cake, 1 serving	2
Cookies, oatmeal, (3 small/1 large)	3
Donuts	0
Fruit Cake, 1 serving	3
Fig Bars, 2	1.3
Muffins, Oat Bran (2 small, 1 large), 4 oz	5
Granola Bars, average, 1 bar	2
Atkins Advantage Bars, average	9
Clif Bars, 2.5 oz	5
Fi-Bar Nectar, 1 bar	4
Health Valley: Fruit/Granola Bars	3
Cereal Bars	7
Luna Bars, avg., 1.7 oz	3

Chocolate, Chips, Popcorn	Fiber
Cheese Balls/Curls/Twists	0
Chocolate, Hard Candy, Cheese Balls	0
Chocolate with nuts/fruit, 2 oz bar	1
Mars Bar, 1.8 oz	1
Potato Chips, corn chips, 1 oz	1
Popcorn, 3 cups	2
Pretzels, Twists, 6	1

Nuts, Seeds	
Almonds: Natural, 25 kernels, 1 oz	3.5
Blanched (skins removed), 1 oz	3
Cashews, Filberts, Pecans, 1 oz	1.7
Peanuts, Mixed Nuts, Coconut, 1 oz	2.5
Peanut Butter, 2 Tbsp, 1 oz	1.8
Pistachio Nuts, dried, shelled, 1 oz	3
Walnuts, Black/English, dried, 1 oz	1.5
Seeds: Amaranth, 2½ Tbsp, 1 oz	3.5
Flax Seeds, 3 Tbsp, 1 oz	7
Psyllium Seed Husks, 5 Tbsp, 1 oz	20
Quinoa Seeds, 3 Tbsp, 1 oz	2.7
Sesame Seeds, whole, 1 oz	3
Sesame Butter/Tahini, 2 Tbsp, 1.1 oz	3
Sunflower kernels, ¼ cup, 1 oz	4.4
Teff Seeds, 1 oz	3.8

Fruit – Fresh	
Apples: 1 medium, 6 oz (whole)	
with skin + core	5.5
with skin, no core	4.5
without skin, no core	3.7
Apricots, 2 medium, 4 oz	2
Avocado, average, ½ medium	3
Banana, 1 medium, 6 oz (w. skin)	2
Blueberries, raw, ½ cup, 2.5 oz	2
Cherries, sweet, raw, 10 fruits, 2½ oz	1.5
Grapefruit, average, ½ fruit, 8½ oz	1
Grapes, 1 medium bunch, seedless, 7 oz	3
Kiwifruit, 1 medium, 3 oz	3
Mango, 1 medium, 11 oz (whole)	1.6
Melons, cantaloup, 4 oz (edible)	1
Nectarine, 1 medium, 4 oz	1.8
Olives, average all types, 7 jumbo, 2 oz	1.5
Oranges, 1 medium (7-8 oz w. skin)	
5½ oz (peeled)	3.8
Passionfruit, 2 medium, 2½ oz	5
Peaches, 1 large, 6 oz	2
Pears, raw, 1 medium, 6 oz	4.5
Pineapple, 1 slice, 3 oz	1.8
Plums, 2 medium, 6 oz	2.8
Strawberries, 6 medium/3 large, 2 oz	1.5
Watermelon, 4 oz (edible)	0.5

Fruit – Dried, Juice	Fiber
Dried Fruit: Apricots, 8 halves, 1 oz	2.2
Dates (3 med); Raisins (2 Tbsp), 1 oz	1.5
Figs, 3 medium, 1½ oz	5
Prunes, 4 medium, 1 oz	2
Fruit Juice: Orange/Apple etc, 1 glass	<0.5
Prune Juice, 5 oz	1.4
Carrot Juice, 8 oz	1.8

Vegetables	
Asparagus, 4 spears	2
Bean Sprouts, ½ cup, 2¼ oz	1.5
Beans: Snap/Green, ½ cup, 2½ oz	2
Baked Beans in Tom Sce, ½ c, 4½ oz	10
Dried Beans, ckd, average, ½ cup	7
Beets, ckd, slices, ½ cup, 3 oz	1.5
Broccoli, cooked, ½ cup, 3 oz	2.2
Brussels Sprouts, ckd, ½ cup, 3 oz	3.5
Cabbage: White, ckd, ½ cup, 2½ oz	1
Red, ckd, ½ cup, 2½ oz	2
Carrots, 1 medium (7½"), ½ cup, 3 oz	2.7
Cauliflower, cooked, ½ cup, 3 oz	2.8
Celery, raw, diced, ½ cup, 2½ oz	1
Chick Peas (Garbanzos), ckd, ½ c., 3½ oz	6
Corn, kernels, ckd, ½ cup, 2½ oz	2.5
Cream-style, ½ cup, 4½ oz	1.5
Cucumber/Lettuce/Mushrooms, 2 oz	0.5
Eggplant, raw, sliced, ½ cup	2.5
Lentils, cooked, ½ cup, 3½ oz	4
Onions, 1 medium, 4 oz	2
Spring Onions, chop., ¼ cup, 1 oz	1.5
Peas: Green, ½ cup, 3 oz	3
Cowpeas (Black-eyed), ckd, ½ cup	10
Split Peas, ckd, ½ cup, 4½ oz	6.5
Peppers, sweet, raw, 1 large, 3½ oz	1.5
Potatoes: 1 medium, with skin, 5 oz	4
without skin	2
½ cup mashed, 3½ oz	1.5
French Fries, 3 oz serving	3
Spinach, cooked, ½ cup, 3 oz	2
Squash: Summer, cookd, 3 oz	1.2
Winter, cooked, 3 oz	2.4
Tomatoes: 1 medium, 5 oz	2
Tomato Sauce, 1 cup	0.3
Frozen: Mixed Vegetables, ckd, ½ cup	3
Soybean Products: Miso, ½ c., 5 oz	7.7
Tempeh, 1 piece, 3 oz	3
Tofu, 4 oz	1.4

Salads: Side Salad, average	
Bean Salad, ½ cup	5
Coleslaw, ½ cup	1
Potato Salad, ½ cup	2

Protein Guide

General Notes

- **Protein has many important body functions.** It builds and repairs muscle, and is the basis of our body's organs, hormones, enzymes, and antibodies to fight infection.

- **Protein is also an emergency fuel** in the absence of sufficient carbohydrate and fats. For this reason, weight loss should be gradual so as to preserve protein levels in muscle, the heart and other body organs.

- **It is easy to obtain sufficient protein,** even if vegetarian. **Plant proteins are not inferior to animal proteins.** In fact, eating more soy and other plant proteins, and less animal protein, may help to build stronger bones and prevent osteoporosis; and may help to control blood cholesterol levels.

- **When changing to a vegetarian diet,** include soybeans, and other dried beans, soy milk drinks (calcium-enriched), lentils, tofu, tempeh, nuts, and wholegrain breads and cereals. Milk, yogurt, cheese and eggs can enhance nutrient intake.

Protein & Muscle

- Although muscles are built of protein, protein is not a special fuel for working muscle cells - carbohydrates and fats are.

- In fact, a diet high in protein (and fat) and low in carbohydrate, can significantly reduce the performance of endurance sports athletes. **Carbohydrate** is the best fuel for muscles exercised for long periods.

- Any **extra protein** required by athletes and body-builders, can easily be obtained from the extra food eaten to satisfy hunger and energy needs.

- Remember, **excessive protein** intake will not build bigger muscles. Any excess is converted and stored as fat. Excess protein can also strain the kidneys which excrete the waste products of protein metabolism.

Elderly people (and dieters) must eat sufficient food to ensure adequate protein intake.

Inadequate protein leads to a drop in immune response with greater susceptibility to illness and infections. Muscle strength and muscle mass also drop.

Protein needs are easily met with sensible eating. Athletes who eat enough food for their energy needs, can obtain sufficient protein.

PROTEIN

RECOMMENDED DAILY PROTEIN INTAKE
~ HEALTHY RANGE ~
(Lower figure is RDA)

		PRO
Children:	1-3 yrs	13g-26g
	4-8 yrs	19g-38g
	9-13 yrs	34g-64g
Males:	14-18 yrs	52g-120g
	19+	56g-120g
Females:	14+	46g-110g
Pregnancy:		71g-120g
Breastfeeding:		71g-120g

Note: On lower calorie diets, aim for higher amounts of protein within the Healthy Range.

Iron & Anemia Guide

- **Iron deficiency** is one of the most common nutritional deficiencies in women. The risk is increased in dieters who do not eat well-balanced meals. Chronic shortage of iron leads to anemia.

- **Women** between 11 and 50 years of age are at greater risk because of the monthly loss of menstrual blood. Pregnancy, growth, and endurance sports also demand extra iron.

- **In red blood cells,** iron combines with protein to form **hemoglobin** - the red pigment which carries oxygen in the blood. A lack of iron limits the production of hemoglobin and hence the amount of vital oxygen delivered to body cells.

Note: A blood test will tell you if your Hb and Iron stores (ferritin) are adequate. (Iron stores can be low even when Hb is normal.)

- **Vitamin C** (in fruits/veges/salads) enhances absorption of 'non-heme' iron in bread, cereals, milk, vegetables, nuts, eggs and iron supplements. Small amounts of meat, fish or poultry also help. (They contain 'heme' iron).

- **Iron absorption is lessened** by up to 60% when high calcium foods are consumed with iron-rich main meals. Tea, coffee, phytates (in bran) and oxalates lessen absorption of non-heme iron.

- **For infants to 1 year,** use iron-fortified milk/soy formula if not breast-feeding. Introduce iron-fortified baby cereals at 4-6 mths.

Note: Iron deficiency in children (even without anemia), can result in lethargy, irritability, repeated infections, and developmental problems.

Iron Supplements

- **Most people** can obtain adequate iron from their diet. **A wide variety** of animal and plant foods contain iron. (See Iron Counter)

- **Iron supplements** are only recommended for women with heavy menstrual blood losses, during pregnancy (if tests show a low-iron status), endurance athletes with low blood ferritin (iron stores) and for persons with diagnosed anemia. Check with your doctor.

- While the 5 mg of iron in multi-vitamin/mineral supplements is safe for most people, large amounts can be toxic, (especially in persons with hemochromatosis iron-overload condition).

A nutritious diet with adequate iron is important - particularly for women and athletes.

RECOMMENDED DAILY IRON INTAKE (mg)

			Iron
Infants (0-6 mths):			
	Breastfed	~	0.5mg
	Bottlefed	~	3mg
	6-12 mths	~	11mg
Children:	1-11 yrs	~	7-10mg
Males:	12-18 yrs	~	11mg
	19+ yrs	~	8mg
Females:	12-18yrs	~	15mg
	19-50yrs	~	18mg
	51+ yrs	~	8mg
	Pregnancy	~	27mg
	Breastfeeding	~	12-16mg

Protein & Iron Counter

Pro ~ Protein (grams)

Meat

	Pro	**Iron**
Steak: Average all cuts, lean (no fat)		
Small (4 oz raw/3 oz ckd)	23	2.3
Medium (6 oz raw/4¼ oz ckd)	34	3.4
Large (10 oz raw/7¼ oz ckd)	57	5.7
Roast Beef, lean, 2 slices, 3 oz	24	2.5
Ground Beef patty, lean, ckd, 3 oz	21	2
Lamb chop, broiled, 3 oz	22	1.5
Liver, cooked, 3 oz	23	5.5
Veal cutlet, 1 medium	23	1
Pork, cooked, lean, 3 oz	24	1
Bacon, 3 medium slices	6	0.3
Ham, roasted, 2 pieces, 3 oz	18	1
Ham, luncheon, 2 slices, 1½ oz	7	0.3
Pastrami (Oscar Mayer), 3 sl., 1¾ oz	10	1.3
Sausages: Bologna, 2 sl., 2 oz	7	1
Braunschweiger, 2 sl., 2 oz	8	5.3
Pork link, thick, 2 oz	6	0.4
Frankfurter, 1⅓ oz	5	0.5
Salami, hard, 3 slices, 1 oz	7	0.5
Vegetarian (BocaBurger), 1 pattie	13	2

Chicken/Turkey

Chicken, ckd; Breast portion, 3 oz	27	1
Leg/Thigh, lean, 3 oz	24	1
½ Whole Chicken	60	2.5
Drumstick, 1 medium, 3 oz	12	0.6
Turkey, cooked: Light meat, 3 oz	24	2
Dark meat, lean, 3 oz	24	2

Fish

Fresh Fish: Per 4 oz, cooked		
Cod, Flounder/Sole, Pollock	28	0.5
Catfish, Haddock, Halibut, M/Mahi	28	1.3
Ocean Perch, Swordf., Orange Roughy	28	1.3
Canned Fish: Tuna, Light, 3 oz	25	1.5
White, 3 oz	23	0.5
Salmon, pink, 3 oz	17	0.7
Salmon, red, 3 oz	17	1
Sardines, 3 whole (3"), 1¼ oz	9	1
Anchovies, 1 can, 1½ oz	13	2
Shellfish: Crabmeat, 3 oz	17.5	0.7
Clams, raw, 4 large/9 sml, 3 oz	11	12
Crayfish, cooked, 3 oz	20	2.7
Lobster, cooked, 3 oz	17	0.5
Oysters, raw, 6 medium, 3 oz	7	5
Scallops, 2 lge/5 small, 1 oz	5	0.1
Shrimp, raw, 6 large, 1½ oz	8.5	1
Fish Products: Fish Sticks, 4 sticks	10	0.5
Fish Portions, in batter, 4 oz	13	0.6
Gefilte Fish, 1 medium ball, 2 oz	8	1

Iron ~ Iron (mg)

Eggs

	Pro	**Iron**
1 Large Egg, whole	6	0.7
Egg Yolk	3	0.7
Egg White	3	0
Omelet: Plain, 2 eggs	13	1.7
Ham & cheese	17	3
Egg Substitutes (liquid):		
Eggbeaters, 1 egg equiv.	4.5	1
Scramblers, ¼ cup, 2 oz	6	0.7

Milk, Yogurt, Icecream

Milk: Whole/Lowfat/Skim, 8 fl.oz cup	8	0.1
Protein Enriched, 1 cup	10	0.1
Carb Countdown (2% or Fat Free), 1 c.	12	0.1
Chocolate Milk, 1 cup	8	0.6
Thick Shake, Chocolate, 10 oz	9	1
Vanilla, 10 oz	11	0.3
Soymilk (fortified), average, 1 cup	7	1
Yogurt: Plain, 6 oz	10	0.1
Fruit flavors: 6 oz	8	0.3
8 oz	11	0.5
Ice-Cream: Rich, ½ cup	2	0
Regular, Vanilla, ½ cup	2.5	0
Sherbet, ½ cup	1	0
Custard, baked, ½ cup	7	0.5

Cheese

Hard Cheeses, average, 1 oz	7	0.2
4 oz piece	28	0.8
Cottage Cheese, ½ cup	13	0.3
Ricotta, part skim, ½ cup	14	1

Bread, Bagels, Biscuits

Bread (w. enriched flour): 1 slice, 1 oz	2	1
4 slices, 4 oz	8	4
4 thick slices, 6 oz	1.2	6
Bagel, plain 2 oz	6	1.5
Biscuits, 1 oz	2	0.7
Pita Bread, 1 pita, 1½ oz	4	1
Pumpernickel, 1 slice, 1 oz	3	1

Infant/Baby Foods

	Pro	**Iron**
Infant Formula Milk:		
Enfamil/Gerber/Similac, 5 fl.oz		
Regular/Low Iron	2.2	0.2
With Iron	2.2	1.8
Isomil/Nursoy/ProSobee	3	1.8
Baby Cereals: *Average All Brands*		
Dry, 4 Tbsp, ½ oz	1	7
Jars (w. fruit), 4½ oz	1	7

Breakfast Cereals	Pro	Iron
Hot Type, cooked:		
Bulgur, cooked, 1 cup, 5 oz	9	2
Oatmeal: Reg., non-fortified, 1 cup	6	1.5
Instant, fortified, average, 1 pkt	4	18
Quaker, all flavors, ½ cup	5	18
McCann's, Steelcut, ¼ cup dry	4	18
Corn/Hominy Grits: Reg., 1 cup	3	1.5
Quaker: Reg., 3 Tbsp, 1 oz	2	0.8
Instant White, 1 packet	2	8
Cream of Wheat, 1 cup	4	10
Ready-To-Eat: *Per 1 oz Serving Unless Shown*		
Arrowhead: Average, all varieties	3	1
General Mills: Basic 4, 1 cup, 2 oz	4	3.8
Cheerios, regular, 1 cup, 1 oz	3	6.8
Cocoa Puffs, 1 cup, 1 oz	1	3.8
Kix, 1⅓ cups, 1 oz	1	6.8
Multi-Bran Chex, 1 cup, 2 oz	4	16
Total Corn Flakes, 1⅓ cups, 1 oz	2	6.8
Total Raisin Bran, 1 cup, 2 oz	3	18
Wheaties Energy Crunch, 1 cup, 1.95 oz	6	18
Health Valley: Oat Bran O's, ¾ cup	3	0.9
Amaranth Flakes, ¾ cup	3	0.6
Bran Flakes w. Raisins, ¾ cup	5	1.5
Low-Fat Granola, ⅔ cup	5	1.2
Real Oat Bran, ½ cup	5	0.6
Golden Flax, ¾ cup, 2 oz	6	1.2
Kashi GoLean: 1 cup, 1.8 oz	13	2.7
GoLean Crunch!, 1 cup, 1.9 oz	9	1.8
Seven in the Morning, ½ cup, 2 oz	7	1.5
Kellogg's: All-Bran, ½ cup, 1 oz	4	4.5
Complete Oatbran Flakes, ¾ cup, 1oz	3	8.5
Cocoa Krispies, ¾ cup	1	1.8
Corn Flakes, 1 cup	2	8.4
Just Right, ¾ cup, 2 oz	4	16
Nutri-Grain, ¾ cup, 1 oz	3	1.2
Product 19, 1 cup, 1 oz	2	18
Raisin Bran, ½ cup, 1 oz	1	3
Rice Krispies, 1¼ cup, 1 oz	2	1.8
Special K: Regular, 1 cup, 1.1 oz	7	8
Low Carb, ¾ cup, 1 oz	10	8
Post: Raisin Bran, ⅔ cup, 2 oz	8	11
Grape Nuts, ½ cup, 1 oz	7	2.5
Quaker: Crunchy Corn Bran, 1 cup, 1 oz	1	8
100% Natural Granola, ⅔ cup, 2 oz	5	2.2
Life, ¾ cup, 1 oz	3	4.5
Puffed Rice/Wheat, 1¼ cup, ½ oz	2	0.8
Shredded Wheat, 3 biscuits	7	3

Brans & Wheatgerm	Pro	Iron
Oat Bran, raw, 1 Tbsp	2	0.5
Rice Bran, raw, 2 Tbsp	1	1
Wheat Bran, unprocessed, 2 Tbsp	1	1
Wheat Germ, 2 Tbsp, ½ oz	4	1.3

Grains & Flours	Pro	Iron
Amaranth, 1 cup, ½ oz	10	3
Barley, ½ cup, 3½ oz	8	2
Buckwheat Flour: Dark, 1 cup	11.5	2.7
Light, 1 cup	6	1
Carob Flour, 1 cup	5	3
Corn Flour, 1 cup, 4 oz	9	2
Corn Meal, enriched, 1 cup	11	3.5
Flour: White, enriched, 1 cup, 4½ oz	13	6
Wholegrain, 1 cup, 4¼ oz	16	5
Millet, wholegrain, 1 cup, 3½ oz	10	7
Rye Flour: Dark, 1 cup, 4½ oz	21	6
Light, 1 cup, 3½ oz	10	1
Soy Flour, full fat, 1 cup, 3 oz	32	5.5
Yeast: Brewer's, dry, 1 Tbsp	3	1.5

Rice, Spaghetti	Pro	Iron
Rice: Brown/White, average		
1 cup cooked, 6½ oz	5	1
Spaghetti/Macaroni/Noodles (enriched):		
Cooked, 1 cup, 4½ oz	7	2
Canned: in Tomato Sauce, ½ cup	2	0.5
w. Meatballs, 1 cup, 8 oz	9	2

Soups	Pro	Iron
With Noodles/Vegetables, 1 cup	3	0.5
With Meat/Beans/Peas, 1 cup	8	1.5

Fruit	Pro	Iron
Fresh/Canned: Average, all types, 1 serving		
1 medium/2 small fruit	1	0.5
Avocado, ½ medium	2	1
Dried Fruit: Apricots, 8 halves, 1 oz	1	1.3
Dates, 6 dates, 2 oz	1.5	0.7
Figs, 4 medium figs, 2 oz	2	1.7
Prunes, 5 medium, 1½ oz	1	1
Raisins, 1 oz	1	0.7
Fruit Juice: Average, 1 cup	0.5	0.5
Prune Juice, 6 fl.oz	1	2.5
Tomato Juice, 6 fl.oz	0.5	1

King Kong was a vegetarian!

Protein & Iron Counter

Vegetables	Pro	Iron
Beans: Snap/green, ½ cup	1	0.8
Dried: Average all types, cooked, ½ cup	7	2.5
Baked Beans, ½ cup 4½ oz	5	2
Bean Sprouts, mung, 1 cup	3	1
Broccoli, ¾ cup pieces, 4 oz	4	1.4
Cabbage; Cauliflower, 1 cup	1	0.6
Corn, ½ cup kernels, 3 oz	2.5	0.3
1 ear trimmed to 3½"	2	0.4
Lentils, cooked, ½ cup, 3½ oz	9	3.3
Mushrooms, raw, ½ cup, sliced	0.5	0.5
Peas: Green, ½ cup, 3 oz	4	1.2
Split Peas, cooked, 1 cup	16	2.5
Potatoes, cooked:		
1 medium, with skin, 5 oz	3.3	2
without skin, 4 oz	2.3	1
French Fries, 3 oz	3	1
Potato Salad, ½ cup	3.5	2.5
Pumpkin, ½ cup mashed	1	2.5
Seaweed, kelp, 1 oz	<1	2.5
Spinach, cooked, ½ cup, 3 oz	2.7	2.5
Squash, ckd, all types, ½ cup	1	0.3
Tomatoes, 1 medium, 4½ oz	1	0.6
Vegetables, mixed, ckd, 1 cup	2.5	0.7
Soybeans, cooked, ½ cup, 3 oz	14	4.4
Tofu, Tempeh, Miso		
Tofu, raw, firm, ½ cup, 4½ oz	10	1.5
Tempeh, ½ cup, 3 oz	16	2
Miso, ½ cup, 5 oz	16	4
Miso Soup, 1 cup	3	0.4
Soybean Protein (TVP), 1 oz	18	3
Cakes, Pastries, Pies		
(Made with enriched flour)		
Carrot w. cream cheese frosting, 4 oz	4	1.3
Cheesecake, 1 piece, 3½ oz	5	0.5
Chocolate, 1 piece, 2 oz	2	2
Fruitcake, 1 piece, 1½ oz	2	1.2
Plain, 1 piece, 2 oz	4	1.2
Croissant, plain, 2 oz	5	2
Danish Pastry, 1 pastry, 2¼ oz	4	1.3
Donuts, average, 2 oz	4	1.2
Muffins, average, 1 medium, 1½ oz	3	1
Pancakes, 4" diam., two, 2 oz	4	1
Pies: Fruit, 1 piece, 5½ oz	4	1.5
Pecan, 1 piece, 5 oz	7	4.5
Puddings, average, ½ cup, 4½ oz	4	0.3
Waffles, 1 large, 2½ oz	7	1.5

Sugar, Honey, Jam	Pro	Iron
Sugar: White	0	0
Brown, 1 Tbsp	0	0.3
Molasses: Light/Medium, 1 Tbsp	0	1
Blackstrap, 1 Tbsp, ¾ oz	0	3
Corn Syrup, 1 Tbsp, ¾ oz	0	1
Honey, Jams, Jelly	0	0.2
Candy, Chocolate, Carob		
Candy, sugar-based	0	0
Chocolate: Plain, 2 oz bar	4	0.8
with nuts, 2 oz bar	6	0.8
Carob, plain, 2 oz	6	0.7
Cookies, Crackers, Chips		
Cookies, average, 4 cookies	2	1
Crackers, Graham, 2½" sq., (2)	1	0
Rice Cakes, average, one	1	0
Corn/Potato Chips, 1 oz	2	0.3
Nuts: Almonds, shelled, 20-25 nuts	6	1
Brazil Nuts, 7-8 medium nuts, 1 oz	4	1
Cashews, 12-16 nuts, 1 oz	5	1.5
Macadamias, 1 oz	2	0.5
Peanuts, dry roasted, 40 nuts, 1 oz	6	0.6
Pecans, 24 halves, 1 oz	2	0.5
Walnuts, 15 halves, 1 oz	4	0.7
Peanut Butter, 1 Tbsp	1	0.5
Seeds: Sesame Seeds, dry, 1 Tbsp	2	0.6
Pumpkin Kernels, dry, hulled, 1 oz	7	4.2
Sunflower Seeds, dried, hulled, 1 oz	6	2
Tahini, 1 Tbsp, ½ oz	2.5	1.4
Granola & Food/Protein Bars		
Granola Bars, average, 1 bar, 2 oz	2	0.5
Atkins Advantage Bar, 2 oz	20	1
Balance Bars, Original, 1.76 oz	14	4.5
Bariatrix Proti-Bars (1), 1.4 oz	15	3.6
Carb Sense Bar	30	2
Choice Bar, 1.23 oz	6	3.6
Dr Soy Protein Bars, 1.76 oz	11	18
Ensure Nutrition Energy Bar, 2.1 oz	9	3.6
GeniSoy Bar, 1.5 oz	14	4.5
Jenny Craig Bars, 1.97 oz	10	3.6
Met-Rx "Big 100", 3.5 oz	27	7.2
Planters Peanut Bar, 1.6 oz	6	0.7
PowerBar: 1 bar, 2.3 oz	10	6.3
ProteinPlus, 1 bar, 2.75 oz	24	7.2
Slim-Fast Bar, 2 oz	8	2.7

Nutritional & High Protein Drinks

	Pro	Iron
Atkins Shakes, 11 fl.oz can	20	2.7
Bariatrix Shakes, dry, 1 oz	15	3.6
Very High Protein, 1 pkt	35	6.3
Boost Ready To Drink, 8 oz can	10	3.5
Carnation Instant Breakfast, 10 oz	13	4.5
Curves Protein Drink, 2 scoops, dry	15	18
Ensure Plus, 8 oz can	13	2.3
GeniSoy Shake, 1 scoop, 1 oz	25	3.6
Kashi GoLean Shake (RTD), 11 oz can	15	2.7
Kindercal, 8 fl.oz	7	2.5
Met-Rx Protein Shake, 11 oz	35	4.5
Myoplex (EAS), Nutrition Shake, 1 pkt	42	5.4
Nature's Best, Protein Shake, 1 scoop	22	3.6
Optifast 800, made-up, 8 oz	14	3.6
Resource (Novartis) Standard, 8 fl.oz	9	4.5
Revival Soy, Plain, 58g pkt	20	3
Slim-Fast Shakes, 325 ml can	10	3.6
Ultra Slim-Fast, 1 can	7	6.3
Usana Soya Max, 2 scoops, 1 oz	24	6
Walgreens Slim For Less, 11 oz can	10	2.7
Weider Lean Pro, 2 scoops	20	6

Coffee, Tea, Soda

	Pro	Iron
Coffee, Coffee Substitutes, 1 cup	0	0.1
Tea (all types); Soft Drinks/Soda	0	0
Hot Chocolate, 6 fl.oz	2	2.2

Beer, Wine, Spirits

	Pro	Iron
Beer, 12 fl.oz	1	0
Wines, red/white, 1 glass	0	0.4
Spirits/Liquor	0	0

Fast-Foods/Burgers

For extra listings ~ see CalorieKing.com

	Pro	Iron
Pancakes: Average all outlets, 3	8	2
Shakes, Chocolate	12	0.4
Sundaes: Average all outlets	7	0.3
Arby's: Roast Beef Sandwich, reg.	21	4
Giant Roast Beef S/wich	32	6
Roast Chicken Club	27	3
Burger King: Whopper S/wich	31	2.5
Hamburger	17	1.5
Bacon Double Cheeseburger	35	2.5
BK Big Fish Sandwich	23	2
Carl's Jr: Famous Star Hamburger	24	2
Ranch Crispy Chicken	24	2
Super Star Hamburger	41	3
Charbroiled Chicken Club Sandwich	42	3

Fast Foods/Burgers (Cont)

	Pro	Iron
Domino's Pizza: Deep Dish (12"), 2 sl.		
Cheese, 2 slices	42	4
Pepperoni, Sausage, Ham	41	4
X-tra Cheese & Pepperoni	50	4.5
KFC: Original, Wing & Breast	51	0.4
3-Pce. Dinner, Original	72	0.6
Crispy Strips, 3	29	0.4
Original Recipe Sandwich	29	1.5
McDonald's: Big Mac	25	4
Cheeseburger	15	3
Chicken McNuggets (6)	15	1
Crispy Chicken Burger	24	3
Filet-O-Fish	14	2
Grilled Chicken Caesar Salad	28	2
Hamburger	13	3
Quarter Pounder w. Cheese	29	5
French Fries: Small, 2.6 oz	2	0.4
Large, 6 oz	4.5	1
Breakfast: Egg McMuffin	17	3
Bacon, Egg & Cheese McGriddles	20	2
Ham, Egg & Cheese Bagel	28	4
Sausage McMuffin w. Egg	20	3
Pizza Hut: Per Medium, 2 slices		
Pan Pizzas, average	26	4
Thin 'n Crispy, Supreme	22	2
Hand Tossed, Pepperoni	24	3
Personal Pan Pizza, Meat	35	4
Subway (6" Subs): Average	20	2
Meatball	25	6
Roast Chicken Breast	24	3.5
Steak & Cheese, 6"	23	6
Subway Club	22	3.5
Taco Bell: Bean Burrito	14	3.5
Beef Burrito Supreme	17	3.5
Tostado	11	1.5
Chicken/Steak Enchirito	23	2
Taco Supreme	10	2
Gordita Baja Beef	13	2.5
Chicken Quesadilla	28	4
Wendy's: Single Sandwich w.mayo	25	3
Big Bacon Classic Sandwich	35	3
Hamburger (Kid's Meal)	15	2
Chicken Club Sandwich w. mayo	31	4

High Blood Pressure

High Blood Pressure

Many American adults have hypertension (high blood pressure), and are unaware of it. It is generally symptomless, so **have your blood pressure checked annually** - particularly if it runs in the family.

Untreated hypertension overworks the heart, damages arteries and promotes atherosclerosis. This in turn greatly increases the risk of heart disease, stroke, blindness, kidney disease and impotence. The earlier hypertension is detected, the sooner it can be brought under control.

BLOOD PRESSURE CLASSIFICATIONS

National High Blood Pressure Educ. Prog. (2003)

	DIASTOLIC		SYSTOLIC
Normal ➤	Below 80	and	Below 120
Prehypertension			
➤	80-89	or	120-139
Stage 1 ➤	90-99	or	140-159
Stage 2 ➤	100 or more	or	160 or more

Treating Hypertension

Prehypertension (in the chart above) means you don't have high blood pressure now but are likely to develop it in the future.

You can take steps to prevent it with healthy lifestyle habits: reducing sodium intake, eating adequate fruit and vegetables, losing weight if overweight, limiting alcohol to 2 drinks or less daily, quitting smoking, exercising regularly, and managing stress.

Stage 1 hypertension can often be treated with the above lifestyle changes.

Stage 2 hypertension usually requires drug therapy. However, salt restriction, abstaining from alcohol and the above lifestyle changes will improve the success of drug therapy, and enable smaller drug doses to be prescribed.

HYPERTENSION DAMAGES ARTERIES & PROMOTES ATHEROSCLEROSIS

STROKE (Brain)
Artery blockage or rupture

NECK ARTERIES
Artherosclerosis can limit blood flow to brain

HEART ATTACK
Coronary artery blockage

STROKE
KNOW THE WARNING SIGNS!

If you notice one or more of these signs, **call your doctor immediately**. They may be signalling a possible stroke or transient ischemic attack:

- **Sudden weakness** or numbness in your face, arm or leg on one side of your body.
- **Sudden dimness**, blurring or loss of vision, particularly in one eye.
- **Loss of speech**, or trouble talking or understanding speech.
- **Sudden severe headache** - 'a bolt out of the blue' - with no apparent cause.
- **Unexplained dizziness**, unsteadiness or a sudden fall, especially if accompanied by any of the other symptoms.

Salt & Sodium

- **Sodium is a mineral element** most commonly found in salt (sodium chloride). It also occurs naturally in much smaller amounts in animal and plant foods, and water - normally sufficient for our needs without having to add salt.

- **Sodium is required** for nerve and muscle function as well as to balance the amount of fluid in our tissues and blood.

  Sodium acts like a sponge to attract and hold fluids in body tissues.

- **Excess sodium** can cause water retention, and increase the risk of developing hypertension. Very high salt intake may also increase the risk of stomach cancer.

- **Too little sodium** may cause low blood pressure (hypotension), and decrease blood flow to the heart, brain and kidneys - especially during exercise. (A certain blood volume is required to sustain the blood pressure needed for adequate blood flow in the capillaries.)

Salt-Sensitive Persons

- **Normally, our kidneys** excrete excess dietary sodium. The thirst we feel after a salty meal is the body calling for water to dilute the sodium, and enable the kidneys to flush out excess sodium.

- **However, 'salt - sensitive' persons** (up to 50% of adults) tend to retain excess sodium (above approximately 3000mg daily) instead of excreting it. Such persons are more likely to develop hypertension and would most benefit from sodium restriction. Assume you are susceptible if there is a family history of hypertension.

- **Although not everyone will benefit**, all Americans are being asked to moderate their salt and sodium intake as a public health measure - particularly that so many do not know whether or not they have hypertension; and also because we do not know just who is salt-sensitive.

SAFE SODIUM LEVELS

The American Heart Association recommends a **maximum sodium intake of 2300mg per day** for adults with normal blood pressure. However, people who consume less than 1500mg sodium have the lowest blood pressure levels.

Persons with hypertension and kidney ailments are usually restricted to as little as **1000mg sodium per day**. Your doctor will discuss the correct sodium level for you.

Persons engaged in prolonged strenuous work or exercise may lose sodium through heavy sweating - especially in hot, humid weather. Adequate salt (and fluids) is necessary to avoid dehydration. A little extra salt at mealtimes is usually sufficient to satisfy any extra need. Do not take salt tablets.

FINDING HIDDEN SODIUM

On average, **less than one third of our sodium intake comes from the salt shaker.** The rest is hidden in processed foods that have salt added during manufacture.

Sodium compounds added to food or medicinals can also contribute significant sodium.

Sodium bicarbonate in particular is widely used in antacid tablets and powders, and saline drink powders (such as Alka Seltzer). Sodium bicarbonate contains 27% sodium by weight. Each gram contributes 270mg sodium. Large amounts of sodium can be unwittingly consumed – up to 600mg per tablet.
(See Antacids ~ Page 293)

Other sodium compounds include mono-sodium glutamate (MSG), sodium ascorbate, sodium nitrite, and sodium citrate.

ALCOHOL DANGER

Excessive alcohol intake contributes to hypertension. Susceptible persons should limit alcohol intake to 1-2 drinks per day.

Salt Sodium Guide

Sodium accounts for only 40% of the weight of salt (sodium chloride). Examples:
1 gram (1000mg) Salt has 400mg Sodium
1 teaspoon (5g) Salt has 2000mg Sodium

Hints to Reduce Sodium

- **Watch the salt shaker.** Start with an easy 50% cut in sodium by using Lite Salt (*Morton*) or *Cardia* Salt. Then gradually cut back until you can leave the salt shaker off the table.

- **Taste your food before salting.** Use the pepper shaker (small holes) for more controlled sprinkling of salt.

- **Choose low sodium,** sodium free, and reduced sodium products in place of regular salted products.

- **Check food labels for sodium levels.** FDA Guidelines for sodium descriptors are:
  - **Reduced Sodium:** At least 25% less sodium than the original product
  - **Low Sodium:** 140 mg or less/serving
  - **Very Low Sodium:** 35mg or less/serving
  - **Sodium Free:** Less than 5mg/serving
  - **No Salt Added:** Made without the salt normally added, but still contains the sodium that is a natural part of the food

- **Use reduced-sodium breads,** butter and margarine. Regular varieties contain up to 2% salt. This is considered high in view of their significant contribution to our diet.

- **Go easy on condiments and sauces** such as tomato ketchup, mustard, soy sauce and spaghetti sauces, plus salad dressings. Use low sodium varieties.

- **Limit pizzas and salty fast-foods.** Check *CalorieKing.com* food database.

- **Avoid salty snack foods** such as potato chips, corn chips, salted nuts, pretzels and cheesy-flavored snacks. **Choose unsalted** popcorn, nuts or seeds. Eat more fruit.

- **Don't salt children's food** to your taste.

- **Limit or avoid antacids and saline powders with** sodium bicarbonate (such as *Alka-Seltzer*). They are high in sodium.

FOODS HIGH IN SODIUM

- Cheese, Butter, Margarine
- Pickles, Sauerkraut, Olives
- Condiments, Sauces
- Salad Dressings
- Canned vegetables/salads/beans
- Deli Salads (with dressing)
- Frozen/Packaged Meals/Entrees
- Soups: Canned/dry; bouillon cubes
- Meats: Ham, bacon, sausage, luncheon meats, smoked meats
- Canned Fish (in brine/salt)
- Sea Salt, Garlic/Celery Salt
- Snack Foods (potato chips, pretzels)
- Tomato Juice (Canned), V8 Vegetable Juice
- Fast Foods: Pizza, Burgers, Chicken
- *Alka-Seltzer* Antacid

MODERATE SODIUM

- Bread (Reduced Salt)
- Meat, Fish, Poultry - Unprocessed
- Milk, Yogurt, Soy Drinks, Eggs
- Peanut Butter
- Breakfast Cereals (less than 200mg/serving)
- Chocolate Candy, Fruit/Nut Bars
- *Reduced Sodium & Low Sodium Products*

FOODS LOW IN SODIUM

- Products labelled *Very Low Sodium,* or *Sodium Free*
- Fresh fruits and vegetables
- Canned and Dried Fruits
- Potatoes, Rice, Pasta
- Dried Beans & Lentils, Tofu
- Nuts & Seeds (unsalted)
- Corn & Popcorn (unsalted)
- Pepper, Spices, Herbs
- Jam, Honey, Syrup
- Candy, Gum
- Hard & Jelly Candy
- Coffee, Tea, Alcohol
- Fresh Fruit Juices, Water

Sodium ~ Sodium (mg)

Milk & Dairy Products

	Sodium
Milk: Whole/lowfat/skim, average	
1 cup, 8 fl.oz	120
Whole, low sodium, 1 cup	5
Choc Milk (Hershey's), 1 cup	130
Soy Milk, 8 fl.oz	30
Buttermilk, cultured, 8 fl.oz	250
Dry/Powder, skim, ¼ cup, 1 oz	110
Yogurt, with fruit average, 8 oz	130
Cheese: Blue, 1 oz	330
Parmesan, 1 oz	450
Kraft Cheddar, 2% milk, 1 oz	230
Philadelphia Cream Cheese, 1 oz	90
Process Cheese., average,1 oz	430
Swiss, 1 oz	40
Cottage Cheese, ½ cup, 4 oz	450
Ricotta Cheese, ½ cup, 4 oz	150

Icecream, Frozen Yogurt

Icecream, average,½ cup	50
Frozen Yogurt, ½ cup	50

Fats/Oils

Butter/Margarine:	
Regular, 2 Tbsp, 1 oz	230
Unsalted, reg., 2 Tbsp, 1 oz	5
Mayonnaise, aver., 2 Tbsp, 1 oz	160
Oils/Lard/Dripping	0
Cream, average, 1 Tbsp	6
Coffee-Mate: Powdered, 1 tsp	2
Liquid, 1 Tbsp	5

Eggs

Whole, 1 large	70
Omelet, 2 egg, plain	220
w. cheese	400
Egg Beaters (Fleischmann's), ¼ cup	115

Meats

Meat, average all types, cooked	
(Beef/Lamb/Veal/Pork), 4 oz	80
Corned Beef, cooked, 3 oz	800
Bacon, cooked, 2 slices, ½ oz	270
Ham, 3 oz	1100

Chicken & Turkey

Chicken/Turkey, cooked, unsalted, 4 oz	80
Stuffing Mixes, average., ½ cup	500

Sausages & Meats

	Sodium
Bologna, 1 oz	280
Frankfurter, 2 oz	640
Ham, chopped, ¾ oz slice	290
Liverwurst (Braunschweiger), 1 oz	320
Pepperoni, 5 slices, 1 oz	570
Salami, cooked, 1 oz	350
dry/hard, 1 oz	600
Sausage, 1 oz link	220
Pork, 2 oz patty	260
Turkey Roll, 1 oz	160

Fish:

Fish: Fresh Fish, average, plain	
Cooked, 4 oz (no bone)	60
Broiled w. butter, 4 oz	150
Breaded & fried, 4 oz	320
Fish fillets, batter-dipped 3 oz	350
Fish sticks, 1 oz stick	160
Gefilte Fish (w. broth), 1 pce, 1½ oz	220
Herring, pickled, 2 pces, 1 oz	260
Lobster, meat only, 4 oz	180
Oysters, fresh, 6 med., 3 oz	95
Salmon: Canned, 3 oz	460
No Salt Added, 3 oz	65
Smoked fish, average, 3 oz	650
Tuna: Canned, 3 oz	330
No Added Salt, 3 oz	40

Entrees & Meals

Frozen Meals, average	600-900
Lean Cuisine, average	700
Stouffer's, average	580
Dinners, average	900-1200
Side Dishes, average	400-600
Pizza, frozen, ¼ large, 6 oz	800-1200
Microwave Cup Meals	900-1200
Cup O'Noodles, average	1500

Fast-Foods & Restaurants

Cheeseburger	750
Chicken Dinner (3 piece)	2200
Chicken Nuggets w. Sauce	800
Fish/Chicken Sandwich	1000
French Fries, small, 2½ oz	150
Hamburger: Regular	500
Large with cheese	1100
Hot Dog (Frankfurter)	800
Pizza, 2 medium slices	1200
Shake, chocolate	250
Taco	400

Extra Listings ~ see CalorieKing.com

Sodium Counter

Sodium ~ Sodium (mg)	**Sodium**
Soups: Condensed, 1 c., 8 oz	800-1000
Low Sodium	70
Chicken Noodle, 1 cup	900
Bouillon Cube, average	950
Cup-A-Soup: Average	850
Lite, average	450
Soup Mixes, average, 1 cup	900

Condiments, Sauces, Dressings

A-1 Sauce, 1 Tbsp	280
Barbecue Sauce, 1 Tbsp	130
Bragg Liquid Aminos, 1 tsp	220
Chili Sauce, 1 Tbsp	230
Ketchup: Tomato, 1 Tbsp	180
Low Sodium, 1 Tbsp	20
Mayonnaise, 1 Tbsp	80
Mustard, 1 tsp	70
Pizza Sauce, ½ cup	700
Salad Dressings, 2 Tbsp, 1 oz	160-400
Spaghetti Sauce, ½ cup	500
Soy Sauce: 1 Tbsp	900
Lite *(Kikkoman),* 1 Tbsp	600
Sweet & Sour, ½ cup	250
Tabasco, 1 tsp	25
Vinegar, Lemon Juice	0
Worcestershire, 1 Tbsp	200
Tomato: Sauce, 1 cup	1200
Paste/Puree (salted), ½ cup	1000
No Salt Added, ½ cup	25

Salt & Salt Substitutes

Table Salt: 1 teaspoon, 6g	2400
Single Serve package, 1 g	400
Cardia Salt, 1 teaspoon	1080
Lite Salt *(Morton),* 1 teaspoon, 6g	1200
Morton Salt Substitute	5
No Salt Salt Substitute, 1 teaspoon	5
Garlic/Seasoned Salt 1 teaspoon, 4g	1300
Sea Salt, 1 teaspoon, 5g	2250

Seasonings, Herbs & Spices

Baking Powder, 1 tsp, 3g	340
Baking Soda (Sodium bicarb), 1 tsp, 3g	810
Accent (Flavor Enhancer), 1 tsp	600
Chili Powder, 1 tsp, 3g	25
Curry Powder	0
Lemon Pepper *(Lawry's),* 1 tsp	340
Meat Tenderizer, 1 tsp, 5g	1750
MSG (Monosodium glutamate), 5g	500
Mrs Dash (Herb/Spice Blend), 1 tsp	0
Pepper, Mustard (dry), 1 tsp	1
Yeast, Nutritional, 1 Tbsp	10

Breakfast Cereals

Kellogg's:	**Sodium**
All-Bran, ½ cup, 1 oz	80
Oatbran Flakes, ¾ cup, 1 oz	210
Corn Flakes, 1 cup, 1 oz	200
Just Right, ¾ cup, 2 oz	240
Mini Wheats Frosted, 24 bisc., 1.8 oz	5
Health Valley Cereals, 1 serving	5
Quaker: Cap'n Crunch, ¾ cup, 1 oz	200
Crunchy Corn Bran, ¾ cup, 1 oz	230
100% Natural Granola, ½ cup, 1 oz	15
Puffed Rice/Wheat, 2 cups, 1 oz	1
General Mills: Total, ¾ cup, 1 oz	190
Oatmeal: Regular, ¾ cup	1
Instant *(Quaker),* ⅔ cup (1 pkt)	270

Breads, Bagels, Crackers

Bread: Average all types, 1 oz	140
Low Sodium, 1 oz	10
Bagels: Plain, 2 oz	200
Sara Lee, 3 oz	500
Biscuits, average, 1 oz	180
Bun/Roll, 1 medium, 1½ oz	200
Crackers: Saltine, 2 crackers	70
Low Salt *(Premium),* 2	25
Graham, 2 regular	50
Croissant, average, 2 oz	280
Rice Cakes, average	25
Ry-Krisp Crispbread, Sesame, 2	100

Cookies, Cakes, Desserts

Cookies: Average, 2-3 cookies, 1 oz	100
Mrs Fields', average, 2½ oz	180
Baked Custard, ½ cup	100
Brownie, ¼ oz piece	75
Cake, average, 3 oz piece	250
Cinnamon Sweet Roll, 2 oz	250
Danish, Apple	250
Donut, average	150
Muffins: 1 medium, 2 oz	150
Pancakes, 3 x 4"	360
Pie, average 1/6 of 9" pie	300
Pudding: Average, ½ cup	160
Jell-O (Mix), Instant, ½ cup	400
Waffles:	
Home-made, 7", 2½ oz	350
Frozen: Average, 1¼ oz	260
Aunt Jemima, avg, 2½ oz	565

Fruit & Juices	Sodium
Fresh Fruit, average all types, 1 serving	1
Dried/Canned Fruit, ½ cup	1
Fruit Juice: Fresh, sqz'd, 6 fl.oz	1
Commercial, aver., 6 fl.oz	20
Carrot Juice *(Ferraro's)*, 8 fl.oz	230
Tomato Juice *(Campbell's)*, 6 fl.oz	570
Low Sodium (No Salt Added)	20
V8 Vegetable *(Campbell's)*, 6 fl.oz	600
(No Salt Added) 6 fl.oz	45

Vegetables	
Fresh/Frozen (No Salt Added): Per ½ Cup	
Asparagus, Bean Sprouts, Corn	3
Beets, Carrots, Celery, ½ cup	40
Broccoli, Cabbage, Cauliflower	10
Cucumber, Green Beans, Mushroom, Okra	3
Onions, Peas, Potato, Pumpkin, Squash	3
Peppers, Hot Chili, raw, each	3
Spinach, Turnips, ½ cup, ckd	40
Tomato, 1 medium, 5 oz	10
Canned: Asparagus, 4 spears	300
Beans, baked in tomato sauce	450
Beets, ½ cup, 3 oz	240
Corn Kernels, ½ cup, 3 oz	190
Creamed, ½ cup, 4½ oz	330
Mushrooms w. butter sce, 2oz	550
Peas, ½ cup, 3 oz	250
Sauerkraut, ½ cup, 4 oz	750

Pickles, Olives	
Olives, pickled: Green, 1 large	90
Ripe/black, 1 large	40
Pickles: Bread & Butter, 4 sl., 1 oz	200
Dill, 1 pickle, 2½ oz	900
Sweet, 1 gherkin, ½ oz	130

Soybean Products	
Miso (Soy Paste), ¼ c., 2½ oz	2500
Soybean Protein Isolate, 1 oz	280
Tempeh, ½ cup, 3 oz	5
Tofu, average, ½ cup, 4 oz	5

Jam, Honey, Syrups	
Jam/Jelly, 1 Tbsp	2
Honey/Maple Syrup, 1 Tbsp	1
Log Cabin Syrup, 1 fl.oz	35
Lite, 1 fl.oz	90

Peanut Butter	
Peanut Butter, regular, 1 Tbsp	70
Unsalted, 1 Tbsp	1

Snacks, Nuts	Sodium
Cheese Balls/Curls, 1 oz	280
Corn/Tortilla Chips, average, 1 oz	220
Granola bars, average, 1 bar	80
Nuts: Plain, unsalted, 1 oz	1
Lightly salted, 1 oz	80
Salted or Honey Roasted, 1 oz	160
Popcorn: Plain (unsalted), 1 cup	1
Flavored, average, 1 cup	60
Salt added, 1 cup	180
Potato Chips: Plain, 1 oz	160
Flavored, average, 1 oz	250
Pretzels, regular, 3, 1 oz	450

Candy, Chocolate	
Chocolate, milk, 1 oz	30
Carob Milk Bar, 1 oz	55
Fudge, chocolate, 1 oz	55
Candy Bars, average, 1½ oz	60
Hard Candy, Jelly Beans, 1 oz	10
Licorice, 1 oz	30

Beverages, Alcohol	
Coffee (& Substitutes), Tea, 1 cup	1
Cocoa, dry, plain, 1 Tbsp	0
Mix, average, 1 envelope	120
Quik (Nestle), 2 tsp	35
Soft Drinks, average, 8 fl.oz	20
Mineral Water, Perrier, 8 fl.oz	5
Gatorade Thirst Quencher, 8 fl.oz	110
Water: Average, 1 cup, 8 fl.oz	5
Drier regions, 1 cup	20+
Alcohol: Beer, average, 12 fl.oz	15
Wines, average, 4 fl.oz	10
Spirits (distilled), 1½ fl.oz	1

Antacids – Alka-Seltzer	Sodium
Alka-Seltzer (Per Tablet):	
Alka-Seltzer P.M., 1 tablet	500
Original (Light Blue Box)	570
Extra Strength (Dark Blue Box)	590
Flavored Lemon/Lime & Cherry	500
Antacid (yellow Box)	310
Gelatine Capsule, 1	0
Alka-Mints, chewable	0
Bromo Seltzer, ¾ capful	760
Rolaids, All types	0
Tums, Regular/Extra Strength	0
Sodium Bicarbonate (27% sodium), 1g	270

Index A - B

FAST-FOOD RESTAURANTS INDEX
~ SEE PAGE 183 ~

Index C - E

Index H - L

Index P - S

FAST-FOOD RESTAURANTS INDEX
~ SEE PAGE 183 ~

Index U - Z